Dedicated to

# Joan Ryan Volk

for her help and encouragement during

the writing of this text.

# Essentials of
# Medical Microbiology

## WESLEY A. VOLK

*Professor of Microbiology*

*University of Virginia School of Medicine*

*Charlottesville, Virginia*

## J. B. Lippincott Company

*Philadelphia   New York   San Jose   Toronto*

PROJECT EDITOR:   Carl May
DESIGN AND PRODUCTION:   Rick Chafian
ILLUSTRATOR:   Judith McCarty
COPYEDITOR:   Jean Frazier
COMPOSITOR:   Typothetae
PRINTER:   Halliday Lithograph

**Library of Congress Cataloging in Publication Data**

Volk, Wesley A
  Essentials of medical microbiology.

  Bibliography: p.
  Includes index.
  1.  Medical microbiology. I.  Title.
QR46.V64          616.01          77–17564
ISBN 0–397–47374–5
ISBN 0–397–47369–9 pbk.

1   3   5   7   9   8   6   4   2

# Essentials of
# Medical Microbiology

# Contents

# Preface

The advent of a new medically-oriented microbiology text to compete with what seems to be an abundance of such texts may seem foolhardy, indeed. But this book, like many other texts, was written with a specific objective and for a fairly specific audience. The objective was a comprehensive text containing the essentials of medical microbiology that could be read in its entirety during a one-term course. Within the confines of this objective every effort has been made to support scientific facts with experimental data, explanations, and illustrations. This text is directed to a reader who has had at least an elementary introduction to biochemistry, but it does not require a background in microbiology.

Who, then, are the expected readers? This text is modeled, in part, after the microbiology course taught to medical students at the University of Virginia, in which the author has taught for over a quarter of a century. It is also designed for upper-level undergraduates and graduate students who wish to complete a one-term course in medical microbiology.

The book is divided into five units. Unit One provides an introduction to the microbial world, and for those individuals who are not new to the field it should provide an easy review of basic microbiology. Unit Two is concerned with immunology and contains a detailed discussion of nonspecific host resistance as well as humoral and cellular immune reactions. This unit describes the structure and synthesis of antibodies, and the role of antibodies, complement, and cells in host protection, allergy, and autoimmune reactions. Unit Three is devoted to the medically important bacteria and fungi, while Unit Four describes the structure, growth, and characteristics of animal viruses. Both of these units emphasize the epidemiology, mechanism of disease production, and laboratory diagnosis for the etiologic agents of human disease. Unit Five contains a brief survey of human disease caused by protozoa and worms. All chapters include a list of current references which direct the reader to additional information on the material covered.

Throughout this book, illustrations and tables are used to illuminate the text. These could not have been included without the generosity of individuals and publishers who provided photographs and permissions, and deepest thanks are extended for them. All but a few figures make their textbook debut here, and the quality of the micrographs should result in a level of interest and attractiveness unattainable by words alone. To maintain a crisp, student-oriented presentation, acknowledgments do not accompany each figure or table; rather, the reader is encouraged to refer to the complete list of credits after the last chapter.

During the writing of this text none of my colleagues escaped my questions, but final responsibility for any errors that may appear must be my own. I would like to acknowledge especially the following persons from the University of Virginia, who read entire units or large portions thereof: D. C. Benjamin, S. U. Emerson, R. J. Kadner, G. L. Mandell, and D. E. Normansell. In addition, the following individuals from other institutions read single chapters or parts of chapters of the manuscript: C. G. Alexander, San Francisco State University; D. F. Bainton, University of California, San Francisco; P. Bodel, Yale University; M. D. Little, Tulane University; S. Madoff, Massachusetts General Hospital; L. A. McGonagle, University of Washington; G. E. Michaels, University of Georgia; L. A. Page, National Animal Disease Center; J. T. Sinski, University of Arizona; E. J. Stanbridge, University of California, Irvine; and H. S. Wessenberg, San Francisco State University. Blocks of chapters were reviewed by J. W. Goodman, University of California, San Francisco, and J. L. Pate, University of Wisconsin, Madison. Entire units were read by C. Albin, Stanford University; A. A. Blazkovec, University of Wisconsin; C. R. Goodheart, Biolabs; R. C. Johnson, University of Minnesota; C. E. Schwerdt, Stanford University; M. Stone, Stanford University; and M. Voge, University of California, Los Angeles. The entire manuscript was reviewed by E. D. Weinberg, Indiana University. My warmest appreciation is extended to all of these reviewers who contributed to this text by their comments.

*Wesley A. Volk*

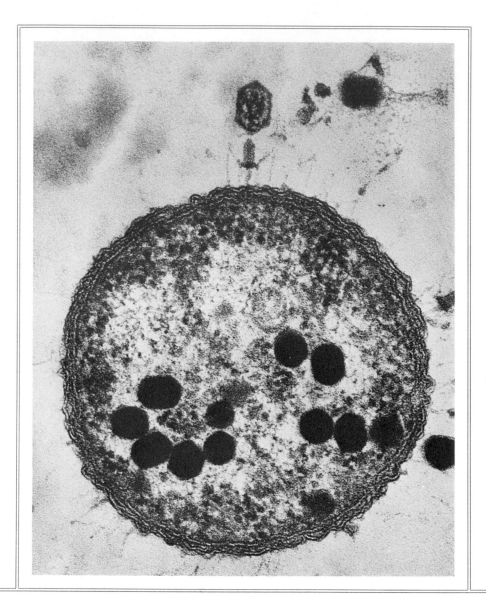

# UNIT ONE

# Introduction to Medical Microbiology

WHERE, when, and how did life originate? How can a single cell divide and differentiate into the incredible complexity of the human body?

Is disease a random event, a punishment, or a result of something real, something solid, something controllable? Is there a general unity or theme of life that is essentially the same in a tree, a human, a bacterium, a virus? Can we learn about ourselves from knowledge of the metabolism and genetic inheritance of organisms so small that literally millions of them could "dance on the head of a pin"?

These questions have occupied the minds of philosophers and scientists for centuries. A number have been answered, others are well on the way toward a solution, and a few seem destined to remain forever unknown.

But we now know that many diseases are caused by microorganisms, and we are continually learning how such organisms cause disease at the molecular level and how the diseases can be prevented, treated, and controlled. Furthermore, we can see a biochemical unity in the world to allow us to extrapolate our knowledge of bacterial genetics toward a better understanding of the regulation and control of human physiology.

The growth of biological knowledge during the past century is analogous to the advances in physics that have taken us off the horse and to the moon. This knowledge allows us to question the role of viruses in human cancer, it permits us to discuss the feasibility of genetic engineering to correct heritable defects, and it brings us closer to an understanding of many hitherto mysterious maladies such as multiple sclerosis, juvenile diabetes, and autoimmune diseases.

Is this what microbiology is all about? In part, yes. Microbiology is that part of biology set aside as a separate science because it deals primarily with the biology of organisms too small for the naked eye to see. Medical microbiology is simply a subdivision concerned with the biology of the microorganisms that cause disease. Thus, medical microbiology includes a study of microorganisms that can grow on or in a host organism and produce disease. It encompasses the responses the host makes to the infection, and it seeks answers to questions concerning the control of infectious diseases as well as diseases resulting from genetic disorders.

This text will not concern itself with a detailed classification of microorganisms. Rather, its objective will be to describe the characteristics of those organisms that cause disease, to discuss (insofar as possible) how they produce the disease in question, and to outline protective measures available to us. However, before these objectives can become comprehensible, we must learn about what bacteria are, how they grow, and how they can be controlled. Unit One is designed to provide some of the answers to these questions.

## GENERAL REFERENCES

Brock, T. D. 1974. *Biology of Microorganisms*, 2nd ed. Prentice-Hall, Englewood Cliffs, New Jersey.

Burrows, W. 1973. *Textbook of Microbiology*, 20th ed. W. B. Saunders Co., Philadelphia.

Davis, B. D., R. Dulbecco, H. N. Eisen, H. S. Ginsberg, W. B. Wood, and M. McCarty. 1973. *Microbiology*, 2nd ed. Harper & Row, New York.

Hayes, W. 1969. *The Genetics of Bacteria and their Viruses*, 2nd ed. John Wiley & Sons, New York.

Jawetz, E., J. L. Melnick, and E. A. Adelberg. 1976. *Review of Medical Microbiology*, 12th ed. Lange Medical Publications, Los Altos, Calif.

Joklik, W. K., and H. P. Willett, eds. 1976. *Zinsser Microbiology*, 16th ed. Appleton-Century-Crofts, New York.

Lamanna, C., M. F. Mallette, and L. N. Zimmerman. 1973. *Basic Bacteriology. Its Biological and Chemical Background*, 4th ed. The Williams and Wilkins Co., Baltimore.

Pelczar, M. J., R. D. Reid, and E. C. S. Chan. 1977. *Microbiology*, 4th ed. McGraw-Hill, New York.

Stanier, R. Y., E. A. Adelberg, and J. L. Ingraham. 1976. *The Microbial World*, 4th ed. Prentice-Hall, Englewood Cliffs, New Jersey.

Stent, G. S. 1971. *Molecular Genetics: An Introductory Narrative*. W. H. Freeman & Co., San Francisco.

# 1

# The Microbial World

The word "microbiology" is a broad term meaning the study of living organisms that are individually too small to be seen with the naked eye. It includes the study of bacteria (bacteriology), viruses (virology), yeasts and molds (mycology), protozoa (protozoology), and algae (phycology). Such minute forms of life are given the name microorganisms, and sometimes they are called microbes or, in the vernacular, germs.

Considering the vast knowledge we now possess concerning microorganisms, it is difficult to imagine that hardly more than a century ago Louis Pasteur and a few of his colleagues were trying to convince the medical profession that these little organisms actually cause disease or even that one kind of microorganism turns fruit juice to wine while a different organism turns it to vinegar. Once a few such seminal ideas were proven and accepted, the study of microorganisms and their metabolic processes has grown rapidly into an important science.

The information acquired from microbiology has made possible great advances in our ability to control many infectious diseases. In addition, many biochemical processes first understood in microorganisms have subsequently been shown to occur in higher forms of life. Thus, many metabolic pathways of human metabolism were first observed in microorganisms. The field of molecular genetics and current models of gene action and gene regulation had much of their origin in the study of microorganisms.

It is therefore clear that the field of microbiology includes more than just a study of disease-producing microorganisms; it is the study of all biological activities of microbes. Perhaps the time is not far distant when we can both understand and control diseases such as cancer and those resulting from genetic defects, and it is certain that the continued study of microbiology will contribute to that knowledge.

## PRACTICAL APPLICATIONS OF MICROBIOLOGY

A practical knowledge of microbiology is immediately and vitally important in medicine and related fields. For example, at a most basic level a primary responsibility of hospital personnel is to safeguard patients, and a large part of this responsibility is to protect the patient from the injurious effects of microorganisms. Under normal hospital conditions, a patient is always in some peril of microbial invasion, and in fact hospital-acquired infections have become so commonplace that they have been given the specific designation of nosocomial infections.

The individual who knows something of the peculiar attributes of each medically important species of microorganism will be able to take advantage of its vulnerabilities. By understanding microorganisms, their anatomy and physiology, something of what they can do, and how they produce disease, we can know much more of how they can be controlled.

## EVOLUTION OF THE STUDY OF MICROORGANISMS

The existence of microorganisms had long been suspected when their presence was verified by microscopic observation in about 1683 through the investigations of the Dutch merchant Antony van Leeuwenhoek (1632–1723). Leeuwenhoek was an amateur scientist who devoted a great deal of time to his hobby of grinding lenses (see Figure 1-1).

With his lenses he observed everything he could think of and described microorganisms in rainwater, seawater, scrapings from between the teeth, fermenting mixtures, and many other materials. Many of the minute organisms, including protozoa, yeast, and bacteria, were seen in motion, and he referred to them as "animalcules." His drawings were remarkably accurate, particularly when one realizes that the highest magnification possible with his lenses was about 300 times, in contrast with today's compound microscope which provides a magnification of 1000 times. As judged from his drawings, Leeuwenhoek's lenses were the best of his time, and although he kept his lens grinding techniques secret, he shared his observations in great detail in voluminous letters to the Royal Society of London.

### The Theory of Spontaneous Generation

At the same time as Leeuwenhoek's observations, a challenge was beginning to be made to the theory of spontaneous generation. This

**Figure 1-1.** *a.* Leeuwenhoek's microscope utilized a single biconvex lens to view bacteria suspended in a drop of liquid placed on a moveable pin. *b.* Although his microscope was capable of only 200 to 300-fold magnification, Leeuwenhoek was able to achieve these remarkable drawings submitted to the Royal Society of London.

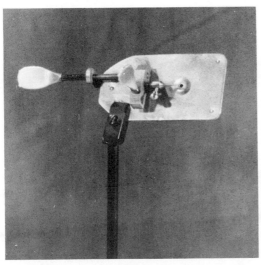

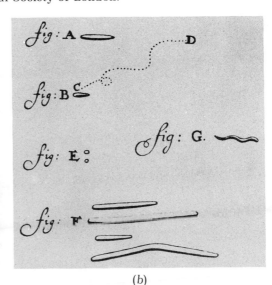

(a)                    (b)

theory proposed the spontaneous origin of living organisms, particularly from decaying organic matter. Over time the theory was not too difficult to disprove for large multicellular organisms such as mice, snakes, and flies; by the middle of the eighteenth century the concept of spontaneous generation of visible and complex forms of life had been largely laid to rest. But it was still widely believed that microorganisms arose spontaneously. John Needham, an English biologist and priest (1713–1781), published a paper in 1749 in support of spontaneous generation in which he claimed that microorganisms arose in his infusions, or broths, whether he boiled them, covered them, or took any other precautions. The controversy was defined when an Italian naturalist and priest, Lazzaro Spallanzani (1729–1799), claimed that Needham had not taken sufficient precautions to prevent microorganisms in the air from entering heated infusions after they had cooled. However, many of Spallanzani's contemporaries found it difficult to accept his totally new concept that putrefaction or decay was initi-

ated by microorganisms floating on dust particles in the air, and so his arguments were widely ignored. These critics felt that by sealing the solutions so completely, Spallanzani was eliminating material necessary to life. The controversy concerning the spontaneous generation of microorganisms continued until the middle of the nineteenth century.

The experiments of two men, Louis Pasteur, a French chemist, crystallographer, and "father of modern microbiology" and the English physicist John Tyndall, provided the final disproof of spontaneous generation. Pasteur poured meat infusions into flasks and then drew the top of each flask into a long, curved neck that would admit air but not dust (see Figure 1-2a). He found that after the infusions were heated they would remain sterile indefinitely unless he broke the neck of the flask, thus allowing dust to enter the infusion. He further demonstrated that if he placed a series of these flasks along a dusty road, opened them, and then resealed them a few minutes later, microorganisms would grow in nearly all flasks. On the other hand,

**Figure 1-2.** *a.* Pasteur's swan-necked flasks remained sterile because the bend in the neck excluded dust particles. *b.* Similarly, broth remained sterile in Tyndall's dust-free incubation chamber. In both cases the broth was exposed to air, but dust was excluded.

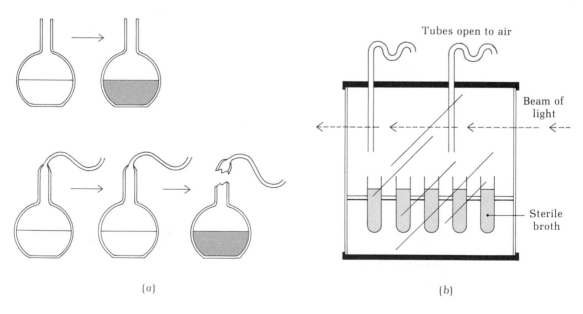

(a)                                                            (b)

if he performed the same experiment on the top of a mountain where there was little dust, practically none of his flasks became contaminated.

Pasteur's experiments appeared to end forever the controversy of spontaneous generation, but the idea was not laid to rest until the work of John Tyndall became known. Tyndall had observed that the pathway of a bright beam of light through air is visible because it is refracted by dust particles in the air. When, however, the air is completely free of dust, the beam cannot be seen. Tyndall constructed a specially designed box (Figure 1-2b), and after the dust in the box had settled (verified by the observation that he could no longer see a beam of light pass through the air) he carefully placed tubes of sterile infusions into the box. As long as the air was not disturbed, the infusions remained sterile even though open to the air, again demonstrating that microorganisms exist on dust particles in the air and that they are not spontaneously generated.

## Fermentation

Although Pasteur's early training was as a chemist and crystallographer, his efforts to disprove the theory of spontaneous generation stimulated his interest in the biological activities of microorganisms. One of his first tasks as a microbiological troubleshooter was to find out why the production of wine would occasionally result in the formation of large amounts of lactic acid. He soon observed that more than one type of microorganism was involved. The undesirable lactic acid fermentation resulted from contamination with rod-shaped bacteria; the ethanol production resulted from the activity of yeast cells. This observation was followed by others in which Pasteur proved that each type of bacterium is able to carry out the conversion of glucose or other carbohydrates to specific end products. Thus, one type of bacterium forms lactic acid from sugar, another forms butyric acid, and so on. Pasteur observed that these fermenta-

tion processes took place in the absence of air, and he coined the terms aerobic and anaerobic to describe respectively those organisms requiring air and those unable to grow in the presence of air. Pasteur's discoveries were soon utilized in industrial fermentation, but the idea that microorganisms could affect humans and animals was less readily accepted.

## Germ Theory of Disease

The contagious nature of certain diseases has been recognized since Biblical times. However, one of the first specific cases of the association of a microorganism with disease was made in 1834 when the Italian Agostino Bassi proved that a disease in silkworms was the result of a fungus infection. In a similar problem Pasteur was called upon in 1865 to study a silkworm disease that was destroying the silk industry in France. He established criteria to identify infected silkworm moths microscopically, and by using female silkworms free of infection, the disease could be eliminated. Joseph Lister (1827–1912), an English physician, soon put to practical use the emerging concept that disease and infection were the result of invading microorganisms. He is credited with the first attempt to prevent infection following surgery by using an antiseptic technique; he used dilute phenol for cleaning hands and instruments, wound dressings, and as an aerosol during surgical procedures. Crude as this practice may have been, it marked the beginning of our effort to control infectious microorganisms.

Once the microbial etiology or cause of infectious diseases was accepted, research activity was directed toward the isolation and identification of the causative agents of the many severe diseases of the day. Thus, the last quarter of the nineteenth century was a time of great activity resulting in tremendous, exciting discoveries. A German physician, Robert Koch (1843–1910), introduced a scientific approach to the field of medical microbiology. He established certain rules (now known as Koch's postulates) that must be followed to establish a cause-and-effect relationship between a microorganism and a disease. We shall discuss these postulates in detail in Chapter 11; working from these postulates, Koch was able to isolate and grow the etiological agents of such diseases as anthrax, cholera, and tuberculosis.

Another important contribution from Koch's laboratory was the use of agar (a complex polysaccharide isolated from seaweed) to solidify culture media. Agar is valuable to the microbiologist because it will melt at about the temperature of boiling water and once melted will not resolidify until it is cooled to approximately 43°C. Thus, if 2% agar is added to a liquid medium and the mixture is then heated to melt the agar and sterilize the medium, it can be dispensed in tubes or petri dishes where it will solidify when cooled. A solid surface is essential for separating mixtures of bacteria to obtain pure cultures; Koch's use of agar for this purpose proved to be a major advance in bacteriological technique.

Many other scientists earned recognition in the history of microbiology—in fact, some died after being infected by the organisms they were studying (for example, Howard Taylor Ricketts and Stanislas von Prowazek from typhus). Today, a little over a hundred years after Pasteur, research in microbiology is aimed at understanding many complex problems, including the etiology and control of cancer, the genetic control of biochemical syntheses, and the potential use of viruses for the correction of genetic defects. We shall begin by discussing the structure of microorganisms and how this structure may influence the properties of the cell.

## PROCARYOTIC AND EUCARYOTIC CELLS

If the biochemical activities of cells derived from such diverse sources as bacteria, spinach, and rat liver were compared, one would find amazing similarities. All the cells would be found to have their heritable characteristics coded in deoxyribonucleic acid (DNA); all would utilize one general mechanism for the storage of energy; all would have essentially identical methods of protein synthesis, nucleic acid synthesis, and polysaccharide synthesis. This incredible biochemical unity exists throughout the living world, with only minor variations on a major theme. When we examine cells morphologically, we find two distinct types, termed eucaryotic and procaryotic.

The eucaryotic cell, found in most animals and plants, is surrounded by a plasma membrane that regulates the movement of substances into and out of the cell, and it possesses a true nucleus that is separated from the cytoplasm of the cell by a well-defined, two-layered nuclear membrane, or, better, nuclear envelope. Within this nucleus, the DNA along with several kinds of proteins is organized into linear strands called chromosomes. The number of chromosomes in a eucaryotic nucleus is fixed for a given species. For certain fungi it may be 1 or 2; it is 46 for humans, and is other numbers for other plants and animals. When a eucaryotic cell divides, it goes through a rather elaborate process to provide each daughter cell with a full set of chromosomes. During this process, called mitosis, the strands of DNA replicate and the chromosomes condense by supercoiling. The replication of DNA provides each chromosome with two identical sets of genetic information visible as two sets of arms or chromatids on the chromosome. The nuclear envelope disintegrates and a spindle forms with the chromosomes on a plane halfway between the poles of the spindle. Fibers of the spindle attach to the chromosomes and the chromatids are pulled apart, each chromatid now becoming a new chromosome and being pulled to one pole or the other of the spindle, where a new nucleus forms. This nuclear division, or karyokinesis, is usually followed by cytokinesis, a division of the material outside the nucleus (the cytoplasm) somewhere between the two new nuclei. Mitosis results in two daughter cells with chromosomal complements and, therefore, genetic information identical to the parent cell.

Eucaryotic cells also contain within their cytoplasm organelles that carry out metabolic activities to provide energy for the cell. These structures are called mitochondria, and their principal function is the generation of adenosine triphosphate (ATP). In plant cells involved in photosynthesis, the light-trapping pigment, chlorophyll, is contained in an organelle called a chloroplast. In general, the process of photosynthesis converts light energy into chemical-bond energy. Many other organelles, most defined by membranes, take part in metabolic activi-

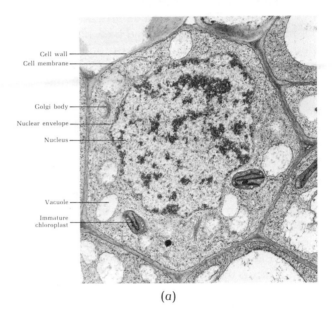

(a)

**Figure 1-3.** a. Section of cell from stem of a young pea plant, *Pisum sativum* (×9,945). b. Section of an animal cell, in this case a macrophage from a mouse (×6,240).

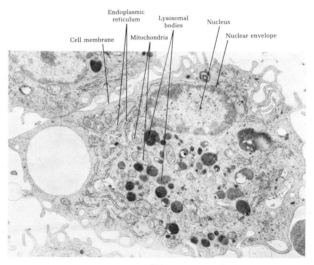

(b)

ties, motility, and other functions of eucaryotic cells. Some eucaryotic organelles may be seen in the micrographs of plant and animal cells in Figure 1-3; however, a complete review is better left to textbooks of cell biology.

The distinctions between eucaryotic and procaryotic cells probably represent the only major example of dichotomy in the evolution of the cell. The type of cell represented by the bacteria, including actinomycetes, spirochetes, rickettsiae, chlamydiae, and mycoplasmas, and the blue-green algae, the procaryotic cell, is bounded by a plasma membrane (cytoplasmic or protoplasmic membrane), but it does not possess a true nucleus, since its DNA is not separated from the cytoplasm by a nuclear envelope. Also, the DNA of the procaryotic cell does not exist in multiple distinct chromosomes as in the eucaryotic cell but in a single continuous thread; however, as we shall learn later, many procaryotic cells possess small pieces of extrachromosomal DNA which control some of the activities of the cell. In any event one can see that the procaryotic cell does not require a mechanism as elaborate as mitosis for the distribution of its DNA to daughter cells. Rather, the DNA of a procaryotic cell appears to be attached to the plasma membrane which is just inside the cell wall, and as the cell divides into two cells (binary fission), a new membrane is formed between the newly divided copies of DNA, extending across the cell to form two identical daughter cells. Unlike eucaryotic cells, procaryotic cells do not possess mitochondria and, if photosynthetic, do not possess chloroplasts. Cytoplasmic streaming, a flow of contents often seen in eucaryotic cells, is not seen in procaryotic cells, but one might expect it is not necessary in a cell sufficiently small for simple diffusion to move material around inside the cytoplasm. Procaryotic cells, other than the mycoplasmas and extreme halophils, possess a cell wall containing muramic acid, a compound not found in eucaryotic cells. Procaryotic cells also possess smaller ribosomes (70S; S represents Svedberg units,

a unit of measurement for the rate at which a particle will sediment during high speed centrifugation) than found in the cytoplasm of eucaryotic cells (80S); however, this difference does not apply to the mitochrondrial ribosomes of eucaryotes, since they also are 70S. And, although many eucaryotic cells

**Figure 1-4.** *a.* Section of bacterium *Klebsiella aerogenes* (×20,730). *b.* Bacterium *Bacillus mucroides* (×26,000).

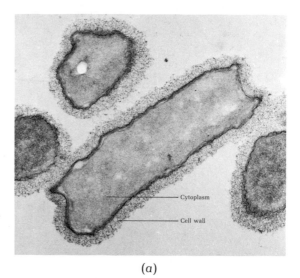

(a)

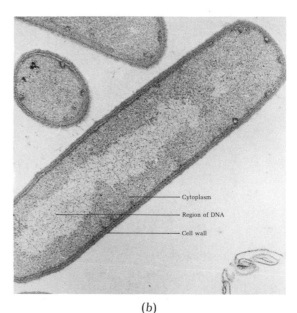

(b)

can engulf particulate material by a process called phagocytosis, procaryotic organisms are not able to take any material inside their cells unless it is first solubilized. Figure 1-4 shows two procaryotic cells with prominent features labeled.

## CLASSIFICATION OF MICROORGANISMS

Exactly where and how do microorganisms fit into the hierarchy of living things? We can find the answer to this question by reviewing some elementary principles of biological classification.

For many years most biologists assigned every form of life to one of two great kingdoms: the animal kingdom and the plant kingdom. The members of each kingdom were then arranged in order of their complexity using a phylogenetic, or natural, classification. Such a classification requires knowledge of fossil forms for the purpose of grouping organisms into an evolutionary tree composed of phyla, classes, orders, tribes, families, genera, and species (plus numerous intermediate levels in some schemes). However, not only were fossils of microorganisms not available until very recent times, but it was not even possible to decide into which kingdom they should be placed. Some possess certain characteristics commonly associated with animals, as the ability to move. Others have chlorophyll and obtain their energy from photosynthesis, as do the green plants. Still others possess characteristics of both plants and animals. Thus, it was necessary to make some rather arbitrary decisions on how microorganisms should be classified, and early schemes placed all microorganisms, except those complex microbes called protozoa, in the plant kingdom.

As more and more was learned about microorganisms, many biologists believed that they should be placed in a separate kingdom. As a result, a third kingdom, called the Protista, was proposed by Haeckel in 1866 to include the bacteria, fungi, algae, and pro-

tozoa. Subsequently, this kingdom was divided into two large divisions in which the eucaryotic Protista were considered as higher protists and the procaryotic Protista as lower protists. Within these divisions, microorganisms were assigned to classes, orders, tribes, families, genera, species, and subspecies. However, insofar as procaryotic cells are concerned, there is no known evolutionary relationship upon which to base such a system of classification, and the schemes in use were really keys attempting to group similar organisms together. It is not surprising, therefore, that the classification of microorganisms is constantly changing, as illustrated by a recent suggestion for a five-kingdom scheme. Because of the great difference between procaryotes and eucaryotes, this recent proposal places all procaryotes in a separate kingdom, the Monera. Unicellular eucaryotes, algae and protozoa, are considered Protista, and fungi receive their own kingdom (Fungi). Plants and animals are, of course, still around as plants and animals. Thus, classification of microorganisms is artificial, and one can only wonder how many kingdoms the future will bring. On the other hand, these schemes are useful in our attempt to give some semblance of order to the endless array of living forms involved in disease.

### The Classification of Bacteria

The system for classification of bacteria routinely used in the United States is outlined in *Bergey's Manual of Determinative Bacteriology*. This manual was first published in 1923, and has undergone periodic revisions, with the eighth edition published in 1974.

*Bergey's Manual* is concerned only with the bacteria, and the current edition has deviated considerably from its predecessors in its approach to classification. The editors of this edition have placed all of the procaryotic organisms into a new kingdom called the Procaryotae. However, the authors of this new classification have felt no compulsion to place microorganisms into orders, families,

## Table 1-1. Key to the Bacteria

| Identifying feature* | Classification |
|---|---|
| I. Phototrophic | Part 1 |
| II. Chemotrophic | |
|    A. Chemolithotrophic (chemoautotrophic) | |
|      1. Derive energy from the oxidation of nitrogen, sulfur or iron compounds, do not produce methane from carbon dioxide | |
|        a. Cells glide | Part 2 |
|       aa. Cells do not glide | |
|          b. Cells ensheathed | Part 3 |
|         bb. Cells not ensheathed | Part 12 |
|      2. Do not oxidize nitrogen, sulfur or iron compounds, produce methane from carbon dioxide | Part 13 |
|    B. Chemoorganotrophic (chemoheterotrophic) | |
|      1. Cells glide | Part 2 |
|      2. Cells do not glide (exceptions in Part 19) | |
|        a. Cells filamentous and ensheathed | Part 3 |
|       aa. Cells not filamentous and ensheathed | |
|          b. Products of binary fission not equivalent (have appendages other than flagella and pili or reproduce by budding). | Part 4 |
|         bb. Not as above | |
|           c. Cells not rigidly bound | |
|             d. Cells spiral-shaped, have cell wall | Part 5 |
|            dd. Cells not spiral-shaped, no cell wall | Part 19 |
|          cc. Cells rigidly bound | |
|            d. Gram negative | |
|             e. Obligate intracellular parasites | Part 18 |
|            ee. Not as above | |
|              f. Curved rods | Part 6 |
|             ff. Not curved rods | |
|               g. Rods | |
|                 h. Aerobic | Part 7 |
|                hh. Facultatively anaerobic | Part 8 |
|               hhh. Anaerobic | Part 9 |
|              gg. Cocci or coccobacilli | |
|                 h. Aerobic | Part 10<br>Part 7 |
|                hh. Anaerobic | Part 11 |
|            dd. Gram positive | |
|             e. Cocci | |

| Identifying feature* | Classification |
|---|---|
| f. Endospores produced | Part 15 |
| ff. Endospores not produced | Part 14 |
| ee. Rods or filaments | |
| f. Endospores produced | Part 15 |
| ff. Endospores not produced | |
| g. Straight rods | Part 16 |
| | Part 17 |
| gg. Irregular rods (coryneform) or tend to form filaments or filamentous | Part 17 |

*See Chapters 3, 4, and 5 for definitions of unfamiliar terms.

or tribes, but have divided the bacteria into various parts (also called hierarchies) based on morphological and metabolic characteristics. Since each part or hierarchy was discussed by specialists in that area, the decision to use orders or families was left to the individual authors. Thus in some cases these taxonomic divisions are used but in many cases they have been omitted. Moreover, there are many genera that did not seem to fit well into any of the parts. Such cases are labeled "Genera of Uncertain Affiliation" and are included as an appendix to the group of organisms to which they seem to be most closely related. As our knowledge of these Genera of Uncertain Affiliation increases, they will undoubtedly acquire a more permanent taxonomic position. Furthermore, it is now known that even though the rickettsiae and chlamydiae are obligately intracellular organisms, this does not in any way relate them to the intracellular viruses. They are merely variations of gram-negative bacteria, and as a result are placed in Part 18 of the kingdom Procaryotae. Similarly, the mycoplasmas are now recognized as a special form of procarotic bacterium, and they now make up Part 19 of the Procaryotae. Thus, the overall philosophy of the editor and authors of the new edition of *Bergey's Manual* is for the manual to serve as a determinative guide to the naming of genera and species, but they

do not provide a phylogenetic classification of bacteria in the sense that higher biological organisms are classified. Table 1-1 pro-provides a simplified key for selecting the correct part for the identification of an unknown bacterium.

Many specific properties are used to show relatedness between various groups of bacteria. The more obvious of these include cell morphology, cell arrangement, colony form, physiology or growth characteristics, nutrition, and antibiotic sensitivities. In addition, the percentage of DNA homology as measured by the amount of base pairing when DNA from two strains of bacteria is mixed under experimental conditions gives good evidence of relatedness (see Figure 1-5 and Table 1-2). One may also determine the percentage of guanine plus cytosine (G + C) by merely determining the temperature at which the paired strands of DNA separate ("melting point" of DNA) or by measuring the buoyant density by high-speed centrifugation of the bacterial DNA in a gradient of cesium chloride. A large difference in G + C content between two strains certainly indicates unrelatedness, but a similar G + C content does not by itself prove any similarity between bacterial strains.

In recent years there has been an increasing tendency to use a type of numerical analysis in which 100 to 300 characteristics of an

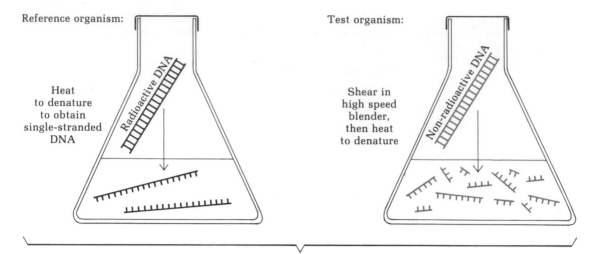

Reference organism: Heat to denature to obtain single-stranded DNA — Radioactive DNA

Test organism: Shear in high speed blender, then heat to denature — Non-radioactive DNA

Combine and cool to reanneal

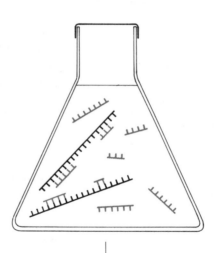

Hydrolyze residual single-stranded DNA with pancreatic DNase

Collect and count radioactivity remaining in double-stranded DNA

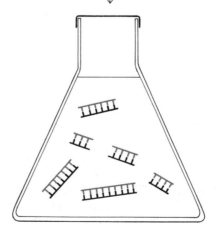

organism are determined and each characteristic is assigned an equal number. This type of taxonomic analysis, called numerical taxonomy, would be essentially impossible without the aid of a computer, but with a computer hundreds of strains of bacteria can be compared to each other. Simply stated, one calculates a similarity index (S) for each pair of organisms being compared using the following formula: $S = NS/(NS + ND)$, where S is the similarity index, NS represents the number of characters common to both organisms, and ND stands for the number of characters not common to the pair being compared. Starting with the highest values of S, one can prepare a matrix such as shown in Figure 1-6. If one then shades each square according to the degree of similarity, clusters of similarity become obvious. These data can also be plotted on bar-type graphs called dendrograms or phenograms. The references at the end of this chapter suggest additional reading on the use and interpretation of numerical taxonomy.

### The Classification of the Fungi

The fungi, considered as a kingdom by some biologists, comprise organisms known as yeasts and molds. Some grow exclusively as single-celled yeasts, others solely as multicellular molds, and a few (particularly some fungi producing human disease) exist as either yeasts or molds depending on their conditions of growth. The exceedingly complex classification of the fungi is based, in part, on the appearance and method of formation of their sexual spores, the type and appearance of their asexual spores, and the overall appearance of the entire organism.

**Table 1-2. *Escherichia coli* and *Klebsiella pneumoniae* DNA Reactions with *Erwinia* Species**

| DNA reaction[a] | Relative percent binding, 60°C | Relative percent binding, 75°C |
|---|---|---|
| Escherichia coli/ Escherichia coli | 100 | 100 |
| Escherichia coli/ Erwinia amylovora | 27 | 5 |
| Escherichia coli/ Erwinia dissolvens | 34 | 7 |
| Escherichia coli/ Erwinia aroideae | 16 | 3 |
| Escherichia coli/ Erwinia carotovora | 17 | 4 |
| Escherichia coli/ Erwinia carnegieana | 32 | 6 |
| Escherichia coli/ Salmonella typhimurium | 45 | 13 |
| Escherichia coli/ Proteus mirabilis | 9 | 0.7 |
| Klebsiella pneumoniae/ Klebsiella pneumoniae | 100 | |
| Klebsiella pneumoniae/ Erwinia dissolvens | 34 | |
| Klebsiella pneumoniae/ Erwinia carotovora | 17 | |

[a]The first organism is the source of labeled DNA.

YEASTS. The microscopic one-celled fungi known as yeasts characteristically reproduce by forming buds on the mother cell which, when mature, pinch off to become new single yeast cells. (Rare exceptions exist as in the genus *Schizosaccharomyces*, which divides

**Figure 1-5.** Relatedness can be determined by measuring the degree of DNA homology existing between two organisms. The reference organism is grown in a medium containing tritiated thymidine so that all its DNA will be radioactively labeled with tritium. The test organism is grown in a medium containing no radioactively labeled components. The DNA is isolated from each organism and treated as described. Only those fragments of DNA from the test organism possessing sequences complementary to the reference DNA will reanneal to form double-stranded DNA.

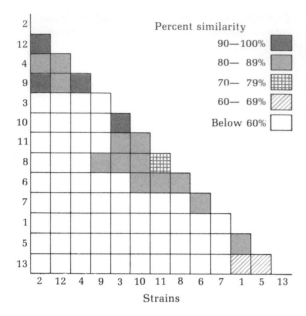

**Figure 1-6.** Thirteen different strains of bacteria are arranged according to their similarity index. Each intersecting square is then shaded to show the degree of similarity existing between each pair. With this type of matrix one can readily see clusters of similarity such as shown here among strains 2, 12, 4 and 9 and among strains 3, 10, 11, 8, 6, and 7.

by fission much like a bacterium). The majority of yeasts also produce sexual spores following the fusion of two separate cells. Many yeasts convert carbohydrates to ethyl alcohol, and by virtue of this characteristic have contributed to the amenities of civilization through their use in the manufacture of alcoholic beverages (*Saccharomyces cerevisciae* and *Saccharomyces carlsbergensis*). Some strains of *Saccharomyces cerevisciae* also are used to raise (leaven) bread through their ability to produce large amounts of gaseous carbon dioxide in the bread dough. Only a few yeasts produce disease in humans.

MOLDS. The multicellular fungi known as molds are considerably more complex than yeasts. Although individually they are microscopic organisms, many molds become read-ily visible as "mildew" on clothes, food, and leather goods during damp weather. Molds grow characteristically as branching hairlike growths, and most form both sexual and asexual spores. Some are responsible for the flavor of certain fine cheeses (Roquefort, Camembert, and Brie), and one, *Penicillium chrysogenum,* is the source of the antibiotic penicillin. On the other hand, a few molds (and yeasts) cause serious diseases in humans. These pathogenic fungi will be discussed in Chapter 29.

**Viruses**

The viruses are the smallest organisms known; indeed, to some biologists it is a moot question whether they actually possess all the attributes of living matter. Viruses are ultramicroscopic, too small to be seen with the conventional light microscope, although they can be visualized with the electron microscope.

As you will learn in Chapter 32, viruses require living host cells for growth and reproduce within these host cells by mechanisms different from bacterial fission. As a result, they cannot be classified with any other organisms and are separated as described in Unit Four into families on the basis of viral shape, presence or absence of a membrane, type of nucleic acid (DNA or RNA), and the form of the viral nucleic acid (double-stranded, single-stranded, linear, circular, and single or multiple pieces within the virion).

Few (if any) cells are not susceptible to viral infections. Thus, in addition to animal viruses, there are numerous plant viruses as well as viruses that infect bacteria (bacteriophage). Because of the many infections caused by viruses, Unit Four of this text is devoted exclusively to these agents and the diseases they cause in humans.

**OVERVIEW**

Although we cannot construct a single phylogenetic classification for procaryotic cells, they certainly represent a primitive type of cell and a major dichotomy in biological evolution. Taxonomy of such cells is an ever-changing field, and the most recent classification scheme in *Bergey's Manual* has placed the bacteria into a key which, though somewhat arbitrary, is designed to lead to their identification with a minimum of required information.

It is possible to come much closer to a phylogenetic classification of the higher eucaryotic protists, since they have more complicated structures and methods of reproduction. Viruses are really not cells at all, and so cannot be grouped with any other form of life. Because they must grow within host cells, it would seem probable that their position on the evolutionary scale is somewhat more recent than either the eucaryotic or procaryotic cell types.

## REFERENCES

Bergan, T. 1971. Survey of numerical techniques for grouping. *Bacteriol. Rev.* **35**:379–389.

Brock, T. D. 1961. *Milestones in Microbiology.* Prentice-Hall, Englewood Cliffs, New Jersey.

Bullock, W. 1938. *The History of Bacteriology.* Oxford University Press, London.

Dobell, C. 1960. *Antony van Leeuwenhoek and His "Little Animals."* Dover, Harcourt Brace, New York.

Doetsch, R. N. 1976. Lazzaro Spallanzani's Opusculi of 1776. *Bacteriol. Rev.* **40**:270–275.

Dubos, R. 1950. *Louis Pasteur. Free Lance of Science.* Little, Brown & Co., Boston.

Kennell, D. E. 1971. Principles and practices of nucleic acid hybridization. *Progr. Nucl. Acid Res.* **11**:259–301.

Lechevalier, H. A., and M. Solotorovsky. 1965. *Three Centuries of Microbiology.* McGraw-Hill, New York.

Lockhart, W. R., and J. Liston, eds. 1970. *Methods for Numerical Taxonomy.* Amer. Soc. Microbiol., Washington, D.C.

Lwoff, A. 1957. The concept of a virus. *J. Gen. Microbiol.* **17**:239–253.

Moore, R. L. 1974. Nucleic acid reassociation as a guide to genetic relatedness among bacteria. *Current Topics in Microbiol. and Immunol.* **64**:105–128.

Penn, M., and M. Dworkin. 1976. Robert Koch and two visions of microbiology. *Bacteriol. Rev.* **40**:276–283.

Porter, J. R. 1976. Anthony van Leeuwenhoek: Tercentenary of his discovery of bacteria. *Bacteriol. Rev.* **40**:260–269.

Tyndall, J. 1882. *Essays on the Floating Matter of the Air in Relation to Putrefaction and Infection.* Appleton & Co., New York.

# 2

## Laboratory Equipment and Procedures

The student of microbiology must learn to use certain basic techniques in the laboratory. These techniques are utilized in growing microorganisms, isolating them in pure culture, observing them, and finally in identifying them.

### THE MICROSCOPE

Accounts in seventeenth-century scientific literature convey the excitement with which the Royal Society of London awaited Antony van Leeuwenhoek's descriptions of microscopic material seen through his remarkable lenses. Since Leeuwenhoek, the use of microscopes in the study of microorganisms has progressed as we have learned that the smallest detail we can distinguish (resolving power) is limited not only by the lens of the microscope but also by the wavelength of the light used to illuminate the specimen. Thus, our current increased resolution can be attributed not only to better lenses but to new types of microscopes using shorter wavelengths of light and some limited only by the wavelength of electrons.

### Light Microscope

The microscope most students use in the laboratory is called a compound microscope because it has two sets of lenses. One set, called the objective, is next to the object to be studied, while the other set, the ocular, is next to your eye. Since the ocular magnifies the image passing through the objective lens, the over-all result is the product of the individual magnification of the two lenses. Thus, a 44-fold objective used in combination with a 10-fold ocular lens will give an over-all magnification of $440\times$ (read "440 times").

The light microscope used most commonly has three objective lenses: low power ($10\times$), high power ($44\times$), and oil immersion ($97\times$). In the study of bacteria, the latter lens is generally required. A drop of clear oil is placed directly on the specimen or on the cover glass over the specimen, and the oil-immersion objective is lowered into the oil. The light rays traveling from the specimen through glass and oil do not bend as much as they would if they were to pass through glass and air, resulting in a clearer image. Since the limit of resolution of a microscope is about one-half the wavelength of light used, the finest resolution that can be seen with a light microscope (using visible light with a minimum wavelength of about 400 nm) is approximately 200 nm (0.2 $\mu$m), and the best lenses in the world will not let you see something smaller unless a shorter wavelength of light is used.

## Ultraviolet Microscope

A variation on the ordinary light microscope is the ultraviolet microscope. Because ultraviolet light is about one-half the wavelength of visible light (200–300 nm), its use can increase the limit of resolution to about 100 nm. However, ultraviolet light is invisible to the human eye, and the image must be recorded on a photographic plate. These microscopes require quartz lenses and are very intricate and expensive for routine use.

## Fluorescence Microscope

For visualization using the fluorescence microscope, bacteria are stained with a fluorescent dye. They will then be a different color from that seen under the ordinary light microscope, because the fluorescent dye will absorb ultraviolet light and then emit light at a longer wavelength visible to the human eye. For example, the tubercle bacillus *Mycobacterium tuberculosis* stained with the fluorescent dye auramine will appear bright against a dark background. Since most bacteria will not take up auramine, this procedure is useful in identifying the tubercle bacillus in sputum samples.

Fluorescence microscopy may also be used to detect or identify various microorganisms by coupling a fluorescent dye to a specific antibody that will react only with the target bacterium. Since antibody-antigen reactions are specific, fluorescence will occur only if the organism in question is present.

## Dark-Field Microscope

The dark-field microscope is particularly useful for viewing living bacteria whose dimensions approach the limit of resolution of the compound microscope. Many pathogenic spirochetes fall into this category,

particularly the syphilis spirochete *Treponema pallidum*.

The dark-field microscope differs from the ordinary compound light microscope in possessing a special condenser which produces a hollow cone of visible light. The rays of light from this hollow cone do not go directly up into the objective lens, and only those rays that are reflected by the bacteria in the specimen will be reflected directly into the objective, with the result that the specimen appears completely white against a dark background. If no specimen were in the field, the field would appear dark since there would be nothing to cause the light to be reflected up into the objective.

## Phase-Contrast Microscope

The ideal way to observe a living cell is in its natural state: unstained and alive. As a rule, however, a microscopic fragment of living matter (such as animal tissue or bacteria) is practically transparent, and individual details do not stand out. This difficulty can be partially overcome with the use of the phase-contrast microscope.

The mechanics of this instrument are complicated, but in essence it measures small differences in density in the material being observed. For example, the nucleus or inclusions within a cell may be invisible when viewed with a light microscope. However, a phase-contrast microscope illuminates the specimen with light that is all in the same phase; those rays of light passing through a more dense part of the cell will be thrown slightly out of phase, and through a series of filters and diaphragms the microscope will translate this phase difference into differences in brightness discernible by the eye, making these structures visible.

## ELECTRON MICROSCOPE

### Transmission Electron Microscope

One of the great boons to microbiologists in the past 30 years has been the development of the transmission electron microscope. This microscope uses a beam of electrons rather than visible or ultraviolet light. Since the wavelength of the electron beam is much shorter (approximately 0.005 nm) than that of even ultraviolet light, the resolving power of the microscope is increased tremendously. With a resolving power greater than 1 nm (0.001 $\mu$m) magnifications of as much as one million diameters are possible. The image produced by the electron microscope is visible when projected onto a fluorescent screen.

There are several major problems involved in using a transmission electron microscope: (1) it requires a skilled technician for operation; (2) it is a very expensive piece of equipment; (3) it requires the use of very thin specimens (which may be easily distorted); (4) the specimen being examined must be contained in a very high vacuum in order for the electrons to move effectively; (5) live specimens cannot be examined; and (6) objects show no color. This means preparations must be dried and fixed with chemicals prior to study, and the drying and fixing process also may result in distortion of some of the cellular components.

An important development in electron microscopy is the use of phosphotungstic acid as a negative stain. Phosphotungstic acid is electron-dense, and structural details of the cell can be observed while the background and empty areas remain opaque.

Shadow casting is a technique for revealing surface details. An electron-dense metal such as platinum or chromium is vaporized under high vacuum and deposited at an angle on the preparation. The uncoated area on the opposite sides acquires a shadow, and the resulting electron micrograph shows a three-dimensional effect (see Figure 2-1).

### Scanning Electron Microscope

The scanning electron microscope also employs a beam of electrons, but instead of being simultaneously transmitted through the entire field, the electrons are focused as a very fine probe or spot which is moved back and forth over the specimen. As the probe electrons strike the surface of the specimen, secondary electrons are emitted which are collected by a cathode ray tube. The strength of the signal will be seen as dark or light areas on the collector, providing an image of the specimen's surface. Photographs taken of the cathode ray tube appear as three-dimensional micrographs, as shown in Figure 2-2.

**Figure 2-1.** Electron micrograph of the spirochete *Spirochaeta stenostrepta* shadowed with platinum ($\times$12,100).

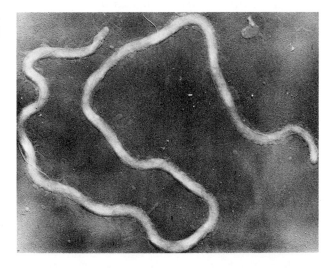

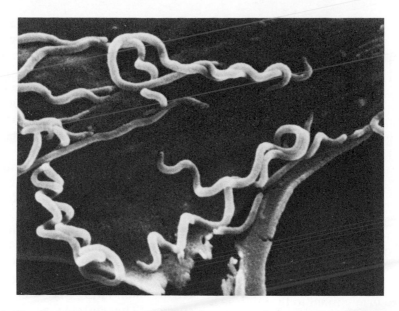

**Figure 2-2.** The three-dimensional qualities of scanning electron microscopy clearly reveal the corkscrew shape of cells of the syphilis-causing spirochete *Treponema pallidum*, attached here to rabbit testicular cells grown in culture (×8,000).

## TECHNIQUES FOR MICROSCOPIC STUDY OF BACTERIA

### Living Bacteria

Living bacteria are difficult to see with the average light microscope because they appear almost colorless when viewed individually, even though the culture as a whole may be highly colored. However, it is often necessary and desirable to look at living bacteria under the microscope, particularly to determine if they are motile.

One satisfactory method of observing living bacteria is in a hanging-drop preparation (see Figure 2-3). A drop of liquid culture (or organisms suspended in water or a solution of physiological saline) is placed in the center of a cover glass. A special slide with a hollow depression in the center is ringed with a thin layer of petrolatum, and then turned upside down over the cover glass so that the drop of organisms is in the center of the depression. The entire slide with the cover glass then is quickly turned over so that the drop of organisms actually hangs from the cover glass down into the depression. The slide is placed on the stage of a microscope and the organisms are observed using the high dry or oil-immersion objective.

Keep in mind that a bacterium is considered motile only if it seems to be going in a definite direction. Even nonmotile bacteria will bounce back and forth due to the bombardment from molecules of water (Brownian movement).

**Figure 2-3.** This side view of a hanging-drop preparation shows the drop of culture hanging from the center of the cover glass above the depression slide.

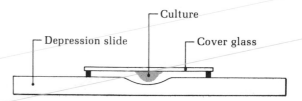

### Stained Bacteria

Bacteria are far more frequently observed in stained smears than in the living state. By staining bacteria, we color the organisms with a chemical stain to make them easier to see and study. In general, stained smears of bacteria reveal size, shape, and arrangement of the cells and the presence of certain internal structures such as granules or spores. Special stains are used for observing certain internal cellular details as well as capsules or flagella. Stains that reveal chemical differences in bacterial structure also may be used.

In order to prepare bacteria for staining, a small amount of culture is spread in a drop of water on a glass slide. This is called a smear. The smear is dried at room temperature, and the bacteria are firmly fixed to the slide as it is passed quickly through a flame. When cool, the smear is ready to be stained. The following sections outline a few of the more common procedures used to stain bacteria.

### Staining

STAINING REACTIONS.  Stains are salts composed of a positive and a negative ion, one of which is colored. In basic dyes, the color is in the positive ion; in acid dyes it is in the negative ion.

The marked affinity of bacteria for basic dyes is due primarily to the large amount of negative charge in the cell's protoplasm. Thus, when a bacterium is stained, the negative charges in the nucleic acid and the cell wall of the bacterium react with the positive ion of the basic dye. Crystal violet, safranin, and methylene blue are examples of the basic dyes commonly used.

In contrast, acid dyes are repelled by the overall negative charge of a bacterium. Thus, when a bacterial smear is stained with an acid dye (such as Congo red or nigrosin), only the background area is colored. Since the bacterial cell is colorless against a colored background, this technique of negative staining is valuable for observing the overall shape of extremely small cells.

SIMPLE STAIN.  This, as the name implies, is the simplest type of staining. One merely covers the smear with a basic dye, and after 30 to 60 seconds, the slide is washed under the water tap, and the smear is gently blotted dry. It is now ready to be observed under the microscope. To observe it with the oil-immersion lens, a drop of oil is placed directly on the stained smear, and the oil-immersion objective is lowered into the oil.

GRAM STAIN.  In 1884, the Danish physician Christian Gram devised a special stain which is probably the most important one used in the identification of bacteria. This is a differential stain, so called because it divides bacteria into two physiological groups, thereby greatly facilitating the identification of a species. The staining procedure has four steps: (1) the smear is flooded with gentian or crystal violet; (2) after 60 seconds, the violet dye is washed off and the smear is flooded with a solution of iodine; (3) 60 seconds later, the iodine is poured off and the slide is washed with 95% ethanol for 15 to 30 seconds; and (4) the slide is counterstained for 30 seconds with either safranin (a red dye) or Bismarck brown. (Bismarck brown may be used by persons who are colorblind to red.)

The violet dye and the iodine form a complex compound. Some genera of bacteria readily lose the stain when washed with ethanol, while other organisms resist decolorization by the ethanol wash. Organisms that do not retain the dye complex after the 95% alcohol wash are called gram-negative organisms; those that retain the complex are called gram-positive organisms. Because gram-negative bacteria are colorless after the alcohol wash, one always counterstains with a different color dye before looking at the smear under the microscope. The usual counterstain is the red dye safranin, and gram-negative bacteria appear red. Alcohol does not wash out the blue dye complex from gram-positive cells, and the safranin counterstain therefore has no effect. Thus, gram-positive cells appear blue or bluish-purple.

Many theories have been proposed to explain why some bacteria are gram-positive and others gram-negative. The most logical explanation is that the cell walls of gram-positive organisms are considerably thicker than those of gram-negative bacteria (as discussed in Chapter 3). The dye-iodine complex appears to become trapped between the cell wall and the plasma membrane of the gram-positive organisms; it can be washed out of the gram-negative organisms.

It is essential to know the gram reaction as positive or negative as well as the overall appearance of a bacterium to identify it. In addition, other general characteristics of an organism are associated with the gram reaction. For example, most gram-positive bacteria are easily killed by low concentrations of penicillin G, gramicidin, or gentian violet, whereas gram-negative bacteria are much more resistant to those compounds but are more sensitive to some antibiotics such as polymyxin. We shall discuss the reasons for these differences in more detail in Chapter 10.

ACID-FAST STAIN. This stain (also called the Ziehl-Neelsen stain) is used specifically to help identify organisms in the genus *Mycobacterium*. This genus contains several virulent pathogens, including the ones causing tuberculosis and leprosy. The mycobacteria are called acid-fast, because once they are stained with carbol fuchsin their unique chemical properties cause the stain to remain even after washing the stained smear with 95% ethanol that contains 3% hydrochloric acid. This property sets the acid-fast organisms apart from other bacteria and makes it possible to stain mixtures of large numbers of bacteria (such as those present in sputum) and still recognize the acid-fast bacteria.

OTHER STAINS. A number of additional specialized staining procedures are used to stain parts of the bacterial cell and some will be seen in the micrographs throughout this book. They include techniques for staining capsules, cell walls, chromatin, flagella, endospores, and other structures. All these staining procedures involve the use of two or more special dyes, but none are used routinely in the identification of a bacterium.

## PREPARATION OF A PURE CULTURE

Suppose that you have a specimen of material (for instance, feces) that contains many different types of bacteria, and you wish to isolate a specific bacterium that is causing a disease, such as typhoid fever. Since it is impractical to try to pick out individual bacterial cells from the material, one must resort to a less direct method of isolation.

This can be accomplished by using a solid or semi-solid medium containing nutrients which the bacteria can use as food. If a dilution of the fecal material is spread out (streaked) on solid nutrient medium in a sterile petri dish, each bacterial cell, theoretically, will reproduce and, within a day or two, the medium will be covered with colonies of microorganisms. Assuming individual cells were well separated in the initial streaking, each isolated colony will have arisen from a single bacterium and will therefore be composed of many identical organisms.

If a colony is touched with a sterile needle and the adhering cells transferred to another sterilized medium, the bacteria will reproduce as a pure culture, a culture composed of only one kind of bacterium.

### Pure-Culture Techniques

To obtain the bacterial colonies from which pure cultures are made, two techniques are employed: the streak-plate and the pour-plate methods.

In the streak-plate method, the sterile nutrient agar medium is melted, cooled to about 45°C, poured into a sterile petri dish, and allowed to solidify. Then, with the wire inoculating loop full of the mixed culture, streaks are made across the surface of the agar. There are several different methods for streaking, but in all methods, the object is to deposit most of the organisms in the first few streaks. Thus, as one continues to streak the loop back and forth from one section of the petri dish to another, fewer bacteria will remain on the loop. If done properly, the last streaks should leave individual bacteria separated sufficiently from each other so that after growth, colonies that develop from individual bacteria will be well separated from each other (see Figure 2-4a). A single colony can then be transferred to a sterile medium, and a pure culture is obtained.

The pour-plate method consists of inoculating a dilution of the mixed culture into a test tube containing a melted agar medium that has been cooled to 45°C. The tube is then agitated to disperse the organisms throughout the medium before being poured into sterile petri dishes and allowed to solidify. A culture from this method should result in evenly dispersed colonies (see Figure 2-4b).

The object in both procedures is obviously to separate individual bacterial cells from each other so that they will grow into isolated colonies in the solid medium. Dilutions for

**Figure 2-4.** *a.* The streak-plate technique is used to isolate bacterial colonies for pure cultures. Each individual colony represents the progeny of a single cell. Note how the number of cells decreases as one goes from the heavy part of the plate to an area of isolated single colonies. *b.* Pour plate prepared from dilution of a bacterial culture. Plates are prepared by inoculating tubes of melted and cooled nutrient agar with various dilutions of bacterial culture. The melted inoculated agar tubes are then poured into petri dishes and allowed to solidify. As with the streak plate, each colony represents the progeny of a single bacterial cell.

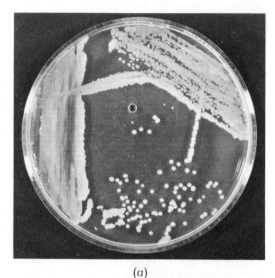

(a)

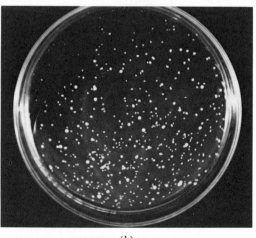

(b)

the pour-plate method must contain enough organisms to provide a number of separate colonies on each plate without covering the petri dish with colonies that have grown together, and this may require several different dilutions to be plated.

## Culture Media

The media on which bacteria are grown will vary in composition according to the requirements of various species. Some bacteria will grow well on a very simple medium containing only inorganic salts plus an organic carbon source such as a sugar. Others may require a very complex medium to which blood or other complex materials are added. Almost all commonly used media can be purchased commercially as dry powders. Thus, to prepare a medium, one need only weigh out the desired amount of powder, add water, dispense, and sterilize before use (or, in some cases, sterilize first and then dispense into sterile petri dishes).

INFUSION MEDIA. One of the most common media used for the routine cultivation of bacteria is called nutrient broth. This is prepared by boiling ground beef with water and filtering off the solid material to yield a clear liquid known as an infusion. Partially degraded peptone and frequently 0.5% NaCl are added to the liquid. After the pH is adjusted, the medium is ready for sterilization and subsequently for bacterial growth. Usually an infusion medium is dispensed into screw-cap test tubes.

To grow bacteria on a solid surface rather than suspended in a liquid broth, 1.5–2% agar is added to any medium. Once the agar has been melted in the medium, it can be dispensed while hot into tubes, capped, and sterilized. After sterilization and while the mixture is still melted, the tubes may be slanted so that after solidification there will be a larger surface area to use for bacterial growth (see Figure 2-5).

A medium that contains complex substances of biological origin such as beef ex-

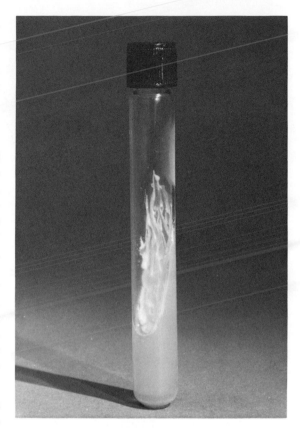

**Figure 2-5.** Agar slants are used to culture bacteria. Because the screw cap prevents desiccation of the agar medium, many bacteria can be kept for weeks or months on slants before it is necessary to transfer them to fresh medium.

tract, yeast extract, tryptones, or blood is called a complex medium. In contrast, one for which we can write the chemical formula of each ingredient in the medium is called a synthetic medium. Synthetic media may contain many chemicals and will vary widely according to the particular organism that one wishes to grow; for the most part, they are used primarily for growing microorganisms for research purposes.

There are many other infusion media similar to nutrient broth or nutrient agar. A few of these include veal infusion, trypticase soy, and brain-heart infusion.

SELECTIVE AND DIFFERENTIAL MEDIA. Dyes may be added to a medium to inhibit the growth of certain bacteria while not interfering with the growth of others. This is called a selective medium, because it will allow only certain types of organisms to grow. The addition of bile salts to a medium can make it selective for the pathogenic enteric organisms, or the addition of dyes such as thionine or basic fuchsin to the growth medium will inhibit certain species of *Brucella* while allowing others to grow.

An acid indicator such as phenol red may also be added to a solid medium so that a colony of bacteria that forms acid can be differentiated from one that does not. This type of medium is called a differential medium. Blood is often added to differentiate hemolytic from nonhemolytic organisms. Both selective and differential media are particularly useful in the identification and the isolation of enteric and urogenital pathogens (see Chapter 20).

ENRICHMENT CULTURES. Bacteria present in very small numbers in some natural environments are frequently isolated with difficulty from the mixed population. If a suitable substrate and other conditions are provided that favor the growth of these rare organisms but are unsuitable for others, one can enrich the growth of one organism so that it will become the dominant organism. Thus, a medium containing citrate as a sole carbon source would greatly favor the growth of *Enterobacter* over that of *Escherichia* because organisms of the latter genus cannot transport citrate into their cells. Another example would include the addition of selenite to enrich for the growth of species in the genus *Salmonella* over the nonpathogenic enteric organisms.

CONTROL OF PH AND TEMPERATURE. Most bacteria grow best at or near neutrality, and most media are adjusted to a pH near 7 before use. A few bacteria grow better at slightly higher or lower pH values, so pH must be adjusted according to the purpose for which a particular medium will be used.

Temperature, too, must be adjusted for the growth of bacteria. Some bacteria will grow at temperatures below 10°C, while others will grow at temperatures as high as 70°C. However, the organisms that cause disease usually grow best at or near normal human body temperature, 37°C, and most disease producing organisms are, in fact, killed when exposed to a temperature of 60°–65°C for more than a few minutes.

OXYGEN REQUIREMENTS. Bacteria can be divided into three or four general groups on the basis of their oxygen requirements. The first group, the strict or obligate aerobes, requires free oxygen in order to grow. Since our atmosphere is approximately 20% oxygen, growing these organisms is no problem as long as the bacteria are exposed to air.

The strict (obligate) anaerobes are organisms that not only will not grow in the presence of free oxygen, but are actually killed by its presence (see Chapter 4). A number of techniques have been devised to grow anaerobic bacteria. One common method is to add a reducing agent such as sodium thioglycollate that will react with the free oxygen in the medium. In other cases, special cultural equipment is employed to remove the oxygen mechanically and replace it with hydrogen (see Figure 2-6).

A subgroup of the obligately anaerobic bacteria are those organisms that grow best with reduced oxygen tension but not necessarily under obligate anaerobic conditions. Such organisms are designated as microaerophilic, but no single explanation for their oxygen requirement is available.

Finally, a large number of organisms are designated as facultative anaerobes or facultative aerobes. These organisms can grow anaerobically and under such conditions will ferment carbohydrates to form stable fermentation products such as lactic acid, acetic acid, and so forth. When they are grown in the presence of air, however, the facultative organisms will change their metabolism to an aerobic one in which carbohydrates are oxidized to $H_2O$ and $CO_2$.

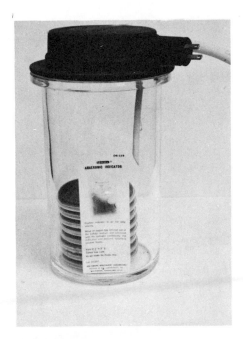

**Figure 2-6.** Petri dishes are placed inside this anaerobic jar, and the air is removed with a vacuum pump. The jar is then refilled with hydrogen gas and evacuated several times. After the final evacuation, the jar is filled with hydrogen and tightly sealed. The plug on the top is then connected to an electric circuit. This heats a palladium screen in the lid that catalyzes the chemical reaction of any residual oxygen with the hydrogen to form water. An oxidation-reduction indicator that changes color when all oxygen has been removed is usually included to insure that anaerobic conditions are present. Other jars with minor modifications accomplish this same objective.

Lactic-acid organisms are referred to as aerotolerant, since they grow in the presence of oxygen but they do not possess an oxidative metabolism and carry out a fermentative degradation of carbohydrates even in the presence of oxygen.

## HOW BACTERIA ARE IDENTIFIED

We shall have occasion to return to this subject later in the text—throughout Unit Three and particularly in Chapter 30—but even at this early point the reader may well wonder how one could ever possibly identify an unknown organism. We have already referred to the classification system in *Bergey's Manual of Determinative Bacteriology,* and Table 1-1 gave a brief key to the various major groups of bacteria. From what you now know, it is possible to think in terms of the minimal amount of information needed before any identification would be possible. This would include: (1) size and shape of the organism, (2) gram-staining reaction, (3) the type of flagellation, if motile, and (4) the overall size and appearance of the bacterial colony. With these minimal observations, it is usually possible to decide to which part (or family) the organism belongs, and sometimes even the correct genus can be chosen.

Further identification of genus and species requires biochemical information. The specific biochemical information needed may vary from group to group. You may have to determine which sugars are metabolized, or whether the organism can utilize gelatin or urea, or even whether the organism can grow on a medium that contains citrate as a sole source of carbon. It is not possible to know how much of this specific information will be required for a complete identification until one has decided to which part or family an unknown organism belongs.

Immunological tests also help in the final identification of certain bacteria, and we shall discuss many of these techniques in Unit Two.

### REFERENCES

Barer, R. 1974. Microscopes, microscopy and microbiology. *Annu. Rev. Microbiol.* **28:**317–389.

Basu, P. S., B. B. Biswas, and M. K. Pal. 1969. Molecular mechanism of gram staining. *J. Gen. Appl. Microbiol.* **15:**365–373.

Everhart, T. E., and T. L. Hayes. 1972. The scanning electron microscope. *Sci. American* **226:**54–69.

Murohashi, T., E. Kondo, and K. Yoshida. 1969. The role of lipids in acid-fastness of mycobacteria. *Annu. Rev. Respir. Dis.* **99:**794–798.

Norris, J. R., and D. W. Ribbons, eds. 1969–1977. *Methods in Microbiology* (nine volumes). Academic Press, New York.

Wilkins, T. D., C. B. Walker, and W. E. C. Moore. 1975. Micromethod for identification of anaerobic bacteria: Design and operation of apparatus. *J. Appl. Microbiol.* **30:**831–837.

# 3

# Bacterial Morphology

## SHAPES OF BACTERIAL CELLS

The word morphology designates the study of form and structure; we shall begin our study of bacterial morphology by discussing the various shapes of bacterial cells. Three distinct forms are generally recognized: (1) cocci, or spherical cells, (2) bacilli, or cylindrical or rod-shaped cells, and (3) spiral forms, curved rods or spiral cells.

### Cocci

The cocci (singular: coccus, meaning "berry") look like miniature berries under the microscope. They exist in several different patterns or groupings, some of which are characteristic for a specific genus. Some cocci characteristically exist singly, others in pairs, cubes, or in long chains, depending upon the manner in which they divide and then adhere to each other after division (see Figure 3-1a). For example, most streptococci form long chains of cells, since they divide in only one plane and do not easily break apart. Cocci which divide into two planes to form tetrads of cells belong to the genus *Gaffkya,* and those that divide into three planes at right angles to each other form cubical packets and belong to the genus

*Sarcinia.* Cocci that divide into two planes to form irregular clusters are classified in either the genus *Staphylococcus* or *Micrococcus.*

### Bacilli

Bacilli (singular: bacillus, meaning "little staff") are shaped like rods or cylinders. Some resemble cigarettes, while others (fusiform bacillus) form tapered ends more like a cigar. Some bacilli are almost as broad as they are long and as a result are called coccobacilli. All bacilli divide across their narrow axes and may be seen as single cells, pairs, or in short or long chains (see Figure 3-1b). However, unlike the cocci, the length of bacilli chains is not an identifying characteristic.

### Spiral Forms

This group comprises a large variety of cylindrical bacteria which are convoluted in varying degrees rather than straight like bacilli (see Figure 3-1c). The spiral bacteria are divided as follows:

1. Vibrios are curved rods resembling commas. Sometimes they adhere together in serpentine or S-shaped strands.

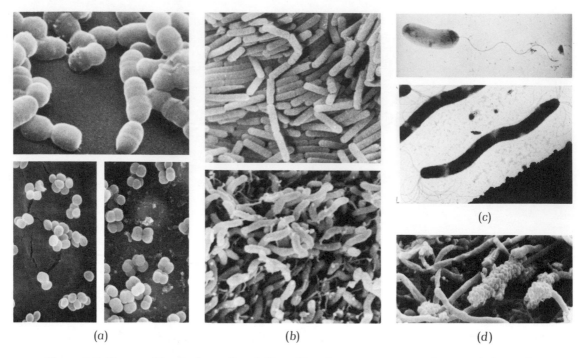

(a)  (b)  (c)  (d)

**Figure 3-1.** Forms of bacteria. *a.* Cocci. Top: *Streptococcus mutans,* demonstrating pairs and short chains (×9,400). Bottom left: single cells and small clusters of *Staphylococcus epidermidis* (×3,000). Bottom right: pairs, tetrads, and regular clusters of *Micrococcus luteus* (×3,000). *b.* Bacilli. Top: single cells and short chains of *Bacillus cereus* (×1,700). Bottom: flagellated bacilli (unnamed) associated with peridontitis (×3,700). *c.* Top: a cell of *Vibrio cholerae;* note curved cell and single flagellum (×8,470). Bottom: the spirillum *Aquaspirillum bengal;* note polar tufts of flagella (×2,870). *d.* Variety of organisms in dental plaque after 3 days without brushing (×1,360).

2. Spirilla (singular: spirillum) are actual spirals, like corkscrews.

3. Spirochetes are also spiral bacteria, but they differ from spirilla by possessing flexible cell walls. Spirochetes are also different from other bacteria in that their flagella, also called axial filaments, are wound tightly around the protoplasmic cylinder in a spiral fashion. The entire protoplasmic cylinder, including the flagella, is enclosed in a fragile external sheath (see Figure 3-2).

## BACTERIAL CELL STRUCTURE

If you keep in mind what you already know about animal or plant cells, you will find that you know something about bacterial cells; also, the features peculiar to bacteria will stand out all the more clearly by contrast. Let us consider the principal parts of a bacterium: appendages (flagella and pili), the surface layers (capsule, cell wall, and plasma membrane), the cytoplasm (nuclear material, ribosomes, inclusions, and chromatophores), and special structures.

### Flagella

Many types of bacteria are able to swim about by themselves, often at remarkable speeds for their size. This motility is typical of almost all spiral bacteria and about half of the bacilli. On the other hand, cocci are nonmotile. The propulsive mechanism of most of the bacteria with which we shall be concerned in this text is a threadlike appendage called a flagellum (plural: flagella), not to be confused with the entirely different flagella or cilia of eucaryotic cells.

Flagella are long and slender, generally several times the length of the cell. Their diameters may vary from 12–20 nm; however, since this size is below the limit of resolution of the light microscope, flagella are not visible in routine stained smears of bacteria. They can be seen with the light microscope only if a special substance, called a mordant, is used to increase the diameter of the flagellum before applying the stain.

The positions at which flagella are inserted into the bacterial cell are characteristic for a genus. Figure 3-3 presents a schematic representation of the various types of bacterial flagellation as well as a micrograph of a cell showing a number of flagella.

If one enzymatically removes the cell wall from a bacterium, the flagella can be seen to originate in the protoplasmic membrane. As shown schematically and by electron microscopy in Figure 3-4, the flagellum is attached to the bacterium by means of a hook and a series of plates or rings which appear to anchor the flagellum to each layer of cell membrane and cell wall. Each flagellum has a wavy structure (the wavelength of which is characteristic for each genus), and actual motility appears to result from the rotation of the flagellum in a manner similar to that of a boat propeller.

The mechanism by which the cell provides the energy for the rotation of its flagella is not known, but the fact that bacteria exhibit chemotaxis, that is, they will move toward a gradient of various attractants (usually nutrient substrates) clearly demonstrates that movement is not entirely random. When the flagellum is rotating in one direction, the bacterium will travel in a more or less straight line, but if the direction of flagellar movement is reversed, the organism will tumble aimlessly. When moving up a gradient of a chemotactic

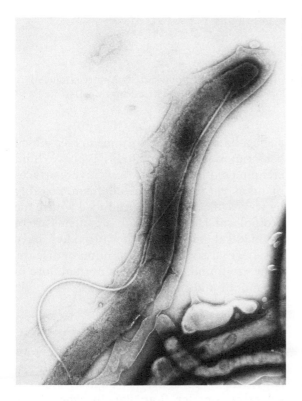

**Figure 3-2.** One end of a free-living spirochete. The protoplasmic cylinder, axial filament, and external sheath are clearly visible in this negatively-stained preparation ($\times 25{,}920$).

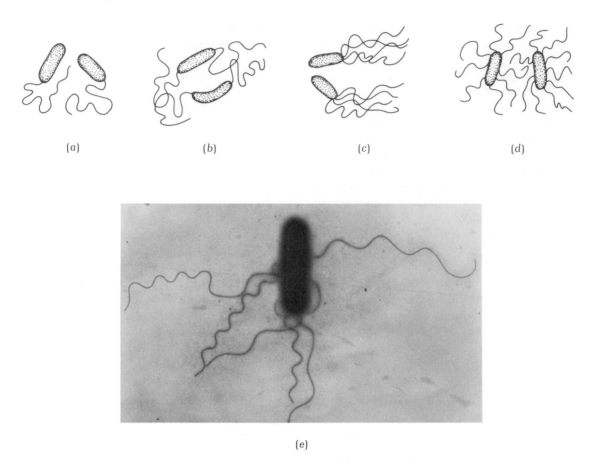

(a)           (b)           (c)           (d)

(e)

**Figure 3-3.** Types of bacterial flagellation. *a.* Monotrichous (polar). *b.* Amphitrichous. *c.* Lophotrichous. *d.* Peritrichous. *e.* Cell of *Salmonella* sp. showing peritrichous flagellation.

attractant, the straight line movements last longer, and the tumbling occurs only briefly. However, if the bacterium is moving away from an attractant or accidentally toward a repellant, the tumbling occurs frequently until the net movement is properly redirected.

If a solution of isolated flagella is made mildly acidic (pH 3), the flagella will dissociate into a large number of identical protein subunits called flagellin. Neutralization of this solution will result in a spontaneous reaggregation of the flagellin to form the intact flagellum. One might assume, then, that during growth the bacterium synthesizes the smaller subunits of flagellin and that these smaller subunits spontaneously aggregate to form flagella.

Flagella are not the only means by which bacteria move about. Some types exhibit creeping motility; they "crawl" over surfaces by an as yet unknown mechanism, possibly by waves of contraction produced within the protoplasm. However, such organisms are of no medical importance because they have not been associated with human disease. They are found, however, as normal flora of the mouth and intestinal tract.

## Pili or Fimbriae

Pili, also called fimbriae, are filamentous appendages, visible only by electron microscopy, which are shorter, straighter, and considerably smaller than flagella (see Figure

3-5). Occurring only on gram-negative bacteria, they are composed of protein which can be dissociated into smaller identical subunits called pilin. We actually know very little of the function of pili, but it does appear that bacteria possessing pili have a greater tendency to stick to each other and to animal cells than do those without pili. In fact, the ability of *Neisseria gonorrhoeae,* as well as some other bacteria such as the enteropathic *Escherichia coli,* to cause disease is thought to be associated with the possession of pili, since mutation to avirulence is accompanied by the loss of pili.

Some enteric bacteria have one or two special pili, called F pili, which are necessary for bacterial conjugation resulting in the transfer of DNA from one cell to another. It is also interesting that a number of bacterial viruses infect only those bacteria possessing an F pilus. This occurs because the F pilus has a specific receptor site to which these viruses can attach and proceed to infect the cell.

**Capsule or Slime Layer**

Many bacteria secrete large polymers that adhere to their external cell walls. In cases where the organisms appear to be randomly embedded in the material, it may be referred to as a slime layer; in other cases it is seen as a discrete, thickened material around each cell or pair of cells and is then called a capsule.

The composition of the capsule is constant within a particular bacterial strain (organisms arising from a single cell) but varies widely even between organisms classified in the same genus and species. For example, capsules from the various types of *Streptococcus pneumoniae* are all composed of large molecules with molecular weights approach-

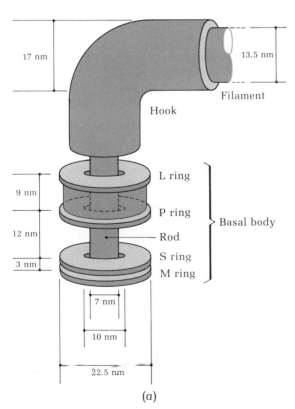

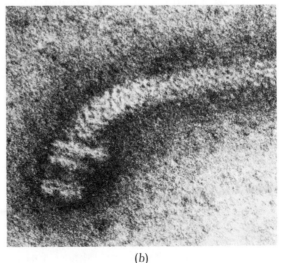

**Figure 3-4.** The electron micrograph and accompanying drawing illustrate the detailed structure of a flagellum and suggest how it is anchored to the bacterial cell. It is proposed that in *Escherichia coli* the L and P rings are anchored to the outer membrane and the S and M rings are anchored to the inner membrane. Flagella from *Bacillus subtilis* (which is gram-positive and has no outer membrane) lack the L and P rings.

(a) (b)

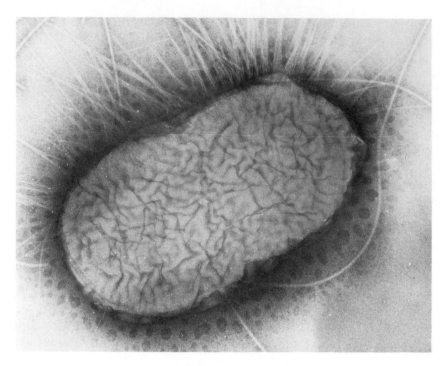

**Figure 3-5.** Pili are the shorter, straight structures on this cell of the bacterium *Proteus vulgaris*. Several longer, curved flagella are also visible in the field (×44,780).

ing 1,000,000 daltons. However, if one isolates the capsular material and hydrolyzes the polysaccharides to their component monosaccharides, one obtains various results as shown by a few examples in Table 3-1. Capsules are often complex polysaccharides which tend to have a low affinity for dyes and as a result are usually not seen in stained smears; they may, however, be visible in wet mounts (suspensions in a liquid) of the organisms.

The actual value of the capsule to the bacterium is not always evident, although it does appear to prevent desiccation of the organism under adverse conditions. However, the presence of a capsule can be of great importance in medical microbiology since its possession may tremendously increase the ability of a bacterium to cause disease. This occurs because the capsule acts as a protective layer that resists ingestion by host's phagocytic cells (cells that engulf and digest foreign

material). Furthermore, since the resistance provided by the capsule can be negated in the presence of specific antibody, immunity to

**Table 3-1. Monosaccharide Components from *Streptococcus pneumoniae* Capsules**

| Type | Constituent monosaccharides |
|------|------------------------------|
| I | Galacturonic acid and amino sugars |
| II | L-Rhamnose, D-glucose, D-glucuronic acid |
| III | Glucose, glucuronic acid |
| IV | Glucose, N-acetylamino sugar |
| VI | Galatose, glucose, rhamnose |
| VII | Galatose, glucose, rhamnose, amino sugar |
| VIII | Glucose, glucuronic acid, galactose |
| IX | Glucose, amino sugar, uronic acid |
| XIV | Galactose, glucose, N-acetylglucosamine |
| XVIII | Rhamnose, glucose |

some infectious agents is directed against the organism's capsule. In fact, prior to the availability of antibiotic therapy, it was frequently necessary to determine exactly which type of encapsulated organism (Streptococcus pneumoniae, Neisseria meningitidis) was causing the disease so that the correct antiserum could be administered.

## Cell Wall

The bacterial cell wall is essential to the integrity of the bacterium. Because it is chemically unlike any structure present in animal tissues, it is an obvious target for drugs that kill bacteria without harming the animal host. It is not surprising, then, that some antibiotics used in the treatment of disease inhibit the synthesis of the bacterial cell wall.

The primary and undoubtedly most necessary function of the cell wall is to provide a rigid structural component that can withstand the strong osmotic pressures caused by the high chemical concentration of inorganic ions and nutrients within the cell. Without the cell wall, a bacterium under normal environmental conditions would take on water and burst. All procaryotic cells (except the mycoplasmas and the extreme halophils— salt requiring) have in common a structural cell wall component called mucopolysaccharide, peptidoglycan, or murein. This component provides the support necessary to maintain the integrity of the cell. Peptidoglycan is a very large molecule, covering the entire cell, consisting of backbones of N-acetylglucosamine and N-acetylmuramic acid. To each molecule of N-acetylmuramic acid is attached a tetrapeptide, and to provide necessary additional strength to this molecule bridges of amino acids (or, in some cases, direct peptide bonding between the tetrapeptides) cross-connect the tetrapeptides from one molecule of N-acetylmuramic acid to the tetrapeptide linked to another molecule of N-acetylmuramic acid. Thus, the completed peptidoglycan molecule consists of many molecules of the repeating disaccharide of N-acetylglucosamine and N-acetyl-

muramic acid cross-linked to each other to form a strong, rigid structure enclosing the fragile protoplast (the cell devoid of its cell wall). Figure 3-6a illustrates the chemical structure of one repeating unit of the bacterial peptidoglycan, and Figure 3-6b shows how the linear polysaccharide strands are cross-linked to provide the completed peptidoglycan molecule.

Interestingly, N-acetylmuramic acid is unique to procaryotic cells, the bacteria and the blue-green algae. It is also unusual in that two of the amino acids involved in the peptidoglycan structure possess the D-configuration; proteins, in general, are synthesized only from L-amino acids.

As discussed in Chapter 2, bacteria can be divided into two large groups on the basis of the differential staining technique called the Gram stain, one group called gram-positive and the other gram-negative. Because these two groups differ in the composition of their cell walls, each will be discussed separately.

GRAM-POSITIVE BACTERIA. The cell walls of gram-positive organisms are quite thick (20–80 nm) consisting of from 60–100 percent peptidoglycan (see Figure 3-7). All gram-positive cells possess a linear polymer of N-acetylglucosamine and N-acetylmuramic acid, but there is variation in the length and composition of the peptide bridge linking the tetrapeptides from one N-acetylmuramic acid to the adjoining polymer.

Some gram-positive organisms also contain cell-wall substances called teichoic acids linked to the muramic acid of the peptidoglycan layer. The teichoic acids occur in two major forms, ribitol teichoic acid and glycerol teichoic acid. In general, they are long polymers of either ribitol (a 5-carbon sugar alcohol) or glycerol (a 3-carbon sugar alcohol) linked to each other through phosphodiester bridges (see Figure 3-8). However, all of the hydroxyl groups are substituted with various mono-, di-, or trisaccharides, or with D-alanine. Also, some organisms possess teichoic acids in which every other glycerol or ribitol is replaced with N-acetylglucosamine or

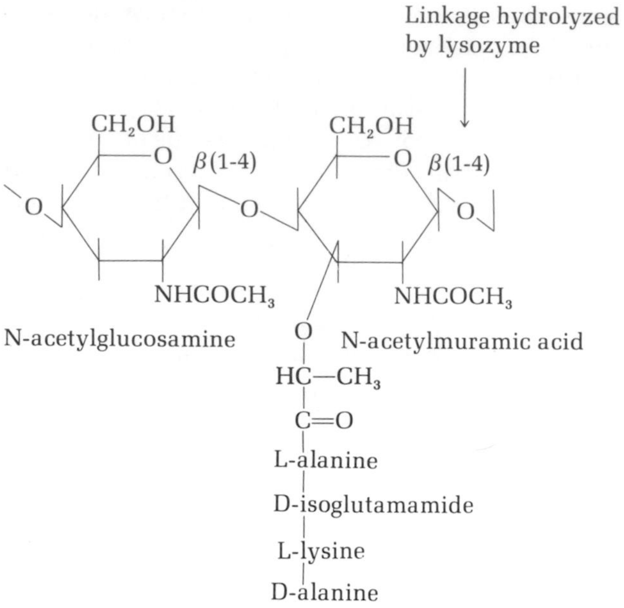

Linkage hydrolyzed
by lysozyme

$CH_2OH$      $CH_2OH$

$\beta(1\text{-}4)$      $\beta(1\text{-}4)$

NHCOCH$_3$     NHCOCH$_3$

N-acetylglucosamine       N-acetylmuramic acid

HC—CH$_3$

C=O

L-alanine

D-isoglutamamide

L-lysine

D-alanine

(a)

**Figure 3-6.** a. Structure of the repeating unit of cell wall peptidoglycan as it exists in *Staphylococcus aureus*. One can visualize the long chains of N-acetylglucosamine and N-acetylmuramic acid to be analogous to the staves of a barrel. The terminal D-alanine is linked to the L-lysine of an adjacent chain by a pentapeptide bridge of L-glycines, thus providing the hoops for the "barrel." b. Schematic structure of the overall peptidoglycan of the cell wall of *Staphylococcus aureus*. In this representation X represents N-acetylglucosamine and Y represents N-acetylmuramic acid. Open circles represent the four amino acids of the tetrapeptide, L-alanyl-D-isoglutaminyl-L-lysyl-D-alanine. Closed circles are pentapeptide bridges that interconnect polymers of N-acetylglucosamine and N-acetylmuramic acid. The shaded portion represents that part of the molecule that is transported to the cell wall. The arrow points to the peptide bond, the formation of which is inhibited by penicillin.

some other sugar molecule. Since these teichoic acids are highly antigenic, it seems that they extend through the peptidoglycan layer and, as a result, provide the antigenic determinants used in the serological identification of many groups and species of gram-positive bacteria.

In addition to this bound peptidoglycan-teichoic acid (which is found in some gram-positive bacteria), all gram-positive bacteria contain a teichoic acid bound to the membrane of the cell. This membrane-bound teichoic acid is always of the glycerol type,

and since it is bound to a glycolipid in the membrane, it is also called lipoteichoic acid.

The function of the teichoic acids is still unresolved, but it has been proposed that since these acids are highly charged, they may have some role in regulating the passage of ions through the thick peptidoglycan layer. However, mutants of *Bacillus subtilis, Lactobacillus plantarum,* and *Staphylococcus aureus* have been isolated that lack teichoic acids, and these mutants seem perfectly viable but may be defective in cell separation. This defect has also been observed when the

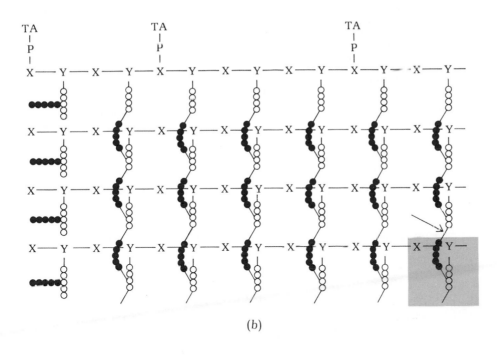

(b)

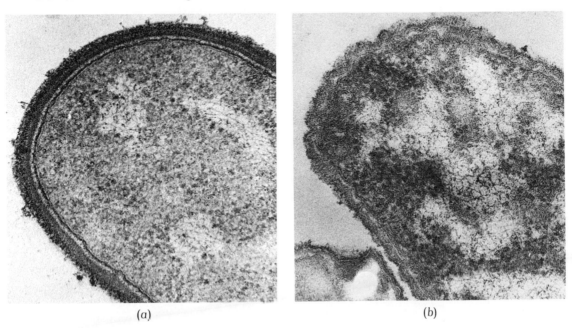

**Figure 3-7.** *a.* A portion of the gram-positive bacterium *Bacillus fastidiosus;* note the cell wall's thick peptidoglycan layer underlaid by the cytoplasmic membrane. *b.* The gram-negative bacterium *Enterobacter aerogenes;* both the cytoplasmic membrane and the outer membrane are visible along some sections of the cell wall.

(a)          (b)

normal choline constituent of *Streptococcus pneumoniae* teichoic acid is substituted with ethanolamine, a close structural analog. Such cells will not separate into normal diplococci but grow in long chains.

A few gram-positive bacteria possess polysaccharides in their cell walls, but very little is known about how the polysaccharides are bound to the cell wall or if they serve any function to the cell.

For the most part, protein is not found as a constituent of the gram-positive cell wall. However, the M protein of the Group A streptococci provides an exception to this rule.

GRAM-NEGATIVE BACTERIA.  The cell walls of gram-negative bacteria are chemically more complex than those of the gram-positive organisms. For example, the gram-negative cell walls contain less peptidoglycan (10–20% of the dry weight of the cell wall), but exterior to this cell-wall layer they possess a second membranous structure (see Figure 3-7b) composed of protein, lipids, and lipopolysaccharides (fatty acids that are ester-bound to polysaccharides). The lipopolysaccharide or LPS component is especially important from a medical viewpoint because of its toxicity. This material is responsible for the high fevers that occur with infections of gram-negative organisms, and because this molecule is an integral part of the bacterial cell, it is also called endotoxin. Structural studies have disclosed that the lipopolysaccharide is composed of two major components: lipid A, which consists of a series of disaccharide units of glucosamine completely esterified with long-chain fatty acids that are bound to each other through pyrophosphate linkages (see Figure 3-9a), and a long chain of sugars and sugar phosphates that are linked to the lipid A moiety. It is known that the toxicity of the molecule resides in the lipid A portion, although the mechanism of the toxicity remains unclear. When an individual is infected (or artificially immunized) with gram-negative bacteria, antibodies are made that will react with the polysaccharide chain of the lipopolysaccharide, and the polysaccharide is called the O or somatic antigen. Figure 3-9b shows the structure of a typical lipopolysaccharide from a species of *Salmonella*. This general structure is similar for all gram-negative bacteria, but the types of fatty acids and the type and arrangement of sugars in the polysaccharide varies from species to species. Moreover, there is now good evidence that the outer leaflet of the outer membrane from gram-negative bacteria is composed exclusively of LPS. This means that the nonpolar region of this leaflet consists solely of those fatty acids that are bound to the lipid A portion of LPS. On the other hand, the inner leaflet of the outer membrane as well as both leaflets of the cytoplasmic membrane contain phospholipids. It has been proposed that this highly charged lipopolysaccharide may function in the regulation of ions passing into the cell.

Immediately beneath the lipopolysaccharide of a gram-negative cell is a thin monomolecular peptidoglycan layer. This

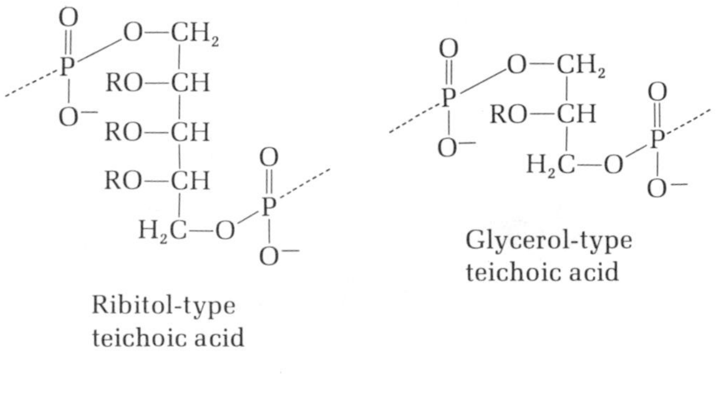

Ribitol-type teichoic acid

Glycerol-type teichoic acid

**Figure 3-8.** Teichoic acids are usually long chains of glycerol or ribitol joined together with phosphodiester bridges. The R group for glycerol teichoic acid is frequently D-alanine, while for the ribitol-type teichoic acid it may be glucose, succinate, N-acetylglucosamine, D-alanine or short oligosaccharides. Substitutions may vary considerably even within a species.

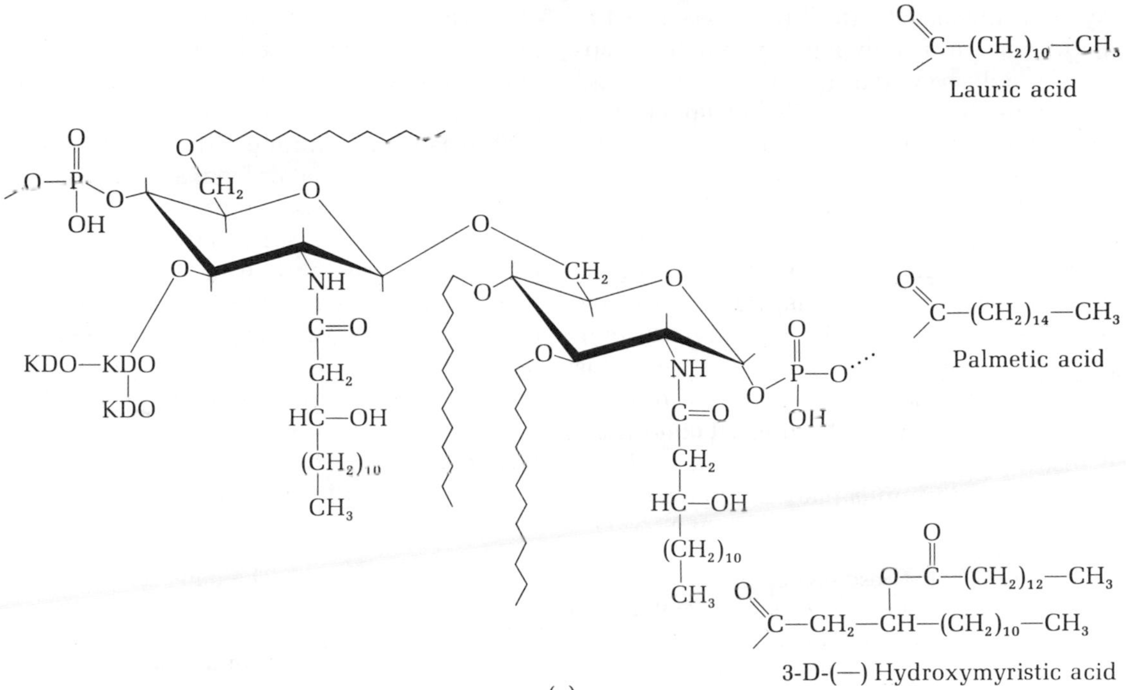

O
‖
C—(CH$_2$)$_{10}$—CH$_3$

Lauric acid

O
‖
C—(CH$_2$)$_{14}$—CH$_3$

Palmetic acid

O
‖
O—C—(CH$_2$)$_{12}$—CH$_3$
C—CH$_2$—CH—(CH$_2$)$_{10}$—CH$_3$

3-D-(—) Hydroxymyristic acid

(a)

lipid A—KDO—KDO—hep—hep——glu—gal—glu—(gal—mann—rham)$_x$

KDO—P—EA  P—P—EA  gal  NAcGlm

Core polysaccharide      O—Antigen
                                 x may be 10 to 20

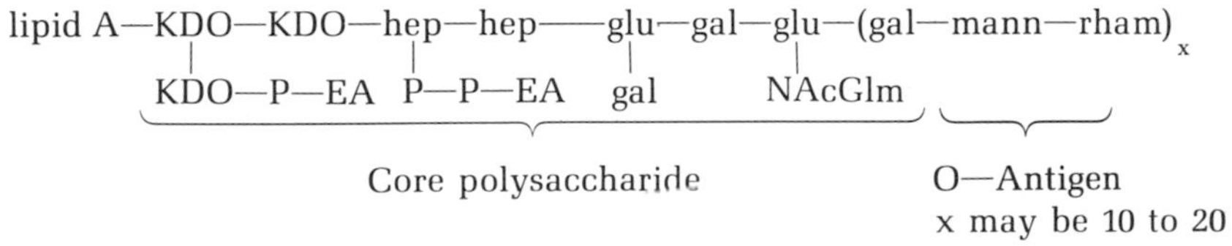

| | |
|---|---|
| KDO | 2-Keto-3-deoxyoctonic acid |
| hep | Heptose |
| glu | Glucose |
| gal | Galactose |
| NAcGlm | N-acetylglucosamine |
| mann | Mannose |
| rham | Rhamnose |
| EA | Ethanolamine |
| P | Phosphate |
| P—P | Pyrophosphate |

(b)

**Figure 3-9.** *a.* Proposed unit structure of lipid A from *Salmonella minnesota* R595 lipopolysaccharide with an attached KDO trisaccharide. The three fatty acid residues shown on the right are linked in an unknown distribution to the hydroxyl groups of the glucosamine residues available at positions 3, 4, and 6′ as shown by the wavy lines. Each amino group is linked to a molecule of 3-hydroxymyristic acid. *b.* The core polysaccharide is identical in all species of *Salmonella*. The O-antigen consists of a repeating sequence of three or four different sugars. The sugars involved and the sequence vary for each species of *Salmonella*.

layer is attached to the lipopolysaccharide membrane by a polypeptide that links approximately every tenth diaminopimelic acid (replacing the L-lysine in the tetrapeptide of gram-negative cell wall peptidoglycan) to the outer membrane (see Figure 3-10).

It is possible to enzymatically dissolve the peptidoglycan portion of the cell wall of both gram-positive and gram-negative organisms with an enzyme (lysozyme) that hydrolyzes the linkage between the N-acetylmuramic acid and the N-acetylglucosamine. This causes the cell wall to break into a number of small pieces and under normal conditions it results in the rupture of the cell. If, however, the bacterium is placed into a solution of sucrose having a higher osmotic strength than the inside of the cell, the removal of the peptidoglycan results in the liberation of the cell contents surrounded by a thin, fragile protoplasmic membrane. When one removes the peptidoglycan layer from a gram-positive organism in the presence of 10–20% sucrose, the remaining cell, surrounded by only the protoplasmic membrane, is called a protoplast. However, when the same procedure is carried out on a gram-negative cell, the outer membrane remains attached to the cell, and the resulting structure is called a spheroplast. In either case, removal of the peptidoglycan layer results in the formation of a rounded-up, osmotically fragile structure.

**Figure 3-10.** Cross-section of cell wall of a gram-negative bacterium. The outer leaflet of the outer membrane is composed of lipopolysaccharide whereas the other leaflets of both membranes are made up of phospholipids. Proteins are inter-dispersed in both the outer and inner membranes. The periplasmic space is the area between the cytoplasmic membrane (inner membrane) and the peptidoglycan.

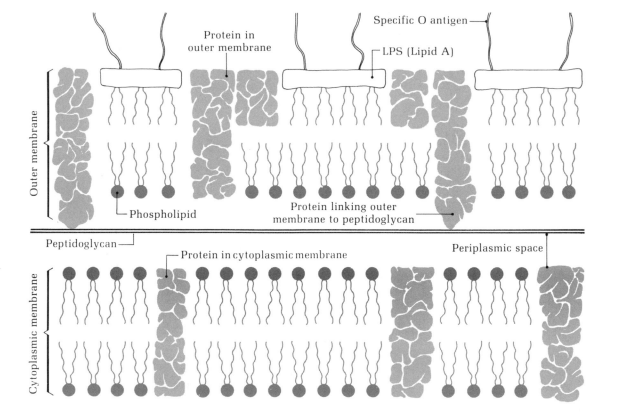

## Plasma Membrane

The fragile plasma or protoplasmic membrane, located just inside the rigid cell wall, has a number of major functions: (1) it carries out electron transport through the cytochrome system, resulting in oxidative phosphorylation; (2) it contains some of the enzymes for the synthesis and transport of peptidoglycan, teichoic acids, and outer membrane components; (3) it secretes extracellular hydrolytic enzymes; (4) it ensures the segregation of DNA to daughter cells during cell division; and (5) it controls transport of most compounds entering and leaving the cell.

Chemically, the protoplasmic membrane is a typical bilayer composed of phospholipids with proteins embedded in the membrane. Figure 3-11 shows a schematic "fluid-mosaic" model of the phospholipid orientation, in which the circular areas represent the hydrophilic ends, and the wavy lines the internal hydrophobic fatty acids. Interspersed throughout this phospholipid membrane are proteins which carry out the various transport and enzymatic functions associated with the membrane.

MESOSOMES. Electron micrographs of bacterial membranes show many areas where the plasma membrane is invaginated, resulting in an increased area of membrane extending into the cytoplasm of the cell (see Figure 3-12). The specific function of such structures, called mesosomes, is not always known, and in all likelihood they may have different functions in different organisms. It has been postulated that septal mesosomes may provide a site for chromosomal attachment to the membrane, and that at the time of cell division cross walls form between the daughter cells in such a manner that one molecule of DNA ends up on each side of the newly formed septum. Lateral mesosomes may occur all along the protoplasmic membrane. One function that has been ascribed to these structures is the excretion of extracellular

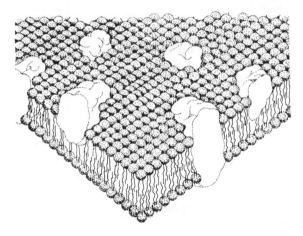

**Figure 3-11.** Fluid-mosaic model for membrane structure. The solid bodies represent the globular integral proteins, which at long range are randomly distributed in the plane of the membrane. The small circles represent the hydrophilic ends of the membrane phospholipids and the wavy lines represent the component fatty acids of the phospholipids.

**Figure 3-12.** A number of mesosomes have invaginated from the cytoplasmic membrane in this section of a *Bacillus fastidiosus* cell. A larger mesosome not continuous with the membrane in the plane of this section is located to the right.

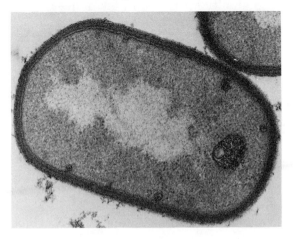

enzymes such as penicillinase, an enzyme that hydrolyzes the $\beta$-lactam bond in the antibiotic penicillin. In all probability future research will unearth new functions for these membrane structures.

TRANSPORT.    Very few substances are able to enter a cell in the absence of a specific membrane-transport system. These systems move substances across the protoplasmic membrane by one of three mechanisms: active transport, the phosphotransferase system, and facilitated transport.

①  Active transport provides the ability to carry a substrate across the protoplasmic membrane to an intracellular environment in which it can be several hundred times more concentrated than in the external environment. Inasmuch as work must be done to move a molecule against a concentration gradient, such transport requires energy, supplied by the metabolic activities of the cell. A model for the mechanism of active transport proposes that the substrate reacts with a specific carrier protein in the membrane which then undergoes an energy-dependent conformational change that brings the substrate across the membrane and, at the same time, decreases the affinity of the carrier protein for its substrate. This releases the substrate into the cytoplasm, after which the freed protein regains its original conformation and again acquires an external binding site with a high affinity for the substrate in question.

②  Phosphotransferase transport is an energy-dependent mechanism for carrying certain sugars and sugar alcohols across the protoplasmic membrane. However, in this system the substrate enters the cell as a phosphorylated compound, and the process is referred to as group translocation. Like active transport, group translocation requires energy, but unlike active transport, the compound is modified by phosphorylation during transport. The overall translocation process requires two different enzymes plus a small heat-labile membrane protein (HPr) which accepts a high-energy phosphate bond from phosphoenolpyruvate and transfers it to the sugar being translocated. The reaction sequence can be depicted as follows:

$$\text{Phosphoenolpyruvate} + \text{HPr} \xrightarrow{\text{Enzyme I}} \text{HPr} \sim \text{P} + \text{pyruvate}$$

$$\text{HPr} \sim \text{P} + \text{sugar} \xrightarrow{\text{Enzyme II}} \text{sugar-P} + \text{HPr}$$

The fact that the phosphorylation occurs as part of the transport process can be demonstrated using small, artificial, membrane-bounded vesicles. If one encloses a sugar and the phosphotransferase enzymes inside such vesicles, no phosphorylation occurs. If, however, the sugar is placed on the outside of the vesicles, it is transported to the inside as a phosphorylated sugar. Glucose, mannose, fructose, sorbitol, and mannitol constitute the best studied systems, but other sugars may also be taken into the cell by group translocation. It should be emphasized that the mechanism of transport for any specific substrate varies for different bacteria. For example, one species of bacteria may transport simple sugars by the phosphotransferase system, while another species may take the same sugars into the cell by active transport. Enzyme I is the same for all substrates, but there is a specific enzyme II for each sugar. Purines and pyrimidines can also cross the cell membrane by a different type of group translocation.

③.  Facilitated transport also requires a specific membrane-bound carrier protein to move a substrate into the cell. However, in this case, no energy is required nor is the substrate transported from a lower to a higher concentration as in the case of active transport. The carrier merely moves back and forth across the membrane transporting its specific substrate (for example, the penetration of glycerol into *Escherichia coli*) into the cell. The over-all end result would be the same as simple noncarrier mediated diffusion except that facilitated transport is specific and much more rapid than simple diffusion.

Simple passive diffusion also takes place across the protoplasmic membrane, but this process would be effective only when the cell is immersed in high concentrations of the substance involved (such as water) or, perhaps when only a low concentration of a substance is required for the metabolism of a cell (such as the requirement for molybdenum for nitrogen fixation). Passive diffusion could not therefore supply a metabolic substrate from a dilute solution at a sufficiently rapid rate to sustain the biosynthetic activities of the cell.

### Bacterial Cytoplasm

In addition to water, inorganic ions, and a few low-molecular-weight compounds, the cytoplasm contains primarily high-molecular-weight polymers of nucleic acid, food-storage reserves, and proteins. Also, all cells contain ribosomes, some form internal endo-

spores, and others may contain cytoplasmic vacuoles.

BACTERIAL CHROMOSOMES.    Even though procaryotic cells lack a nuclear membrane, their heritable properties are encoded in DNA in a manner essentially identical to that seen in eucaryotic cells. This chromosomal DNA exists in the bacterium as a single circular molecule, although smaller, extrachromosomal molecules of DNA called plasmids are also frequently present.

Because of the basophilic nature of the cytoplasm, it is not easy to see the stained DNA unless the cells are first subjected to mild acid hydrolysis to remove the cytoplasmic RNA (see Figure 3-13).

RIBOSOMES.    Observation with the electron microscope shows that the cytoplasm carries a high concentration of ribosomes. Bacterial ribosomes are similar in size to those found

**Figure 3-13.** In this cell of *Corynebacterium parvum* the chromatin making up the bacterial nucleoid is the fibrous skein filling most of the cell. It is attached to the membrane of the large mesosome. (×113,000).

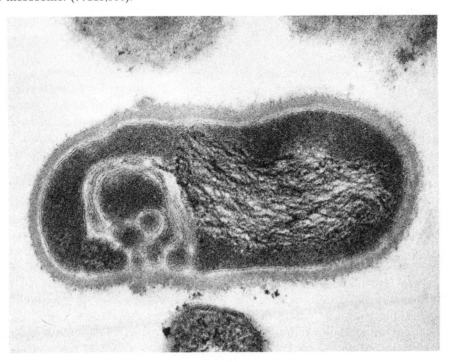

in the mitochondria of eucaryotic cells but smaller than the cytoplasmic ribosomes of eucaryotic cells. Measured in terms of sedimentation values, single procaryotic ribosomes are 70S, and, if placed in a solution with a low $Mg^{++}$ concentration, will dissociate into two particles, a 50S subunit and a 30S subunit. In contrast, cytoplasmic eucaryotic ribosomes are 80S and will dissociate into 60S and 40S subunits.

The ribosome is composed of 23S, 16S, and 5S RNA in close association with a large number of small-molecular-weight proteins. The 23S and 5S molecules of RNA are in the 50S subunit, and the 16S RNA is in the 30S subunit of the ribosome. The 30S subunit of ribosomes in the bacterium Escherichia coli contains 21 different proteins, and the 50S subunit has 34 separate proteins. As we shall discuss in Chapter 10, certain antibiotics possess a selective bactericidal effect as a result of their ability to combine specifically with the structural proteins of bacterial ribosomes.

INCLUSIONS. Bacterial cytoplasm may also contain cellular inclusions of various kinds that serve as reserve food or energy sources. One of the most common storage compounds is a long polymer of β-hydroxybutyric acid. Inclusions of poly β-hydroxybutyric acid can be easily seen with a light microscope as bright refractile bodies. Other bacteria accumulate granules of glycogen which are composed primarily of α-1-4 linked glucose units. Members of one group of bacteria, known as the sulfur bacteria, oxidize sulfur-containing compounds as a source of energy and stores granules of elemental sulfur in their cytoplasm. These granules can subsequently be oxidized to provide energy for the cell.

One common inclusion is composed of a high-molecular-weight polymer of polymetaphosphate. These particular granules, which serve as a reserve source of high-energy phosphate, are called metachromatic granules because they show a reddish color when stained with methylene blue or toluidine blue. Meta-chromatic granules are also given the name of volutin.

ENDOSPORES. Only two genera of bacteria of medical importance (Bacillus and Clostridium) are capable of endospore formation. However, endospores are also formed by the members of the genera Sporolactobacillus, Sporosarcina, and Desulfotomaculum.

An endospore is a minute, highly durable body which under appropriate growth conditions will germinate to form a new vegetative cell. The process of endospore formation is, in general, as follows: after the active growth period, or under conditions of inadequate nutrition, a chromosome (probably attached to a mesosome) migrates to one end of the cell. The bacterial membrane then invaginates so as to completely enclose the nuclear material within a double membrane, as shown in Figure 3-14. This structure, called a forespore, synthesizes a thin peptidoglycan spore wall adjacent to the inner membrane, and deposits a thick layer of peptidoglycan between the two membranes. The peptidoglycan in this latter area, called the cortex, is poorly crosslinked; the peptidoglycan in the spore wall is like that in the vegetative cell. At the same time the cortex is being synthesized by the inner spore membrane, the outer membrane forms an external spore coat composed of a tough keratin-like protein. Some species surround the entire spore in a thin covering called the exosporium. The residual vegetative cell eventually lyses, and the mature spore is liberated (see Figure 3-15).

Because of the impervious spore coat, endospores cannot be stained by the usual staining procedures. Thus, in a Gram-stained preparation, the endospore appears as a clear, refractile body within the vegetative cell. However, special spore stains may be used in which the spore is heated with the stain, or the stain is mixed with a surface-active detergent that allows the stain to penetrate the cell wall.

The most obvious property possessed by an endospore that is not characteristic of a

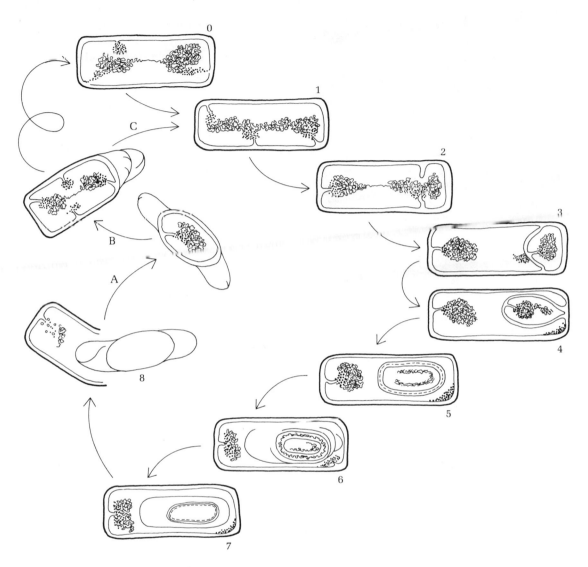

**Figure 3-14.** Diagrammatic summary of sporulation in a *Bacillus* species. Stages 1 through 4 represent steps in forespore development. Note the inversion of the cytoplasmic membrane resulting in the outer leaflet of this membrane becoming the inner leaflet of the spore membrane. At stage 5 cortex development commences (dotted line) and continues through 6 when the coat protein is deposited. Stage 7 is characterized by a dehydration of the spore protoplast and an accumulation of dipicolinic acid and calcium in the spore. At stage 8 the spore is completely refractile and a lytic enzyme acts to release the spore. Also shown are germination A; outgrowth to a primary cell B; from which the cell may, under special conditions, enter sporulation by a shortcut C, "the microcycle," but normally undergoes logarithmic growth (spiral arrow).

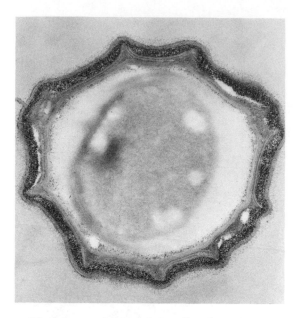

**Figure 3-15.** Spore of *Bacillus fastidiosus* (×53,590).

**Figure 3-16.** Structural formula of the calcium salt of dipicolinic acid.

vegetative cell is its resistance to heat and chemicals. For example, an endospore may remain viable for many years, perhaps centuries, under normal soil conditions. Furthermore, while most vegetative cells are killed by temperatures beyond 60–70°C, endospores may survive in boiling water for an hour or more. There is no simple explanation for this resistance, but the fact that endospores contain very little free water undoubtedly is a major reason for their thermal stability, and the impermeability of the spore coat may account for their resistance to chemical disinfectants.

Endospores are unique in that they normally contain quite large amounts of calcium dipicolinate (Figure 3-16), a compound rarely found elsewhere in the biological world. In fact, even the vegetative cell in which the endospore was formed does not contain detectable amounts of dipicolinic acid. Early experiments using endospores obtained from *Bacillus cereus* indicated that the heat resistance of the spores was directly correlated with the content of calcium dipicolinate in the spore; however, more recently, endospores obtained from mutants of *Bacillus subtilis* have been shown to be devoid of calcium dipicolinate, but they still possess essentially the same heat resistance shown by the endospores containing calcium dipicolinate.

As long as environmental conditions are adverse to the growth of the bacterium, the endospore remains dormant. If conditions become favorable for growth, several changes may occur. The refractility and heat resistance disappear, and the endospore "sprouts" or germinates and once again becomes a vegetative bacterial cell, reproducing in the normal manner. Sporulation (the formation of an endospore) is not part of the reproductive process of endospore-forming bacteria since one cell forms one endospore which, after germination, is again only one cell.

Most endospore-forming bacteria are inhabitants of the soil, but bacterial endospores exist almost everywhere. The fact that they are difficult to destroy is the principal reason for the lengthy and elaborate sterilization procedures employed in hospitals, canneries, and other places where absolute freedom from bacteria is required.

## REFERENCES

Adler, J. 1976. The sensing of chemicals by bacteria. *Sci. American* **234**:40–47.

Adler, J. 1975. Chemotaxis in bacteria. *Annu. Rev. Biochem.* **44**:341–356.

Archibald, A. R. 1974. The structure, biosynthesis and function of teichoic acid. *Adv. Microbiol. Phys.* **11**:53–95.

Aronson, A. I., and P. Fitz-James. 1976. Structure and morphogenesis of the bacterial spore coat. *Bacteriol. Rev.* **40**:360–402.

Berg, H. C. 1975. How bacteria swim. *Sci. American* **233**:36–44.

Beytia, E., and J. W. Porter, 1976. Biochemistry of polyisoprenoid biosynthesis. *Annu. Rev. Biochem.* **45**:113–142.

Christensen, H. N. 1975. *Biological Transport*, 2nd ed. W. A. Benjamin, Inc., London.

Cordaro, C. 1976. Genetics of the bacterial phosphoenolpyruvate: glycose phosphotransferase system. *Annu. Rev. Genetics* **10**, 341–359.

Costerton. J. W., J. M. Ingram, and K. J. Cheng. 1974. Structure and function of the cell envelope of gram-negative bacteria. *Bacteriol. Rev.* **38**:87–110.

DePamphilis, M. L., and J. Adler. 1971. Fine structure and isolation of the hook-basal body complex of flagella from *Escherichia coli* and *Bacillus subtilis*. *J. Bacteriol.* **105**:384–395.

Gould, G. W., and G. J. Dring. 1974. Mechanisms of spore heat resistance. *Adv. Microbial Phys.* **11**:137–164.

Greenawalt, J. W., and T. L. Whiteside. 1975. Mesosomes: Membranous bacterial organs. *Bacteriol. Rev.* **39**:405–463.

Hamilton, W. A. 1975. Energy coupling in microbial transport. *Adv. Microbial Phys.* **12**:2–53.

Henning, U. 1975. Determination of cell shape in bacteria. *Annu. Rev. Microbiol.* **29**:45–60.

Ottow, J. C. 1975. Ecology, physiology and genetics of fimbriae and pili. *Annu. Rev. Microbiol.* **29**:79–108.

Pace, N. R. 1973. The structure and synthesis of ribosomal ribonucleic acid of prokaryotes. *Bacteriol. Rev.* **37**:562–603.

Salton, M. R. J., and P. Owen. 1976. Bacterial membrane structure. *Annu. Rev. Microbiol.* **30**:451–482.

Schleifer, K. H., and O. Kandler. 1972. Peptidoglycan types of bacterial cell walls and their taxonomic significance. *Bacteriol. Rev.* **36**:407–477.

Shively, J. M. 1974. Inclusion bodies of prokaryotes. *Annu. Rev. Microbiol.* **28**:167–187.

Simoni, R. D., and P. W. Postma. 1975. The energetics of bacterial active transport. *Annu. Rev. Biochem.* **44**:523–554.

Slater, M., and M. Schaechter. 1974. Control of cell division in bacteria. *Bacteriol. Rev.* **38**:199–221.

Smit, J., Y. Kamio, and H. Nikaido. 1975. Outer membrane of *Salmonella typhimurium*: Chemical analysis and freeze-fracture studies with lipopolysaccharide mutants. *J. Bacteriol.* **124**:942–958.

Smith, R. W., and H. Koffler. 1971. Bacterial flagella. *Adv. Microbiol. Phys.* **6**:219–339.

Tso, W. W., and J. Adler. 1974. Negative chemotaxis in *Escherichia coli*. *J. Bacteriol.* **118**:560–576.

Wicken, A. J., and K. W. Knox. 1975. Lipoteichoic acids: A new class of bacterial antigen. *Science* **187**:1161–1167.

# 4

# Bacterial Nutrition

All organisms, whether procaryotic or eucaryotic, require food to live and grow. How an organism assimilates its food is called its nutrition, and the specific cellular requirements are its nutrients.

Precisely what nutrients do bacteria need to synthesize the materials that comprise a bacterial cell? Here is a basic list:

1. A carbon source (for example, a carbohydrate)

2. A nitrogen source (for example, protein or ammonia)

3. Certain inorganic ions

4. Essential metabolites (vitamins; possibly amino acids)

5. Water

The cell also requires a source of energy for the synthesis of cellular constituents and for other life processes such as motility and transport. The mechanisms by which bacteria obtain this energy will be discussed in the following chapter.

## GROWTH

Practically everyone working with bacteria is involved with the growth of microorganisms. Clinical laboratories must grow the organisms from an infected patient so a diagnosis can be made. For the patient to be properly treated, bacteria must also be grown in the presence of drugs or antibiotics to determine if they are sensitive or resistant. A bacteriologist in a food-processing plant must grow the bacteria present on finished food products (such as frozen dinners) so the safety of such foods can be evaluated. The biochemist interested in microbial metabolism must grow bacteria so the cells can be studied. Growth is one of the fundamental activities concerning the bacteriologist.

What is growth? Growth of an animal or plant means increasing the number of constituent cells, and this is also the case with microorganisms. If you place ten bacterial cells in 1 milliliter of a favorable medium, and 24 hours later find ten million bacteria per milliliter, you have had bacterial growth. In fact, you have had a million-fold bacterial growth. This increase in bacterial numbers takes place by a process called binary fission, whereby each bacterium forms a new cell wall across its short axis (transversely) and then breaks apart into two cells. Each of these may then divide into two more cells, and on and on. The over-all result of this type of growth is an exponential, or logarithmic, increase in bacterial numbers. Hence, the progeny of a single bacterium will double with each division, yielding progressively 2, 4, 8, 16, and finally 32 cells over five divisions. The potential for the production of large numbers of cells by binary fission in a short period of time is demonstrated in Figure 4-1.

## Measurement of Growth

How would you measure bacterial growth to know that there are ten million bacteria present in 1 milliliter of medium? Quite obviously, one could not count ten million bacteria. But, the number can be estimated by diluting the culture with sterile water until 1 milliliter of the dilution contains a number of bacteria that can be counted (preferably between 30 and 300). A measured quantity of the dilution is mixed with a melted nutrient agar medium. The mixture is poured into a petri dish and incubated for one or two days to allow each individual cell to multiply until it forms a colony (a mass of bacteria) visible to the naked eye. The colonies can be counted and this number multiplied by the amount the culture was diluted to obtain the number of organisms present per milliliter in the original culture. For example, if one diluted this culture 100,000-fold and subsequently counted 100 colonies in a plate count of 1 milliliter of this dilution, the original culture could be calculated to contain 100,000 times 100, or 10,000,000 bacteria per milliliter (see Figure 4-2 for method of preparing dilutions).

Other techniques that may be used for the quantitation of bacterial growth are the determination of the dry weight of the cells, the measurement of the amount of tubidity, the determination of total nitrogen, or even the direct microscopic count of cells from a diluted culture on a slide. Also, organisms can be electronically counted using a Coulter counter as they pass through a small orifice. However, much of the time you will not be concerned with exactly how much growth occurred, but rather with the prob-

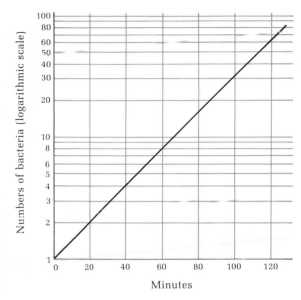

**Figure 4-1.** Because bacteria divide by binary fission, their growth occurs exponentially. In the above logarithmic plot, one bacterium divided into two cells during the first 20 minutes. However, during the sixth generation, 32 bacteria divided to become 64 organisms during the same 20-minute generation time.

lem of whether or not growth took place at all. To determine this, you have only to look at the culture; a liquid medium will have become turbid, and a solid medium will have visible growth either on the surface or down in the medium.

## Phases of Growth

Under favorable conditions, most bacteria are able to reproduce rapidly. The time it takes for one bacterium to divide into two is referred to as the generation time. For some bacteria, such as *Escherichia coli,* the average generation time may be as little as 20 minutes, whereas in others, for example *Mycobacterium tuberculosis,* it is about 15 to 20 hours. The generation time during active growth varies with each species of bacterium, although for the majority it will be less than one hour. The generation time of bacteria has

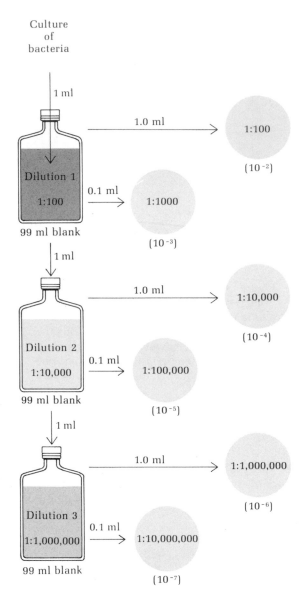

Culture
of
bacteria

1 ml

Dilution 1
1:100

99 ml blank

1.0 ml → 1:100 (10⁻²)

0.1 ml → 1:1000 (10⁻³)

1 ml

Dilution 2
1:10,000

99 ml blank

1.0 ml → 1:10,000 (10⁻⁴)

0.1 ml → 1:100,000 (10⁻⁵)

1 ml

Dilution 3
1:1,000,000

99 ml blank

1.0 ml → 1:1,000,000 (10⁻⁶)

0.1 ml → 1:10,000,000 (10⁻⁷)

**Figure 4-2.** Serial dilutions for counting bacteria. Circles represent platings, and all dilutions are expressed as the dilution per ml of the original culture. Thus, when 0.1 ml of a $10^{-2}$ dilution is plated, this is expressed as a $10^{-3}$ dilution, since it represents one-tenth as many cells as would be used by plating 1.0 ml of the $10^{-2}$ dilution.

great practical importance. Suppose that a urine sample contaminated with only 500 *E. coli* per milliliter is left in the hospital ward for a few hours before it is taken to the diagnostic laboratory. Assuming a generation time of 20 minutes, those 500 *E. coli* could become 256,000 organisms in three hours, and over two million in four hours. What started off as a small contamination could now be incorrectly interpreted as a serious infection in the patient.

If one determines the rate of growth of a bacterial culture, these results can be plotted as the logarithm of the number of cells versus the time of growth. In this manner, a growth curve (see Figure 4-3) is obtained that can be divided into four major phases.

LAG PHASE. When bacteria are inoculated into a new medium, reproduction usually does not begin immediately. The lag phase is a period of adaptation to the environment, and it may last from an hour to several days. The length of time depends on the kind of bacteria, the age of the inoculum culture, and the available nutrients in the medium provided.

The lag phase is a lag in multiplication only, for the cells are metabolically active. Inclusions are consumed and there is active synthesis of enzymes and other essential constituents. In the latter part of the lag phase there is some increase in over-all cell size, with some bacilli increasing two or three times their original length.

LOG PHASE. This is the period of most rapid reproduction and the one in which the typical characteristics of the active cells usually are observed. During this phase the generation time is relatively constant, and if one plots the logarithm of the number of organisms against time, the log phase appears as a straight line.

The generation time of an organism can be determined during the log phase. As noted earlier, each generation results in a doubling of the cell number. With this information, the following equation can be used to calculate the generation time.

$$B_t = B_0 \times 2^n$$

$B_0$ = number of bacteria at beginning of time interval

$B_t$ = number of bacteria at end of any interval of time ($t$)

$g$ = generation time, usually expressed in minutes

$t$ = time, usually expressed in minutes

$n$ = number of generations

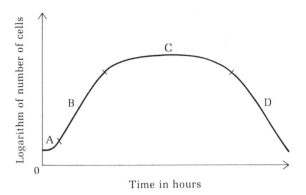

**Figure 4-3.** Typical growth curve illustrating the phases of growth occurring when bacteria are inoculated into a culture medium. (A) Lag phase: cells begin to synthesize inducible enzymes and use stored food reserves. (B) Logarithmic growth phase: the rate of multiplication is constant. (C) Stationary phase: death rate is equal to rate of increase. (D) Death phase: cells begin to die at a more rapid rate than they reproduce. The slope of this phase varies from one genus to another and may last from less than one day to several months.

We take the logarithm (to the base 10) of both sides of the equation.

$$\log B_t = \log B_0 + n \log 2$$

Then we solve for $n$.

$$n = \frac{\log B_t - \log B_0}{\log 2}$$

Since by definition $t/n = g$ and $n = t/g$ we can, by substitution, get the following equations.

$$\frac{t}{g} = \frac{\log B_t - \log B_0}{\log 2}$$

$$g = \frac{t \log 2}{\log B_t - \log B_0}$$

Let us take an example to illustrate the use of this equation.

$B_0 = 2.83 \times 10^7$ cells per ml; or $\log B_0$ = 7.45

$B_t = 4.5 \times 10^8$ cells per ml; or $\log B_t$ = 8.65

$t = 135$ minutes

$\log 2 = 0.301$

Plugging in the above figures,

$$g = \frac{(135)(0.301)}{8.65 - 7.45} = 33.9$$

The generation time for this organism is 33.9 minutes.

The generation time varies with the species of organism, the concentration of available nutrients in the medium, and the temperature of incubation. Other conditions such as pH and, for aerobes, oxygen availability also influence the rate of fission.

One important concept concerning the log growth of bacteria is that at any point in time during this period some cells are just beginning to divide, others are half-finished, and still others are finishing division. Researchers who want to learn the stage in reproduction during which certain enzymes are synthesized must have all cells at the same stage of division simultaneously. This can be accomplished by several techniques, such as chilling a culture for a short period followed by returning to the normal growth temperature, or limiting an essential metabolite during early growth and then supplying additional amounts of this metabolite. When all cells of a culture are dividing at almost the same time, the condition is referred to as synchronous growth.

Bacteria can be maintained in the logarithmic phase by continually transferring them to fresh medium of the same composition. This state can be maintained automatically using a special device called a chemostat (see Figure 4-4). The chemostat consists of a growth chamber connected to a reservoir of fresh medium, which is continually supplied to the bacteria in the growth chamber. One particular nutrient of the medium may be provided in limited concentration to control the rate of growth. As fresh medium enters the growth chamber, the grown culture is pumped out. The chemostat is valuable for providing large amounts of bacteria for use in physiological studies.

STATIONARY PHASE.  As the culture grows older and approaches the maximum population that the medium present can support, the rate of reproduction slows down and some cells die. When the rate of reproduction equals the rate of death, the over-all number of bacteria remains constant.

This stationary phase results from the exhaustion of nutrients in the medium and the presence of waste products of bacterial metabolism, which may be toxic to the organisms; for aerobic organisms, the rate of oxygen diffusion into the medium may be inadequate for a large number of cells. Endospores develop in spore-forming genera, and granular inclusions are usually observed.

DEATH PHASE.  When the rate of death exceeds the rate of reproduction, the actual number of bacteria declines. With certain species, it may take weeks or months before the end of this phase is reached. During this period, abnormal shapes called involution forms are frequently seen, making it difficult to identify an organism in an old culture.

## BACTERIAL NUTRIENTS

We have already discussed the fact that nutrients must be water soluble in order to enter the bacterial cell. Let us now briefly concern ourselves with the scope of required nutrients.

### Carbon Source

With the exception of some synthetic plastics, there is probably no carbon-containing compound that cannot be used by some bacterium as a carbon source for the synthesis of its protoplasm. Carbon sources even include wood, asphalt, and gasoline. However, most disease-producing organisms obtain their carbon by metabolizing simple carbohydrates or proteins.

### Nitrogen Source

Since all proteins and nucleic acids contain nitrogen, it is obvious that growth requires substantial amounts of nitrogen. Some organisms can obtain the required nitrogen by

**Figure 4-4.** Chemostat used for continuous cultures. Rate of growth can be controlled either by controlling the rate at which new medium enters the growth chamber or by limiting a required growth factor in the medium.

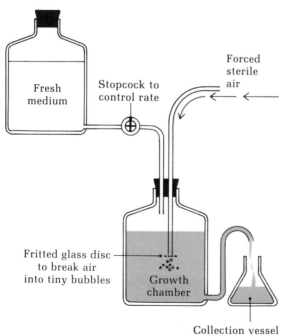

fixing nitrogen gas in the air; others can utilize inorganic sources of nitrogen, such as ammonium salts; some may require organically-bound nitrogen, such as glutamine, asparagine, or peptide digests.

## Inorganic Ions

All organisms require phosphate, both to take part as a component of cellular structures and for the storage of energy. Sulfur, usually as sulfate, can be used by most bacteria to produce the many sulfhydryl (—SH) groups in proteins (cysteine and methionine). Other ions that act as cofactors for certain enzymes and must be added to a growth medium include $Mg^{++}$, $K^+$, and $Ca^{++}$. Some ions are required in such minute amounts that contaminants in tap water and other ingredients in a medium may provide adequate supplies.

One ion that deserves special consideration is iron. Many bacteria form compounds (given the general name of siderophores) that will chelate and solubilize iron so it can be brought into the bacterial cell. Interestingly, since essentially all the host's iron is bound to either lactoferrin, transferrin, or ferritin, the growth of a bacterium within a host may well depend on the ability of the infecting organism to produce siderophores that can successfully compete with the iron-binding protein in the host. It has been postulated that one major difference between virulent and avirulent tubercle bacilli may be the possession of a tightly-bound iron-binding siderophore (mycobactin) which permits the virulent organisms to compete with the host for available iron.

Finally, some ions may be required under certain conditions. For example, molybdenum is necessary only when an organism capable of the process is fixing atmospheric nitrogen.

## Essential Metabolites

It is readily apparent that to reproduce all bacteria must synthesize their own proteins, carbohydrates, fats, nucleic acids, cell-wall constituents, and other biological molecules. But the diversity of the raw materials that bacteria utilize to accomplish these syntheses varies from one species to another. Some organisms have extraordinary powers of synthesis and are able to reproduce using only carbon dioxide and inorganic compounds for cellular nutrition. On the other hand, some pathogenic (disease-causing) bacteria cannot be grown in the laboratory unless they are supplied with complex organic materials such as whole blood. Such dependent bacteria have a limited enzymatic endowment and hence an equally limited ability to synthesize. Many must be provided with precursors such as purines, pyrimidines, amino acids, and vitamins. Such requirements are collectively termed essential metabolites or growth factors. Since all cells use these metabolites for biosynthetic reactions, any organism that cannot synthesize an essential metabolite must have it supplied for growth to occur.

## Necessary Conditions for Bacterial Growth

A number of conditions other than adequate nutrition must be met in order to grow bacteria. The medium must have the correct pH; most bacteria do not grow under alkaline conditions, and with the exception of *Vibrio cholerae* (cholera bacillus), essentially none do well above pH 8. Most of the pathogens of concern to us grow best at a neutral or slightly alkaline pH (pH 7.4). However, some bacteria grow well at pH 6, and not infrequently one finds organisms (for example, fungi) that grow well at a pH of 4 to 5.

Temperature is also a variable that must be controlled. Bacteria, in general, may be placed into one of three groups according to the temperature range in which they grow best. By far the largest number, including those that concern us, are called mesophiles because their optimum growth temperature falls between 15° and 40°C. Psychrophiles are another important group of organisms; they have optimum growth temperatures below 15°C and may grow, though slowly, at temperatures as low as 2°–3°C. Such organisms continue to multiply even at temperatures in refrigerators. This fact is extremely important for medical personnel to know and remember, because placing material into a refrigerator (2°–8°C) does not ensure that microbial growth will not take place. Thermophiles form the third category of bacteria based on optimum growth temperature. These organisms are certainly not a health problem inasmuch as their optimum growth occurs above 40° or 50°C. Some are even found growing in hot springs at temperatures above 95°C or in rotting compost piles that have generated considerable internal heat as a result of their metabolic activities.

The requirement for oxygen (or its absence) was discussed in Chapter Two, and we shall return again to this subject in defining its role as a final electron acceptor in the metabolism of aerobic organisms. Oxygen's lethal effect on obligate anaerobes, however, puzzled microbiologists for many years, and only recently has an explanation for this phenomenon come to light. In brief, it is now known that in the presence of oxygen, all organisms produce miniscule amounts of a free radical of oxygen ($O_2^-$) called superoxide. Superoxide is very unstable in an aqueous medium, but because of its extreme cytotoxicity, aerobically-respiring cells survive only by possessing the enzyme superoxide dismutase, which scavenges the superoxide radical as follows:

$$O_2^- + O_2^- + 2H^+ \longrightarrow H_2O_2 + O_2$$

Obligate anaerobes lack superoxide dismutase and cannot tolerate the presence of molecular oxygen; they therefore must use a different final electron acceptor. The range and type of electron acceptors will be discussed in Chapter Five.

## REFERENCES

Dawes, E. A., and P. J. Senior. 1973. The role and regulation of energy reserve polymers in microorganisms. *Adv. Microbiol. Phys.* **10**:136–266.

Fridovich, I. 1975. Superoxide dismutase. *Annu. Rev. Biochem.* **44**:147–159.

Guirard, B. M., and E. E. Snell. 1962. Nutritional Requirements of Microorganisms. In I. C. Gunsalus and R. Y. Stanier, eds., *The Bacteria,* IV, 33. Academic Press, New York.

Morris, J. G. 1975. The physiology of obligate anaerobiosis. *Adv. Microbiol. Phys.* **12**:169–246.

Tempest, D. W. 1970. The continuous cultivation of microorganisms. I. Theory of the chemostat. In J. R. Norris and D. W. Ribbons, eds., *Methods in Microbiology,* II, 259. Academic Press, New York.

# 5

## Bacterial Metabolism

Metabolism is the word that sums up all the chemical processes that occur within a cell. One can think of metabolism as consisting of two opposite and, paradoxically, simultaneous processes. The first, anabolism, comprises the synthesis of cellular constituents and thus requires energy; the second, opposite process, called catabolism, entails the oxidation of a substrate accompanied by the release of energy and the formation of degradation products. Anabolic reactions are, in general, similar for all types of cells since the synthesis of nucleic acids, proteins, polysaccharides, and lipids show only minor variations among all cells. Catabolic reactions among bacteria, however, are exceedingly diverse, and vary from the oxidation of inorganic compounds such as sulfides, ferrous salts, or hydrogen to the oxidation of carbohydrates or even hydrocarbons for a source of energy.

This chapter will be concerned with some of the catabolic reactions carried out by bacteria and the subsequent storage of the released energy. It must be emphasized, however, that it includes only a brief orientation to bacterial metabolism; a more comprehensive and detailed coverage will be found in the references listed at the end of this chapter.

### ENERGY LIBERATION AND STORAGE

When chemical oxidations are carried out in a test tube, the energy liberated is usually lost as heat. A prerequisite of living cells, however, is that the energy liberated by the oxidation of a metabolite be trapped and stored for use for the many vital processes that require energy.

Consider the oxidation of glucose to carbon dioxide and water as shown in the following general equation:

$$C_6H_{12}O_6 + 6\,O_2 \longrightarrow 6\,CO_2 + 6\,H_2O$$

Although this may be written as a single reaction, biochemically it represents the end result of 20 to 30 individual reactions and the liberation of a considerable amount of energy. Much of the released energy is captured and stored by the cell in the form of high-energy phosphate bonds in adenosine triphosphate (ATP).

The energy released as a result of catabolic reactions can be trapped as ATP by either of two basically different processes. In the first case, the energy released through oxidation is localized in a high-energy phosphate bond in the oxidized substrate. This is exemplified by one of the oxidations occurring in glycolysis (the stepwise conversion of glucose to two molecules of lactic acid) in which one molecule of glyceraldehyde 3-phosphate is oxidized in the presence of inorganic phosphate ($P_i$) to form a molecule of 1,3-diphosphoglyceric acid as shown below.

$$
\begin{array}{c}
\text{HC}=\text{O} \\
| \\
\text{HCOH} \\
| \\
\text{CH}_2\text{OPO}_3^{=}
\end{array}
\quad + \text{ } P_i \quad
\xrightarrow{\text{NAD} \quad \text{NADH}}
\quad
\begin{array}{c}
\text{O} \\
\| \\
\text{C}-\text{O}-\text{PO}_3^{=} \\
| \\
\text{HCOH} \\
| \\
\text{CH}_2\text{OPO}_3^{=}
\end{array}
$$

Glyceraldehyde 3-phosphate      1,3-Diphosphoglyceric acid

In the above case, the carboxy-linked phosphate is linked to the glyceric acid via a high-energy bond that can be transferred directly to ADP to form a molecule of ATP as shown below.

$$
\begin{array}{c}
\text{O} \\
\| \\
\text{C}-\text{O}-\text{PO}_3^{=} \\
| \\
\text{HCOH} \\
| \\
\text{CH}_2\text{OPO}_3^{=}
\end{array}
\quad
\xrightarrow{\text{ADP} \quad \text{ATP}}
\quad
\begin{array}{c}
\text{O} \\
\| \\
\text{C}-\text{OH} \\
| \\
\text{HCOH} \\
| \\
\text{CH}_2\text{OPO}_3^{=}
\end{array}
$$

1,3-Diphosphoglyceric acid      3-Phosphoglyceric acid

This direct transfer of a high-energy linked phosphate bond to ADP is known as substrate-level phosphorylation, but as we shall see, this process accounts for the release and biological trapping of only a small percentage of the total energy available in the glucose molecule.

The other process of ATP formation, known as oxidative phosphorylation, occurs as electrons released from oxidation are passed through a series of intermediate carriers to arrive eventually at a final electron acceptor—frequently oxygen. If we look back at the equation depicting the oxidation of glyceraldehyde 3-phosphate to 1,3-diphosphoglyceric acid, it can be seen that in addition to forming a high-energy phosphate bond, released electrons were accepted by a molecule of nicotinamide adenine dinucleotide (NAD)

to form a molecule of reduced nicotinamide adenine dinucleotide (NADH). The reoxidation of the NADH by the passage of electrons from the NADH through a series of electron acceptors to oxygen results in the formation of three additional high-energy phosphate bonds which are trapped as ATP. It can therefore be seen that the metabolism of glucose to lactic acid (an anaerobic process) results in the formation of considerably fewer molecules of ATP (net of two high-energy phosphate bonds per molecule of glucose) than does the complete oxidation of glucose to carbon dioxide and water in which four molecules of ATP are formed by substrate-level phosphorylation, and 36 additional high-energy bonds are formed by oxidative phosphorylation during transport of the electrons released by oxidative reactions (see Figure 5-1).

The exact mechanism by which high-energy phosphate bonds are formed during oxidative phosphorylation is still not completely clear. It was believed for many years that during electron transport a high-energy phosphate bond was formed in a third component, perhaps a protein, that could subsequently transfer that energy to phosphorylate ADP to form ATP. However, such an intermediate has never been found, and current concepts of oxidative phosphorylation are based on a chemiosmotic hypothesis in which the suggestion is made that the orientation of the electron-transport chain in the cell membrane results in an outward flow of protons, which cannot re-enter the membrane except at specific sites in the membrane. This creates a pH gradient across the membrane which, in the presence of a

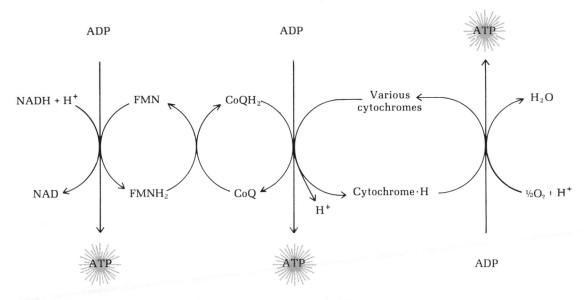

**Figure 5-1.** The passage of electrons from NADH occurs in a stepwise fashion through flavin mononucleotide (FMN), coenzyme Q (CoQ) and various cytochromes to eventually react with oxygen to form water. The detailed steps vary among bacteria, but most organisms appear capable of synthesizing three high-energy phosphate bonds for each pair of eletrons passed from NADH to oxygen.

membrane-bound ATPase, drives the following reaction.

$$ADP + P_i + \xrightarrow{\text{ATPase}} ATP + H_2O$$

Regardless of the precise mechanism of oxidative phosphorylation, the aerobic degradation of a carbohydrate such as glucose yields about 12 times more energy for the bacterial cell than does the anaerobic metabolism of the same sugar-forming products such as lactic acid.

## CARBON AND ENERGY SOURCES FOR BACTERIA

Microorganisms may be placed into one of four possible groups based on their source of carbon and the method by which they obtain their energy. Those organisms that gain energy from light are called phototrophs; those that obtain energy from chemical oxidations are called chemotrophs. Organisms whose sole source of carbon is carbon dioxide are called autotrophs, while those requiring an organic source of carbon are heterotrophs. As shown in Table 5-1, these terms may be combined to produce photoautotrophs, photoheterotrophs, chemoautotrophs, and chemoheterotrophs.

## PHOTOSYNTHETIC BACTERIA

Although it is not within the scope of this text to present a detailed discussion of photosynthesis, it is significant to note that even though the energy for photosynthetic organisms comes from light, the usable biochemical form to which it is converted, the high-energy phosphate bond of ATP, is in general the same for all types of cells. Thus, when light is absorbed during photosynthesis by a molecule of the pigment chlorophyll, the chlorophyll becomes excited and emits an electron. The emitted electron is accepted by an iron-containing electron acceptor called ferredoxin and is then passed down through an electron-transport chain to return eventually to a chlorophyll molecule (see Figure 5-2). During this transport of electrons from ferredoxin back

### Table 5-1. Classification Based on Energy and Carbon Source

| Group | Energy Source | Carbon Source |
|---|---|---|
| Chemoheterotrophs | Oxidation of organic compounds | Organic |
| Chemoautotrophs | Oxidation of inorganic substances such as ammonia, sulfides, and ferrous compounds | $CO_2$ |
| Photoheterotrophs | Light | Organic |
| Photoautotrophs | Light | $CO_2$ |

to chlorophyll, two molecules of ATP are formed from ADP for each pair of electrons passed. Thus, in energy terms this process is analogous to the oxidative phosphorylation of ADP occurring during electron transport.

Like green plants, photoautotrophic bacteria utilize carbon dioxide as their source of carbon for the synthesis of cellular constituents. All organic carbon compounds, however, are more reduced than carbon dioxide, and all photoautotrophs must have a reductant (NADPH) to reduce the carbon dioxide when it is fixed by the cell. Green plants possess a second photosystem in series with the one described in the previous paragraph that generates NADPH from the photolysis of water; photoautotrophic bacteria, however, lack this second photosystem and must chemically oxidize substances such as $H_2S$, $S$, or $H_2$ to provide electrons to generate the required NADPH. Some bacteria are photoheterotrophs which, like the photoautotrophs, lack the photosystem that forms NADPH. But photoheterotrophs can directly assimilate or oxidize various organic compounds and thus do not oxidize inorganic compounds for a source of reducing potential.

## CHEMOAUTOTROPHIC BACTERIA

Chemoautotrophs (also called chemolithotrophs) obtain their energy from the oxidation of inorganic compounds and their

**Figure 5-2.** Schematic diagram depicting cyclic photophosphorylation. Note that the energy for the formation of the high-energy phosphate bonds comes from light as it excites the chlorophyll and releases an electron. However, after the energy is converted to chemical energy, the electron returns to chlorophyll; hence, the designation cyclic.

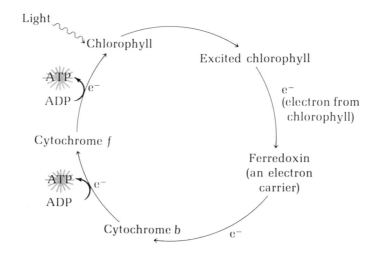

carbon from carbon dioxide. Even though such organisms do not constitute a health hazard, their ability to reproduce in an entirely inorganic environment places them in a unique niche in the scheme of things. These bacteria have been assigned to genera based on the type of inorganic substance oxidized as an energy source. The following are a few representative examples of chemoautotrophs and their energy-yielding reactions.

*Thiobacillus thiooxidans* (oxidation of sulfur and sulfur-containing compounds)

$$2\,S + 3\,O_2 + 2\,H_2O \longrightarrow 2\,H_2SO_4$$

*Thiobacillus ferrooxidans* (oxidation of iron compounds)

$$4\,FeCO_3 + O_2 + 6\,H_2O \longrightarrow$$
$$4\,Fe(OH)_3 + 4\,CO_2$$

*Nitrosomonas* species (oxidation of ammonia)

$$2\,NH_4Cl + 3\,O_2 \longrightarrow 2\,HNO_2 + 2\,HCl + 2\,H_2O$$

*Nitrobacter* species (oxidation of nitrites)

$$2\,NaNO_2 + O_2 \longrightarrow 2\,NaNO_3$$

It should be noted that the over-all mechanism by which chemoautotrophic bacteria trap the released energy is as described for oxidative phosphorylation. Thus, when an inorganic substance is oxidized, the electrons are transported stepwise through a series of electron acceptors. At various steps during this passage, the released energy is trapped as high-energy phosphate bonds by the phosphorylation of ADP to ATP.

## CHEMOHETEROTROPHIC BACTERIA

Bacteria that are unable to use carbon dioxide as their sole source of carbon and must obtain their energy from the oxidation of organic compounds are called chemoheterotrophs, which include the bacteria with which the medical microbiologist is concerned. However, the over-all method of obtaining and trapping chemical energy still requires either the oxidation of a phosphorylated com-

pound, with the concomitant formation of high-energy phosphate bonds, or the passage of electrons through a series of electron acceptors resulting in oxidative phosphorylation and synthesis of ATP. Many microorganisms metabolize organic substances anaerobically and synthesize ATP solely by substrate-level phosphorylation. This type of metabolism is called fermentation, as contrasted with respiration, in which ATP is formed also by oxidative phosphorylation.

## MICROBIAL FERMENTATION

During fermentation the intermediate products formed by the catabolism of an organic substrate serve as final electron acceptors, resulting in the formation of stable fermentation products. For example, some microorganisms metabolize sugars to acetaldehyde and carbon dioxide. In such a case, however, NADH is also formed and it must be reoxidized if the organism is to continue to metabolize. This is accomplished by using the acetaldehyde as a final hydrogen acceptor, which as a consequence is reduced to ethyl alcohol. This particular type of fermentation is vital to the brewing and distilling industries. Some other examples in which an intermediate degradation product can serve as a final electron acceptor in fermentation reactions are the reduction of pyruvic acid to lactic acid, glyceraldehyde to glycerol, fumaric acid to succinic acid, acetone to isopropyl alcohol, and crotonic acid to butyric acid. Other end products of fermentation reactions which are not necessarily formed as a direct reduction include acetic acid, formic acid, propionic acid, hydrogen, and carbon dioxide. As can be seen, many end products of fermentations are organic acids, and it is therefore a simple procedure to determine whether or not a particular bacterium can ferment a specific sugar. One merely adds an acid-base indicator to the medium containing the specific sugar being tested; after growth, the medium changes color if acid is produced. A small inverted vial can also be added to trap any gas that is produced. Thus, one has only to glance at the inoculated tubes to see whether or not fermentation has taken place.

Gas-liquid chromatography also is used for the rapid identification of some of the obligate anaerobes (*Bacteroides, Fusobacterium,* *Leptotrichia,* and *Bifidobacterium*) since the injection of a few microliters of liquid culture medium (which has been methylated to make the organic acids volatile) provides a rapid means for identifying the end products of fermentation.

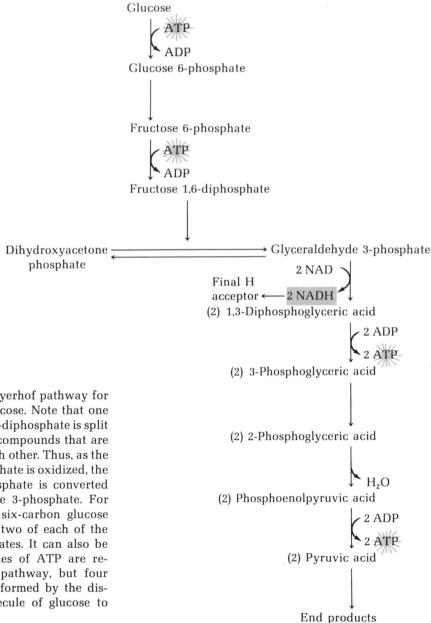

**Figure 5-3.** Embden-Meyerhof pathway for the dissimilation of glucose. Note that one molecule of fructose 1,6-diphosphate is split into two three-carbon compounds that are in equilibrium with each other. Thus, as the glyceraldehyde 3-phosphate is oxidized, the dihydroxyacetone phosphate is converted to more glyceraldehyde 3-phosphate. For each molecule of the six-carbon glucose metabolized, there are two of each of the three-carbon intermediates. It can also be seen that two molecules of ATP are required to initiate the pathway, but four molecules of ATP are formed by the dissimilation of one molecule of glucose to pyruvic acid.

## Pathways of Fermentation

The Embden-Meyerhof pathway is a common mechanism for the conversion of glucose to pyruvic acid. As can be seen in Figure 5-3, two molecules of ATP are required per molecule of glucose to initiate this pathway, but four molecules of ATP are obtained through substrate phosphorylation by the conversion of glucose to pyruvic acid, giving a net yield of two moles of ATP per mole of glucose metabolized. (Note that the six-carbon fructose 1,6-diphosphate is broken into two three-carbon molecules—dihydroxyace- tone phosphate and glyceraldehyde 3-phosphate. Since dihydroxyacetone phosphate is constantly converted to glyceraldehyde 3-phosphate as the latter is further metabolized, every step following glyceraldehyde 3-phosphate occurs twice for each original glucose molecule.) Furthermore, although Figure 5-3 indicates that pyruvic acid is the final product of this pathway, there are still two molecules of NADH that must be reoxidized. Thus, depending on the type of microorganism, pyruvic acid ($CH_3COCOOH$) will be additionally metabolized to yield final fermentation products as shown in the boxes below.

1. Homolactic-acid fermentation (some streptococci and lactobacilli)

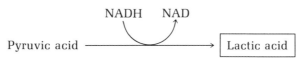

2. Alcoholic fermentation (yeast)

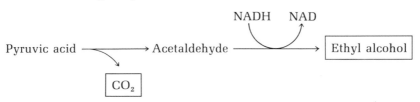

3. Mixed-acid fermentation (*Escherichia coli* and some other enteric bacteria)

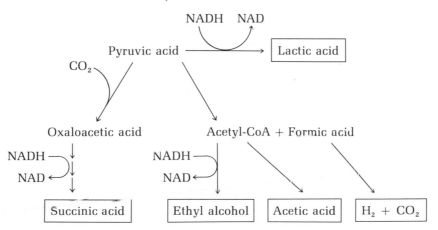

4. Butylene-glycol fermentation *(Enterobacter, Bacillus, Pseudomonas)*

This fermentation produces small amounts of the same end products as the mixed acid fermentation, but, in addition, a large part of the pyruvic acid is converted to 2,3-butylene glycol as shown below.

$$2\ CH_3COCOOH \longrightarrow CH_3COHCOOH + CO_2$$

Pyruvic acid

with the substituents:
$$C=O$$
$$CH_3$$

Acetolactic acid

$$CH_3CHOHCHOHCH_3 \longleftarrow CH_3CHOHCOCH_3$$

NAD   NADH     $CO_2$

2,3 Butylene glycol          Acetoin

Also, as will be discussed in Chapter 20, the presence of a small amount of acetoin in the growth medium is used as a criterion for differentiating *Enterobacter* and *Escherichia.*

5. Propionic-acid fermentation *(Propionibacterium* and *Veillonella)*

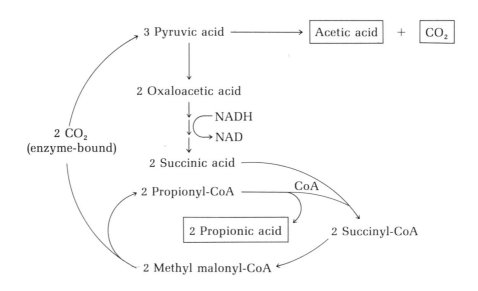

The energy incorporated into the propionyl-CoA bond is preserved by the reaction
of propionyl-CoA with succinic acid to
form succinyl-CoA and free propionic acid.
Furthermore, the $CO_2$ arising from the decarboxylation of methyl malonyl-CoA remains bound to a biotin-containing enzyme
which transfers the $CO_2$ directly to the pyruvic acid to form oxaloacetic acid. In addition
to this mechanism for the formation of oxaloacetic acid, these organisms can also form
oxaloacetic acid by a reaction of phospho-
enolpyruvic acid with free $CO_2$.

6. Butyric-acid, butanol, acetone fermentation (Clostridium)

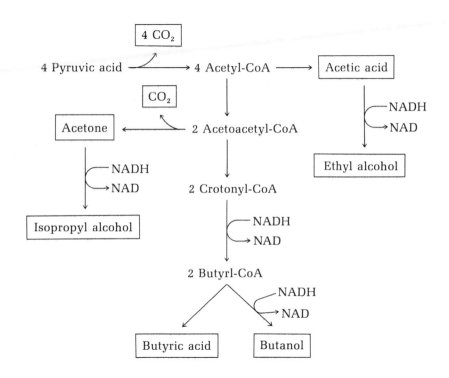

### Alternative Pathways from Glucose to Pyruvic Acid

Some bacteria do not use the Embden-Meyerhof pathway for the dissimilation of glucose
and use alternate pathways that are variations of the hexosemonophosphate shunt involving pentose phosphates as intermediates.

1. Heterolactic-acid fermentation (*Leuconostoc* and some strains of lactobacilli)

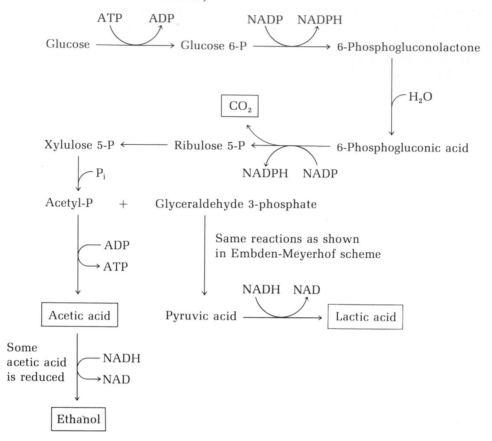

Thus, the end products of the heterolactic acid fermentation are lactic acid, ethanol, acetic acid, and carbon dioxide.

2. Entner-Doudoroff fermentation (*Zymomonas*, enterics, *Acinetobacter*)

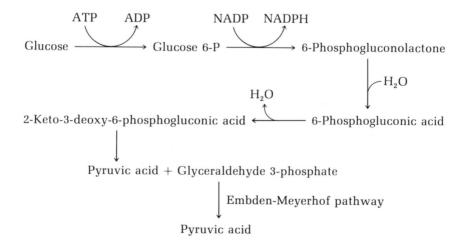

The ultimate fate of the pyruvic acid will vary for each genus. In one case, *Zymomonas mobilis* decarboxylates the pyruvic acid to form acetaldehyde and $CO_2$ and then reduces the acetaldehyde to ethyl alcohol. Thus, the over-all result reached by a different pathway is identical to the alcoholic fermentation by yeast. *Zymomonas mobilis* is used for the fermentation of a cactus sap resulting in the Mexican drink, pulque.

## RESPIRATION

Respiration in animal cells may be defined as metabolic oxidations in which molecular oxygen serves as a final electron acceptor. Thus NADH becomes reoxidized by the stepwise passage of electrons through the electron-transport chain (see Figure 5-1) to ultimately reduce molecular oxygen to water, and the energy released during this process is trapped as ATP by oxidative phosphorylation. Thus, NADH becomes reoxidized by passing its electrons to an external acceptor (oxygen) and stable fermentation products are not formed.

The citric-acid cycle (Krebs tricarboxylic acid cycle, see Figure 5-4) and the pentose phosphate pathway (see Figure 5-5) provide pathways by which bacteria are able to aerobically oxidize carbohydrates to carbon dioxide and water. Occasional obligately aerobic organisms lack both of these pathways and carry out incomplete oxidations, resulting in the accumulation of partially oxidized intermediates. One familiar example is the oxidation of ethyl alcohol present in wine or apple cider to acetic acid by *Gluconobacter suboxydans*, producing vinegar.

Some bacteria are able to pass electrons through an electron-transport chain (including the flavoproteins and at least some of the cytochromes) and use a final electron acceptor other than oxygen. Because this occurs anaerobically but yet results in oxidative phosphorylation, microbiologists have termed this process anaerobic respiration. The final electron acceptors used in anaerobic respiration may be sulfate, nitrate, or carbon dioxide, which are reduced, respectively, to hydrogen sulfide, nitrite, and methane.

## DISSIMILATION OF NONCARBOHYDRATE SUBSTRATES

Bacteria are versatile in the diversity of compounds they can degrade; in fact, there is probably no biological substance that a bacterium of one kind or another cannot degrade.

### Protein Dissimilation

Only rarely or under unusual circumstances can proteins be taken into a bacterial cell. However, some bacteria are able to excrete a variety of proteases which will enzymatically hydrolyze proteins into their component amino acids. The amino acids can then enter the cell, usually by means of a specific energy-requiring active-transport mechanism.

After entering the cell, amino acids may be incorporated into bacterial proteins, or they may be degraded by decarboxylases, deaminases, or both, allowing the amino acids to be further degraded to yield energy or to serve as building blocks for biosynthetic reactions.

### Fat Dissimilation

The hydrolytic breakdown of fats occurs through the action of fat-splitting enzymes called lipases. Simple fats are degraded to glycerol and fatty acids as shown in the following example:

$$\begin{array}{l} CH_2OOC_4H_7 \\ | \\ CHOOC_4H_7 \\ | \\ CH_2OOC_4H_7 \end{array} + 3\ H_2O \longrightarrow \begin{array}{l} CH_2OH \\ | \\ CHOH \\ | \\ CH_2OH \end{array} + 3\ CH_3(CH_2)_2COOH$$

Tributyrin                          Glycerol                    Butyric acid

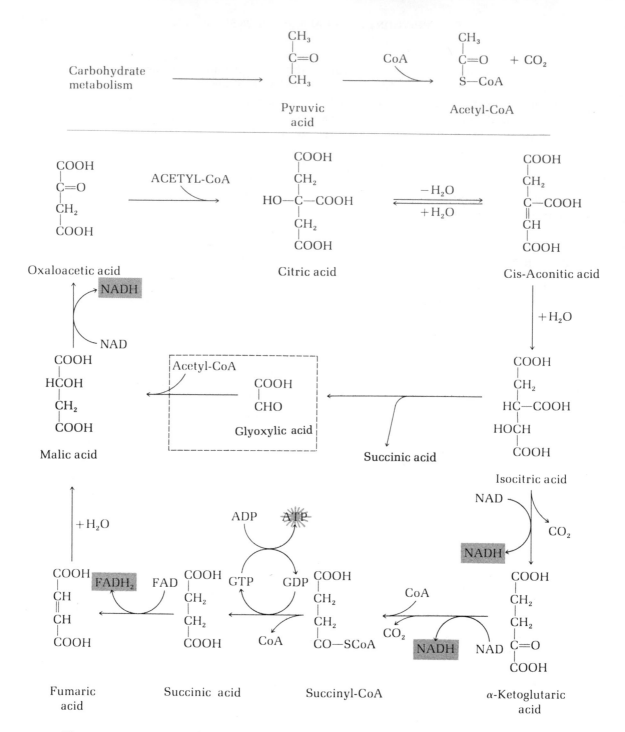

**Figure 5-4.** The citric acid cycle. Each turn of the cycle results in the oxidation of one two-carbon compound, which enters the cycle as acetyl-CoA. In addition, some organisms can cleave isocitric acid to yield glyoxylic acid and succinic acid. As shown in the box, the glyoxylic acid can combine with a molecule of acetyl-CoA to form malic acid. The glyoxylic acid cycle thus formed provides a continual source of intermediates for the synthesis of carbohydrates and proteins for an organism using acetic acid as its sole source of carbon, which, as before, enters the cycle as acetyl-CoA.

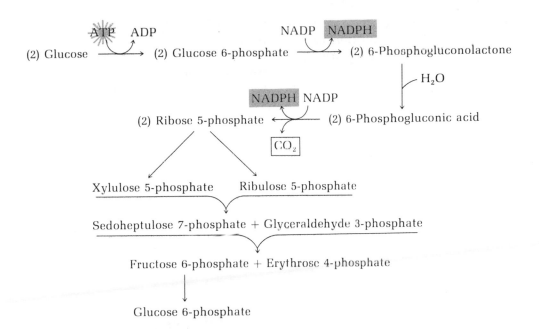

**Figure 5-5.** Pentose phosphate pathway. Note that the erythrose 4-phosphate can accept a two-carbon intermediate from a molecule of sedoheptulose 7-phosphate to form fructose 6-phosphate and ribulose 5-phosphate. The complete oxidation of one molecule of glucose requires six revolutions of the cycle with each revolution liberating one molecule of $CO_2$ and forming two molecules of NADPH. This pathway thus provides a pathway for the formation of ribose 5-phosphate for nucleic acid biosynthesis, a source of NADPH for many biosynthetic reactions, and a second pathway for the aerobic oxidation of glucose to $CO_2$ and $H_2O$.

The liberated glycerol can then be phosphorylated, oxidized to glyceraldehyde 3-phosphate, and metabolized via the Embden-Meyerhof pathway. The fatty acid can be degraded by a series of reactions similar to those occurring in mitochondria.

## BIOSYNTHESIS OF MICROBIAL INTERMEDIATES

Bacteria vary widely in their growth requirements; some can reproduce in a completely inorganic medium, others require a number of preformed compounds such as amino acids, purines, pyrimidines, and vitamins. These requirements are inversely proportional to an organism's synthetic abilities—one that can synthesize its own amino acids, coenzymes, and so forth will grow in a sim-

pler medium than one which has lost these abilities. Most biosynthetic pathways are identical in procaryotic and eucaryotic cells; however, all bacteria must synthesize certain key intermediates and structural components that are peculiar to procaryotic cells.

### Glyoxylate Cycle

Many intermediates of the tricarboxylic-acid cycle (see Figure 5-4) are used for the biosynthesis of amino acids, nucleic acid, polysaccharides, and other important constituents of cells. Thus, an organism using acetate as a sole carbon source requires a mechanism to synthesize a four-carbon compound which will replace those intermediates of the TCA cycle that are used for biosynthetic reactions. This is accomplished by a modification of the

TCA cycle known as the glyoxylate cycle, in which two molecules of acetyl-CoA can be converted into a four-carbon dicarboxylic acid as shown in Figure 5-4.

### Amino-Acid Biosynthesis

Many microorganisms are able to synthesize all of the amino acids necessary for protein synthesis. Intermediates of both fermentation pathways and the TCA cycle serve as sources for their biosynthesis, and based on the pathways by which they are made, the amino acids can be divided into five families.

1.

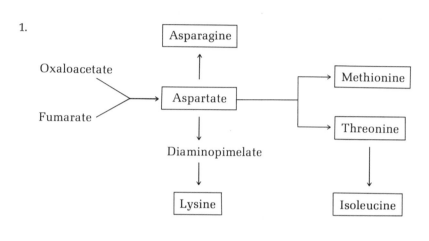

2.

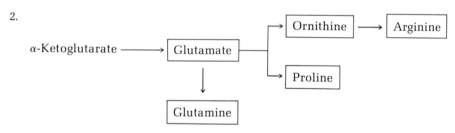

3.

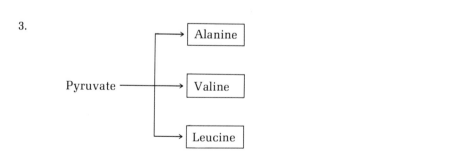

4.

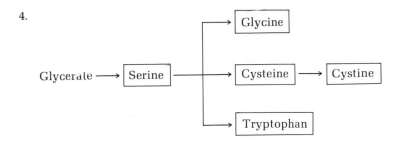

5.

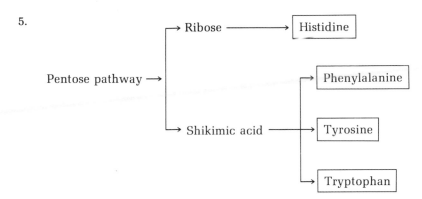

## Carbon-Dioxide Fixation in Bacteria

Both chemoautotrophs and photoautotrophs use an identical pathway for the fixation of $CO_2$. They differ only in that the chemoautotrophs obtain their energy and reducing power by the oxidation of inorganic compounds, while the photoautotrophic bacteria receive their energy from the reaction of chlorophyll with light and their reducing power by the oxidation of inorganic or organic compounds. After synthesizing ATP and NADPH, the fixation of $CO_2$ takes place as shown below:

1. Ribulose 5-phosphate + ATP $\longrightarrow$
       Ribulose 1,5-diphosphate + ADP
2. Ribulose 1,5-diphosphate + $CO_2$ $\longrightarrow$
       2 (3-phosphoglyceric acid)
3. 2 (3-phosphoglyceric acid) + 2 NADPH
       + 2 H$^+$ $\longrightarrow$
   2 (glyceraldehyde 3-phosphate) + 2 NADP$^+$
4. 2 (glyceraldehyde 3-phosphate) $\longrightarrow$ $\longrightarrow$
       $\longrightarrow$ Glucose

It should be noted that many if not all heterotrophic organisms may fix small amounts of $CO_2$, but they lack the $CO_2$-fixation pathway used by the chemoautotrophic and photoautotrophic organisms, and are, thus, unable to grow with $CO_2$ as their sole source of carbon. Heterotrophic $CO_2$ fixation occurs as an energy-dependent reaction with pyruvate or phosphoenolpyruvate to yield oxaloacetate or malate. In addition, $CO_2$ fixation occurs in the pathway leading to the biosynthesis of purines and pyrimidines.

## REFERENCES

Bartsch, R. G. 1968. Bacterial cytochromes. *Annu. Rev. Microbiol.* **22**:181–200.

Becker, W. M. 1977. *Energy and the Living Cell.* J. B. Lippincott, Philadelphia.

Doelle, H. W. 1975. *Bacterial Metabolism,* 2nd ed. Academic Press, New York.

Forrest, W. W., and D. J. Walker. 1971. The generation and utilization of energy during growth. *Adv. Microbial Phys.* **5**:213–274.

Fraenkel, D. G., and R. T. Vinopal. 1973. Carbohydrate metabolism in bacteria. *Annu. Rev.
Microbiol.* **27:**69–100.

Glenn, A. R. 1976. Production of extracellular proteins by bacteria. *Annu. Rev. Microbiol.* **30:**
41–62.

Vogel, N. J., J. S. Thompson, and G. D. Schockman.
1970. Characteristic metabolic patterns of pro-
karyotes and eukaryotes. In *Organization and
Control in Prokaryotic and Eukaryotic Cells.*
Symp. Soc. Gen. Microbiol. 107–119, Cambridge
University Press.

Yoch, D. C., and R. C. Valentine. 1972. Ferredoxins
and flavodoxins of bacteria. *Annu. Rev. Microbiol.* **26:**139–162.

# 6

# Bacteriophage

Viruses that infect bacteria are called bacteriophages, or merely phages. Although the spectrum of bacteria that any one kind of phage can infect is limited, the enormous number of phages in existence makes it likely that there is at least one phage for every type of bacterium.

## CHEMICAL COMPOSITION AND STRUCTURE OF BACTERIOPHAGES

Bacteriophages occur in assorted shapes, but all have a protein coat, called a capsid, which encloses the phage nucleic acid. Some also possess complex structures that are used to attach the phage to a susceptible cell. Figure 6-1 is a drawing of a T2 phage (which infects certain strains of *Escherichia coli*) and an electron micrograph of this phage isolated from a culture.

The phage head, which contains the nucleic acid, is frequently icosahedral (20-sided), but there are several other shapes, including round or cylindrical. Also, there may be considerable variation in the tail structure even between related phages. For example, the tail of the T-even phages (T2, T4, and T6) infecting coliform bacteria con-

sists of a hollow core surrounded by a contractile sheath which extends from an end plate to a collar immediately below the head. Attached to the base of the tail are six pins and six tail fibers that react with the specific receptor sites on the bacterium to attach the phage to the bacterial cell wall. In contrast, coliphages T1 and T5 do not possess a contractable sheath, and T3 and T7 have tails considerably shorter than those of the T-even phages.

## BACTERIOPHAGE MULTIPLICATION

The sequence of events occurring during replication is similar for most phages; however, the following steps apply more specifically to the T-even phages.

### Adsorption

Phage adsorption occurs tail first because of a reaction between the organs of attachment on the phage and specific receptor sites in the bacterial cell wall (see Figure 6-2). Infection cannot occur in the absence of adsorption, and thus a bacterial mutation which results in the inability to synthesize specific recep-

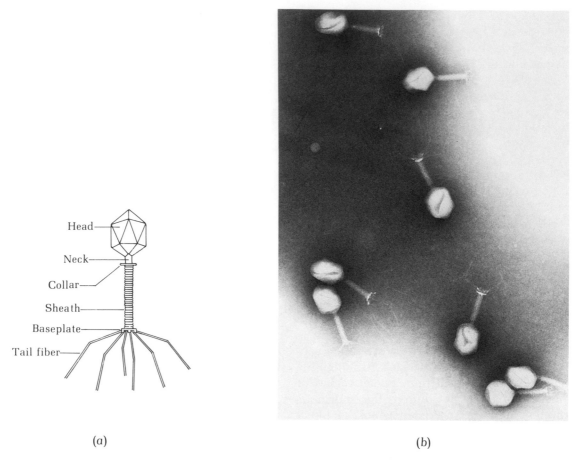

(a)                                          (b)

**Figure 6-1.** *a.* Anatomy of a T2 bacteriophage. *b.* Isolated, negatively-stained T2 phages.

tors will render a bacterium resistant to infection by the respective phage. In some cases the phage receptor is part of the bacterial lipopolysaccharide, while for others it is part of the cell wall protein.

### Penetration

Following adsorption, the phage injects its nucleic acid into the bacterial cytoplasm, while the protein capsid remains outside the bacterium. (The only exception appears to be the filamentous rod-shaped DNA phages such as fd and M13 which, like animal viruses, enter the bacterial cell prior to uncoating.) In the case of the T-even phages, the sheath contracts, forcing the hollow interior tail tube

through the bacterial cell wall. However, since phages such as T1 and T5 that do not possess a contractible sheath also inject their nucleic acid through the cell wall (possibly at adhesion sites between the inner and outer membranes), contraction is not a general prerequisite for phage infection. Some idea of the magnitude of the injection task can be gained from the length of the T2 DNA molecule in Figure 6-3.

### Phage DNA Transcription

The steps involved in the transcription of phage DNA will vary from one phage to another, but a brief description of the sequence of events that occur after the entrance of coliphage T4 DNA into the bacterial cytoplasm will illustrate how this phage takes over the metabolic control from the infected bacterium.

Phage T4 transcription occurs in several stages, resulting in the formation of immediate early, delayed early, and late gene products. The total transcription and subsequent translation of T4 DNA produces approximately 200 different proteins, but we shall be concerned here primarily with those gene products involved in the control of T4 reproduction.

Immediate early genes are transcribed using the existing bacterial DNA polymerase, and, for the most part, code for nucleases that hydrolyze host DNA and for enzymes that alter the bacterial transcriptase so that it will preferentially transcribe delayed early phage genes.

Delayed early genes code for phage enzymes that produce a new nucleotide base, 5-hydroxymethylcytosine (5-HMC) that replaces cytosine in the phage DNA and an enzyme that transfers a molecule of glucose to the hydroxyl group of the 5-HMC. An

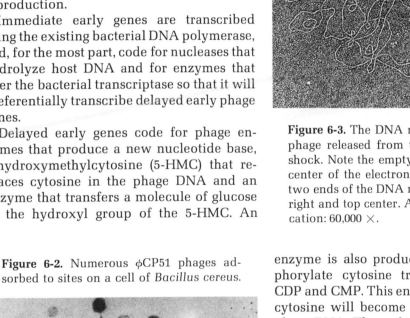

**Figure 6-3.** The DNA molecule of a T-even phage released from the head by osmotic shock. Note the empty phage capsid in the center of the electron micrograph and the two ends of the DNA molecule at the lower right and top center. Approximate magnification: 60,000 ×.

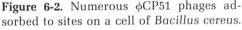

**Figure 6-2.** Numerous φCP51 phages adsorbed to sites on a cell of *Bacillus cereus*.

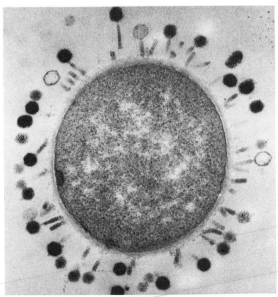

enzyme is also produced that will dephosphorylate cytosine triphosphate (CTP) to CDP and CMP. This ensures that no bacterial cytosine will become incorporated into the phage DNA. These alterations are important because bacterial nucleases (called restriction enzymes) are unable to degrade the phage DNA modified by substitution of 5-HMC for cytosine and by glucosylation of this substituted base. Moreover, a phage nuclease will degrade any DNA that contains unsubstituted cytosine. Delayed early genes also code for polymerases and ligases to replicate the phage DNA and for a second altered RNA polymerase that will transcribe the late genes.

Late T4 gene products include the structural components of new phage particles, such as heads, tails, and fibers. Late products also include a phage lysozyme which, when present in sufficient amounts, will lyse or rupture the bacterial cell, liberating the mature phage particles.

### Assembly and Release

Only after the synthesis of both nucleic acid and structural proteins is well underway does the phage begin to assemble into mature particles. This assembly for the T4 phage is schematically illustrated in Figure 6-4. After the assembly of 100 to 200 phage particles, the bacterial cell lyses as a result of membrane alterations and the formation of the previously mentioned phage-coded lysozyme.

The over-all multiplication of a phage such as T4 can be plotted as a one-step multiplication cycle as shown in Figure 6-5. Here one can see that during the first 10 minutes, no phage can be recovered either externally or by disrupting the infected bacterium. However, at the end of this eclipse period, mature phage particles begin to accumulate intracellularly until their numbers are sufficient to cause lysis. Thus, if one plots the formation of intracellular phage, an increase in numbers can be seen to occur from about 12 minutes until 34 minutes, but extracellular phage cannot be seen until lysis begins. The yield of phage per bacterium is called the burst size (100 to 300 phages), and the time from infection until lysis is the latent period (20 to 40 minutes).

### RNA PHAGES

Several RNA phages attach only to the F pili of male bacteria (See conjugation, Chapter 8). The phage RNA enters the bacterium and, after attachment to host ribosomes, is translated into proteins. The resulting RNA polymerase replicates the phage RNA by first forming a double-stranded RNA (replicative form or RF), and then producing multiple

**Figure 6-4.** The morphogenic pathway of phage maturation has three principal branches leading independently to formation of heads, tails, and tail fibers, which then combine to form complete phage particles. The numbers refer to the T-even phage genes whose products are involved at each step. The solid arrows indicate the steps that have been shown to occur in extracts.

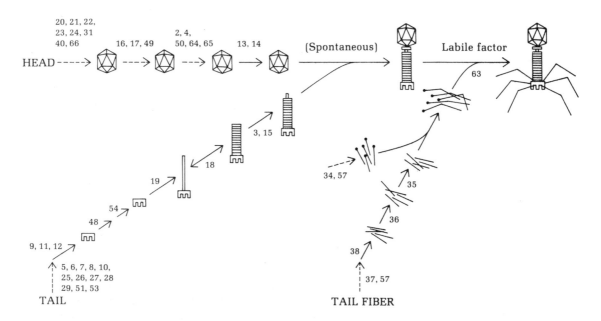

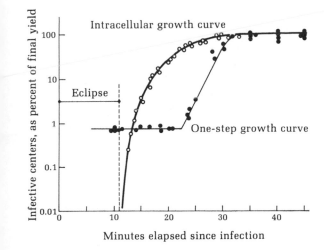

**Figure 6-5.** Intracellular growth kinetics of phage T4. Note that during the eclipse no intact phage exists, but, as shown by the open circles, intracellular phage particles can be detected by disruption of the bacterium after about 12 minutes. Without artificial disruption to release intracellular phages, the number of infective centers available outside the cell follows the one-step growth curve, showing a sharp rise at the end of the burst time, when the bacterium is lysed and the phage liberated.

parental single strands of RNA using the RF as a template. As the newly formed strands of RNA are released from the replicative intermediate, they assemble into capsids and the completed phages are eventually released by lysis of the host bacterium.

## ASSAY OF PHAGES

Bacteriophages can be counted by mixing a dilution of the phage with a large excess of susceptible bacteria and then, after adsorption has taken place, plating the entire mixture on a suitable solid medium to form a bacterial lawn. As each phage reproduces and lyses its host bacterium, the progeny infect adjacent bacteria on the plate. The result is a clear area, or plaque, occurring for each phage present in the original dilution (See Figure 6-6). By counting these plaques

and multiplying by the dilution factor, the number of phages in the original material can be calculated. The large excess of bacteria is necessary so that each cell is infected by only one phage.

## PHAGE GENETICS

Since the genetic control of a bacteriophage is contained in its DNA, any change in DNA can result in mutant phage with different properties such as plaque size, latent period, host range, and other variables. If one simultaneously infects a bacterium with two different but closely related phage mutants, the progeny are found to consist of each parental type plus recombinants possessing properties of both parental types. Such recombinants arise from the base pairing and crossing over between the nucleic-acid genomes from both parental phages. This is particularly evident if neither parental phage can replicate alone due to some genetic defect, but

**Figure 6-6.** Plaques, caused by lysis of adjacent bacteria on a medium at sites originally infected by single bacteriophages, are the clear areas in this photograph.

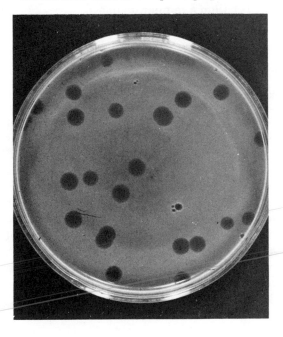

when simultaneous infection of a susceptible bacterium occurs, some normal phages will be produced. This latter phonemenon involves a crossing-over between the defective genomes of the two parental types so as to produce a nondefective DNA molecule as well as a molecule with both genetic defects. Of course, it is the nondefective DNA that results in normal phage.

## LYSOGENY

As previously described, the liberation of mature phage particles always results in the lysis and death of the infected bacterium. Those phages whose infection is followed by reproduction and lysis are called virulent bacteriophage. However, many phages are able to infect a bacterium without inducing the production of more phage or the lysis of the infected cell. In such cases, the phage DNA can become a part of the genetic material of its host bacterium. Phage DNA that exists and replicates along with the bacterial DNA is called prophage. A bacterium that carries a prophage is called a lysogenic bacterium, indicating it possesses the potential to lyse, and a phage that can produce lysogeny is called a temperate phage.

### Nature of the Prophage

Genetic experiments have now established that the prophage from some temperate phages is integrated into the bacterial chromosome, whereas the prophage from other temperate phages exists in the bacterium as extrachromosomal DNA.

INTEGRATED PROPHAGE. The most thoroughly studied temperate phage giving rise to an integrated prophage has been given the name of lambda phage ($\lambda$ phage). The DNA of $\lambda$ phage exists in a linear double strand in which the 5′ ends of both strands are 20 base pairs longer than the 3′-hydroxyl terminus. These extended ends are composed of complementary bases, and within minutes after

entering an E. coli cytoplasm, they pair to form a molecule of double-stranded circular DNA. The circular $\lambda$ DNA appears to possess a very small region which is complementary to a $\lambda$ attachment site on the bacterial chromosome. After site-specific recombination, the $\lambda$ prophage becomes integrated into the bacterial chromosome as shown schematically in Figure 6-7. The integration of the $\lambda$ DNA is catalyzed by a specific integration protein which is encoded by a $\lambda$ gene.

NONINTEGRATED PROPHAGE. Many temperate phages are unable to integrate their DNA into the bacterial genome, and in such cases the prophage exists and replicates as extrachromosomal DNA. Since integration requires both an integration site and a specific integration enzyme, any phage lacking either of these properties would be unable to integrate into the host DNA. The observation that this extrachromosomal DNA is faithfully passed on to daughter cells suggests that the prophage is attached to the bacterial plasma membrane in a manner analogous to that of the host DNA. Such extrachromosomal, self-duplicating DNA is referred to as a plasmid, and it is now established that many bacteria may be multiply lysogenic for several phages at one time, and hence contain several plasmids. Figure 6-8 shows an electron micrograph of plasmid DNA from a bacterial cell.

### Mechanism of Lysogeny

As previously noted, the infection of a susceptible bacterial culture with a virulent phage always results in the reproduction of the phage and lysis of the infected cells. Infection with a temperate phage also results in phage reproduction and the lysis of most of the culture, but a small percentage of infected cells survive as lysogenic bacteria. Quite obviously, the temperate phage possesses the potential to cause lysis but, unlike a virulent phage, does not always do so.

An explanation for this phenomenon was formulated in 1953 by Jacob and Wollman,

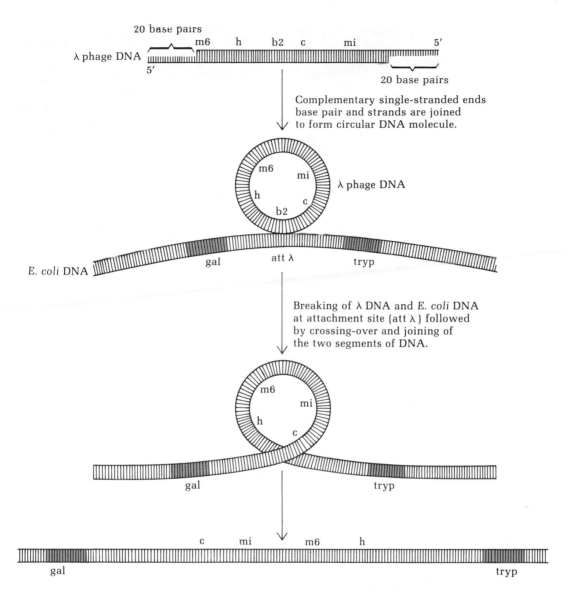

**Figure 6-7.** Insertion of λ phage into the *Escherichia coli* chromosome. Immediately after entering the bacterial cell, the single-stranded ends of the linear λ phage DNA base-pair to form a molecule of circular DNA. This molecule binds to a λ attachment site on the E. coli DNA in the b2 region of the λ DNA and is incorporated into the E. coli DNA as shown. The λ genes are shown to indicate the change in gene order that occurs during cyclization and integration. Note that in the linear λ DNA m6 and mi are near the ends of the molecule whereas c and h are found at the ends of the integrated λ DNA.

who proposed that temperate phages possess a gene that codes for a repressor protein which prevents the formation of mature phage particles. Furthermore, it is now known that this repressor protein (also called immunity repressor) is specific for its own temperate phage, so that the repressor for λ phage will bind only to certain operator

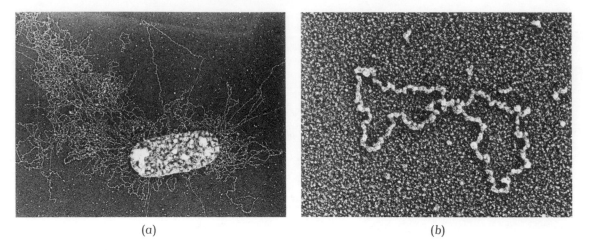

(a)                                                          (b)

**Figure 6-8.** *a.* Disrupted cell of *Escherichia coli*; the DNA has spilled out and a plasmid can be found slightly to the left of top center. *b.* Enlargement of a plasmid (about $1\mu$ from side to side); this plasmid provides the *E. coli* cell bearing it with resistance to the substance colicin.

genes in the $\lambda$ genome to prevent their transcription. When a bacterium is infected with a temperate phage, the phage begins to reproduce in a manner identical to that described for virulent phage. However, in a small percentage of cases, sufficient repressor is synthesized to stop phage reproduction, resulting in a lysogenic state. This immunity repressor from $\lambda$ phage has now been purified; it reacts with two different operator genes on the $\lambda$ phage genome to prevent their transcription and the eventual formation of mature phage. Thus, as described by Jacob, the initial establishment of a lysogenic condition is a "race between the synthesis of the immunity repressor and that of the early proteins required for vegetative multiplication." Once the repressor protein is formed, the bacterium is resistant to lysis from both the prophage and from externally infecting phage, hence the name "immunity repressor."

Of course, unless a prophage occasionally becomes virulent and produces mature phage particles, it would be very difficult to know whether or not any particular bacterium is lysogenic. However, an occasional lysogenic bacterium does go through the lytic cycle, and the liberated phage particles can be assayed by plating the bacterium-free supernatant fluid on a second nonlysogenic strain, which is lysed by the liberated phage particles. Better yet, in most cases if one treats a lysogenic culture with very small doses of ultraviolet light (wavelength about 250 nm), the result will be maturation of all of the prophage and lysis of the lysogenic bacterial culture. Both spontaneous lysis and ultraviolet light-induced lysis of a lysogenic bacterium probably result from the inactivation of phage immunity repressor. It is also apparent that any mutation which results in the loss of an effective immunity repressor will permit a temperate phage to complete the lytic cycle.

**Lysogenic Conversion**

Even though a lysogenic bacterium is unable to transcribe part of its DNA because of the presence of immunity repressor, all phage genes are not so blocked. As a result, part of the phage DNA may be transcribed to eventually form proteins new to the bacterium. These products may be enzymes that change the structure of the bacterium's lipopolysaccharide, causing a change in the cell wall antigens, or toxins which are excreted by the bacterium into the surrounding environment. These excreted proteins, called exotoxins, are the basis for such serious diseases as diphtheria, scarlet fever, and botulism. The acquisition of new phenotypic characteristics coded for by prophage DNA is called lysogenic conversion. The details of the biological action of exotoxins will be discussed in Unit Three.

## REFERENCES

Barksdale, L., and S. B. Arden. 1974. Persisting bacteriophage infections, lysogeny, and phage conversions. *Annu. Rev. Microbiol.* **28**:265–299.

Butler, P. J. G. 1976. Filamentous phage assembly. *Nature* **260**:283–284.

Cairns, J., G. S. Stent, and J. D. Watson, eds. 1966. *Phage and the Origins of Molecular Biology.* Cold Spring Harbor, New York.

Couturier, M. 1976. The integration and excision of the bacteriophage Mu-1. *Cell* **7**:155–163.

Douglas, J. 1975. *Bacteriophages.* Chapman and Hall, London.

Eoyang, L., and J. T. August. 1974. Reproduction of RNA bacteriophages. In H. Fraenkel-Conrat and R. R. Wagner, eds., *Comprehensive Virology,* Vol. 2. Plenum Press, New York.

Hershey, A. D., ed. 1971. *The Bacteriophage Lambda.* Cold Spring Harbor, New York.

Jacob, F., and E. Wollman. 1953. Induction of phage development in lysogenic bacteria. *Cold Spring Harbor Symp. Quant. Biol.* **18**:101–121.

Lindberg, A. A. 1973. Bacteriophage receptors. *Annu. Rev. Microbiol.* **27**:205–241.

Signer, E. R. 1968. Lysogeny: The integration problem. *Annu. Rev. Microbiol.* **22**:451–488.

# 7

# Bacterial Genetics:
# Gene Function and Mutation

In this chapter, we shall be concerned with the role of DNA in the control of cellular activities; however, since this control is mediated through the proteins and enzymes synthesized by the cell, we shall discuss first how the information present in the DNA is translated into specific proteins.

## THE NATURE OF DNA

Deoxyribonucleic acid is composed of two purines—adenine and guanine—and two pyrimidines—cytosine and thymine (see Figure 7-1). To each of these bases is attached the five-carbon sugar, 2-deoxyribose. The purine and pyrimidine bases are joined by phosphodiester bonds which link the number-five carbon of one molecule of 2-deoxyribose to the number-three carbon of the adjacent 2-deoxyribose. Thus, in brief, DNA is a large molecule consisting of a chain of 2-deoxyribose molecules connected by phosphodiester bridges; bound to the number one carbon of each 2-deoxyribose is one of the purine or pyrimidine bases. The specific arrangement or sequence of these nucleotide bases carries the genetic information in the cell. A brief discussion of the physical struc-ture of the DNA molecule will show how it is able to copy itself accurately as it is passed to progeny cells.

The DNA within the cell exists as long strands wound together in a configuration referred to as a double helix. The two strands are united in such a manner that each pyrimidine and purine base of strand 1 is joined through hydrogen bonds to a complementary base on strand 2. Obviously, the complementary bases must be structurally compatible so that hydrogen bonding can occur. The compatible complementary pairs are adenine (A) with thymine (T), and guanine (G) with cytosine (C). Thus, within the double helix each A on one strand is across from and hydrogen-bonded to a molecule of T on the other strand, and each G is across from and hydrogen-bonded to C (see Figure 7-2).

Synthesis of the DNA to be passed to progeny cells provides the mechanism for making an exact copy through the use of complementary bases. Thus, an enzyme in *Escherichia coli* called DNA polymerase III uses an existing strand of DNA as a template to line up the correct complementary bases and join them together. Two additional enzymes from *Escherichia coli* that have been designated

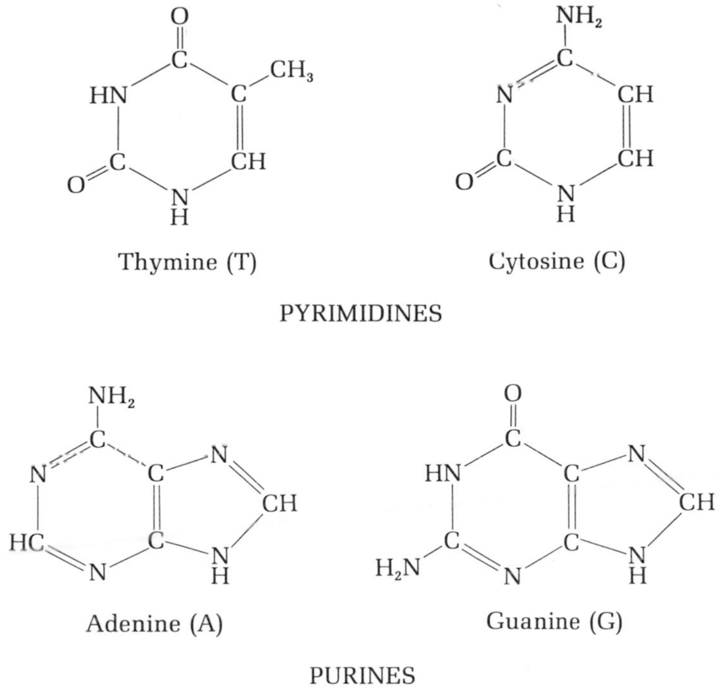

Figure 7-1. The purine and pyrimidine bases of DNA.

DNA polymerases I and II are also capable of catalyzing the *in vitro* replication of DNA. However, since mutants defective in these two enzymes (but not DNA polymerase III) are still able to grow, it is believed that DNA polymerases I and II are used for the repair of DNA, and that DNA polymerase III is the enzyme involved in the replication of bacterial DNA. When one strand is replicated, it is paired with a strand identical to the original second strand, and when the original strand is replicated, it is paired with a strand indentical to the first. The final result is two double helixes, each of which contains one original template strand and one new strand, as shown in Figure 7-3. This type of replication in which each new double helix consists of one strand of parental DNA and one newly synthesized strand is referred to as semiconservative replication.

The actual mechanism of replication of the circular bacterial chromosome begins at a specific origin, and, except for replication during conjugation, the growing point proceeds in both directions to complete the biosynthesis of the DNA (see Figure 7-4). One of the parental strands is enzymatically broken or nicked, and the 5′ end reattaches to a new site on the bacterial membrane. As DNA synthesis proceeds, the two mesosomal sites at which the DNA is attached become separated by newly synthesized membrane, so that by the time the chromosome is replicated and the free ends joined to form a circle, the two chromosomes are well isolated from each other.

## TRANSCRIPTION OF DNA TO RNA

Although the above mechanism explains how DNA copies itself, it does not explain how DNA controls cellular activity through the synthesis of protein. This is done indirectly, through the synthesis of RNA. RNA is

**Figure 7-2.** A schematic representation of the double-helical DNA molecule. The double helix may be discerned by letting your eye follow the black and grey atoms in the sugar-phosphate backbones. The stacked bases of the interior are also easily recognized.

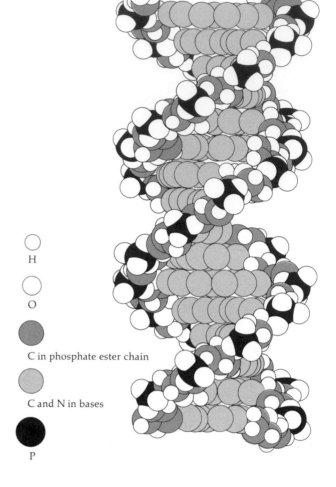

H

O

C in phosphate ester chain

C and N in bases

P

very similar in structure to DNA, but differs in that it contains the pyrimidine uracil (U) instead of thymine (T), and contains the five-carbon sugar ribose instead of deoxyribose (see Figure 7-5). Furthermore, except in the case of double-stranded RNA viruses, RNA does not exist in the cell as a double helix like DNA. In RNA synthesis DNA is used as the template, and an enzyme, DNA-dependent RNA polymerase, joins together the bases of RNA as each base binds to its complementary base on the DNA template. It should be noted that only one strand of DNA along any given

segment of the double helix (called the positive strand) is used as a template for RNA synthesis. Thus, a segment of DNA having a base sequence of AGTCTGACT would result in an RNA sequence of UCAGACUGA. This process is called transcription, since the message carried in the DNA is transcribed to the RNA through complementary base pairing of the RNA nucleotides with the template DNA. Since the resulting RNA now carries the "message" formed by the precise sequence of bases in the positive strand of DNA, it is called messenger RNA (usually written

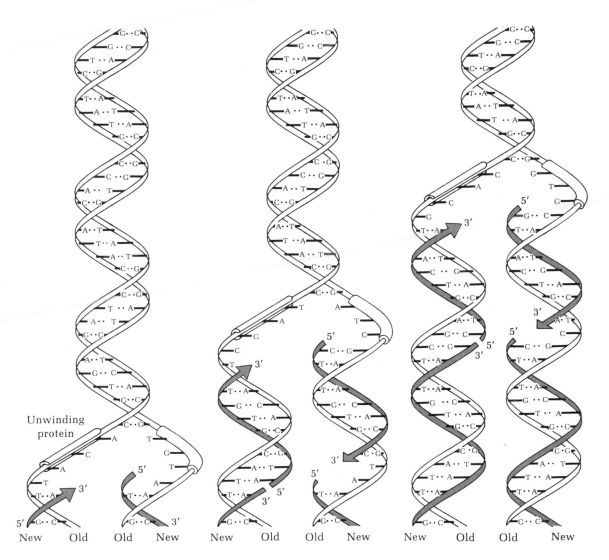

**Figure 7-3.** Highly schematic representation of the replication of DNA. As strands of the parent molecule unwind—most likely with the aid of unwinding proteins, which are more numerous and cover more bases than shown here—complementary nucleoside-5'-triphosphates are bound to the exposed bases. The triphosphates react with 3'-hydroxyl groups of the preceding nucleotide in the growing strands with the formation of a new 3', 5'-phosphodiester linkage and the loss of inorganic pyrophosphate. Thus, the new chains are formed in the 5' → 3' direction along both parental strands. As the new chains grow, sections of new double helices (each with many more bases than shown here) are formed on each of the parent strands. The daughter strands in each new double helix are stitched together at their ends with the enzyme DNA ligase.

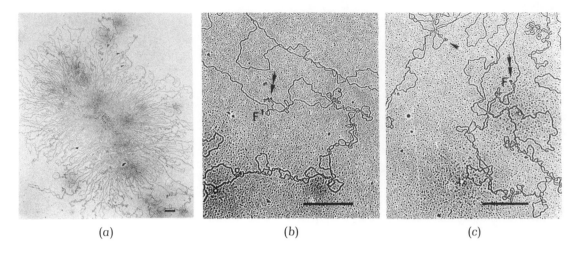

(a)                              (b)                              (c)

**Figure 7-4.** *a.* Electron micrograph of membrane-free folded chromosome from *E. coli;* two replication forks are shown at F and F′ in *b* and *c*. (All bars = 1μm.)

mRNA) and it is capable of dictating the specific protein which was coded in the DNA segment.

### TRANSLATION OF RNA TO PROTEIN

The process by which the mRNA uses its message to direct the synthesis of a specific protein (or more precisely, a polypeptide) is called translation, because the message carried up to this point in the base sequence of nucleic acids must be translated into the amino-acid sequence of the polypeptide. This message is encoded in the RNA according to the order in which the nucleotide bases occur in the mRNA molecule. Each series of three nucleotides is called a codon and codes for one specific amino acid. For example, a segment of DNA which was AAC would be

transcribed into mRNA as UUG, and this is a codon for the amino acid leucine.

Let us briefly review the series of events that must occur to translate the mRNA into protein, as illustrated in Figure 7-6. First, a ribosome, a small body made up of RNA (rRNA) and protein, attaches itself to an initiation site on the mRNA. Amino acids to be joined together to form a polypeptide must be activated by enzymes which join them to specific small molecules of yet another kind of RNA to form an amino acid-RNA complex. Because this RNA then carries the amino acid to the mRNA on the ribosome, it is called transfer RNA, written tRNA. There is a different tRNA and a different activating enzyme for each of the 20 amino acids that can make up polypeptides. Also, each tRNA contains a specific anticodon that will react through

**Figure 7-5.** Structural components of RNA that differ from those occurring in DNA. RNA contains the pyrimidine base uracil rather than thymine, and ribose takes the place of deoxyribose as the sugar component.

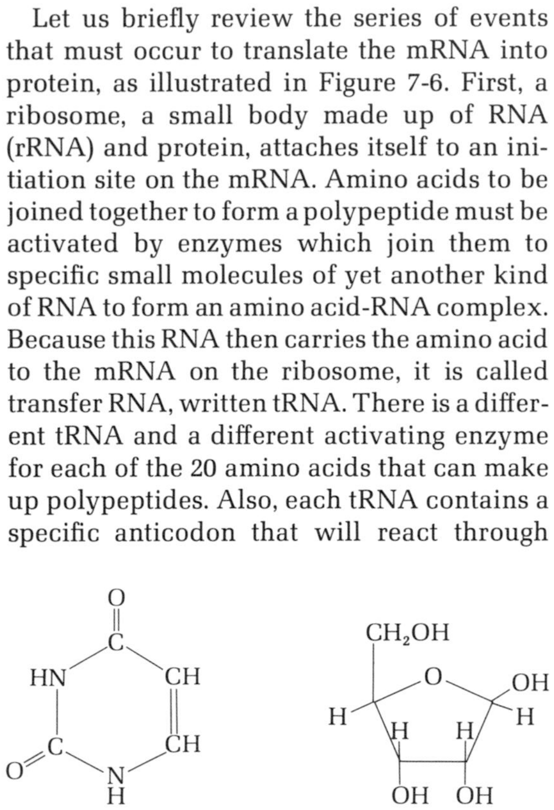

Uracil (U)

Ribose

base pairing only with a codon on the mRNA specifying the amino acid carried by that tRNA. In other words, if the mRNA codon is UUG (the codon for leucine), only the specific tRNA carrying leucine can pair with this codon, and the anticodon on the tRNA in this case would be AAC. Pairing takes place at a particular codon on the mRNA when a "reading" site on the ribosome moves to that codon. As soon as the peptide bond is formed between the incoming activated amino acid and the partially formed polypeptide, the tRNA that carried the previous amino acid is released and the ribosome moves down the mRNA molecule so as to expose the next codon. The ribosome is now ready to accept the activated amino acid called for by the next codon. When the polypeptide is finished, the ribosome reaches a termination codon, at which point the newly synthesized polypeptide is liberated. Actually, as soon as a ribosome moves away from the initiation site on the mRNA, another ribosome joins the mRNA, and so on, until there are ribosomes all along the length of the mRNA, each directing the synthesis of a molecule of the

**Figure 7-6.** Summary of protein synthesis. Formation of a polypeptide takes place on the surface of a ribosome, across which moves a molecule of messenger RNA (mRNA) in the 5′ → 3′ direction. Using energy from ATP, specific activating enzymes attach particular amino acids to their appropriate tRNAs with high-energy bonds. As the ribosome shifts to a new three-base codon on the mRNA, it releases a tRNA from the vacated codon (tRNA 1). In the diagram this places the tRNA bearing the growing polypeptide chain (tRNA 2) in the left-hand binding site on the ribosome, and a tRNA with an anticodon complementary to the codon in the newly "read" right-hand position (tRNA 3) assumes its place by base pairing. The next events will be the formation of a peptide bond between the growing polypeptide and the amino acid on tRNA 3 (using the energy acquired during activation), the release of tRNA 2, the shifting of the mRNA one more codon to the right, and the attachment of tRNA 4 bearing its associated amino acid. These steps are repeated until a stop codon on the mRNA is reached; the completed polypeptide, which has been spontaneously folding into a precise three-dimensional configuration as it is synthesized, is then freed with the aid of a release factor.

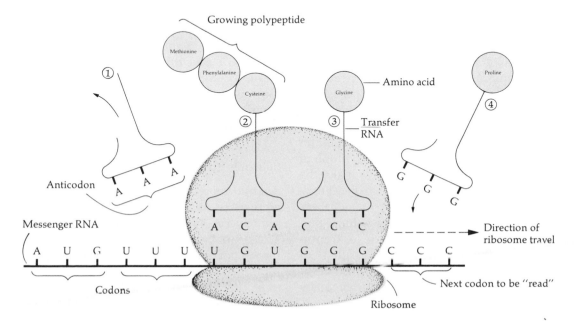

polypeptide coded for by that segment of mRNA. In this way a single molecule of mRNA can be simultaneously translated into many copies of the polypeptide. A single polypeptide may by itself form a protein, or several different polypeptides may need to join before a functional protein is completed. Of course, most proteins find roles in the cell as enzymes or as parts of structures.

## REGULATION OF PROTEIN SYNTHESIS

If all of the cellular DNA were continually being transcribed and subsequently translated into protein, the cell would undoubtedly find itself in such an utterly chaotic situation that it would not long survive. In actual fact, only a small amount of DNA is transcribed at any one time, and then only when a polypeptide coded by a particular segment of DNA (called a gene) is needed. This section will be concerned with the molecular regulation of polypeptide synthesis by the cell.

### The Nature and Repression of an Operon

Genes governing the synthesis of enzymes involved in a common metabolic pathway are sometimes adjacent to each other on the chromosome. For example, there are four enzymes involved in the synthesis of the amino acid tryptophan, and the five genes that control the ultimate synthesis of these four enzymes are along one single stretch of a DNA strand; such a stretch is known as an operon. If a bacterium that is synthesizing its own tryptophan, and so transcribing these five genes, is transferred to a growth medium that already contains sufficient tryptophan for growth, the cells will cease to make the enzymes necessary for tryptophan synthesis. In other words, the presence of sufficient tryptophan turns off the transcription of that entire portion of DNA responsible for tryptophan biosynthesis. This has been called coordinated enzyme repression, because all of the enzymes involved are simultaneously repressed.

An explanation of this enzyme repression became clear when it was shown that the addition of tryptophan to the growth medium results in the activation of a repressor that can then bind to a specific region of the chromosome known as the operator site. The operator is located adjacent to the sequence of structural genes coding for the synthesis of the enzymes involved in tryptophan biosynthesis. This entire sequence of genes, the operon, is transcribed into a single strand of mRNA. However, for the operon to be transcribed, the operator site must be free. Thus, if the repressor has been activated by binding to tryptophan, the operon cannot be transcribed and is repressed (see Figure 7-7).

We know that much of the genetic material of a bacterium is located within various operons that are similarly turned off by the presence of a repressor. Thus, there are many cases in which a product of the metabolic reactions catalyzed by the enzymes produced by an operon (like an excess of tryptophan in the case of the tryptophan operon) will react with some repressor molecule, allowing it to bind to the operator site of that operon. This prevents transcription of the operon and thus the synthesis of enzymes coded for by its genes. In the case of the tryptophan operon, the active repressor is a product of tryptophan and a protein produced by a specific regulating gene. If tryptophan levels fall and the cell needs more tryptophan, tryptophan is not available to activate the repressor, the operator site is freed, and the tryptophan operon is thus derepressed and again transcribed.

### Inducible Enzyme Synthesis

A situation which, at first glance, seems to be almost the opposite of enzyme repression is seen in the synthesis of inducible enzymes. These enzymes are not synthesized unless the bacterium is placed into a medium containing the substrate for the enzymes. For example, *Escherichia coli* which has been growing using glycerol as a carbon source

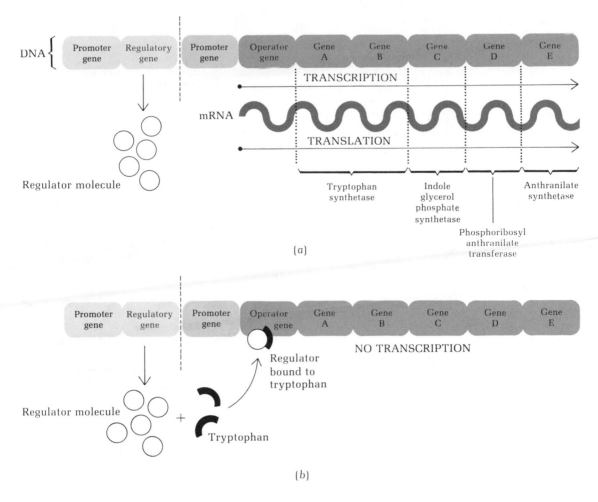

**Figure 7-7.** A simplified scheme for the regulation of tryptophan biosynthesis. *a.* Regulator molecules are unable to bind to the operator gene, so transcription may take place. *b.* Regulator molecules become activated after binding to tryptophan, resulting in blockage of the operator gene and preventing transcription.

does not contain the enzymes necessary for the degradation of the sugar lactose. If, however, these cells are placed into a medium containing lactose, they will immediately begin to synthesize the enzymes necessary to transport lactose into the cell and to hydrolyze the disaccharide into glucose and galactose. Lactose, then, induces the synthesis of the enzymes making up the lactose operon. In fact, other β-galactosides in addition to lactose, some of which cannot be metabo-

lized, have also been found to cause the induction of this operon.

This phenomenon is the result of a regulatory gene (gene i) which produces a soluble repressor that reacts with the operator gene to prevent its transcription (see Figure 7-8a). In the case of the lactose operon, this regulator gene is adjacent to the operon; however, regulator genes for other operons may be considerably removed from the operon they are regulating. When an inducer (in this case,

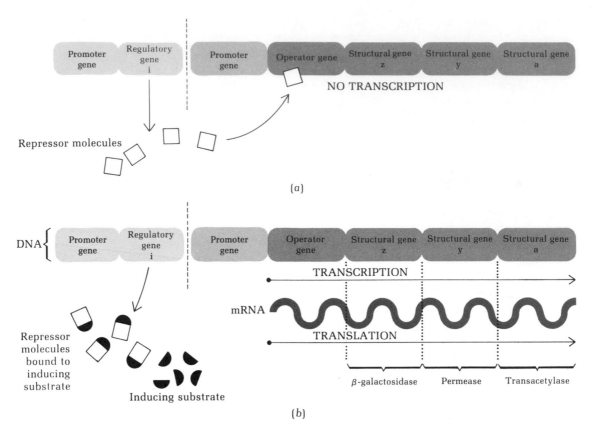

**Figure 7-8.** Jacob and Monod operon theory for the regulation of inducible enzyme synthesis. *a.* The regulatory gene produces a repressor that reacts with operator gene to prevent transcription of the operon. *b.* The inducer (usually the substrate) binds to the repressor and thus allows transcription to occur.

lactose or related β-galactosides) enters the cell, it binds to the soluble repressor, as shown schematically in Figure 7-8*b*, and prevents the repressor from reacting with the operator gene. The operator gene is thus free, and the operon can be transcribed.

On the other hand, some inducible operons are derepressed by the reaction of inducer with the regulating protein forming a new molecule which then binds to the operator gene. For example, when arabinose combines with its regulator protein, the resulting product reacts with the arabinose operator gene and only then can the arabinose operon be transcribed; in the absence of arabinose, the regulatory protein acts as a repressor.

What appear at first to be opposing processes—enzyme repression and enzyme induction—are in reality different manifestations of similar mechanisms. In the one case, an excess of a product reacts to form a repressor for the transcription of the operon, while in the other case, a substrate (or structural analogue) reacts with a repressor or regulator already present in the cell to allow the operon to be transcribed.

### Catabolite Repression

If one adds a substrate such as lactose to a culture of *E. coli* that is rapidly growing with glucose as a carbon source, no inducible enzymes for lactose metabolism are synthesized until the glucose in the medium has been metabolized. Or, if one adds glucose to a culture that is already metabolizing lactose, there is a repression of the synthesis of the inducible enzymes for lactose metabolism; in other words, the lac operon is no longer transcribed (see Figure 7-9). In the latter case, an initial transient repression may be followed by a period in which the lac operon is again being transcribed, but at a slower than normal rate until the glucose is depleted. This over-all phenomenon, called catabolite repression, has been observed most frequently using glucose as a substrate, but it appears to occur any time there is simultaneous availability of a carbon source that will support better or faster growth than does the inducer.

An explanation for these observations unfolded when it was found that rapid growth of E. coli on glucose lowered the cellular

**Figure 7-9.** Catabolite repression. Curve A illustrates the synthesis of the enzyme, $\beta$-galactosidase, by *Escherichia coli* when growing in a medium containing lactose as the sole source of carbon. Curve B illustrates the catabolite repression of the lac operon that occurs after adding glucose to the lactose-containing medium.

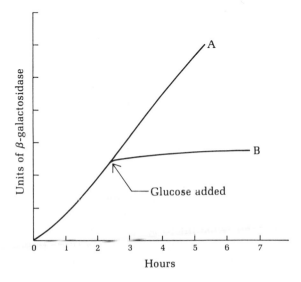

level of adenosine 3',5'-monophosphate (cyclic AMP or cAMP) and that catabolite repression could be terminated by the addition of cAMP to the culture. The role of cAMP appears to be as follows: (1) cAMP combines with a protein which has been called the cAMP receptor protein (CRP); (2) this cAMP-CRP complex then combines with a gene, called the promotor, which lies adjacent to the operator gene; (3) the promotor gene is the binding site for the RNA polymerase, and, for those operons that show catabolite repression, the binding of the cAMP-CRP complex to the promotor gene is necessary before the polymerase can bind to transcribe the operon. Thus, whenever glucose is being used, cAMP levels will fall during the period of rapid metabolism, and inducible enzyme synthesis will not occur until sufficient cAMP is again available to form a complex which can react with the promotor gene in the inducible operon. Catabolite repression, therefore, occurs even though there has been a mutation in the regulatory or operator gene converting the inducible operon to a constitutive operon (one not under the control of a repressor).

It should be noted that even in the absence of catabolite repression, the normal affinity, great or small, of a promotor gene for the RNA polymerase provides a mechanism for the rate of gene expression; some promotors under normal conditions bind poorly to the polymerase, resulting in the synthesis of only a small amount of gene product.

## REGULATION OF ENZYME ACTIVITY

As might be surmised, enzyme repression is somewhat coarse control; it responds only when there are rather large changes in substrate availability. There is a much finer enzyme control in which the end products of a pathway will react directly with the enzyme catalyzing an early reaction (usually the first) and temporarily inactivate it so that substrate does not enter the pathway, intermediates are not formed, and more end pro-

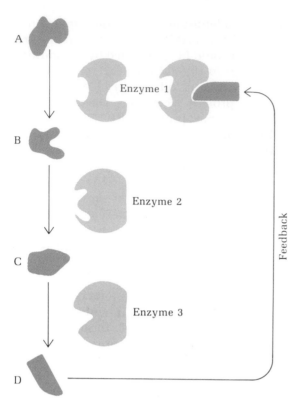

**Figure 7-10.** Feedback inhibition. Product D, resulting from a series of enzymatic reactions beginning with substrate A, reacts with enzyme 1, causing the enzyme to become inactive. This prevents the conversion of A to B. As the concentration of D falls, enzyme 1 and product D disassociate allowing enzyme 1 to become active again. Feedback inhibition represents a much finer control than enzyme repression.

duct cannot be made (see Figure 7-10). This mechanism, called feedback inhibition, does not prevent synthesis of an enzyme; it only inhibits its activity. As the end product of the pathway is used by the bacterium, the enzyme is freed to catalyze its reaction and more end product soon results.

Enzymes that are subject to feedback inhibition possess two binding sites, one that binds to the normal substrate and a second site that binds to the inhibiting end product. Such enzymes are called allosteric enzymes, and when they react with their end-product inhibitor, the substrate binding site undergoes a conformational change so that the substrate binds to the enzyme much less effectively.

## MUTATIONS IN MICROORGANISMS

Mutation means genetic change, and it is manifested by changes in cellular DNA. Many microbiologists believe that the myriad microorganisms that exist in the world today evolved from a common ancestor that lived billions of years ago. This evolution would have resulted from chemical changes in the DNA that occur occasionally and cause errors during replication. If such changes are not too extensive, the cell continues to grow, but with an altered genotype. If this altered genotype results in the appearance of a new characeristic or in the loss of an old characteristic, the cell has a changed phenotype. In other words, the genotype tells us what genes are present in a cell, and the phenotype is the expression of the genes. When such changes in DNA occur during normal growth, they are called spontaneous mutations.

The time scale for mutation rates is not expressed in terms of hours or days, but rather in terms of generations. Even though the number of mutations per generation (typically $10^{-6}$ to $10^{-8}$) is no larger than that seen in higher organisms, the number of mutations occurring in a single bacterial culture may be large, since many bacteria may reproduce in as little as 30 minutes. The microbiologist is not always immediately able to tell whether an organism has mutated or merely adapted to a new situation, since a large number of mutations do occur. Also, under appropriate conditions bacteria can adapt to many situations by forming inducible enzymes.

To be more specific, suppose one wishes to isolate mutants of *Escherichia coli* that have become resistant to lysis by a virulent bacteriophage. The only way to determine that a particular organism is resistant is to add the bacteriophage to the culture and isolate the survivors. One is then faced with the question of whether the resistant survivors are true spontaneous mutants, or if, as a result of the bacteriophage's presence, a certain percentage of the bacteria were able to adapt by inducing enzymes that result in phage resistance.

## Tests That Identify Spontaneous Mutants

Spontaneous mutants may be difficult to identify because, for example, the only way to ascertain if an organism is phage resistant is to add the bacteriophage. A clever test, called the fluctuation test, was designed by Luria and Delbruch to answer this question. This test was based on the concept that spontaneous mutation is a completely random event. Thus, in 50 identical cultures, spontaneous mutants will occur very early in some, in others somewhat later, and in some not at all or only near the end of the growth cycle. Obviously, since each mutant continues to reproduce itself, those cultures in which a mutation occurred early in the growth cycle will contain a large number of mutants while those in which the mutation occurred late would contain only a few mutants. In other words, there would be a large fluctuation in the number of phage-resistant organisms in these 50 identical cultures if they arose as a result of a spontaneous mutation. On the other hand, if a certain percentage of the culture was rendered resistant as a result of adding the bacteriophage, one would expect a fairly constant number of organisms in each of the 50 cultures. As seen in Figure 7-11, a large fluctuation in the number of bacteriophage-resistant organisms indicates that these are mutations and not a result of adding the bacteriophage.

A second method to show that mutations are spontaneous and not specifically induced in bacteria is called replica plating. Developed by the Lederbergs, this technique has been used, for example, to isolate penicillin-resistant staphylococci without exposing the

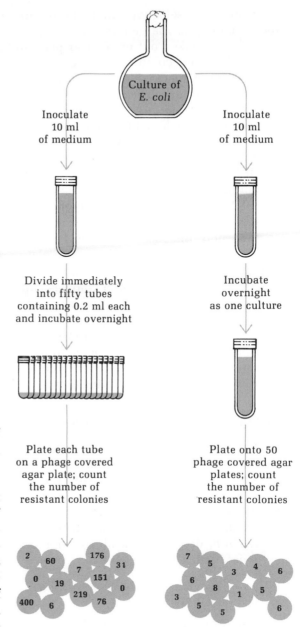

**Figure 7-11.** Fluctuation test. On the left one can see that mutation to phage resistance must have occurred quite early in the tube that provided 400 resistant organisms and quite late in the tube with only two resistant organisms. The control tubes on the right show very little fluctuation.

organisms to the selective action of this antibiotic. To do this, a large number of staphylococci are streaked out on an agar plate so as to yield isolated colonies. After four or five hours, each organism will develop into a microcolony, and a sterile pad of velvet is pressed down gently over the plate. A few bacteria from each colony adhere to the velvet, so that when the velvet is pressed down upon a second sterile plate containing penicillin, it produces an exact copy of the original master plate. However, since the copy plate contains penicillin, only those organisms resistant to penicillin can grow. One can then note the location of the resistant colonies and, going back to the master plate, select the resistant colonies (see Figure 7-12). The demonstration that these colonies contain penicillin-resistant organisms, even though they have never previously been exposed to penicillin, is additional proof that changes (such as resistance to penicillin) are the result of spontaneous mutations and not bacterial adaptations to the testing substance.

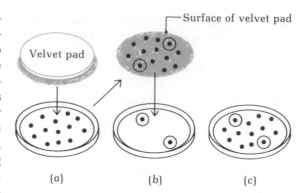

**Figure 7-12.** Replica plating. *a.* A sterile velvet pad is pressed lightly down on a plate containing microcolonies of staphylococci. *b.* The velvet pad is then pressed lightly on a sterile agar plate containing penicillin. Only two colonies grew in this example. *c.* By noting the position of the colonies that grew, it is possible to go back to the original plate and subculture penicillin-resistant colonies that have never been exposed to penicillin.

## MOLECULAR TYPES OF MUTATIONS

Since all information carried in the DNA is eventually converted to specific proteins, any change in the base sequence of the DNA can result in a change in the molecular composition of the resulting protein. In general, such changes are caused by a substitution, an insertion, or a deletion of one or more base pairs in the DNA molecule.

### Base-Pair Substitution

Each amino acid in a polypeptide is coded for by a sequence of three nucleotides in the DNA, and any change in one of these nucleotides may cause a different amino acid to be inserted into the polypeptide. For example, if during DNA replication the triplet GAA (coding for leucine) should be mistakenly replicated as GTA, leucine would be replaced by histidine during subsequent protein synthesis. Mutations of this type, which result in the substitution of one amino acid for another, have been termed missense mutations. Depending upon the function of the resulting protein and the position of the new amino acid in the polypeptide, such a change may or may not result in a detectable change in the ability of the changed protein to function normally. It should also be noted that the four bases in DNA have the ability to code for $4^3$, or 64, different triplet sequences. Many of the 20 amino acids possess more than one triplet code, and if in our example of DNA replication the base substitution from GAA had been to GAT, there would have been no detectable mutation because GAT also codes for leucine.

### Insertion or Deletion of DNA Bases

Insertion or deletion of only one base might appear not to cause a major change in the resulting protein composition. But, since each amino acid requires a triplet code, the loss or gain of a single base in the DNA results in the following type of frame shift:

DNA  AAC GAA CGC TGA
RNA  UUG CUU GCG ACU

Deletion of the first A in the DNA shifts "reading" frame as follows:

DNA  ACG AAC GCT GA?
RNA  UGC UUG CGA CU

This would change the tetrapeptide encoded in this segment of DNA completely, from leucine-histidine-alanine-threonine to cysteine-leucine-arginine-leucine. Unless such a loss is compensated by the insertion of a new base very close to the deleted base, it is obvious that a completely new polypeptide and thus a new protein will be coded for by the segment of DNA following the deletion.

## Nonsense Mutations

There are three codons, UAG, UAA, and UGA, whose normal function is to cause the termination of synthesis of the polypeptide chain. Any mutation resulting in the formation of one of these termination codons will cause the release of an incomplete polypeptide. This is called a nonsense mutation. Two of these codons have been given the trivial names of amber mutation (UAG) and ochre mutation (UAA).

## Suppressor Mutations

A suppressor mutation is the general name given to a change in DNA that compensates for a previous mutation. An obvious example would be a frame-shift suppressor which inserts a new base in place of or very close to one that was lost. However, suppressor mutations may occur in a gene far removed from the original mutation and in such cases function by changing the specificity of the tRNA. Thus, if a UUG (for leucine) mutated to a UAG (for chain termination), no polypeptide chain could be synthesized past the UAG codon because there is no normal tRNA that possesses an anticodon for UAG. This mutation, called an amber mutation, is a nonsense mutation, which can be suppressed if a second mutation results in the formation of a new tRNA that possesses an anticodon to UAG. This second mutation is referred to as an amber suppressor.

Missense mutations which cause the substitution of one amino acid for another may also be suppressed by a missense suppressor in which the correct tRNA has mutated to now possess an anticodon to the mutated triplet. Such suppressors occur much less frequently, however, than do nonsense suppressors.

## Conditional Lethal Mutations

The general term "conditional lethal mutations" is assigned to those mutations that are lethal under one set of circumstances but not lethal under other conditions (permissive conditions). The most common type of conditional lethal mutations are called temperature-sensitive (ts) mutants. These mutant organisms may be able to function normally at 30°C, but cannot grow if an essential protein affected by the mutation is nonfunctional at a higher temperature, such as 42°C. Temperature-sensitive mutants have provided invaluable tools for the study of DNA replication, RNA synthesis, and protein synthesis.

## METHODS OF INDUCING MUTATIONS

Spontaneous mutations will occur during the normal growth of an organism at a usual rate between one in a million and one in 100 million cells; however, there are techniques to increase the "mistakes" a cell makes while its DNA is being replicated. Most such mutations are lethal for the organism, but the use of proper selection methods can frequently result in the isolation of the desired mutant. Agents which increase the over-all incidence of mutants are called mutagens.

One can grow organisms in the presence of unusual pyrimidines which will be incor-

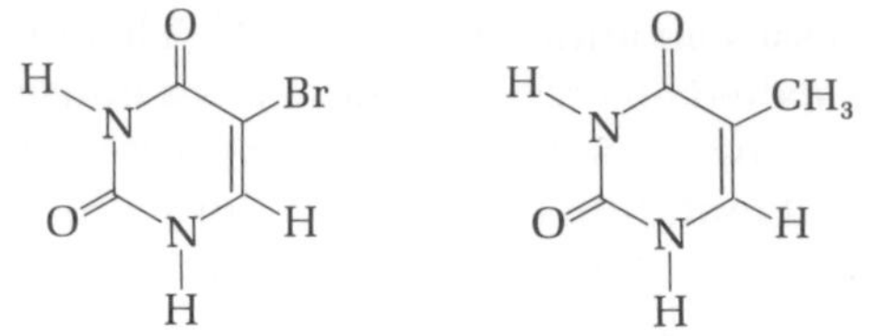

5-Bromouracil                    Thymine

**Figure 7-13.** Bromouracil induces mutations through mispairing when it is incorporated into DNA as a structural analogue of thymine.

porated into their DNA. If 5-bromouracil (a molecule structurally similar to thymine) is used, the organism incorporates some 5-bromouracil where it should have thymine (see Figure 7-13). When this organism reproduces, some of the 5-bromouracil bases will pair with guanine instead of the correct complementary purine, adenine. Thus, the new cell will have a number of guanine residues where it should have had adenine, and as a result the information in the DNA will be changed so that an incorrect or nonfunctional protein may result from the transcription and subsequent translation of that segment of DNA.

Another method of increasing mutation rates is to treat cells with alkylating agents, such as nitrogen mustard, ethylene oxide, or nitrosoguanidine. These agents react with the guanine in the DNA causing an occasional wrong complementary base to pair with guanine during replication of the DNA. This also, of course, changes the information in that segment of DNA.

Finally, treatment of cells with ultraviolet light also results in an increased mutation rate. This treatment causes the formation of a covalent linkage between adjacent pyrimidines, particularly thymine (see Figure 7-14). The presence of these thymine dimers causes distortion of the DNA and results in mistakes during its replication. Visible light will frequently reverse this effect by activating an enzyme which excises the thymine dimers, allowing normal repair to take place. This latter process is referred to as photoreactivation.

Mutant organisms have provided valuable tools for the microbial geneticist to study such things as gene function and gene regulation. They have provided the physician with avirulent organisms that are used as living vaccines, and mutants that will produce more antibiotic or more of a commercially impor-

**Figure 7-14.** Formation of a thymine dimer by ultraviolet light. Repair takes place by one of several routes. In the light a photoenzyme may recognize and bind to the dimer in the strand of DNA. This complex then absorbs a photoreactivating wavelength of light, which results in the splitting of the dimer to restore the monomers. In the dark, excision repair or the less-understood post-replication gap repair may occur. Excision repair consists of the removal from the strand of DNA of the dimer and several bases on either side by an excision enzyme, followed by replacement of the excised bases by DNA polymerase using the information on the complementary strand.

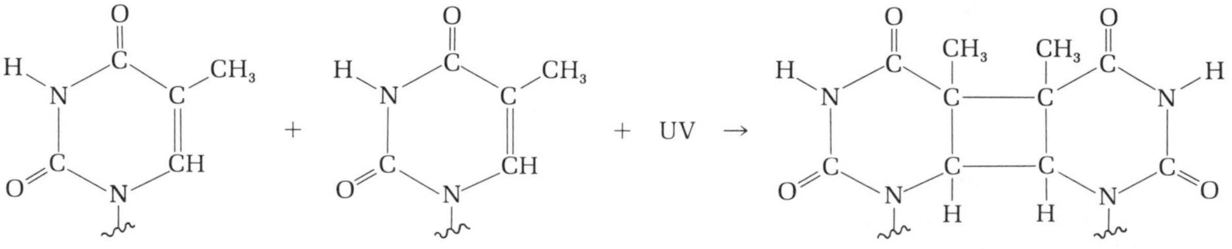

Adjacent thymine residues                              Thymine dimer

tant enzyme are being constantly sought by various industries.

## REFERENCES

Beckwith, J. R., ed. 1970. *The Lactose Operon.* Cold Spring Harbor, New York.

Drake, J. W., and R. H. Balz. 1976. Biochemistry of mutagenesis. *Annu. Rev. Biochem.* **45**:11–37.

Gefter, M. L. 1975. DNA replication. *Annu Rev. Biochem.* **44**:45–78.

Hill, C. W. 1975. Informational suppression of missense mutations. *Cell* **6**:419–427.

Lederberg, J., and E. M. Lederberg. 1952. Replica plating and indirect selection of bacterial mutants. *J. Bacteriol.* **63**:399–406.

Lewin, B. 1974. Interaction of regulator proteins with recognition sequences of DNA. *Cell* **2**:1–7.

Luria, S. E., and M. Delbrück. 1943. Mutations of bacteria from virus sensitivity to virus resistance. *Genetics* **28**:491–511.

Maniatis, T., and M. Ptashne. 1976. A DNA operator-repressor system. *Sci. American* **234**:64–76.

Miller, O. J., Jr. 1973. The visualization of genes in action. *Sci. American* **228**:34–42.

Rich, A., and U. Raj Bhandary. 1976. tRNA: Conformation structure and role. *Annu. Rev. Biochem.* **45**:805–860.

Stahl, F. W. 1969. *The Mechanisms of Inheritance,* 2nd ed. Prentice-Hall, Inc., Englewood Cliffs, New Jersey.

Stein, G. S., J. S. Stein, and L. J. Kleinsmith. 1975. Chromosomal proteins and gene regulation. *Sci. American* **232**:(2)46–57.

# 8

# Bacterial Genetics:
# The Nature and Transfer of Genetic Material

The tremendous advances in biological science of the nineteenth century include a germ theory for disease, a disproof of spontaneous generation at all levels of life, and a biological explanation for fermentation. It was also during this period that Johann Gregor Mendel's studies on the inheritance of various characteristics in the garden pea formed the framework of modern genetics. But, it was not until the middle of the twentieth century that researchers discovered that DNA is the true genetic material by which one generation of organism can pass on information dictating morphological and biochemical characteristics to the next and discovered how this information is coded in the genetic material to be "read" and used by the cell. Many of the discoveries in molecular genetics resulted from study of bacterial genetics.

## TRANSFORMATION

Bacterial transformation (gene transfer using extracted DNA), first described by Griffith in 1928, was perhaps the earliest major discovery in the field of molecular genetics. It not only demonstrated that it is possible to transfer genetic material from one bacterial cell to another but subsequently led to the realization that this genetic material is DNA.

Griffith studied the transformation of one type of pneumococcus into a different type of pneumococcus. As will be discussed in Chapter 18, the pneumococci are divided into about a hundred distinct types based on differences in their capsular material. Encapsulated pneumococci are very virulent for mice. But if the organism loses the ability to produce a capsule, it also loses its virulence, and the injection of these "rough" variants will not usually kill a mouse. What Griffith did was this: he mixed a living culture of nonencapsulated pneumococci that had originally been type II with heat-killed encapsulated type-I pneumococci (see Figure 8-1). This mixture was injected into several mice. The following day, Griffith isolated the pneumococci present in the blood of the mice and found fully encapsulated types I and II. One can explain where the encapsulated type II came from, since his living nonencapsulated type II probably contained a very small percentage of encapsulated type II (maybe one out of a million) which were able to grow and produce disease in the mouse. However,

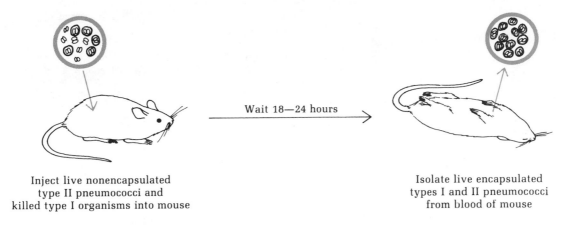

**Figure 8-1.** Griffith's original transformation experiment. The isolation of living encapsulated type I pneumococci from the mouse could occur only if some genetic substance from the killed type I organisms was able to enter the nonencapsulated type II cells. This was subsequently shown to be DNA.

since the type-I organisms had been killed prior to injection into the mouse, their origin could be explained only by assuming that some genetic material from the killed type-I organisms was able to enter the living nonencapsulated type-II pneumococci and transform the type-II cells into living type-I organisms. It was 16 more years before the work of Avery, MacLeod, and McCarty demonstrated, using purified DNA, that the substance transferring the genetic capability from one pneumococcus to another is DNA alone, and protein is not an essential component of this transforming principle. In addition to *Streptococcus pneumoniae* (pneumococcus), transformation has been shown to occur in a number of bacterial genera, including *Haemophilus, Neisseria, Bacillus,* and *Rhizobium*. Since the principles are similar for all genera, our discussion will be confined to transformation in pneumococci.

### Nature of the DNA in Transformation

When DNA is extracted from a donor organism (as shown in Figure 8-2), the bacterial chromosome becomes fragmented into 200 to 500 pieces. Since a recipient bacterium is capable of taking up a maximum of about ten of these pieces of DNA (whose molecular weight ranges from 300,000 to 10,000,000 daltons), the amount of DNA involved in any one transformation represents, at most, 2–5% of the total donor DNA. Moreover, only double-stranded DNA is effective in transformation, even though after entry one strand is immediately degraded while the other strand undergoes base pairing with a homologous portion of the recipient's chromosome. After a double crossover, the portion of the donor strand between the points of crossing over is permanently integrated into the recipient genome. The fact that one strand of the donor DNA must undergo complementary base pairing with an area of the recipient's chromosome undoubtedly explains why only closely related DNA can be used for transformation of an organism.

### Entry of DNA into a Recipient Cell

It was unexpected that such large molecules of DNA as those involved in transformation could gain entrance to a cell, and it was even more surprising to find that only during certain periods of growth is a pneumococcus capable of being transformed. The transitory period during which the cell is capable of

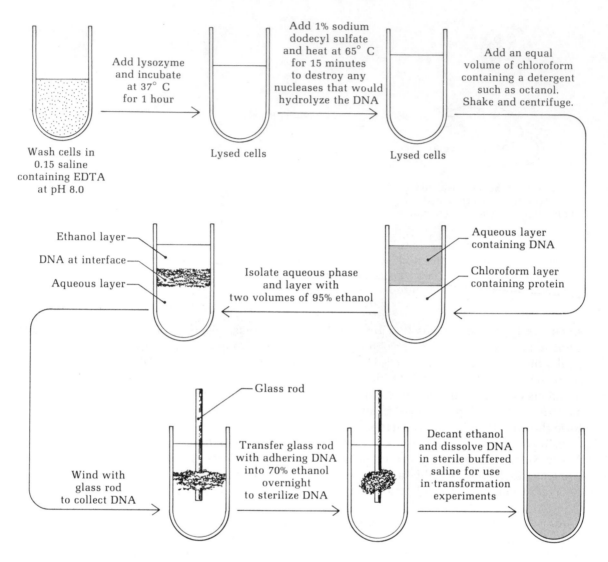

**Figure 8-2.** Isolation of DNA from a donor organism for use in transformation experiments. The addition of sodium dodecyl sulfate in the second step aids in the lysis of the organism.

taking up the transforming DNA is called competence, and cells in this state are referred to as competent cells. The nature of competence is not fully understood, but current data suggest that it results from the synthesis of a surface protein (called competence factor) which interacts in some way to allow the uptake of the transforming DNA. This concept is supported by the observation that the supernatant fluid from a competent culture is capable of inducing competence when added to a noncompetent culture.

## Importance of Transformation

In all likelihood transformation occurs in nature following the lysis of an organism and release of its DNA into the immediate environment. It is difficult, however, to evaluate whether transformation plays an important role in the ability of an organism to cause disease, but it is certainly conceivable that recombinants arising from transformation between strains of low virulence could give rise to highly virulent organisms. Transformation is also valuable in mapping the bacterial chromosome, since the frequency of co-transformation of two characteristics is a measure of their distance apart on the chromosome.

For the research scientist it provides a tool by which DNA can be purified and chemically altered in the laboratory and then reintroduced into a bacterium to ascertain the effect of the *in vitro* alteration. Moreover, as will be discussed later in this chapter, transformation provides the techniques for the production of innumerable genetic hybrids (cells possessing DNA that originated in a different cell), and as such, has become an important tool in the new field of genetic engineering.

## TRANSDUCTION

Transduction is a second method by which the genetic material from one bacterial cell can be transferred to a second bacterium. However, in this case the DNA is not passed naked as in transformation but is carried to a recipient bacterium by a bacteriophage.

When a lysogenic bacterium enters the lytic cycle (either spontaneously or induced by ultraviolet light), occasionally part of the bacterial chromosome is accidentally assembled into the phage head. Thus, when a phage which has incorporated genetic material from bacterium A subsequently infects bacterium B, the part of the chromosome from bacterium A that had been incorporated into the phage head is injected into bacterium B. After complementary base pairing and crossing over, the newly injected genetic material from bacterium A will become a permanent part of the genome of bacterium B.

Depending upon whether the original pro-

phage was integrated into the chromosome of bacterium A or existed as extrachromosomal DNA, two types of transduction may occur: (1) restricted (or specialized) transduction, and (2) general transduction.

### Restricted Transduction

Restricted transduction occurs only in those situations in which the prophage had been integrated into the bacterial chromosome as was described in Chapter 6 for lambda phage (λ phage) in *Escherichia coli*.

In the usual sequence of events when a strain of *E. coli* lysogenic for λ phage enters the lytic cycle, the λ genome forms a loop and is excised from the bacterial chromosome. Subsequent replication and transcription of the excised λ DNA results in the final liberation of mature λ phage. However, about one time in a million, the λ genome apparently loops out improperly, and the excised portion of the chromosome includes the bacterial gene for galactose fermentation but leaves behind part of the λ genome (see Figure 8-3). Since such phages still possess the site necessary for integration into an *E. coli* chromosome and can code for the specific integration protein, a subsequent infection of a gal⁻ *E. coli* will result in lysogenization and integration of the partial λ genome and the gal⁺ gene picked up from the previous bacterium. However, this λ DNA has lost some essential parts of its genome, and it can yield phage only if the cell is also infected with a complete λ phage that can code for the missing functions. Thus, the λ phage which is carrying gal⁺ is defective, and such a transducing phage that has acquired the gal⁺ gene is referred to as λdg (for λ-defective gal). Thus, restricted transduction is limited to genes that lie closely adjacent to the integrated prophage on the bacterial chromosome.

### General Transduction

General transduction is the phage-mediated transfer of bacterial DNA that occurs when

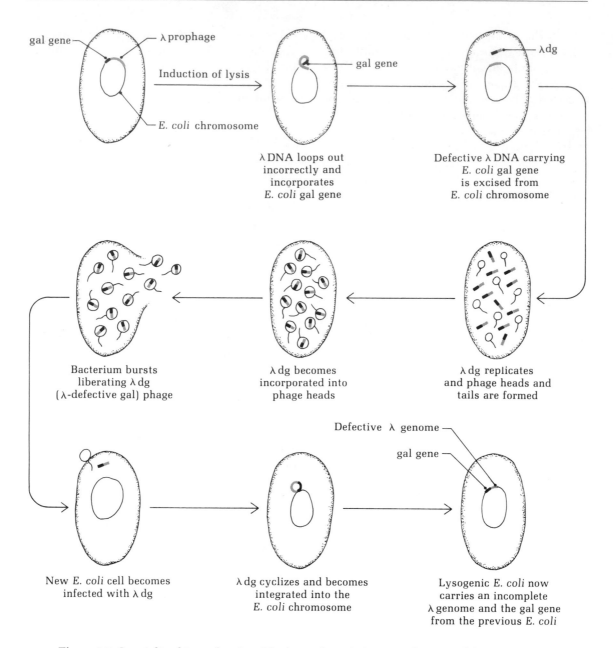

**Figure 8-3.** Specialized transduction. The λ prophage is incorrectly excised from the E. coli chromosome and as a result incorporates the adjacent gal gene from the E. coli into the λ genome. Subsequent infection with this defective λ phage results in the integration of the defective DNA as well as the gal gene into the chromosome of the newly infected E. coli.

prophage not integrated into the bacterial chromosome enters a lytic cycle (see Figure 8-4). As the phage begins the lytic cycle, phage enzymes hydrolyze the bacterial chromosome into a number of small pieces of DNA, and as a result any part of the bacterial chromosome may be incorporated into the phage capsid during final assembly of the phage. Thus, unlike restricted transduction, all characteristics have an equal chance of

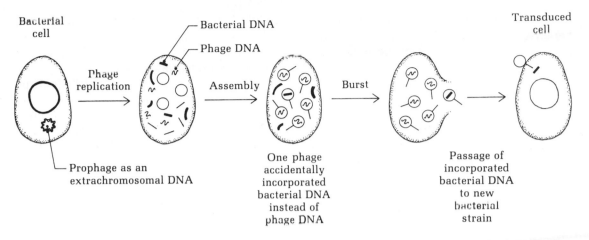

Bacterial cell

Phage replication

Prophage as an extrachromosomal DNA

Bacterial DNA

Phage DNA

Assembly

One phage accidentally incorporated bacterial DNA instead of phage DNA

Burst

Passage of incorporated bacterial DNA to new bacterial strain

Transduced cell

**Figure 8-4.** Generalized transduction. When the extrachromosomally located prophage begins its replicative cycle, the bacterial DNA is hydrolyzed into small fragments which, during assembly, can be accidentally incorporated into a phage head. Subsequent infection of a bacterium with such a phage releases functional bacterial DNA into the newly infected cell.

being transduced. Using phage P1 (which infects *E. coli*), it has been established that about 0.3 percent of the phage will accidentally incorporate bacterial DNA into their capsid during assembly. Since this DNA is wholly bacterial in origin, an organism subsequently infected by the phage carrying it will not become lysogenic for P1 phage, but the injected bacterial DNA can be integrated into the genome of the recipient bacterium. Generalized transduction has been used extensively to map bacterial chromosomes. This is possible because less than 3 percent of the total bacterial chromosome can be incorporated into a phage head. As a result, only closely related genes can be cotransduced by a single phage particle. It is therefore possible to establish close linkage of certain bacterial genes through transduction.

## CONJUGATION

Conjugation is another mechanism for the transfer of genetic material from one bacterium to another (see Figure 8-5). This actual contact of two cells with the passage of genetic material from one cell to another is,

in all likelihood, the least common method of genetic exchange in bacteria. Moreover, conjugation differs from both transformation and transduction in that these latter processes result in the transfer of only very small fragments of the bacterial chromosome to the recipient cell. Conjugation, on the other

**Figure 8-5.** Conjugating *Escherichia coli.* The male cell (with numerous short pili) is connected to the female bacterium by an F pilus, as described in the text. (×3,000.)

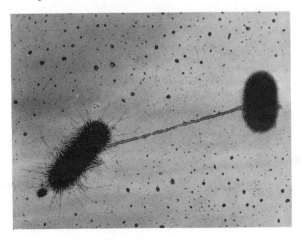

hand, may transfer very large segments of the bacterial chromosome and in special cases the entire chromosome may be transferred.

### Sex Factors

Conjugation in *E. coli* was first described in 1946 by Joshua Lederberg and Edward Tatum. It has since been demonstrated in a number of different gram-negative organisms, but inasmuch as the largest part of the work has been done with *E. coli*, we shall confine our discussion of conjugation to this organism.

Early experiments used various K12 strains of *E. coli*. Each strain was selected so that it required two or three added vitamins or amino acids for growth. Then, for example, a strain requiring methionine and biotin would be grown together with a strain requiring threonine, leucine, and thiamine. After growth, the organisms were plated out on a minimal medium so only organisms that could synthesize all of their amino acids and vitamins could grow. Such organisms were assumed to arise from conjugation, and the resulting strains were called prototrophs or recombinants.

Initial crosses between strains of *E. coli* yielded a very small percentage of recom-

binants, about one from every one to ten million cells. Futhermore, it soon became obvious that when conjugation did occur, it resulted in a one-way transfer and not a cell fusion followed by segregation of the mating cells. Thus, bacterial conjugation occurs between donors (or male cells) and recipients (or female cells). Even more surprising was the observation that, although only a very small percentage of recipients received suficient donor chromosome to become recombinants, a large percentage of recipient cells were rapidly converted to donor cells. Since in this latter case no true chromosomal material appeared to be transferred to the recipient cells, it was postulated that a donor cell possesses a genetic factor in its cytoplasm which is not part of the bacterial chromosome but which is rapidly transferred to a recipient cell converting it to a donor cell. This sex factor is called an F factor, and it is now established that when an F+ (donor) cell conjugates with an F− (recipient) cell there is a rapid transfer of a copy of the nonchromosomally linked sex factor, resulting in the conversion of the F− cell into an F+ cell as diagrammed in Figure 8-6. Furthermore, it was observed that when a cell became an F+ cell, it produced one or more short filaments that have been named F pili. The F pilus

**Figure 8-6.** When an F+ cell conjugates with an F− cell, the F factor is rapidly replicated and a copy is transferred to the F− cell, converting the F− recipient to an F+ donor.

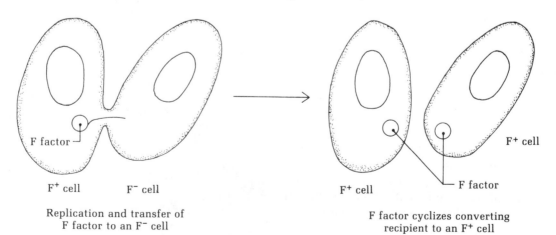

F factor

F+ cell          F− cell

Replication and transfer of
F factor to an F− cell

F+ cell                    F+ cell

F factor

F factor cyclizes converting
recipient to an F+ cell

appears to bind to a receptor on the F⁻ cell and, after binding, the pilus retracts into the F⁺ cell, pulling the F⁻ cell into intimate contact.

## High-Frequency Recombination Strains

The study of bacterial conjugation was facilitated when strains of *E. coli* that produced at least a thousand times more recombinants were isolated from F⁺ cultures. These new donor strains were called Hfr strains, standing for high-frequency mating strains. An initial understanding of what occurs during conjugation resulted from what was termed an "interrupted mating" experiment by Elie Wollman and Francois Jacob. An Hfr strain was mixed with an F⁻ strain, and at various times the conjugation was interrupted by breaking the cells apart in a high speed blender. The cells were then plated out, and a genetic analysis was carried out to see whether donor chromosome material had been transferred to the F⁻ cell. The results, plus those of subsequent experiments, can be briefly summarized as follows:

1. The Hfr chromosome is transferred to the F⁻ cell in a linear fashion.

2. The first genetic marker transferred required about 8 minutes, and the transfer of the entire Hfr chromosome required about 120 minutes. Since the genes are transferred linearly, a map of the Hfr chromosome can be drawn in which the distance between genes is measured in minutes required for their transfer.

3. Conjugation with an Hfr strain did not result in the transformation of an F⁻ strain to an F⁺ strain, but if the entire Hfr chromosome was transferred, the F⁻ strain was converted to an Hfr donor strain.

4. Although the order with which any Hfr strain transferred its genetic markers to the F⁻ recipient was constant, different Hfr strains were observed to initiate transfer with different genetic markers. That is to say, Hfr strain 1 might transfer its genes in the

order ABCDE, while Hfr strain 2 could transfer its genetic material in the sequence CDEAB (see Figure 8-7).

The first two of these observations certainly show that bacterial genes occur in a structure that appears to be a linear chromosome. The third observation shows that Hfr strains do not possess a separate cytoplasmic sex factor like the F⁺ cells, but they do have an Hfr factor, located on the chromosome, which appears to be the last genetic marker to enter the F⁻ cell. The observation that different Hfr strains initiated transfer with different genetic markers can be explained by postulating that the bacterial chromosome exists as a circular structure, and that transfer is initiated in the position of the Hfr factor. Thus, the initial part of the transferred chromosome may contain part of the integrated sex factor, but the majority of this factor does not enter the recipient until the last bit of the chromosome is transferred.

The mystery of why different Hfr strains may begin with the transfer of different genes may be explained by discussing the origin of the integrated Hfr factor. It is proposed that occasionally the cytoplasmic sex factor, F, which is itself a circular structure, becomes integrated into the circular bacterial chromosome in a manner analogous to that of λ phage. Moreover, the F factor appears to possess segments that are complementary to a number of different sectors in the bacterial chromosomes, and as a result may integrate at any one of a number of positions. Thus, different Hfr strains will have the F factor integrated into different locations in the bacterial chromosome, and, since the initial DNA to enter a recipient is part of the Hfr factor, the first bacterial genes to enter will depend on the integrated position of the Hfr factor.

It is also now established that normal F⁺ cells do not transfer their bacterial chromosome to an F⁻ cell. Their apparent very low rate of transfer described previously is believed to be due to the presence of a very small percentage of cases in which the F

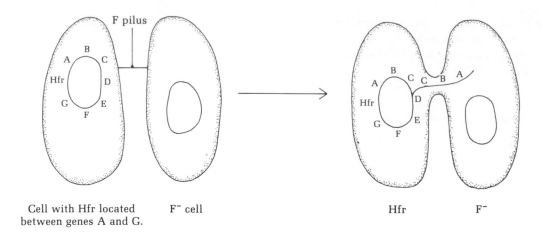

Cell with Hfr located          F⁻ cell                                    Hfr                    F⁻
between genes A and G.

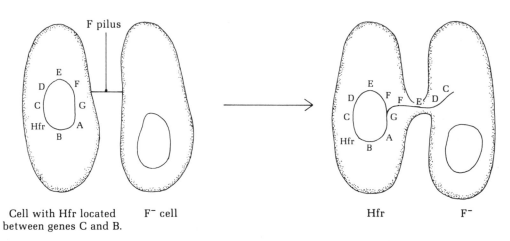

Cell with Hfr located      F⁻ cell                                        Hfr                    F⁻
between genes C and B.

**Figure 8-7.** Conjugation between Hfr strains and F⁻ cells. During conjugation the Hfr chromosome begins replicating at the point of insertion of the Hfr factor. Since Hfr can integrate in different positions of the bacterial chromosome as shown in the two examples here, the first genes to enter an F⁻ cell will vary among different Hfr strains.

factor has integrated into the chromosome in a manner analogous to the integration of λ phage producing an Hfr strain. As we discussed earlier, genetic elements of DNA, such as the F factor, that can exist either extrachromosomally or as integrated genes have been given the name of episomes, whereas those that are restricted to an extrachromosomal existence are called plasmids.

**F Factor as a Carrier
of Genetic Information**

It has been established that on rare occasions the integration of F factor to create an Hfr strain can be a reversible process. Thus, reminiscent of λ prophage entering the lytic cycle, the integrated F factor loops out, is excised, and forms a circular, autonomously replicating unit of extrachromosomal DNA. However, as was described for λ phage, occasionally the looping out may be improper and one or more adjacent bacterial genes may be included in the released F factor, as shown schematically in Figure 8-8. These episomes carry both sex-factor genes and chromosomal genes, and, as a result, are quickly transferred to an F⁻ cell during conjugation as was described for the F factor alone. They are designated as F′ followed by the bacterial gene that is incorporated into the episome. Thus, the F factor episome carrying the genes for lactose utilization is designated F′ lac. Interestingly, and unlike the F factor alone, the reintegration of an F′ into a new bacterial chromosome following conjugation is restricted to the area from which it was originally excised, inasmuch as it is only at this location that the bacterial determinants on the episome can pair with complementary bases on the bacterial chromosome and be integrated.

One extremely important group of episomes, which carry an F-like sex factor, codes for the bacterial resistance to many antibiotics. Because these episomes are so readily transferred to F⁻ cells, they have been specifically designated as resistance transfer factors (RTF). We shall return to RTF in Chapter 10.

## GENETIC ENGINEERING

The ease with which DNA can be transferred to procaryotic cells has given rise to a new science that fits within the term genetic engineering. Briefly, organisms with new genetic features are created in the laboratory by melding the genes from several of many possible sources (viruses, bacteria, eucaryotic cells) to produce hybrid forms with characteristics different from those of the original cells.

At first thought, such experiments would appear to provide a new, exciting approach to remedies for genetic deficiencies or to the production of better cells for use in industry and agriculture. But, many scientists are deeply concerned that the potential hazards of such gene manipulation might far exceed any possible benefits. For example, as will be discussed later in this section, it would not be difficult to put DNA from an oncogenic virus such as SV40 into an E. coli; but since E. coli is a normal inhabitant of the intestinal tract, what would happen if this hybrid should escape from the laboratory and infect millions of persons? Other possibilities of harmful recombinants include the introduction of antibiotic resistance into a pathogen that is routinely sensitive to antibiotic therapy and the transformation of usually benign "normal flora" into toxin producers. Moreover, such experiments are done as "shotgun" experiments in which any portion of the donor DNA may become incorporated into the newly formed hybrid, and it is thought possible that genes which are normally repressed (such as oncogenes—see Chapter 41) could become derepressed within an E. coli cell and be expressed as virulent human cancer viruses.

On the other hand, the potential benefit of this type of genetic engineering is unlimited. Bacterial strains could be made which could inexpensively synthesize vitamins, hormones, or antibiotics. It is within the realm of possibility that the nitrogenase genes which fix atmospheric $N_2$ could be placed into different kinds of soil saprophytes to tremendously increase agricultural production. Such experiments could provide a wealth of information on how genes work and how they are controlled. It is conceivable that in the not too distant future certain genetic diseases such as diabetes and cystic fibrosis could be cured by the insertion of the correct DNA into a eucaryotic cell.

How does one insert a fragment of DNA into a microorganism so that it will continue to replicate with the host organism? The answer is relatively simple if one uses the proper endonuclease—enzymes that cleave DNA at specific sites in a very specific manner. The DNA of the potential host and donor must be cleaved so that each exists as a linear fragment with "sticky" ends. In brief, the

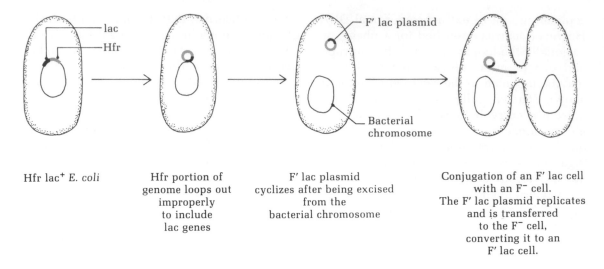

Hfr lac⁺ E. coli

Hfr portion of
genome loops out
improperly
to include
lac genes

F′ lac plasmid
cyclizes after being excised
from the
bacterial chromosome

Conjugation of an F′ lac cell
with an F⁻ cell.
The F′ lac plasmid replicates
and is transferred
to the F⁻ cell,
converting it to an
F′ lac cell.

**Figure 8-8.** Formation and subsequent conjugation of an F′ lac cell. Once the F′ lac exists
as an extrachromosomal plasmid, it is rapidly transferred to an F⁻ cell during conjugation.

sticky ends are on any double-stranded DNA that possesses single-stranded complementary regions at both the 3′ and the 5′ ends. When properly annealed (cooled slowly), the 3′ and 5′ ends will base-pair to form a circular DNA, as illustrated in Figure 8-9. Treatment with a polynucleotide ligase will then join the two DNAs covalently.

To introduce foreign DNA into a bacterium, the following steps are taken:

1. Bacterial plasmids are isolated and cleaved with an endonuclease that leaves the plasmid DNA with sticky ends.

2. Foreign DNA from any source—bacteria, viruses, fruit flies, toads, and so forth—is isolated and treated with the same endonuclease so that it will be cleaved into fragments containing one to ten genes, each possessing the same sticky ends as the cleaved plasmid DNA.

3. Foreign DNA fragments are then mixed with the cleaved plasmid DNA and the entire mixture is annealed so that the sticky ends will pair to form circular DNA. Because both the plasmid and the foreign DNA possess the same sticky ends, various fragments of foreign DNA will pair with the plasmid DNA

and become incorporated into the final circular DNA plasmid. The newly formed circular plasmid with its segment of foreign DNA is treated with polynucleotide ligase, and it can then be reintroduced into the bacterium by transformation. The entire hybrid plasmid will be replicated.

So, what is the current status of experiments in genetic engineering, and what has been done to prevent the creation of a "monster" organism which could cause untold misery in society? Starting in 1974 scientists from around the world have had a series of meetings to establish guidelines to minimize the risks in this virgin field. Safeguards of two general types have been proposed: (1) biological barriers to limit genetic recombinants (such as described above) to those that cannot grow in humans—for example temperature-sensitive strains that could not grow above 30°C or osmotically-fragile organisms that could exist only in an environment of high osmotic pressure; (2) physical barriers for moderate to high-risk experiments to prevent hybrids from infecting laboratory personnel or gaining access to the external environment.

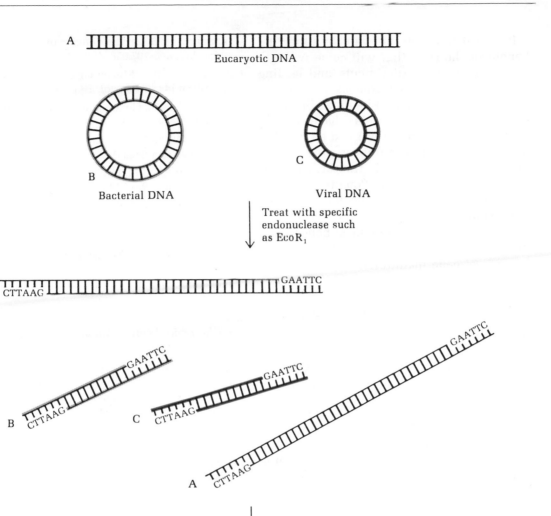

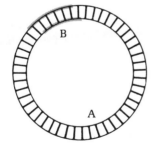
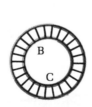
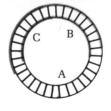

A — Eucaryotic DNA
B — Bacterial DNA
C — Viral DNA

**Figure 8-9.** Endonuclease action resulting in the formation of DNA fragments with sticky ends. DNA from any source is cleaved so as to yield a single-stranded end with a sequence of GAATTC (reading from 5′ to 3′). When slowly cooled any of these fragments can base-pair to form both longer linear strands or circular molecules. Treatment with a DNA ligase will repair the break, resulting in the formation of a new molecule.

It is still too early to evaluate either the benefit or the risks that will come with genetic engineering experiments, and leading scientists strongly disagree as to whether such experiments should be done. But, such experiments done thus far have clearly shown that eucaryotic DNA can be inserted into a bacterium and, moreover, such eucaryotic DNA is replicated, transcribed, and translated into protein. Potential benefits from these experiments include increased understanding of gene function and regulation, and one can hope that these benefits can be gained while minimizing any potential hazards of gene manipulation.

## REFERENCES

Asilomar conference on DNA recombinant molecules. 1975. *Nature* **255**:442–444.

Avery, O. T., C. M. MacLoed, and M. McCarty. 1944. Studies on the chemical nature of the substance inducing transformation of pneumococcal types. Induction of transformations by a deoxyribonucleic acid fraction isolated from pneumococcus type III. *J. Exp. Med.* **79**:137–158.

Bachmann, B. J., K. B. Low, and A. L. Taylor. 1976. Recalibrated linkage map of *Escherichia coli* K-12. *Bacteriol. Rev.* **40**:116–167.

Campbell, A. M. 1969. *Episomes.* Harper and Row, New York.

Chang, A. C. Y., R. A. Langsman, D. A. Clayton, and S. N. Cohen. 1975. Studies on mouse mitochondrial DNA in *Escherichia coli.* Structure and function of the eucaryotic-procaryotic chimeric plasmids. *Cell* **6**:231–244.

Chargaff, E. 1976. On the dangers of genetic meddling. *Science* **192**:938–940.

Clowes, R. C. 1972. Molecular structure of bacterial plasmids. *Bacteriol. Rev.* **36**:361–405.

Cohen, S. N. 1976. Gene manipulation. *New Engl. J. Med.* **294**:883–889.

Cohen, S. N. 1975. The manipulation of genes. *Sci. American* **233**:(1) 25–33.

Hotchkiss, R. D. 1974. Models of genetic recombination. *Annu. Rev. Microbiol.* **28**:445–468.

Jones, D., and P. H. A. Sneath. 1970. Genetic transfer and bacterial taxonomy. *Bacteriol. Rev.* **34**:40–81.

Lappé, M. and R. S. Morison, eds. 1976. Ethical and scientific issues posed by human uses of molecular genetics. *Ann. New York Acad. Sci.* **265.**

Levinthal, M. 1974. Bacterial genetics excluding *Escherichia coli. Annu. Rev. Microbiol.* **28**:219–229.

Novick, R. P., R. C. Clowes, S. N. Cohen, R. Curtiss III, N. Datta, and S. Falkow. 1976. Uniform nomenclature for bacterial plasmids: A proposal. *Bacteriol. Rev.* **40**:168–189.

Sherratt, D. J. 1974. Bacterial plasmids. *Cell* **3**:189–195.

Singer, M. 1976. Summary of the proposed guidelines for genetic engineering. *Amer. Soc. Microbiol. News* **42**:277–287.

Wade, N. 1976. Recombinant DNA: The last look before the leap. *Science* **192**:236–238.

Williamson, B. 1976. First mammalian results with genetic recombinants. *Nature* **260**:189–190.

# 9

## Physical and Chemical Control
## of Microorganisms

Effective control of microorganisms is ideally directed toward the complete exclusion of all microbes from any area where they might do harm. Bandages and surgical instruments are sterilized to avoid infecting a wound. Disinfection procedures are required for contaminated clothing, bedding, and even the floor and walls of rooms that have been occupied by patients with certain contagious diseases such as tuberculosis. The aim of the disinfection process is the destruction of disease agents; sterilization is an absolute term meaning the killing of all forms of life in a given area.

Sterilization procedures vary considerably, depending upon such factors as the material of which the object is made and the circumstances incident to its use. New developments, such as the use of indwelling intravenous polyethylene tubing and open-heart surgery, continue to create new problems in sterilization. For many articles sterilization can be effected by a variety of procedures, while for other objects the choice may be limited.

This chapter is devoted to a description of the major physical and chemical sterilization techniques; the principles which are discussed provide the basic knowledge necessary for success in the control and the elimination of undesirable microorganisms.

## Physical Methods

### HEAT

For most objects, heat is the most practical and efficient method of sterilization; however, the amount of heat required to kill (that is, to denature at least one essential protein) varies from one organism to another. For any organism, one must consider both the degree of heat to be used and the length of time the material to be sterilized must be maintained at a given temperature. In general, the temperature required for sterilization is inversely related to time—the higher the temperature, the shorter the time required.

Sterilization might not be too difficult in most cases if one did not have to contend with bacterial endospores, the most resistant form of life known; some such as those of *Clostridium botulinum* will survive the temperature of boiling water for several hours.

Another important factor to be considered with heat sterilization is the environment of the microorganisms being destroyed, whether they are in a heavy blanket, in pus or feces, in a contaminated bandage, or in blood that has been allowed to clot in a syringe. Environment is important for two reasons: (1) in order to kill, the heat must reach the organisms, and (2) more heat than normal is required to kill organisms embedded in proteinaceous material such as pus, tissue, or tissue exudate.

From these major considerations, it is obvious that no single standard temperature or time for all conditions of sterilization can be set. Certainly, small tubes of media are sterilized more quickly than are heavy blankets or mattresses.

### Methods of Sterilization by Heat

MOIST HEAT. Steam under pressure is the most efficient sterilizing agent and is the chief means used for sterilizing surgical bandages, instruments, media, and contaminated material. The temperature of sterilization is dependent upon the pressure of the steam. Normally, the temperature of steam in an open container at sea level is 100°C; however, if the steam is confined in a closed vessel and its pressure is raised, the temperature of the steam is elevated correspondingly. At 15 pounds per square inch (1.05 Kg per square cm) the temperature reaches 121°C, and this is the temperature routinely employed for sterilization.

It should be stressed that if steam is to reach the expected temperature for a corresponding pressure (e.g., 121°C for 15 lbs/sq in or 1.05 Kg/sq cm), the atmosphere must be free of air and contain only steam. These conditions are fulfilled in an autoclave, a laboratory appliance similar to a large pressure cooker (see Figure 9-1). Most autoclaves are equipped with controls which automatically allow the air to be exhausted before the steam pressure is allowed to rise. In addition, loading involves a certain amount of knowledge and common sense. One must know that to kill all microorganisms, the steam must actually penetrate through the entire load. Thus, no object should be wrapped in a material impermeable to steam (such as rubber sheeting) or sealed in a tight container. Common sense comes into play when one must decide on the length of time for the autoclaving process. Quite obviously, sterilizing a large load of fabric would require a considerably longer time (1–2 hours) than would a load of surgical instruments (15 minutes).

When using an autoclave, one can determine the effectiveness of the sterilization procedure by placing a container of heat-resistant endospores (for example, those of *Bacillus stearothermophilus*) in the center of the load; the endospores are subsequently cultured to see if complete killing has taken place. One may also use temperature-sensitive tapes that change color when the proper temperature (121°C) is reached.

DRY HEAT.    This is accomplished in an oven. In fact, the home oven—with the use of a household oven thermometer to indicate the proper temperature—can be an improvised device for sterilization. Dry-heat sterilizers may or may not have a fan to circulate the air to better distribute the heat.

The effectiveness of dry heat lies in its ability to provide penetration of heat through the object being sterilized; thus, it is possible to sterilize objects such as syringes that have already been assembled and sealed in a container. Dry heat is used to sterilize powders, special or petrolatum gauze dressings, and other items that could be damaged by steam or water. It is also effective for oily substances such as ointments, which are insoluble in water and not permeable to moist heat.

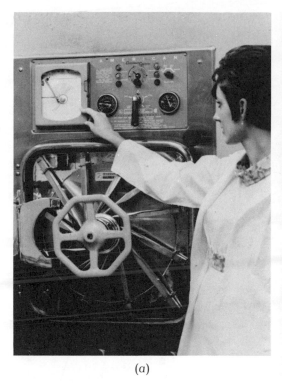

(a)

**Figure 9-1.** *a.* A modern autoclave. *b.* Temperature-sensitive tape changes color at 121°C.

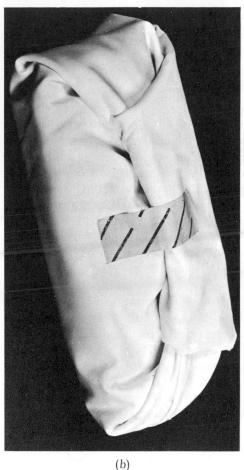

(b)

Dry-heat sterilization requires considerably higher temperatures for complete effectiveness than does steam sterilization. As with steam sterilization, there is no definite standard time, but 160°–170°C for two hours is probably the most common range. However, one must also take into account the weight or bulk of the load to be sterilized.

### Pasteurization

Pasteurization is not a form of sterilization, but is a process designed to destroy disease-producing organisms. It was devised by Pasteur to preserve wine by killing bacteria (such as lactobacilli) that cause wine to sour. We are now more likely to associate pasteurization with milk. The process involves heating the milk to 62.9°C for 30 minutes or to 71.6°C for at least 15 seconds. Both options are followed by rapid cooling. Such techniques reduce the over-all numbers of most bacteria in the milk, but they are specifically designed to eliminate the etiologic agents of tuberculosis, brucellosis, and Q-fever.

### RADIATION

All types of radiation can be injurious to microorganisms, causing mutations or death. The effects of radiation may be explained as alterations of the cell membrane, a change in essential enzymes, or a change in nucleic acids. The two main groups of radiation used for controlling microorganisms are: (1) ionizing radiations (X-rays, gamma rays, and cathode rays), and (2) ultraviolet light.

## Ionizing Rays

X-rays (produced by generating machines and varying in wavelength from 0.1 nm to 40 nm) and gamma rays (originating from radioactive elements such as $^{60}$Co and similar to short X-rays) are much more powerful and penetrating than ultraviolet light. Ionizing radiation causes protein denaturation as well as breaks in strands of DNA. Single-stranded breaks are usually successfully repaired, but if both strands of DNA are broken, the effect is frequently lethal.

One major effect of ionizing radiations results from the formation of free radicals ($^-$OH and $^-$HO$_2$) produced as the high-energy photon travels through water. These free radicals contribute to the lethal action of ionizing radiation by forming peroxides that act as powerful oxidizing agents.

Although to date ionizing radiations have not been used extensively as a means of sterilization, they can be used to sterilize certain pharmaceuticals and stable plastic items such as petri dishes, catheters, and syringes. Foods have been preserved experimentally by treatment with ionizing rays; however, changes in odors, flavors, and other qualities of foods have resulted.

## Ultraviolet Light

The light we call ultraviolet light is, for the most part, invisible to the human eye. Its wavelengths cover a range from the visible range to X-rays, that is, wavelengths of 390 nm to 40 nm, with the maximum killing effect at 260 nm (see Figure 9-2).

Ultraviolet light is lethal because of its absorption by the cell's nucleic acids. When absorbed, cross-links (dimers) in a DNA strand are produced between neighboring thymine molecules (see Chapter 7). Such cross-links inhibit replication of DNA by altering the template DNA.

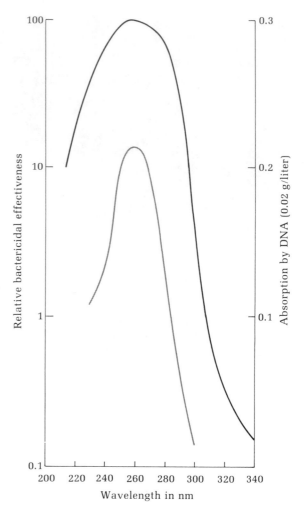

**Figure 9-2.** The black curve shows the bactericidal effectiveness of various ultraviolet wavelengths in killing bacteria. The grey curve represents absorption by DNA. Note that both curves peak at 260 nm, indicating that bacterial death caused by ultraviolet light is due to absorption by DNA.

Ultraviolet light has one major limitation; it does not penetrate ordinary glass, dirt, paper, pus, or more than a few layers of cells. Germicidal lamps, however, have been used to reduce the microbial population of the air in operating rooms, nurseries, communicable disease wards, school rooms, bacteriology laboratories, bakeries, restaurants, and other food establishments. It is important to use special precautions to protect the eyes when exposed to ultraviolet light.

## FILTRATION

Solutions of heat-labile compounds that cannot be subjected to heat or chemical treatment without decomposition or other injury can be sterilized by the process of filtration. Bacteria are not killed during filtration but are physically separated from a fluid by this method. The efficacy of most types of bacterial filters is a function of both filter pore size and an electrostatic attraction between the filter and the bacterium.

SEITZ FILTERS. The filtering unit of these filters is made up of a mixture of asbestos fibers and other filter materials. The pads are several millimeters thick and fluid passes through irregular channels that are formed by the random orientation of the fibers in the pad. It is therefore not possible to assign an exact pore size, although they are in the range of 1 $\mu$m in diameter. This is large enough to allow many bacteria to pass, and the efficiency of these filters is ascribed to the adsorption of the bacteria to the pore walls, probably as a result of an electrostatic positive charge on the asbestos.

BERKEFELD FILTERS. These filters (like the Seitz filters) are depth filters in which fluids are passed through diatomaceous earth. Based on the fineness of the diatomaceous earth, several pore sizes are available, but even the finest Berkefeld filter has pore sizes in the range of 1 $\mu$m and, like the asbestos pads, must rely on adsorption of the bacteria to the filter material.

MEMBRANE FILTERS. These filters are the most widely used in both laboratory and industry. The cellulose ester membranes are made with various pore sizes ranging from 8 $\mu$m to 0.025 $\mu$m (see Table 9-1), and are usually purchased sterile from the manufacturer, although they may be autoclaved satisfactorily at 121°C for 15 minutes. Because of

### Table 9-1. Pore Size and Filtration Rates for Membrane Filters

| Membrane Filter Type | Pore Size | Rates of Flow water[a] | air[b] |
|---|---|---|---|
| SC | 8.0 $\mu$m ± 1.4 $\mu$m | 950 | 55 |
| SM | 5.0 $\mu$m ± 1.2 $\mu$m | 560 | 35 |
| SS | 3.0 $\mu$m ± 0.9 $\mu$m | 400 | 20 |
| RA | 1.2 $\mu$m ± 0.3 $\mu$m | 300 | 14 |
| AA | 0.8 $\mu$m ± 0.05 $\mu$m | 220 | 9.8 |
| DA | 0.65 $\mu$m ± 0.03 $\mu$m | 175 | 8.0 |
| HA | 0.45 $\mu$m ± 0.02 $\mu$m | 65 | 4.9 |
| PH | 0.30 $\mu$m ± 0.02 $\mu$m | 40 | 3.7 |
| GS | 0.22 $\mu$m ± 0.02 $\mu$m | 22 | 2.5 |
| VC | 100 nm ± 8nm | 3.0 | 1.0 |
| VM | 50 nm ± 3 nm | 1.5 | 0.7 |
| VF | 25 nm ± 2 nm | 0.5 | 0.3 |

[a]ml/min./sq. cm     ⎱ Under 70 cm Hg
[b]litre/min./sq. cm  ⎰ differential pressure.

their thinness (approximately 150 $\mu$m) their efficiency is based essentially entirely on pore size, and a pore size of 0.22 $\mu$m is usually effective in removing bacteria. However, viruses and some mycoplasmas (see Chapter 27) will pass through this pore size.

Membrane filtration can be used to quantitate the number of bacteria present in a water or air sample. This is done by placing the membrane (after filtering the sample through it) directly onto a suitable agar medium. The plate is then incubated and each viable bacterium will grow into a visible colony. Figure 9-3 shows a laboratory-size membrane filter and colonies that have grown on the filter after incubating the used membrane on an agar medium.

Membrane filters have also been used to separate toxins from bacterial cells, to sterilize drugs and organic materials such as proteins (serum) and certain sugars, and to filter beer on a large scale, to produce what the industry calls "bottled draft beer."

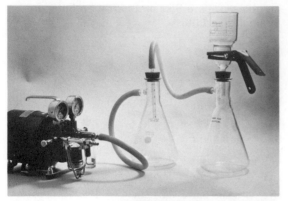

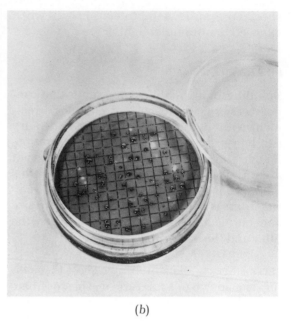

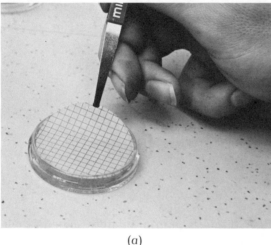

(b)

**Figure 9-3** a. Membrane filter apparatus and membrane being laid on agar medium. b. Typical coliform colonies with metallic "sheen" on a millipore filter.

(a)

# Chemical Agents

Some of the terms used to describe the action of chemical agents on microorganisms have rather vague popular meanings, and the following definitions may help to clarify the subject. The terms antiseptic and disinfectant are usually assigned to chemical substances that are used topically or on inanimate objects, respectively, to specifically destroy potential disease-producing microorganisms. Most are not effective against bacterial endospores or *Mycobacterium tuberculosis*. The suffix -stasis refers to inhibiting, and -cide to a killing effect. So, a bacteriostatic agent acts by inhibiting growth, but does not necessarily kill the organisms. A bactericide is defined as an agent that kills bacteria. In like manner, one can define a sporocide, a viricide, and a fungicide as agents that will kill spores, viruses, and fungi, respectively.

## MECHANISMS OF DISINFECTANT ACTION

The major factors that determine how a disinfectant acts are: (1) concentration of the disinfectant, (2) time during which the disinfectant is allowed to act, (3) temperature of disinfection, (4) number and types of organisms present, and (5) the nature of the material being disinfected.

## Action on the Cytoplasmic Membrane

Injury to the cytoplasmic membrane allows essential inorganic ions, nucleotides, coenzymes, and amino acids to leak out of the cell. In addition, such injury can prevent the concentration of essential materials in the cell since this membrane also controls active transport. Thus, the action of any substance that can inhibit the essential functions of the cytoplasmic membrane will result in either death of the cell or its inability to grow.

Since the cytoplasmic membrane is composed primarily of protein and lipid, surface-active agents such as soaps and detergents are effective for the disorganization of the membrane. All such agents possess a hydrophilic (water-attracting) and hydrophobic (water-repelling) group in their molecular structure. Thus, when they interact with the cell membrane, the hydrophilic part of the surface-active agent associates with the surface of the membrane while the hydrophobic portion of the detergent penetrates into the lipid-rich interior of the membrane. This, of course, causes a distortion resulting in leakage of essential metabolites from the cell.

## Action on Cellular Proteins

Chemical agents that injure the cell through their effect on enzymes or structural proteins include acids, alkalies, phenol, cresol, alcohols, salts of heavy metals, formaldehyde, halogens, and other oxidizing agents such as peroxides. Some of these, such as acids, alkalies, and organic solvents exert their effect by denaturing proteins, that is, by altering the tertiary structure of a protein so that it is unable to function. Other agents are effective disinfectants because they are able to modify functional groups (such as sulfhydryl or amino groups) of essential enzymes. Many disinfectants react first to de-

stroy membrane permeability and then enter the cell to denature or modify cytoplasmic enzymes or structural proteins.

## CHEMICAL AGENTS AND THEIR ACTION ON CELLS

### Phenol

The initial action of phenol is apparently injury to the cell membrane; however, since phenol will precipitate proteins, it also inactivates enzymes, probably by denaturing them.

Phenol is effective against vegetative forms of bacteria, including *Mycobacterium tuberculosis*, as well as fungi. Spores are not destroyed by phenolic action nor are viruses particularly susceptible.

Derivatives of phenol are used as preservatives in wood, paper, paints, and textiles. However, because of the caustic effectiveness of phenol, it is not widely used at the present time.

### Substituted Phenols

Attempts to reduce the toxicity of phenol compounds led to the synthesis of a number of substituted phenolic disinfectants. Two of the most popular were hexylresorcinol and hexachlorophene, and at one time these were incorporated into many soaps and detergents to enhance the germicidal activity of these surface-active agents.

Subsequent research with hexachlorophene indicated that it was absorbed through the skin and in animal models resulted in brain damage. Its use in baby powder is believed to have caused a number of infant deaths in Europe. As a result, the use of hexachlorophene has been prohibited in the United States except by a physician's prescription.

Cresols, also substituted phenols, are effective as bactericidal agents, and their action is not seriously impaired by the presence of organic matter. However, they cause irritation to living tissue and are therefore used primarily as disinfectants for inanimate objects. The action of cresol is similar to that of phenol; however, its germicidal activity is greater. The concentration customarily used is 2–5%. Since cresols are not soluble in water, they are ordinarily mixed with soap solutions. Figure 9-4 shows the structural relationship of these substituted phenols.

## Alcohols

While 70% ethyl alcohol is probably the most familiar and the most commonly used alcohol antiseptic, isopropyl and benzyl alcohol are more germicidal and are also employed. In addition, some alcohols, such as ethylene and propylene glycol, have been used as aerosols for air disinfection.

Because alcohol does not destroy endospores, it is not actually a sterilizing agent. When used on skin, the contact is usually too brief for a substantial germicidal effect. However, it does remove oil and dust particles and with them, no doubt, bacteria as well. The routine for disinfecting the skin prior to injection or withdrawal of blood is to: (1) swab the area with alcohol to remove oil and surface debris; (2) swab the area with a 2–3% solution of iodine in alcohol to kill contaminating organisms; and (3) swab again with alcohol to remove most of the residual iodine.

## Halogens

Of the halogens, chlorine and iodine are the only two used to any extent as antimicrobial agents. There are a number of different disinfectants containing chlorine—ranging from chlorine gas and hypochlorites to organic chloramines. All appear to exert their bactericidal effect by reacting with water to form hypochlorites as shown below:

$$Cl_2 + H_2O \longrightarrow HCl + HClO$$

Hypochlorites are powerful oxidizing agents that undergo the following reaction:

$$HClO \longrightarrow HCl + O$$

The released nascent oxygen oxidizes cell constituents (such as sulfhydryl groups essential for enzymatic activity) causing the death of the cell.

Iodine has been extensively used for skin disinfection and is germicidal against bacteria, fungi, spores, and viruses. Its mode of action is believed to be a reaction with tyrosine which prevents the normal function of tyrosine-containing enzymes. Iodine, however, like chlorine, also reacts with water to form hypoiodite, and in all likelihood the oxidizing ability of this compound exerts a bactericidal activity.

**Figure 9-4.** Structures of phenol and several substituted phenol disinfectants.

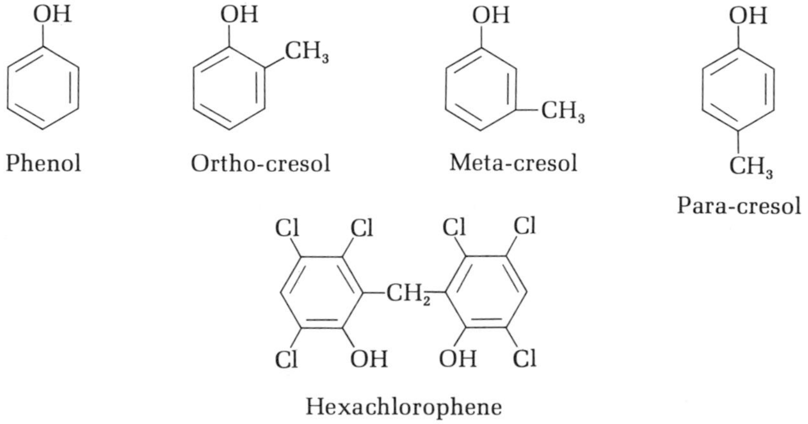

Phenol    Ortho-cresol    Meta-cresol    Para-cresol

Hexachlorophene

## Salts of Heavy Metals

Both silver and mercury-containing compounds have been used as inhibitory agents. The effect of mercury results from its reaction with sulfhydryl (−SH) groups present on many enzymes within the cell. Once mercury has reacted with the —SH groups, the enzymes can no longer function and the cell dies. Mercury poisoning can be reversed by the addition of other compounds such as British anti-lewisite (BAL) rich in sulfhydryl groups. Mercuric chloride is used as a preservative for wood, paper, and leather, as well as for the control of fungal infections in skin. Several mercuric organic compounds are used rather commonly for skin disinfection, namely Merthiolate, Mercurochrome, and Metaphen.

Silver compounds appear to exert their toxic effect by the denaturation of proteins, and, as a result, their effect is irreversible. Weak solutions of silver nitrate have been used for many years in eye drops and lotions.

## Dyes

Certain dyes used for staining bacteria have a bacteriostatic action, particularly against gram-positive bacteria. It is believed that the dyes may combine with proteins or interfere with peptidoglycan synthesis in some manner. Because of their selective inhibition of gram-positive bacteria, a number of dyes have been incorporated into bacteriologic culture media for the selective cultivation of the gram-negative bacteria. This has been especially useful in isolating gram-negative pathogens from the intestinal tract.

## Quaternary Ammonium Detergents

This group of compounds may be either bacteriostatic or bactericidal, depending upon the concentration used. Their action appears to be primarily due to the disruption of the membrane. Although the quaternary compounds are active against both gram-negative and gram-positive bacteria, the gram-positive cells appear to be far more susceptible. The practical use of these compounds is in skin antisepsis and for the control of bacteria on utensils in dairies and restaurants. As shown in Figure 9-5, they consist of a pentavalent nitrogen (like $NH_4Cl$) in which various organic groups are substituted for the hydrogen atoms. Since the functional part of the molecule carries a positive charge, they are classified as cationic detergents.

## Soaps and Detergents

Soaps and detergents act primarily as surface-active agents; they reduce surface tension. This mechanical effect is of tremendous importance, since the bacteria, along with oil and other particles, become enmeshed in the soap or detergent and are removed through the washing process. But, soaps and detergents, as ordinarily used, cannot really be classed as germicides. Even though they are mildly bactericidal, their contact is usually too short to produce much destructive effect. Nevertheless, fragile bacteria such as the gonococcus, the meningococcus, and the pneumococcus may be readily

**Figure 9-5.** Chemical structure of the quaternary ammonium compound, benzalkonium chloride.

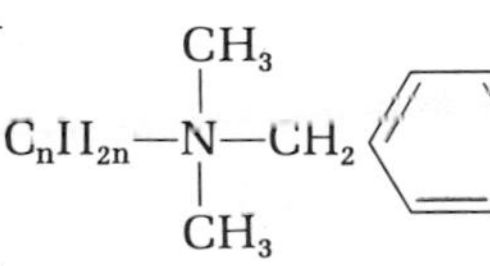

$$\left[ \begin{array}{c} R_1 \\ | \\ R_2-N-R_4 \\ | \\ R_3 \end{array} \right]^+ \quad Cl^-$$

General structure

$$\left[ \begin{array}{c} CH_3 \\ | \\ C_nH_{2n}-N-CH_2 \\ | \\ CH_3 \end{array} \right]^+ \quad Cl^-$$

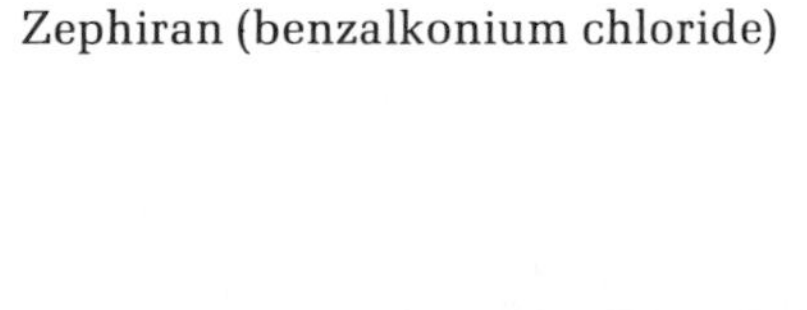

Zephiran (benzalkonium chloride)

killed by the chemical action of these surface-active agents.

### Formaldehyde

Formaldehyde is an excellent disinfectant when used as a gas. It is quite effective in closed areas as a bacteriocide and fungicide. In an aqueous solution of about 37%, formaldehyde is known as formalin. Its microbicidal action results from its reaction with essential sulfhydral groups as shown below:

$$R\text{-}SH + HCHO \longrightarrow R\text{-}S\text{-}CH_2OH$$

Formaldehyde destroys spores of both bacteria and fungi; however, its use is limited by its very irritating vapor. It is used in the preservation of labatory specimens and can be used in disinfecting shoes carrying the fungi causing athlete's foot. In alcohol solutions, it may be used on instruments.

### Hydrogen Peroxide

This agent owes its mild antiseptic properties to its oxidizing ability. It is quite unstable but is frequently used in cleaning wounds, particularly deep wounds in which anaerobes are likely to be introduced. The action of the peroxide is limited because the enzyme catalase, present in tissue fluids, rapidly decomposes peroxide to water and free oxygen. The liberation of oxygen accounts for the foaming noted when peroxide is introduced into the mouth or open wounds. Ordinarily it is used as a 3% solution.

### Ethylene Oxide

Ethylene oxide (see Figure 9-6) boils at 10.8°C, so it exists as a gas unless it is kept cold or tightly sealed. However, whether used as a gas or as a liquid, ethylene oxide is a very effective killing agent for bacteria, spores, molds, and viruses. An important property which makes this compound such a valuable germicide is its ability to penetrate into and through essentially any substance that is not

**Figure 9-6.** Chemical structures of gaseous disinfectants.

hermetically sealed. For example, ethylene oxide is used commercially to sterilize barrels of spices without opening the barrels. The barrels are placed in a large, drumlike apparatus, and after much of the air has been removed with a vacuum pump the ethylene oxide is admitted.

It is not difficult to recognize the value of such an agent for sterilizing certain pieces of equipment used in the hospital operating room, particularly those items which are large, expensive, and delicate, and which cannot be subjected to heat or liquid sterilization. Heart pumps, respirometers, and intravenous catheters are easily sterilized with this gas.

Ethylene oxide has the major disadvantage of being extremely flammable in high concentrations. For safety, it is usually mixed with an inert gas. The most commonly used mixture (called carboxide) consists of 10% ethylene oxide and 90% carbon dioxide. Such mixtures of ethylene oxide and carbon dioxide are used in special autoclaves in which the temperature and the humidity are carefully controlled.

Ethylene oxide is a very active chemical and will react readily with free carboxyl, amino, sulfhydryl, and hydroxyl groups, replacing the labile hydrogen present in each of these groups with a hydroxy-ethyl radical. It is believed that it is this type of reaction with the structural and enzymatic components of the cell that causes the death of the cell.

Bacteriologic culture media also have been sterilized by the addition of liquid ethylene oxide. The ethylene oxide is volatilized by warming, following which the medium may be used.

## Beta-propiolactone

Beta-propiolactone (see Figure 9-6) possesses many properties similar to those of ethylene oxide. In concentrations not much greater than those required for killing vegetative bacteria it kills spores. The effect is rapid, a necessary feature because $\beta$-propiolactone in aqueous solution undergoes fairly rapid hydrolysis to yield acrylic acid. This instability is an advantage, inasmuch as it permits one to add the substance to many materials, knowing that it will disappear spontaneously in a few hours. Consequently, $\beta$-propiolactone may be used to sterilize bone, cartilage, and artery grafts. It may also be added directly to serum to destroy hepatitis virus and can be used to sterilize a culture medium.

Betapropiolactone has also been used as an aerosol. In one report, it is claimed that a two-story building was completely sterilized inside by spraying with 16 liters of the substance.

## THE DISINFECTION PROCESS

For both physical and chemical methods of sterilization, the rate at which a microbial population dies can be plotted as a logarithmic function of the number of survivors at any given time. In other words, if we heat a suspension of vegetative bacterial cells to 55°C, they begin to die, but all do not die instantly.

Let us take a hypothetical example in which we begin with 100 million bacteria and heat the suspension at 70°C. Let us assume that after one minute, 90 percent of the cells are killed, leaving only 10 million viable bacteria in the suspension. At first thought, one might reason that just a few seconds more of heating would result in a complete sterilization of the suspension. Not so! If 90 percent of the viable cells were killed during the first minute, 90 percent of the survivors will be killed during the second minute. Thus, while 90 million bacteria were killed during the first minute, only 9 million

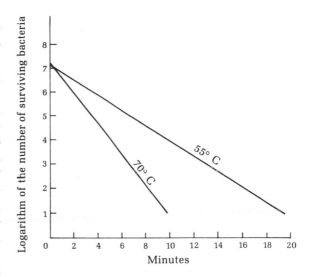

**Figure 9-7.** Curve showing exponential death of bacteria. Death occurs as a first-order reaction and thus the actual rate of killing is a function of the number of survivors at any time.

will be killed during the second minute, and only 900,000 will be killed during the third minute.

This type of reaction is called a first-order reaction because the rate of killing is dependent upon the number of viable cells at any time. When this is plotted on a semi-log graph, one obtains a straight-line death curve that shows death is a logrithmic function. In general, the slope of the line (which will show the speed of the reaction) will vary according to the conditions of killing, as depicted in Figure 9-7. At 55°C, it will require longer to kill a particular number of cells than at 70°C, but both cases will yield a straight-line death curve. In practical cases, the line may deviate from normal as the number of survivors becomes very small. One must always allow a safety margin if sterilization conditions are mild and if complete sterilization is necessary.

## REFERENCES

Benarde, M. A., ed. 1970. *Disinfection.* Marcel Dekker, New York.

Borick, P. M. 1968. Chemical sterilizers (chemosterilizers). *Adv. Appl. Microbiol.* **10**:291–312.

Bruch, C. W. 1961. Gaseous sterilization. *Annu. Rev. Microbiol.* **15**:245–261.

Farrell, J., and A. Rose. 1967. Temperature effects on microorganisms. *Annu. Rev. Microbiol.* **21**:101–120.

Ginoza, W. 1967. The effects of ionizing radiation on nucleic acids of bacteriophages and bacterial cells. *Annu. Rev. Microbiol.* **21**:325–361.

Grossman, L., J. C. Kaplan, S. R. Kushner, and I. Mahler. 1968. Enzymes involved in the early stages of repair of ultraviolet irradiated DNA. *Cold Spring Harbor Symp. Quant. Biol.* **33**:229–234.

Hamkalo, B. A., and P. A. Swenson. 1969. Effects of ultraviolet radiation on respiration and growth in radiation-resistant and radiation-sensitive strains of *Escherichia coli* B. *J. Bacteriol.* **99**:815–823.

Hugo, W. B., ed. 1971. *Inhibition and Destruction of the Microbial Cell.* Academic Press, New York.

Lawrence, C. A., and S. S. Block. 1968. *Disinfection, Sterilization and Preservation.* Lea and Febiger, Philadelphia.

Rahn, O. 1945. Physical methods of sterilization of microorganisms. *Bacteriol. Rev.* **9**:1–47.

Sugiyama, H. 1951. Studies on factors affecting the heat resistance of spores of *Clostridium botulinum. J. Bacteriol.* **62**:81–96.

Sykes, G. 1965. *Disinfection and Sterilization,* 2nd ed. J. B. Lippincott, Philadelphia.

# 10

# Unique Macromolecular Biosyntheses; Antimicrobial Agents in Chemotherapy

Sick people have been treated with herbs, bark, weeds, and uncounted other concoctions for thousands of years. Yet, there was little systematic approach to the practice of chemotherapy until experiments in 1909 carried out by Paul Ehrlich led to the development of an agent which would selectively destroy certain spirochetes without serious injury to the host's cells. This particular "magic bullet" was called by several names —such as arphenamine, salvarson, and 606— and was used for many years for the successful treatment of syphilis.

Since 1935, a multitude of chemotherapeutic agents have become available. Many of these compounds are prepared synthetically in the laboratory, while others occur as by-products of the metabolic activity of bacteria and fungi. This latter group of chemotherapeutic agents has been given the general name of antibiotics. Currently, a very large number of antibiotics have been isolated and characterized. Unfortunately, many lack practical value because they are too toxic to the host to be used for the treatment of infectious diseases.

For any chemotherapeutic agent to be useful against invading microorganisms, several ideals must be sought.

1. The drug should be low in toxicity to the host's cells while destroying or inhibiting the disease agent; in other words it must demonstrate a selective toxicity for the disease agent.

2. The host should not become hypersensitive (allergic) to it.

3. The host should not destroy, neutralize, or excrete the drug until after the latter has performed its function.

4. The organism should not readily become resistant to the drug.

Of course, these criteria comprise an idealized list of properties for a chemotherapeutic drug, and even the best and most widely used drugs do not possess all of the above attributes. For example, many drugs demonstrate some toxicity to the host (upset stomach, diarrhea, fever) and many individuals become allergic to antibiotics such as penicillin. However, since most drugs demonstrate a selective toxicity toward the invading microorganisms, let us examine the mechanisms by which common chemotherapeutic agents exert their killing effect against infectious disease agents.

119

## CHEMICAL SYNTHESIS OF CHEMOTHERAPEUTIC AGENTS

No one would have predicted in 1935 that the discovery of the sulfonamides would usher in a revolutionary era in the treatment of infectious diseases in which many frequently fatal infections would be conquered or that this could happen in such an infinitesimally small fraction of the time that our species has inhabited the earth.

### The Sulfonamides

The preparation which led to the discovery of the sulfonamides was a red dye known as Prontosil. In 1933, Prontosil was reported to cure a normally fatal bloodstream infection caused by staphylococci and to be highly effective against streptococcal infections as well. Subsequent research showed that the active chemical group of Prontosil was actually sulfanilamide. However, even though sulfanilamide was effective against many microorganisms (gram-positive and gram-negative) it produced some toxic side effects, and researchers developed other sulfonamide derivatives by adding different chemical groups to the sulfur-bound amide group, as shown in Figure 10-1. Such synthesis gave rise to a whole family of "sulfa" drugs which vary considerably in the rate at which they are absorbed and excreted by the host.

The action of the sulfonamides is described as competitive inhibition. What actually happens can be explained as follows: for a bacterium to synthesize folic acid (one of the B vitamins necessary for growth) it must syn-

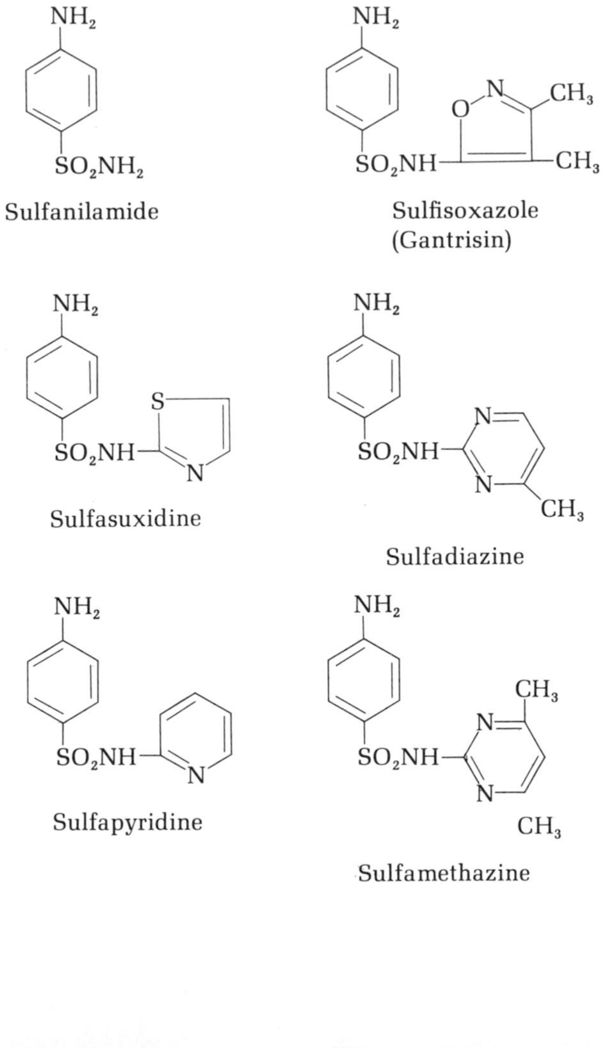

**Figure 10-1.** Structural formulas for some of the representative sulfonamides that are used as chemotherapeutic agents.

thesize and join together several molecules. One of the molecules, which makes up part of the folic-acid molecule, is para-aminobenzoic acid (frequently called PABA). The chemical structure of PABA, as shown below, is similar to that of sulfanilamide.

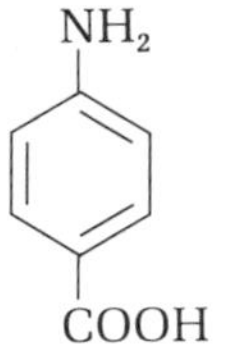

PABA 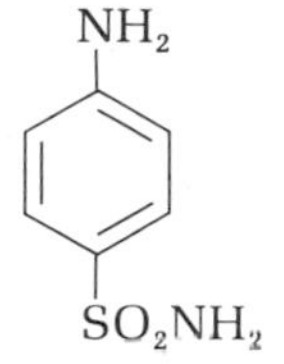          Sulfanilamide

Because of this similarity, the enzyme which normally incorporates PABA into folic acid mistakenly attaches to the sulfanilamide (or other sulfonamide derivative), but then cannot incorporate it into the folic acid molecule. The continued inhibition of growth requires the presence of a large excess of sulfa compound since both the sulfa drug and the true substrate, PABA, compete for a site on the enzyme. As a result, any time the concentration of the chemotherapeutic drug falls below a competitive level, the high affinity of the PABA for its enzyme will permit the synthesis of folic acid. Thus, it can be seen that this is a bacteriostatic effect, and treatment must be continued long enough to allow the body defenses to destroy the infecting organisms. Only organisms that synthesize their own folic acid are affected.

Resistance to sulfonamides occurs frequently—particularly in gram-negative organisms such as *Escherichia coli, Neisseria gonorrhoeae,* and *Neisseria meningitidis.* The mechanism of this resistance is in most cases not understood. Some are mediated by plasmids and may cause a destruction of the sulfonamide or an inability to transport the drug into the cell. Resistance could also occur from a decreased affinity of the PABA-incorporating enzyme for the sulfonamide. This latter hypothesis is theoretical and has yet to be proven.

## Para-Aminosalicylic Acid

Para-aminosalicylic acid (PAS) is weakly active against *Mycobacterium tuberculosis* and has been used for many years concurrently with streptomycin for the treatment of tuberculosis. The rationale for using PAS with streptomycin is that it will reduce the possibility that a streptomycin-resistant mutant might develop to produce serious pathological changes. Its mechanism of action is considered to be the same as that of the sulfonamides, classifying it as a competitive inhibitor of PABA.

## Isonicotinic Acid Hydrazide

This drug is frequently referred to as isoniazid or INH. Like PAS, it demonstrates a highly selective activity against *M. tuberculosis,* although its effect against most other bacteria is negligible. In the treatment of tuberculosis, it is given concurrently with a second drug (rifampin, ethambutol, streptomycin, or PAS) to reduce the development of resistant strains of *M. tuberculosis.* INH is structurally similar to the B vitamin pyridoxine as shown below. As a result, its mode of action has been suggested to be the competitive inhibition of pyridoxine-catalyzed reactions which act as coenzymes for transamination and amino acid decarboxylation reactions.

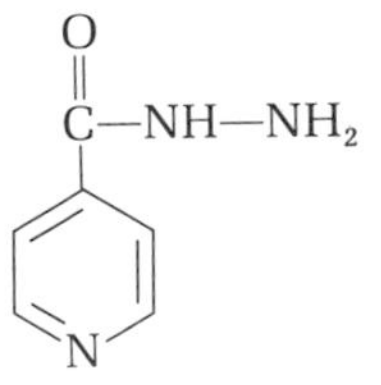

Isoniazid 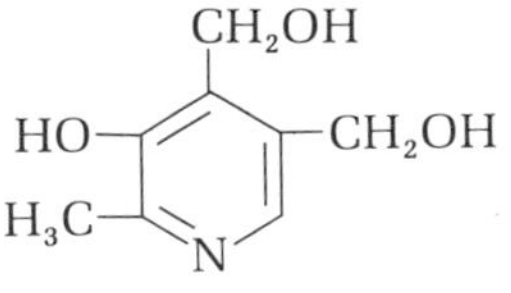          Pyridoxine

## ANTIBIOTICS IN CHEMOTHERAPY

Although it is beyond the scope of this text to discuss all of the antibiotics used for the treatment of infectious diseases, the more commonly used antibiotics will be described in the following passages. For the purpose of describing their mode of action, these antibiotics are divided into four categories based on their bacteriostatic or bactericidal effect on various structures and macromolecules in the bacterial cell: (1) inhibition of cell wall synthesis, (2) injury to cell membrane, (3) inhibition of protein synthesis, and (4) inhibition of nucleic acid synthesis. Major antibiotics in each of these categories are listed in Table 10-1.

### Table 10-1. Target Structures of Major Antibiotics

| Target Structure | Antibiotic |
| --- | --- |
| Cell wall | Penicillins |
| | Cephalosporins |
| | Cycloserine |
| | Bacitracin |
| | Vancomycin |
| | Ristocetin |
| Cell membrane | Polymyxins |
| | Nystatin |
| | Amphotericin B |
| Protein synthesis | Streptomycin |
| | Chloramphenicol |
| | Erythromycin and other macrolide antibiotics such as Oleandomycin, Carbomycin, and Spiromycin |
| | Tetracyclines |
| | Lincomycin |
| | Fucidin |
| | Puromycin |
| Nucleic acid synthesis | Mitomycin |
| | Nalidixic acid |
| | Novobiocin |
| | Griseofulvin |
| | Actinomycins |
| | Rifampicins |

## ANTIBIOTICS THAT INHIBIT CELL WALL SYNTHESIS

### Penicillin

To understand how penicillin exerts its bactericidal effect, it is necessary to know some of the steps involved in the synthesis of the cell-wall peptidoglycan. As discussed in Chapter 3, peptidoglycan is the wall layer that provides the rigidity of the cell, and anything that interferes with peptidoglycan synthesis will weaken the wall and allow the cell membrane to burst, liberating the cell contents. It may help to visualize the structure of peptidoglycan as like that of a barrel. In this analogy, the long staves would be a repeating polymer of N-acetylglucosamine and N-acetylmuramic acid (see Figure 3-6). However, the staves would not be able to hold together unless there were hoops around the barrel. In peptidoglycan, these hoops are composed of short peptides of amino acids, as represented by both the open and closed circles in Figure 3-6.

During growth, the bacterial cell synthesizes units of the cell wall made up of (in the case of *Staphylococcus aureus*) one N-acetylglucosamine (GlmNAc) and one N-acetylmuramic acid (MurNAc) plus ten amino acids which will provide the hoops to the barrel (see Figure 10-2). This unit (marked in Figure 3-6) is then transported to the growing section of the cell wall.

After the incorporation of the GlmNAc-MurNAc decapeptide into the existing wall, the last step is to cross-link these linear polymers with a bridge of amino acids to provide the required rigidity and strength. The mechanism of this cross-linking is shown in Figure 10-3, where it can be seen that the two linear polymers are cross-linked by a process called transpeptidization. In this process, the terminal glycine from one polymer replaces the terminal D-alanine from an adjacent polymer, resulting in a cross-bridge and the liberation of one molecule of D-alanine. This reaction is inhibited by penicillin. Penicillin has a structure similar to the terminal

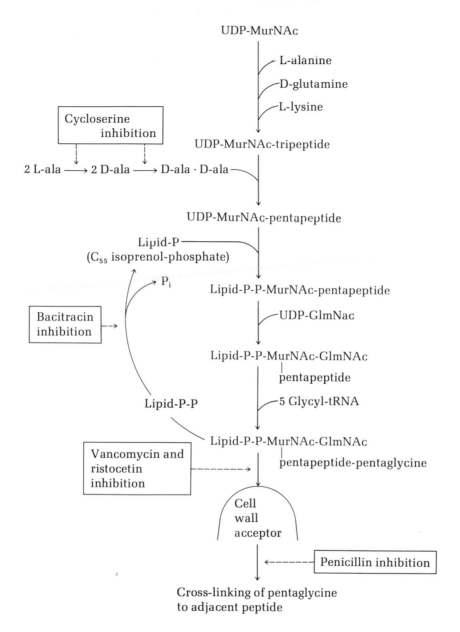

**Figure 10-2.** Biosynthetic steps in the synthesis of one repeating unit of peptidoglycan. Note the steps that are blocked by various antibiotics.

D-alanyl-D-alanine, which must undergo transpeptidization (see Figure 10-4). Thus, the transpeptidase reacts with the penicillin and is not available to complete the pentaglycine bridge between the linear polymers of GlmNAc-MurNAc. As a result, the peptidoglycan cell wall does not possess sufficient strength to withstand the internal osmotic pressure of the cell, and the bacterium bursts.

The amino acids that make up this cross-connecting bridge vary from one genus of bacterium to another (in some cases the pen-

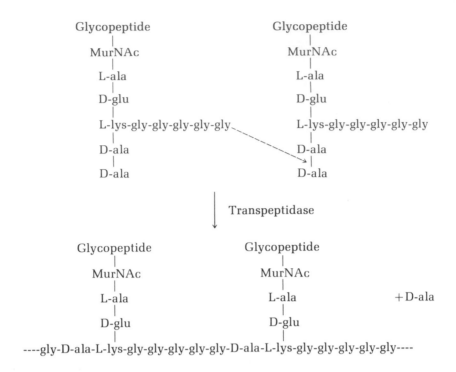

**Figure 10-3.** Transpeptidization to join two linear peptidoglycan strands by forming an interpeptide bridge of pentaglycine.

tapeptides from the MurNAc are joined directly by transpeptidization between the D-alanyl-D-alanine and an amino acid in an adjacent chain) but the mechanism of penicillin action remains the same—no matter how the connection is made, the transpeptidization always occurs to a terminal D-alanyl-D-alanine.

OTHER PENICILLIN-BINDING COMPONENTS. Other penicillin-sensitive enzymes to which penicillin binds have been reported, namely a D-alanine carboxypeptidase, which cleaves the terminal D-alanine from the peptide chain before cross bridging can occur, and an endopeptidase, which in *Escherichia coli* cleaves the peptide bond between the D-alanine and the diaminopimelic acid. As yet, these enzyme sensitivities cannot be correlated with the bactericidal role of penicillin.

CHEMISTRY OF PENICILLIN. Penicillin (as produced by the mold *Penicillium chrysogenum*) has several limitations: (1) it is easily destroyed by acids and therefore is of limited value when taken orally; (2) it is destroyed by penicillinase, an enzyme formed by many bacteria; (3) it is for the most part effective only against gram-positive bacteria (although notable exceptions include the organisms causing gonorrhea, epidemic meningitis, and syphilis).

Over the past several decades, a great deal of research has been directed toward the problem of chemically overcoming some of these disadvantages without losing the desirable features. This has been accomplished, in part, in two different ways. In the first case, one can alter the type of penicillin produced by the mold by controlling the culture medium. For example, the addition of phenoxyacetic acid to the medium results in the production of phenoxymethyl penicillin, or, as it is frequently called, penicillin V. Penicillin V is much more resistant to hydrolysis by stomach acids than is the usual benzyl penicillin and is, therefore, more effective when taken orally.

A second breakthrough came when it was discovered that all penicillins possess the

**Figure 10-4.** Stereomodels of penicillin, *a*, and of the D-alanyl-D-alanine end of the peptidoglycan strand, *b*. Arrows indicate the position of the CO-N bond in the *β*-lactam ring of penicillin (left) and of the CO-N bond in the D-alanyl-D-alanine. Hydrolysis of the *β*-lactam bond of penicillin by penicillinase changes the structure of the penicillin so that it is no longer an analog of D-alanyl-D-alanine.

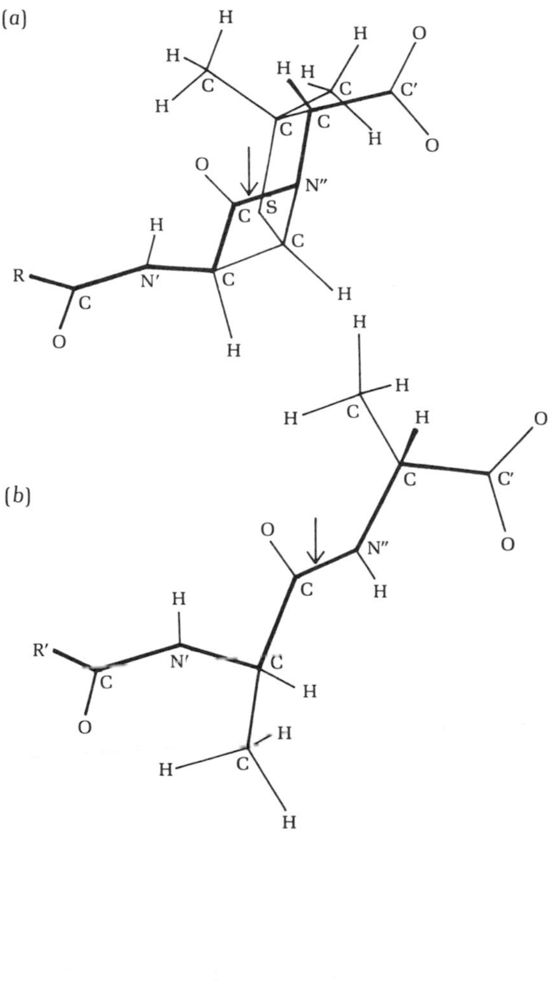

same basic molecular structure. It then became possible to produce semisynthetic penicillins by interrupting the synthesis of penicillin so that only 6-amino penicillanic acid was produced or by enzymatically removing the side groups attached to the 6-amino penicillanic acid. New side groups could then be added which resulted in different properties for the penicillin. The major new advantage was that many of the new semisynthetic penicillins were highly resistant to hydrolysis by the enzyme penicillinase. Figure 10-5 depicts the structures of a few of the natural and semisynthetic penicillins and indicates the N-CO bond of the *β*-lactam ring that is hydrolyzed by penicillinase, destroying the function of the molecule. Several of the semisynthetic penicillins, as illustrated by ampicillin, have overcome the limited spectrum of activity of the normal mold product. Such compounds are called moderate-spectrum antibiotics because they are effective against many gram-negative bacteria as well as gram-positive bacteria (Table 10-2). They are not, however, active against mycoplasmas, rickettsiae, or mycobacteria.

### Cephalosporins

Cephalosporin C was isolated in 1952 as a product of the mold *Cephalosporium*. This antibiotic is less potent than penicillin, although structural similarities to penicillin suggest that its mechanism of action on the bacterial cell is analogous to that of penicillin.

The production of chemical derivatives of the original cephalosporin has resulted in the synthesis of several useful semisynthetic cephalosporins. Their major properties can be summarized as follows: (1) they possess a moderate-spectrum activity against both gram-negative and gram-positive bacteria; (2) although they possess a *β*-lactam ring, they are resistant to hydrolysis by penicillinase; (3) they do not usually cause allergic reactions in individuals who are hypersen-

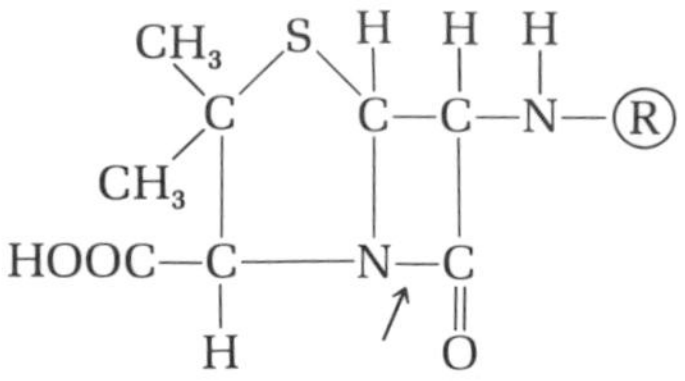

6-Aminopenicillanic acid

| Natural Penicillins | R Prosthetic Group |
|---|---|
| Penicillin G (benzyl penicillin) | 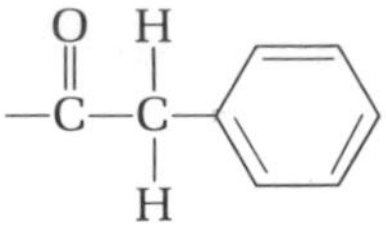 |
| Penicillin V (phenoxymethyl penicillin) | 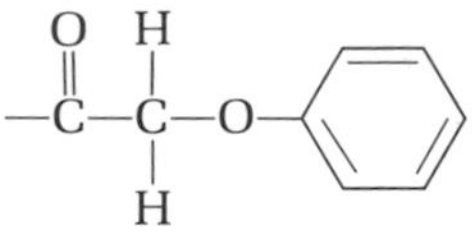 |

Semisynthetic Penicillins

| | |
|---|---|
| Ampicillin (6-[D(—)α amino phenyl acetamido] penicillanic acid) | 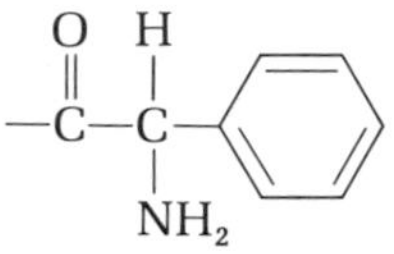 |
| Methicillin (6-[2,6-dimethoxybenzamido] penicillinate monohydrate) | 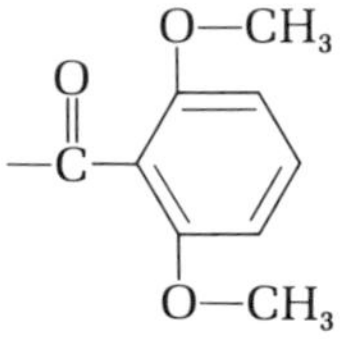 |
| Oxacillin (3-[2-chlorophenyl]-5-methyl-4-isoxazoyl-penicillanic acid) | 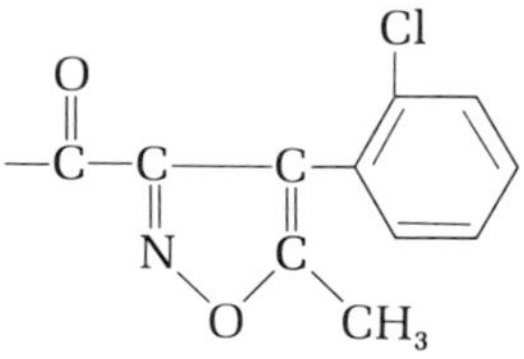 |
| Nafcillin (2-ethoxy-1-naphthyl-penicillanic acid) | 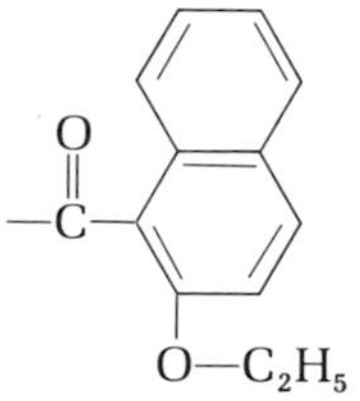 |

**Figure 10-5.** Structures of some natural and semi-synthetic penicillins. Arrow indicates $\beta$-lactam bond that is hydrolyzed by penicillinase and R represents the various side groups present on the different natural and semi-synthetic penicillins.

sitive to penicillin. Their relationship to penicillin can be seen by examining the structure of cephalothin, one of the semisynthetic cephalosporins.

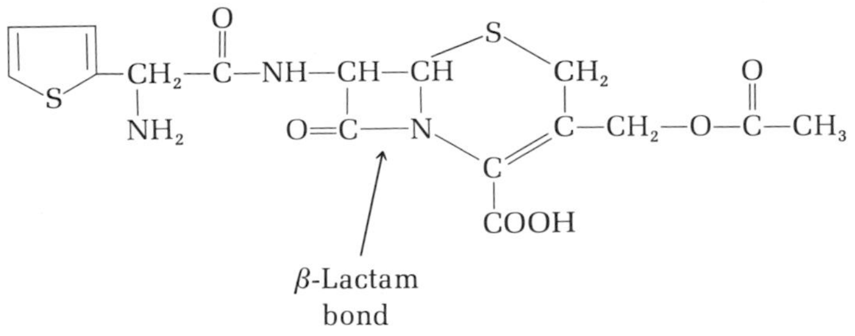

β-Lactam
bond

Cephalothin

## Cycloserine

Cycloserine, also called oxamycin, is structurally related to D-alanine and as such acts as a competitive inhibitor for the following two reactions required for the synthesis of peptidoglycan.

1. L-alanine $\xrightarrow{\text{racemase}}$ D-alanine

2. D-alanine $\xrightarrow{\text{synthetase}}$ D-alanyl-D-alanine

Since cycloserine is a structural analog of D-alanine, its inhibitory effect can be negated by the addition of D-alanine.

## Bacitracin

Bacitracin is a polypeptide antibiotic produced by the spore-forming bacillus *Bacillus*

*licheniformis*. This antibiotic is chiefly bactericidal against gram-positive bacteria, but it is also effective against meningococci and gonococci. However, because of its toxic effect on the kidney, it is administered only under carefully controlled conditions.

Bacitracin inhibits cell-wall peptidoglycan synthesis by blocking the dephosphorylation of the lipid-P-P carrier which transports the newly formed cell wall components from the cytoplasmic membrane to the external wall (see Figure 10-2). When this dephosphorylation is prevented, the lipid can no longer function as a carrier of the cell-wall material and the cell dies in the same manner as does a cell killed by penicillin.

Since this same lipid phosphate carrier is used to transport both the teichoic acids to the cell walls of gram-positive organisms and the specific O antigens to the lipopolysaccharide

**Table 10-2. Major Properties of the Penicillins**

| Antibiotic | Spectrum | Acid Lability | Penicillinase Resistant |
|---|---|---|---|
| Penicillin G | Primarily against gram-positive | Yes | No |
| Penicillin V | Primarily against gram-positive | No | No |
| Ampicillin | Moderate spectrum against both gram-positive & gram-negative | No | No |
| Methicillin | Primarily against gram-positive | Yes | Yes |
| Oxacillin | Primarily against gram-positive | No | Yes |
| Nafcillin | Primarily against gram-positive | No | Yes |

in the outer membrane of gram-negative organisms, bacitracin would also be expected to prevent these reactions. However, neither of these latter cases would be likely to result in a bactericidal effect, since neither cell wall teichoic acid nor specific O antigens appear to be essential to the bacteria in which they are normally found.

### Vancomycin and Ristocetin

Both of these antibiotics are bactericidal against gram-positive bacteria and spirochetes, and both act by inhibiting peptidoglycan biosynthesis. Their modes of action seem to be identical in that they bind tightly to the terminal D-alanyl-D-alanine present in the cell-wall peptidoglycan and thereby prevent transpeptidization but by a different mechanism than penicillin. (see Figure 10-2). Since they appear to possess a strong affinity for this dipeptide portion of the peptidoglycan, it is not surprising that their bactericidal effect can be averted by the addition of D-alanyl-D-alanine.

### ANTIBIOTICS AFFECTING CELL MEMBRANES

The plasma membrane serves as a semipermeable structure that controls the transport of metabolites into and out of the cell. Thus, damage to this structure hampers or destroys its ability to act as an osmotic barrier and also prevents a number of necessary biosynthetic functions from taking place in the membrane. However, many antibiotics that affect bacterial cell membranes are also injurious to mammalian cell membranes. As a result, only a few such agents have been clinically useful.

### Polymyxins

Various polymyxins, designated A, B, C, D, and E, are produced by different strains of *Bacillus polymyxa*. Both B and E may be used effectively against certain gram-negative bacteria, but the other three are too toxic for general use. Polymyxin is a peptide in which one end of the molecule is soluble in lipids and the other end is soluble in water. When it gets into the cell membrane, the water-soluble end remains in the hydrophilic layer, and the lipid-soluble end is dissolved in the hydrophobic part of the membrane. This results in a distortion between the layers of the membrane (see Figure 10-6) allowing substances free passage into and out of the cell.

Polymyxin is particularly effective against infections caused by members of the genus *Pseudomonas*, although it has also been used effectively against infections by *Brucella abortus, Klebsiella pneumoniae,* and *Bordetella pertussis.* Since toxic effects on the kidney, and to a lesser extent the central nervous system, may occur, it is used chiefly when the infective agent is resistant to other less toxic antibiotics.

**Figure 10-6.** Schematic diagram illustrating how polymyxin distorts the cell membrane, destroying its effectiveness as a semipermeable barrier.

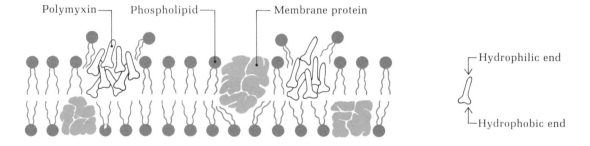

## Nystatin and Amphotericin B

Both of these antibiotics possess large ring structures, and because of the presence of a number of alternating double bonds, they are frequently referred to as the polyene antibiotics.

The polyene antibiotics combine with sterols present in the cell membrane causing disruption and leakage of the cytoplasmic contents. Therefore, they are specifically effective only against the sterol-containing mycoplasmas and the systemic eucaryotic fungal infections. They are ineffective for the treatment of other bacterial infections because bacteria other than mycoplasmas lack sterols in their membranes. Because of their toxicity to the patient, however, they are not used to treat mycoplasma infections.

## ANTIBIOTICS AFFECTING NUCLEIC ACID BIOSYNTHESIS

Any antibiotic that specifically reacts with DNA to prevent its replication or transcription will obviously inhibit cell growth and division. However, many of the antibiotics that possess this potential are not completely selective for the target microorganism and show considerable toxicity to the host's cells.

In general, antibiotics inhibit nucleic-acid synthesis in one of two ways: (1) interaction with the strands of the DNA double helix in a manner that prevents subsequent replication or transcription, or (2) combination with the polymerases involved in these reactions. We shall list here only a few representative antibiotics acting in these ways.

## Mitomycin

This heterocyclic antibiotic is one of a group of compounds that are converted enzymatically in vivo to an alkylating agent that can form cross-links between the two strands of double-stranded DNA. It is believed that mitomycin reacts with the guanine residues and inhibits replication by preventing separation of the DNA strands, thereby preventing them from acting as templates.

Curiously, mitomycin exhibits some selectivity, preventing host-cell DNA replication while permitting viral DNA replication in some instances. It has also been used to cure E. coli of plasmids by allowing bacterial DNA replication while preventing plasmid DNA synthesis. An explanation for these observations is not readily available.

## Nalidixic Acid and Novobiocin

Each of these antibiotics exerts multiple effects on susceptible cells, and the inhibition of DNA replication occurs immediately in the presence of these drugs. Both antibiotics also cause membrane damage and perhaps because the DNA is attached to the membrane, the inhibition of DNA synthesis is a result of the membrane damage.

Nalidixic acid is primarily effective against gram-negative organisms and has been used for the treatment of enteric urinary tract infections. Novobiocin is bactericidal for gram-positive organisms.

## Griseofulvin

Griseofulvin is used to treat superficial dermatophyte infections which destroy the keratin structures in the host. Its mode of action is uncertain, but it has been proposed that griseofulvin inhibits DNA replication. However, it seems surprising that topical application to an infected area is ineffective, and that only after prolonged oral administration, which permits the incorporation of the antibiotic into the newly synthesized keratin, is the antibiotic fungicidal.

## Actinomycin

Within the family of actinomycins, actinomycin D is the best studied and most widely used. Actinomycin D binds to DNA at guanine-cytosine pairs and is inserted into the helix between existing elements. As a result, it prevents both DNA replication and transcription.

Because actinomycin D blocks both eucaryotic and procaryotic DNA functions, it is too toxic for general clinical use. It has been used as a research tool and as a chemotherapeutic drug against cancer.

### Rifampicins and Other Transcription-Inhibiting Antibiotics

Rifampicins form a large family of drugs, of which many have been chemically modified to produce semisynthetic antibiotics. Rifampin, an effective semisynthetic rifampicin, inhibits DNA transcription by binding to the DNA-dependent RNA polymerase. RNA polymerase is composed of five subunits, expressed as $\alpha_2\beta\beta'\sigma$. Different polymerases may possess different sigma factors ($\sigma$), but the core enzyme $\alpha_2\beta\beta'$ appears common in all cases. Rifampin inhibits transcription by binding to the $\beta$ subunit. Once bound, the polymerase can still attach to the promotor region of the DNA, but it is unable to initiate transcription. Mutants resistant to rifampin have been shown to have an altered $\beta$ subunit which no longer binds to rifampin.

Streptovaricin appears to act identically to rifampin, while streptolydigin, which also binds to the $\beta$ subunit of the RNA polymerase, allows initiation but blocks elongation of the chain.

### ANTIBIOTICS AFFECTING PROTEIN SYNTHESIS

Prior to a discussion of specific blocks in protein synthesis caused by antibiotics, a brief review of the major steps in protein biosynthesis may be of value. In general, the sequence of events proceeds as follows:

1. Messenger RNA (mRNA) is transcribed from the DNA.

2. The mRNA binds to the 30S subunit of the ribosome along with GTP and the first amino acid joined to its specific transfer RNA, (formyl-methionyl-tRNA or fMet-tRNA).

3. The 50S subunit of the ribosome joins this complex to produce a 70S ribosome.

4. The fMet-tRNA is transferred from the acceptor site, the A site, to the second site, the peptidyl or P site on the 50S subunit of the ribosome, thus freeing the acceptor site to receive whatever aminoacyl-tRNA (AA-tRNA) is specified on the next mRNA codon. The AA-tRNA recognizes the codon on the mRNA and binds to an acceptor site on the 50S subunit.

5. A peptide bond is formed between the new amino acid in the A site and the amino acid occupying the P site.

6. The ribosome moves along the mRNA to place the next codon in the A site and the last-added AA-tRNA in the P site. This movement is called translocation and requires an elongation factor (EF) plus an energy source derived from the hydrolysis of the terminal high-energy phosphate bond in guanosine triphosphate (GTP).

7. Finally, after all the amino acids for a given polypeptide have been joined by peptide bonds, the ribosome reaches a termination codon on the mRNA, and the completed polypeptide molecule is released from the ribosome.

8. A polypeptide may, by itself, be a complete protein molecule, or it may join with other like or unlike polypeptides to complete a protein such as DNA-dependent RNA polymerase or hemoglobin.

Blockage of any one of these steps (including the activation of each amino acid to form an aminoacyl-tRNA) will result in the cessation of protein synthesis and the eventual death of the cell. Since the steps in eucaryotic protein synthesis are essentially identical to those described for bacteria, one might wonder why so many antibiotics display a selective inhibition of bacterial protein synthesis. The answer appears to lie in the fact that eucaryotic ribosomes are 80S structures made up of 40S and 60S subunits, and many of the protein-inhibiting antibiotics do not react with proteins in these ribosomes. The following section will describe some of the major antibiotics effective in blocking microbial protein biosynthesis.

## Antibiotics Reacting with the 50S Ribosomal Subunit

CHLORAMPHENICOL. This antibiotic is produced by the actinomycete *Streptomyces venezuelae* but due to its comparatively simple structure, chloramphenicol is synthesized chemically rather than isolated as a product of microbial metabolism.

$$O_2N \underset{\phantom{x}}{\overset{\phantom{x}}{\bigcirc}} \overset{OH}{\underset{H}{C}} \overset{CH_2OH}{\underset{H}{C}} \overset{\phantom{x}}{\underset{H}{N}} \overset{O}{C} CHCl_2$$

Chloramphenicol

Chloramphenicol is a broad-spectrum antibiotic, effective against gram-positive and gram-negative bacteria as well as mycoplasmas, rickettsiae, and chlamydiae. Unlike penicillin, its effect is bacteriostatic rather than bactericidal. It exerts this effect by binding to the 50S portion of the ribosome, where it inhibits the enzyme peptidyl transferase. It is this enzyme that catalyzes the formation of a peptide bond between the new amino acid, which is attached via its tRNA to the A site on the ribosome, and the last amino acid, which still occupies the P site of the ribosome. As a result, protein synthesis stops.

The use of chloramphenicol is not, however, without some danger. In some persons it suppresses cells of the bone marrow and produces aplastic anemia (loss of stem cells that are precursors to red blood cells); even though this occurs rarely, it is a serious complication.

MACROLIDE ANTIBIOTICS. Antibiotics of this large family are characterized by the possession of a large lactone ring in their structures. They include such antibiotics as erythromycin, oleandomycin, carbomycin, and spiramycin. All prevent protein synthesis by reacting with the 50S subunit of the ribosome, and all appear to possess a similar mechanism of inhibition. The bacterial spectrum of the macrolide antibiotics is similar to that of penicillin and they are useful in patients allergic to the latter drug. Macrolides are also effective for the treatment of mycoplasma infections.

Erythromycin acts very much like chloramphenicol in that it prevents peptide-bond formation between the two amino acids bound to the 50S subunit of the ribosome. However, other aspects of the action of erythromycin are not completely clear, and there is good evidence that erythromycin also blocks the translocation reaction on the 50S subunit.

LINCOMYCIN. Like some other 50S subunit-binding antibiotics, lincomycin competes with chloramphenicol for a binding site on the ribosome. Thus, it would also appear to inhibit peptide-bond formation. Unlike chloramphenicol, however, lincomycin causes the breakdown of existing polysomes (multiple ribosomes on an mRNA molecule) and the dissociation of the resulting ribosomes into their 30S and 50S subunits.

Lincomycin is most effective against gram-positive bacteria and can replace penicillin for the treatment of some infections in cases of allergy to penicillin. However, it is considerably more toxic than erythromycin and should therefore be reserved for pathogens that are resistant to the macrolides.

PUROMYCIN. This antibiotic prevents protein synthesis by binding to the 50S subunit of the ribosome, causing a premature release of the partially formed protein. It is able to do this because it is a structural analog of the aminoacyl end of tRNA. Thus, a peptide bond is formed between puromycin and the last amino acid. The ribosome then moves so that puromycin occupies the P site, but the binding between puromycin and the ribosome is not sufficiently strong to hold the protein to the ribosome. As a result, the nascent peptide chain is released from the ribosome.

## Antibiotics Reacting with the 30S Subunit of the Ribosome

The 30S subunit of the ribosome provides the attachment site for mRNA and for the aminoacyl-tRNA's. Any substance that inhibits these functions will prevent protein synthesis.

STREPTOMYCIN. Streptomycin exerts a bactericidal effect on a large number of gram-positive and gram-negative organisms, and is widely used for the treatment of tuberculosis (see Figure 10-7 for structure). As a result of its very basic guanidino groups, streptomycin causes a variety of nonspecific effects such as an efflux of potassium from the cells or, in larger amounts, actual agglutination of the bacteria. However, its specific bactericidal effect depends on its ability to specifically bind to one of the proteins in the 30S subunit of the ribosome. This binding results in two major effects on protein synthesis: (1) it causes a misreading of the mRNA; and (2) it prevents the movement of the first aminoacyl-tRNA (which in bacterial systems is always formyl-methionine) from the A site to the P site on the ribosome. The result is that the mRNA can take on only a single ribosome at its initiation site, and that ribosome cannot move.

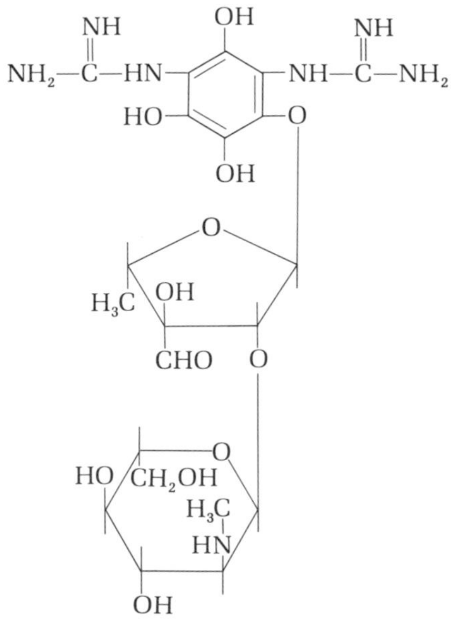

One might wonder which of the above effects exerts the bactericidal action of streptomycin. The misreading has been shown to occur using synthetic polynucleotides as mRNA's; one can show that in the presence of streptomycin an isoleucine is inserted instead of phenylalanine, the correct amino acid. Such misreading undoubtedly occurs in an *in vivo* situation, but one would not ordinarily expect this effect to be completely lethal. Thus, it is generally assumed that the irreversible binding of streptomycin causing the freezing of the initiation complex accounts for most of the bactericidal activity of streptomycin.

Curiously, one can isolate mutant bacteria that are completely resistant to streptomycin or that are dependent upon its presence for growth. The resistant organisms can be shown to have an altered protein that will no longer react with streptomycin in their 30S subunits. The mechanism of streptomycin dependence is not readily apparent, but it is postulated that the ribosome has undergone a configurational change that causes misreading of the mRNA. The addition of streptomycin is thought to correct this malfunction, permitting the correct translation of codons along the mRNA.

**Figure 10-7.** Structure of streptomycin.

OTHER AMINOGLYCOSIDE ANTIBIOTICS. There are a number of antibiotics which, like streptomycin, contain carbohydrates and basic amino groups in their structures. The most common of these aminoglycosides include neomycin, kanamycin, gentamycin, and spectinomycin. All except spectinomycin are bactericidal, and all react with the 30S subunit of the ribosome. Spectinomycin is bacteriostatic, probably because its reaction with the ribosome is reversible and because it does not cause misreading of the mRNA. The other aminoglycosides cause a greater degree of misreading than streptomycin, and since they bind irreversibly with the 30S subunit, it appears their bactericidal effect is similar to that of streptomycin. Unfortunately, the aminoglycosides may be toxic to the eighth cranial nerve and, in some cases, to the kidney.

TETRACYCLINES. There are a half dozen tetracyclines, which differ from each other by modifications of several side groups on the tetracycline structure, as illustrated in Figure 10-8. All are broad-spectrum antibiotics that exert a bacteriostatic effect against all pathogenic procaryotes except the mycobacteria. They inhibit protein synthesis by binding to the 30S subunit of the ribosome, preventing the attachment of the aminoacyl-tRNA to the mRNA.

## MECHANISMS OF DRUG RESISTANCE

Microorganisms become resistant to drugs by one of two general mechanisms: (1) a mutation that alters the cellular target site of the antibiotic, or (2) the acquisition of the ability to chemically modify the antibiotic, thereby destroying its inhibitory effect.

The first type of resistance is often found in laboratory-derived resistant strains but less frequently seen in clinical isolates. On the other hand, resistance based on the ability to modify the antibiotic is seen only in clinical isolates of drug-resistant organisms, and such resistance is normally coded for by extrachromosomal plasmids or episomes. Accordingly this latter type of resistance is readily transferred among related organisms by either conjugation or transduction.

### Resistance Involving Chromosomal Mutations

Many mutations causing resistance to an antibiotic are the result of alterations creating components that no longer bind the antibiotic. For example, a mutation causing the substitution of a single amino acid in protein S-12 of the 30S ribosomal subunit of *Escherichia coli* prevents the binding of streptomycin, thereby conferring resistance to that antibiotic. Similarly, alteration in protein S-5 in the 30S ribosomal subunit provides resistance to aminoglycosides such as neomycin and kanamycin. Alteration of a 50S

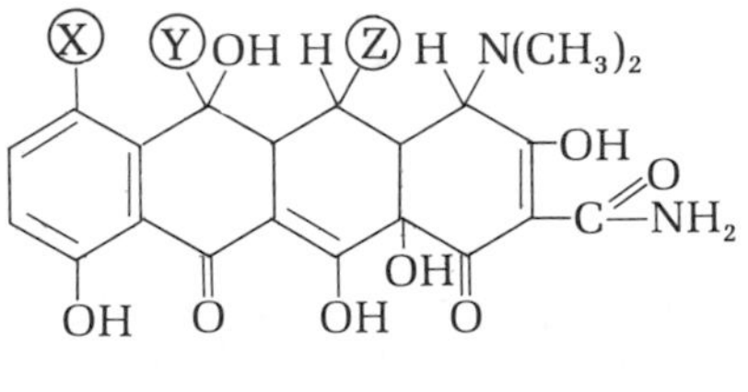

**Figure 10-8.** Structure of several important tetracyclines.

| Antibiotic | X | Y | Z |
|---|---|---|---|
| Tetracycline | —H | —CH$_3$ | —H |
| Oxytetracycline | —H | —CH$_3$ | —OH |
| Chlortetracycline | —Cl | —CH$_3$ | —H |
| Minocycline | —N(CH$_3$)$_2$ | —H | —H |

ribosomal protein provides erythromycin resistance to both *E. coli* and *Bacillus subtilis;* however, erythromycin resistance in *Staphylococcus aureus* is reported to result from an alteration of the ribosomal RNA. Fusidic-acid (produced by the mold *Cephalosporium acremonium*) resistance occurs in mutants with an altered G elongation factor (involved in translocation of the ribosome) which no longer binds the antibiotic, allowing such mutants to function normally in the translocation reaction.

Rifampin and streptolydigin resistance appears to result from an altered $\beta$ subunit in the RNA polymerase which will no longer bind these antibiotics.

In some cases, resistance may result from the inability of the organism to transport the antibiotic into the cell. Cycloserine resistance is reported to occur by this mechanism.

### Resistance Involving Extrachromosomal Plasmids

Plasmid-coded resistance was originally shown in the genus *Shigella* isolated in Japan from cases of bacillary dysentery. These isolates were resistant to multiple antibiotics such as chloramphenicol, streptomycin, tetracycline, and the sulfonamides. When resistant strains of *Shigella* were mixed with antibiotic-sensitive strains of *Escherichia,* the multiple resistance was transferred to the sensitive organisms. This resistance is encoded on extrachromosomal plasmids which, because of their rapid transfer during conjugation to antibiotic-sensitive strains, are called resistance transfer factors (RTF).

This type of infectious drug resistance is worldwide and has been reported to confer resistance to such antibiotics as streptomycin, chloramphenicol, tetracycline, neomycin, kanamycin, ampicillin, and the sulfonamides.

Gram-positive bacteria also possess plasmids that provide multiple antibiotic resistance. A staphylococcus may possess several plasmids capable of conferring resistance to penicillin, erythromycin, chloramphenicol, tetracycline, streptomycin, and others. However, unlike the resistance factors in the gram-negative organisms, these plasmids are transferred to sensitive strains only by transduction.

### Biochemical Mechanisms of Plasmid-Coded Resistance

Most plasmid-coded resistance results from the synthesis of enzymes that modify an antibiotic so that it can no longer react with its normal target site in the cell. The following will illustrate general types of plasmid-coded enzymes involved in antibiotic modification.

PENICILLIN AND THE CEPHALOSPORINS. These drugs are named $\beta$-lactam antibiotics, inasmuch as it is the presence of the $\beta$-lactam ring that makes them structural analogs of D-alanyl-D-alanine. Many gram-positive and gram-negative bacteria produce a $\beta$-lactamase (penicillinase) which hydrolyzes the $\beta$-lactam bond, as shown in Figure 10-5. Gram-positive organisms produce penicillinase as an inducible enzyme which is secreted into the extracellular environment. Gram-negative penicillinase producers constitutively form a penicillinase that remains bound to the cell. Bacterial resistance to methicillin, a penicillinase-resistant semisynthetic penicillin, occurs by a mechanism as yet unknown.

AMINOGLYCOSIDES. There are a number of different enzymes that inactivate the various aminoglycoside antibiotics by the addition of chemical groups to the antibiotic. The three major mechanisms include: (1) acetylation of amino groups, (2) phosphorylation of hydroxyl groups, and (3) adenylation of hydroxyl groups. Table 10-3 lists the modifying enzymes for the aminoglycosides.

CHLORAMPHENICOL. The inactivation of chloramphenicol is catalyzed by an RTF-coded transacetylase that transfers the acetyl group from acetyl-coenzyme A, as shown in

## Table 10-3. Aminoglycoside Modifying Enzymes

| Enzyme | Bacterial source | Modification |
|---|---|---|
| Kanamycin acetyltransferase (KAcT) | R+ E. coli P. aeruginosa | 6-amino group of an amino hexose is acetylated |
| Gentamicin acetyltransferase I (GAcT I) | P. aeruginosa K. pneumoniae E. coli | 3-amino group of 2-deoxystreptamine is acetylated |
| Gentamicin acetyltransferase II (GAcT II) | Providencia | 2-amino group of an amino hexose is acetylated |
| Streptomycin-spectinomycin adenylyltransferase (SAdt) | R+ E. coli | hydroxyl group of a D-threo methylamino alcohol moiety is adenylylated |
| Gentamicin adenylyltransferase (GAdt) | R+ E. coli R+ K. pneumoniae | 2-hydroxyl group of an amino hexose is adenylylated |
| Streptomycin phosphotransferase (SPT) | R+ E. coli S. aureus P. aeruginosa | 3-hydroxy group of N-methyl L-glucosamine is phosphorylated |
| Neomycin-kanamycin I phosphotransferase (NPT) II | R+ E. coli P. aeruginosa S. aureus | 3-hydroxyl group of an amino hexose is phosphorylated |
| Lividomycin phosphotransferase (LvPT) | P. aeruginosa R+ E. coli | 5-hydroxyl group of D-ribose is phosphorylated |

Figure 10-9. Neither the chloramphenicol-3-acetate nor the 1,3-diacetate possesses antibacterial activity.

TETRACYCLINE. The mechanism of plasmid-coded resistance to the tetracyclines is not well understood. The antibiotic does not appear to be chemically altered, and resistance may result from a decreased permeability to the antibiotic by RTF-carrying strains.

SULFONAMIDES. Plasmid-mediated resistance to the sulfonamides also appears to be due to a decreased permeability of R+ strains to the drugs, but this has been shown only for E. coli.

### Control of Resistant Organisms

How may the problem of drug resistance be solved? There is certainly no single answer, but several measures have been proposed for reducing the development of resistant strains. A most significant point is the avoidance of the indiscriminate use of antibiotics. Because antibiotics act as selective agents for resistant organisms, wide and indiscriminate use soon results in the death of all sensitive strains, with only resistant strains left to infect new hosts. Moreover, the dose administered should be adequate to control the microbe population as quickly as possible. The faster the organisms are inhibited, the less chance there is for the emergence of stepwise mutations to high levels of antibiotic resistance.

Another measure sometimes effective is the simultaneous use of a combination of two or more drugs. In this case, a mutant becoming resistant to one drug would still be inhibited by the second antibiotic. However, because certain antibiotics tend to have mutually an-

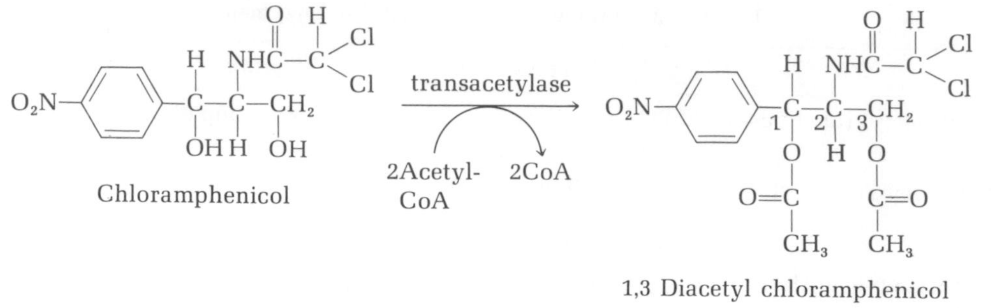

**Figure 10-9.** Inactivation of chloramphenicol by the acetylation of the antibiotic. Chloramphenicol-3-acetate is formed first, and the 1,3-diacetate forms later. Neither the mono- nor the diacetylated antibiotic possesses antibacterial activity.

tagonistic effects, there should be clinical proof of their effectiveness in combination before use. A desirable combination is exemplified by the use of streptomycin and isoniazid or para-aminosalicyclic acid in the treatment of tuberculosis. A third measure that is usually effective is to discontinue the use of the drug for a few months. This enables susceptible strains to replace resistant strains in the environment.

### Laboratory Test for Antibiotic Sensitivity

A physician frequently must know to which antibiotic a particular organism is most sensitive to make a decision concerning the treatment of a patient. Two general techniques are used in clinical laboratories for providing this information. The easiest and most common method is to inoculate a tube of melted agar medium with the organism to be tested and to pour this inoculated medium into a petri dish. After the agar has solidified, a multilobed disc that has been impregnated with different antibiotics is laid on the top of the agar (see Figure 10-10). The antibiotic in each lobe of the disc diffuses into the medium, and if the organism is sensitive to a particular antibiotic, no growth occurs in the zone surrounding the lobe. This test provides a qualitative answer to antibiotic sensitivity of a particular bacterium.

A more quantitative approach is to use the tube-dilution technique. In this procedure, the antibiotic in question is diluted out in a broth growth medium in a series of twofold dilutions. The tubes are then inoculated with a standard number of bacteria, and the minimal inhibitory concentration (MIC) is determined by observing the minimal concentration of the antibiotic that prevents growth.

### COMPLICATIONS OF CHEMOTHERAPY

A serious problem encountered with many of the chemotherapeutic agents is that some patients develop allergies to them. This type of hypersensitivity elicits various reactions, of which skin rashes and fever are the most common manifestations.

Penicillin is one of the least toxic and most potent of the antibiotics, and it can be taken by many people with no undesirable results. However, there are allergic reactions to penicillin, including skin rashes, serum sickness (fever and joint pain), and death.

In addition to the hypersensitivity reactions just described, several chemotherapeutic agents may give rise to severe toxic reactions. For example, the toxic effects of streptomycin taken over a prolonged period of time may result in dizziness or nerve damage (8th cranial nerve) which affects

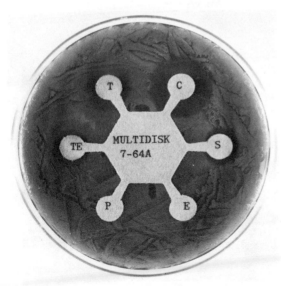

**Figure 10-10.** Multilobed antibiotic sensitivity disc. Note the inhibition around C, lesser inhibition around T, TE, and S, and lack of inhibition around P and E. (C = chloramphenicol, T = oxytetracycline, TE = tetracycline, S = dihydrostreptomycin, P = penicillin, and E = erythromycin.)

hearing. A toxic effect on the kidney has been noted with several agents, particularly the polymyxins.

The long-term use of the broad-spectrum antibiotics provokes another side effect. In these cases, one may find that the normal flora of the body is disrupted and, as a result, yeast such as *Candida albicans* may take over and flourish. Also, when urinary tract infections are treated with broad-spectrum antibiotics, antibiotic-resistant strains of the gram-negative enteric *Proteus* may take over and be very difficult to eradicate. Such infections are sometimes called superinfections.

It is apparent that the availability of antibiotics has drastically changed the relationship between pathogenic microorganisms and the hosts in which they cause disease. However, as will become apparent from reading the following unit of this text, our major defense against infectious diseases lies in our immune system, and antibiotics alone are unable to prevent death in those individuals who are born with or develop a severe defect in their immune system.

## REFERENCES

Benveniste, R., and J. Davies. 1973. Mechanisms of antibiotic resistance in bacteria. *Annu. Rev. Biochem.* **42:**471–506.

Blumberg, P. M., and J. L. Strominger. 1974. Interaction of penicillin with the bacterial cell: Penicillin binding proteins and penicillin sensitive enzymes. *Bacteriol. Rev.* **38:**291–335.

Clowes, R. C. 1973. The molecule of infectious drug resistance. *Sci. American* **228:**18–27.

Corcoran. J. W., and F. E. Hahn, eds. 1974. *Mechanism of Action of Antimicrobial and Antitumor Agents.* Springer-Verlag, New York.

Hamilton-Miller, J. M. T. 1973. Chemistry and biology of the polyene macrolide antibiotics. *Bacteriol. Rev.* **37:**166–196.

Helinski, D. R. 1973. Plasmid-determined resistance to antibiotics: Molecular properties of R-factors. *Annu. Rev. Microbiol.* **27:**437–470.

Kucers, A., and N. McK. Bennett. 1975. *The Use of Antibiotics,* 2nd ed. J. B. Lippincott, Philadelphia.

Nayler, J. H. C. 1973. Advances in penicillin research. *Adv. in Drug Res.* **7:**1–105.

Salton, M. R. J., and A. Tomasz, eds. 1974. Mode of action of antibiotics on microbial walls and membranes. *Ann. New York Acad. Sci.,* **235.**

Sobell, H. M. 1974. How actinomycin binds to DNA. *Sci. American* **231:**82–91.

Wehrli, W. and M. Staehlin. 1971. Actions of the rifamycins. *Bacteriol. Rev.* **35:**290–309.

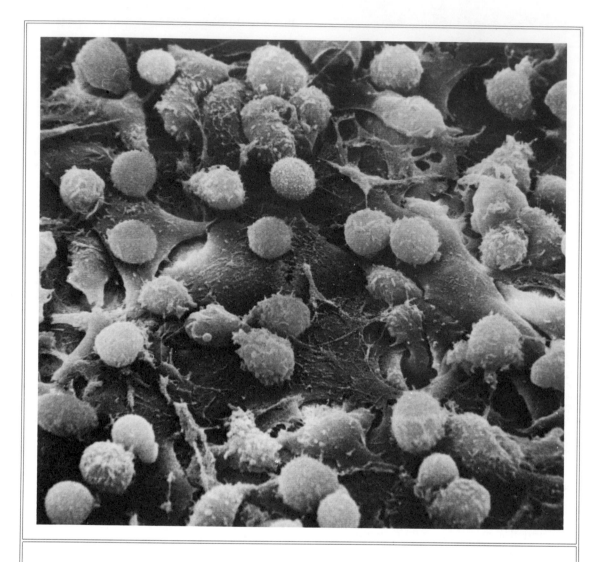

# UNIT TWO

# Immunology

$E$ ARLY medical observations noted that recovery from disease frequently resulted in a "specific immunity" to reinfection. This undoubtedly led to the ancient custom of variolation, in which children were intentionally infected with dried smallpox scabs to "get it over with," for this universal and frequently fatal disease. The first major advance in the control of infectious diseases came with the realization that specific immunity to a serious disease could occasionally be induced by exposing an individual to a related, but milder, disease, as when Jenner noted that milkmaids who had had cowpox did not get smallpox. A practical application of this knowledge took place in 1796 when Jenner injected fluid from an infected cowpox lesion to give a subclinical infection that induced a specific immunity to smallpox.

After Jenner's remarkable discovery about a hundred years elapsed before the germ theory of disease acquired a sufficiently respectable position in the medical profession to permit the scientist to think in terms of disease prevention. Immunology, the study of immunity, truly began when Pasteur discovered that organisms causing diseases such as fowl cholera, anthrax, and rabies could be "altered" in the laboratory so that they would no longer produce serious disease but, like Jenner's cowpox, would induce a specific immune response. We now know that this alteration resulted from the selection of an avirulent mutant—a technique that subsequently gave rise to many successful attenuated vaccines.

The real breakthrough for immunologists followed the discovery that diseases such as tetanus and diphtheria were caused by organisms that secrete powerful toxins and that the injection of minute amounts of these toxins induced immunity to the disease. Moreover, this immunity was found to be the result of antibodies in the serum, which react with and neutralize the toxin. Even more astonishingly, when such an immune serum from one person was injected into another, the recipient exhibited a similar but transient immunity.

These observations opened the entire field of specific serum therapy. Inactivated toxins and vaccines were used to immunize animals, and their sera subsequently were used to treat the corresponding infection in humans. In fact, until the advent of the sulfonamides and antibiotics in the second quarter of the twentieth century, specific serum therapy was the only effective treatment available for many microbial infections.

By the 1930s, it was possible to categorize the various types of specific immunity due to the presence of circulating antibodies, as shown below.

*Passive immunity*

Natural passive:   Antibody crosses the placenta from mother to fetus

Artificial passive:   Antibody is received by the injection of antiserum

*Active immunity*

Natural active:   Antibody is synthesized as a result of an infection

Artificial active:   Antibody is synthesized following the use of a vaccine

It was soon learned that antibody is metabolized by the body and that in the absence of a continued synthesis, effective immunity from passively transferred antibody lasts only about six weeks. The newborn, however, has a lesser ability to metabolize the antibodies passively received from the mother and as a result may possess the

139

mother's specific immunity for a period of three to six months. Long-term specific immunity, however, requires the stimulation of the immune system to synthesize its own antibodies.

A different type of immunity was described by Robert Koch during the 1890's from observations that reinfection of an animal with tubercle bacilli resulted in the localization and killing of the organisms. However, unlike immunity transferred with serum, this immunity could be transferred only with live cells. Only during the past decade has insight been gained into the mechanism of this specific cellular-type immunity.

Last to be appreciated, or at least studied as a major mechanism of defense, are the factors which contribute to nonspecific immunity. Appreciation of some of these factors has followed the study of individuals with either genetic or acquired defects in their nonspecific immune systems.

In this brief introduction we have divided the activities of the immune system into three general types: (1) a specific immunity mediated by soluble factors (antibodies) in the serum; (2) a specific immunity mediated by viable lymphoid cells; and (3) nonspecific immune mechanisms. However, it must be emphasized that nature does not segregate biological systems into isolated units but rather provides a continuum that the scientist artificially dissociates into parts. For our study, we shall proceed to dissect the immune system and when finished, we hope to find that these subunits will reassemble to provide an over-all comprehension of immunity.

## REFERENCES

Abramoff, P., and M. La Via. 1970. *The Biology of the Immune Response.* McGraw-Hill, New York.

Barrett, J. T. 1974. *Textbook of Immunology,* 2nd ed. C. V. Mosby, St. Louis.

Bellanti, J. A. 1971. *Immunology.* W. B. Saunders, Philadelphia.

Bigley, N. J. 1975. *Immunologic Fundamentals.* Year Book Medical Publishers, Chicago.

Borek, F., ed. 1972. *Immunogenicity.* North-Holland Pub., Amsterdam.

Carr, I. 1972. *Biologic Defense Mechanisms.* Blackwell Scientific Pub., Oxford.

Cooper, E. L. 1976. *Comparative Immunology: Foundations of Immunology Series.* Prentice-Hall, Englewood Cliffs, N.J.

Eisen, H. N. 1974. *Immunology.* Harper and Row, New York.

Freedman, S. O., and Gold, P. 1976. *Clinical Immunology,* 2nd ed. Harper and Row, New York.

Gordon, B. L., 1974. *Essentials of Immunology,* 2nd ed. F. A. Davis, Philadelphia.

Guttman, R. D., ed. 1972. *Immunology.* Medcom Press, New York.

Hobart, M. S., and D. McConnell, eds. 1976. *The Immune System.* Blackwell Scientific Pub., Oxford.

Holborow, E. J. 1973. *An ABC of Modern Immunology,* 2nd ed. Little, Brown and Co., Boston.

Hudson, L., and F. C. Hay. 1976. *Practical Immunology.* Blackwell Scientific Pub., Oxford.

Roitt, I. M. 1974. *Essential Immunology,* 2nd ed. Blackwell Scientific Pub., Oxford.

Rose, N. R., F. Milgrom, and C. J. van Oss, eds. 1973. *Fundamentals of Immunology.* Macmillan, New York.

Rose, N. R., and H. Friedman. 1976. *Manual of Clinical Immunology.* Amer. Soc. Microbiol., Washington, D.C.

Sercarz, E. E., A. R. Williamson, and C. F. Fox. 1974. *The Immune System.* Academic Press, New York.

Smith, E. E., and D. W. Ribbons, eds. 1975. *Molecular Approaches to Immunology.* Academic Press, New York.

# 11

## Microbial Invasiveness and Nonspecific Host Resistance

To discuss immunity or, more specifically, the mechanisms by which a host can protect itself from and combat infectious diseases, it is necessary to "put the cart before the horse." In other words, we must know something about microbial invasiveness to delineate what countermeasures may be used by the host, and we must also distinguish between infection and disease. All of us are "infected" from birth until death— our normal flora is actually an infection since these organisms obtain their nutrients from the host on which they live. Disease occurs when an organism invades an area of the body that is normally sterile or if a microbe not part of the normal flora becomes established in a site where it can cause harm to the host. This difference between infection and disease is important, particularly because an individual may harbor organisms which, although they do not harm that person, may provide a source of infection and disease to others. In this chapter, we shall discuss the general properties that enable an organism to cause disease and the nonspecific mechanisms of resistance available to the host to eliminate or control these harmful invaders.

## Microbial Invasion

### HOW PATHOGENS ENTER AND LEAVE THE BODY

In general, infective microbes are carried in secretions and excretions from infected areas. In some illnesses (such as malaria, yellow fever, the viral encephalitides, Rocky Mountain spotted fever, typhus, and plague) the body exit site may not be obvious, since the organisms are present in the blood and require a mosquito, tick, or louse for transmission to another host. However, whether it is obvious or not, each disease-producing organism has its own portal or portals of entry as well as a means of escape from the host.

Microorganisms enter the body through the following areas:

141

1. Respiratory tract via the nose and mouth. This is the portal of entrance for microbes causing respiratory diseases such as the common cold, measles, pneumonia, and tuberculosis.

2. Gastrointestinal tract via the mouth. Examples include agents responsible for typhoid fever, paratyphoid fever, dysentery, cholera, polio, and infectious hepatitis, as well as many foodborne illnesses such as botulism and staphylococcal food poisoning.

3. Skin and mucous membranes. Although the skin provides an effective barrier, some organisms appear capable of penetrating the intact skin; in addition, minor breaks frequently occur, allowing the entrance of many organisms. The staphylococcus that causes boils and furuncles is one of the more frequent organisms entering by this route; however, streptococci may also cause spreading skin infections. Tularemia and anthrax are examples of severe systemic diseases usually contracted through the skin from handling infected animals or animal products.

4. Genitourinary system. The mucous membranes of the genital tract are the site for invasion by agents causing venereal diseases such as gonorrhea and syphilis. In addition, the urinary tract may be infected by microorganisms originating in the blood and infecting the kidney or by the introduction of organisms into the bladder during catheterization.

5. Blood. Those organisms that must be introduced directly into the blood to cause disease usually are transmitted from one individual to another by insects that penetrate the protective skin barrier with their bites. In addition to those mentioned earlier, our advancing civilization has added another way for direct blood inoculation: inadequately sterilized syringes and needles. Also, many cases of hepatitis (particularly serum hepatitis) have been transmitted by using whole blood from individuals who

are asymptomatic carriers of the hepatitis virus in their blood.

The portals of exit for a disease agent are usually the same as their portals of entry. Thus, diseases of the respiratory tract are spread by way of secretions and excretions of the respiratory tract and mouth. Similarly, microorganisms causing enteric infections leave the body by the intestinal tract and are spread through fecal contamination. Skin or wound infections may be spread by drainage from these areas either directly to another person or through contamination of some inanimate object. Blood infections, which are spread by insects or contaminated needles or syringes, usually leave the individual in a similar fashion, through direct contact with a needle or syringe during the withdrawal of blood or by the ingestion of the microorganisms by a biting insect.

## PROOF OF THE ETIOLOGY
## OF A DISEASE

The isolation of a particular organism from an infected person does not establish proof that it is the causative agent of the disease; it may exist in or near a lesion merely as normal flora or as a transient contaminant. In the late nineteenth century, Robert Koch established rules for determining whether or not an isolated organism is indeed the pathogen. These four rules, called Koch's postulates, can be summarized as follows:

1. The same organism must be found in all cases of a given disease.

2. The organism must be isolated and grown in pure culture from the infected person.

3. The organisms from the pure culture must reproduce the disease when inoculated into a susceptible animal.

4. The organism then must be isolated in pure culture from the experimentally infected animal.

Although these postulates have been

effective in establishing the causative agents for most bacterial diseases, there are a few exceptions. For example, neither *Treponema pallidum*, the causative agent for syphilis, nor *Mycobacterium leprae*, the etiologic agent of leprosy, have been grown in pure culture on artificial media. Thus even though there is no doubt as to the etiology of these diseases, only the first postulate is fulfilled.

## Major Properties of Pathogenic Bacteria

Pathogenicity is defined as the ability of a microorganism to cause disease; virulence refers to the extent of pathogenicity. Thus, strictly speaking, virulence is a measure of pathogenicity, although many people tend to use the two words interchangeably. For an organism to be pathogenic or virulent, in other words to invade and cause disease, it must possess certain characteristics or properties not possessed by the saprophytic organisms. In many cases, the properties conferring virulence to an organism are either unknown or unclear. However, some bacteria are known to have special structures that protect them from the host's defenses, while others may secrete substances that contribute to their virulence. Some of the factors believed to contribute to pathogenicity are described below.

**Figure 11-1.** Encapsulated cells of *Streptococcus pneumoniae*. The capsules around the pairs of cells are swollen by use of type-specific antibody (see Chapter 18).

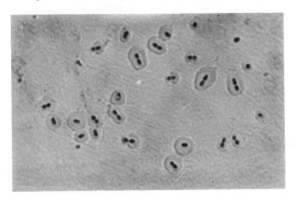

### CAPSULES

Some pathogenic bacteria possess a large capsule surrounding their cell walls (see Figure 11-1). The ability of these organisms to produce disease depends upon the presence of this capsule, and loss of the capsule (as a result of mutation) invariably results in a concomitant loss of the ability to produce disease. The possession of a capsule contributes to an organism's disease-producing potential by preventing phagocytosis, engulfment of the encapsulated organisms by the host's leukocytes (white blood cells). The exact reason for this anti-phagocytic activity is not known, but it seems to be due to surface properties of the capsule which prevent the phagocyte from forming a sufficiently intimate contact with the microorganism to allow phagocytosis to take place. As we shall see later in this unit, the presence of specific antibodies to the capsular material provides receptors for the phagocyte and permits phagocytosis to occur. For example, immunity to infection by *Streptococcus pneumoniae* depends on antibody to the microorganism's capsule, and in the presence of this antibody the invading organism is rapidly engulfed and destroyed by the host's leukocytes. The chemistry of some of these capsules is discussed in Chapter 3.

### PILI OR FIMBRIAE

We shall use the terms pili and fimbriae synonomously—and immediately point out that just as many nonpathogenic bacteria possess capsules, so do many non-disease-producing bacteria possess pili. This obviously demonstrates that neither capsules nor pili are sole determinants for the virulence of microorganisms. However, it is known that the possession of pili endows an organism with an enhanced ability to adhere to other bacteria and to the membranes of the host's cells and phagocytes. Thus, in at least several instances (such as *Neisseria gonorrhoeae,* the cause of gonorrhea, and enteropathic *Escherichia coli,* a cause of gastroenteritis) the possession of pili appears to be associated with virulent strains.

## EXOTOXINS

Many pathogenic organisms do not possess anti-phagocytic structures such as capsules or pili but have other characteristics that permit them to overcome normal host defenses. These include for many microbes the production and secretion of toxic substances. Some of these products, called exotoxins, are responsible for the symptoms of such diseases as diphtheria, tetanus, gas gangrene, scarlet fever, and the staphylcoccal scalded skin syndrome. In addition, certain types of food poisoning, such as those caused by *Clostridium botulinum, Clostridium perfringens,* and *Staphylococcus aureus,* are also due to the presence of exotoxic substances.

There are other pathogenic organisms that neither possess anti-phagocytic capsules nor produce exotoxins. With these it is somewhat more difficult to pinpoint the properties responsible for invasiveness. However, an array of substances (some of which are enzymes) secreted by various bacteria may play an important role in their ability to cause disease. Many of these substances have not been isolated, purified, or chemically characterized, and they have been given names based on observations of the biological or chemical activities of crude materials. A few of the more commonly found extracellular products include various hemolysins, which lyse red blood cells; leukocidins, which kill leukocytes; hyaluronidase, which hydrolyzes the hyaluronic acid of connective tissue; collagenase, which hydrolyzes collagen; coagulase, which coagulates plasma to form fibrin clots; and streptokinase, an enzyme that indirectly lyses plasma clots. Still another type of excreted virulence factor is exemplified by siderophores. These are phenolates or hydroxamates that, in some cases, can successfully obtain microbial growth-essential iron from transferrin or lactoferrin of the host.

## ENDOTOXINS

Endotoxins are large molecules of lipopolysaccharide that are normal components of the cell walls of all gram-negative organisms. They are not excreted by the cell into the surrounding environment like exotoxins, but they are liberated during the lysis of gram-negative cells and are also able to manifest their toxicity while still attached to the bacterial cell wall. The biological effects of endotoxins are manifold, but the two particularly prominent effects of an infection with gram-negative organisms are fever and shock. Humans are particularly sensitive to minute amounts of endotoxins and often a mild gram-negative bacterial infection will cause fever. Larger amounts of endotoxin may cause irreversible shock. This is seen in association with a fulminating, gram-negative bacteremia.

Despite the toxicity of endotoxins, a microbe's pathogenicity is not entirely explained by its content of endotoxin. Undoubtedly, many of the symptoms of infections by organisms such as *Salmonella typhi* or *Neisseria meningitidis* are a result of endotoxins, but the fact that many non-pathogenic gram-negative bacteria possess equally toxic endotoxins and do not normally produce disease indicates that endotoxin by itself is not a major determinant of bacterial virulence.

## FACTORS IN THE DEVELOPMENT OF DISEASE

We now can see that a number of different factors come into play for a disease agent to produce an infection. At the outset the portal of entrance must be suitable for the particular pathogen to cause disease. In many cases, a microorganism is restricted to only one portal of entry—for example, the typhoid fever organism (*Salmonella typhi*) must be swallowed and reach the small intestine in large numbers to cause disease. On the other hand, *Staphylococcus aureus* can use multiple portals of entry; it can cause pneumonia via the respiratory route, boils and furuncles via the skin, internal abscesses via the blood, or food poisoning via the gastrointestinal tract.

The ability to exit from the body and survive in the outside world are also important factors in disease development. Some organisms such as *Neisseria meningitidis* and *Neisseria gonorrhoeae* are extremely sensitive to drying and will die after several hours outside the host. Organisms such as the tubercle bacillus, however, may survive in dried sputum or secretions for months and still maintain their pathogenicity.

### Relationship of Dose to Infection

The number of organisms required to cause disease under different settings is certainly an important variable. For example, it may take thousands of staphylococci to cause infection in a clean cut, but a few hundred may infect a suture. On the other hand, some highly virulent organisms such as *Franciscella tularensis*, the organism causing tularemia, can cause severe disease with invasion of the skin by only three or four cells. Thus, it is easy to see that the division between pathogens and saprophytes is a vague line and that it is only at the extreme ends that one can see clear-cut examples of obligate pathogens (*Franciscella tularensis*, *Treponema pallidum*) or obligate saprophytes (such as *Bacillus megaterium* and *B. cereus*).

When we study specific infections, we shall see that some diseases normally are found only in humans (typhoid fever, cholera, syphilis, meningococcal meningitis), and thus humans are necessary for the continued life of the microorganisms involved. It will also become apparent that there are many infectious diseases humans acquire only as accidental hosts. Examples of diseases in this category include yellow fever and malaria (both carried as an endemic infection in jungle monkeys), endemic typhus, Rocky Mountain spotted fever, tularemia, and brucellosis. A third category of infectious organisms, the soil saprophytes, live and grow in the soil, but, if introduced via a wound into a susceptible host, some may cause serious illness and death. These include such diseases as tetanus, gas gangrene, and the deep-seated mycoses.

## Nonspecific Host Resistance

The complex reactions a host animal undergoes after contact with microorganisms may be grouped under the broadly-defined heading of resistance. We may categorize such resistance as being of two major types: (1) nonspecific or natural resistance, and (2) specific resistance directed against specific microbes.

In the first category, resistance or susceptibility (lack of resistance) to infections may vary from one species of animal to another. For example, mice are extremely susceptible to infection by *Streptococcus pneumoniae*. The intraperitoneal introduction of just a few organisms into a healthy mouse will almost invariably kill it within

24 to 36 hours. Humans, on the other hand, are relatively resistant to *Streptococcus pneumoniae* infections, as evidenced by the large percentage of persons who carry these organisms in their respiratory tract without symptoms of infection (under some conditions as high as 50%). As another example, the guinea pig is extremely susceptible to human tuberculosis, as opposed to our relatively high resistance to the tubercle bacillus.

We often do not know why resistance varies from one species to another or why a disease may be mild in one person and severe in another. In some cases there may be a genetic or racial factor that makes certain races of people more susceptible to a particular infection than other. Examples of increased susceptibility to disease can be seen in the apparent inordinate susceptibility of the American Indian to tuberculosis. Also, statistical data indicate that if one identical twin contracts tuberculosis, there is a 75% chance that the other twin will develop overt tuberculosis. In contrast, for fraternal twins there is only a 33% chance the second twin will contract overt disease. We do not fully understand the genetic determinants that control this increased susceptibility to infection, although there are a few instances where genetically determined resistance to a specific disease can be pinpointed. For example, resistance to infection by *Plasmodium vivax* (a causative agent of malaria) is found among almost all African blacks and is attributed to the lack of a specific membrane factor on their erythrocytes to which the parasite must bind in order to invade and multiply intracellularly. Similarly, persons with hemoglobin AS (sickle-cell trait, also restricted to blacks) have a survival advantage in regions where *Plasmodium falciparum* (also an etiologic agent of malaria) is endemic.

The age of an individual at the time of infection is also an important factor in determining the severity of the disease. Many diseases such as mumps, measles, and chickenpox may be relatively mild during childhood but can frequently be exceedingly severe when contracted during adult life.

It is therefore apparent that susceptibility and resistance to infection varies considerably among various species of animals as well as among persons with different genetic backgrounds.

## MECHANICAL AND CHEMICAL MECHANISMS OF DEFENSE

### Skin and Mucous Membranes

The intact skin and mucous membranes provide a mechanical barrier that prevents the entrance of most microbial species. However, even though the structure of the skin itself undoubtedly gives a great deal of protection, considerably more important are the fatty acids secreted by the sebaceous glands and the propionic acid produced by the normal flora of the skin. Secretions from the sebaceous glands contain both saturated and unsaturated fatty acids that are bactericidal for many bacteria and fungi. A striking example of this type of resistance to infection is seen in the case of the fungi causing ringworm of the scalp (species of *Microsporum* and *Trichophyton*). This infection is difficult to cure in children, but after puberty it disappears without treatment, presumably as a result of a change in the amount and kinds of fatty acids secreted by the sebaceous glands.

Infections through the mucous membranes occur in the conjunctiva, respiratory tract, and genitourinary tract. However, such infections are not commonplace, and it would appear that in many cases organisms able to penetrate the mucous membranes possess special invasive properties. Alternatively, a prior viral infection may have resulted in damage, as in influenza, when destruction of the cilia-bearing epithelial cells allows infection by *Streptococcus pneumoniae* or *Staphylococcus aureus* to occur more readily. Under normal conditions, the beating action of the cilia on the mucous membranes of the respiratory tract provides for the continuous movement of a fluid layer of mucus. Particles of dust or microorganisms adhere to this mucus and are moved to the exterior, in this way keeping the lungs remarkably free of microorganisms.

### Chemical Factors

The body produces many antimicrobial substances that are important in preventing infections. Tears are rich in lysozyme, an enzyme that hydrolyzes the peptidoglycan cell wall of many bacteria. Lysozyme is also present in blood, and, as we shall see, it may also be an important determinant in the killing of some microorganisms by our white cells.

Acids of the stomach, vagina, and skin also provide important resistance to infection. A notable example of this is seen by the greatly reduced number of organisms required to cause typhoid fever if the acid in the stomach is neutralized before ingestion of the organisms. Furthermore, although it is difficult to relate to specific chemical factors, the microbial antagonism of our normal flora is of great value in preventing the growth of potentially pathogenic organisms. This is readily seen following long-term therapy with broad-spectrum antibiotics— therapy which destroys a large part of the normal flora, allowing yeast or staphylococci resistant to the antibiotic to proliferate and cause severe infections of the mucous membranes of the mouth or gastrointestinal tract.

## CELLULAR MECHANISMS OF DEFENSE

In spite of the physical and chemical barriers that normally prevent the entrance of microorganisms into our bodies, probably no day passes when bacteria do not enter the blood stream. This occurs when we cut ourselves, have a difficult bowel movement, brush our teeth, or even chew gum vigorously. One survives these daily attacks of bacteria primarily because such organisms are quickly removed and killed by phagocytic cells. The remainder of this chapter will give a brief description of these cells and describe how they are able to destroy the invading microorganisms.

## POLYMORPHONUCLEAR NEUTROPHILS

Polymorphonuclear neutrophils (also called PMN's, polys, or granulocytes) are the major circulating leukocyte, making up 65–70% of all circulating leukocytes. Their function is to remove debris, including bacteria, from the body's tissues by engulfing and destroying the foreign material. This process of engulfing particulate matter is called phagocytosis.

PMN's contain a nucleus that is divided into several large segments (hence the name polymorphonuclear) and, as shown in Figure 11-2, many granules that stain with neutral dyes (the basis of the name granulocyte or neutrophil). Following many infections there is an early increase in the number of these leukocytes in the blood as a result of an increased rate of release from the bone marrow, a condition known as leukocytosis. In some infections, particularly those caused by viruses or following a severe bacteremia caused by gram-negative organisms, there may be a decrease in the number of circulating leukocytes. This is referred to as leukopenia.

For a PMN to be effective in host defense, it must migrate to the area of the infection, phagocytize the infecting organisms, and finally kill the invader. We shall briefly examine each of these steps.

### Chemotaxis and Migration

PMN's are produced in the bone marrow where, after differentiation into mature granulocytes, they are released into the blood stream (see Figure 11-3). From there they circulate throughout the body and subsequently enter the tissues by squeezing between the cells lining the blood vessels. In the event of an infection (or a local inflammation) large numbers of PMN's will specifically migrate into the infected area of the body. This directed migration is called chemotaxis.

The molecular events which direct the movement of the PMN's toward the inflamed site are not fully understood, but it is well established that a large number of different factors are involved. In general terms chemotactic factors can be categorized as cyto-

taxins (those substances that directly stimulate the directional migration of cells) and as cytotaxigens (those substances which cause a chemical change in a noncytotaxin, converting it to a cytotaxin). Examples of a few cytotaxins include: (1) certain components of the complement system (see Chapter 14) known as C3a, C5a, and C$\overline{\text{5b},6,7}$ (produced during activation of the complement system); these factors activate a proesterase present on the PMN membrane, but the mechanism by which this activated esterase triggers the events directing the movement of the PMN is not known; (2) a number of bacterial products (which are not well characterized); (3) the products from damaged tissue cells (including the supernatants from virus-infected cells) as well as products released from cells engaged in phagocytosis; and (4) a number of compounds that include such things as denatured serum albumin, enzyme-digested collagen, cyclic AMP, whole casein, and peptone medium. Many of the cytotaxigens are enzymes such as trypsin, plasmin, bacterial proteases, collagenase, tissue proteases, and macrophage proteinase. A few nonenzymatic cytotaxigens include antibody-antigen reactions, aggregated proteins, aggregated immunoglobulins, and lipopolysaccharides. From the foregoing it is apparent that the rapid accumulation of PMN's at an infected site follows the release of a variety of chemotactic factors from that site.

## Attachment and Ingestion by the Phagocyte

The act of ingestion of a microorganism requires an initial contact between the cell membrane of the phagocyte and the surface of the microbe. This attachment is usually greatly facilitated by the presence of specific antibodies to the invading microorganism, since PMN's (as well as monocytes and macrophages that are discussed later in this chapter) have specific binding sites for the exposed Fc portion of an antibody molecule

**Figure 11-2.** Electron micrograph of a mature neutrophilic granulocyte (PMN) from rabbit bone marrow, showing two lobes of its dense nucleus and cytoplasmic granules. There are two types of granules: the larger, denser azurophil granules contain peroxidase, lysozyme, and lysosomal enzymes; the smaller, less dense specific granules lack lysosomal enzymes but contain alkaline phosphatase, lysozyme, and lactoferrin. (×25,000)

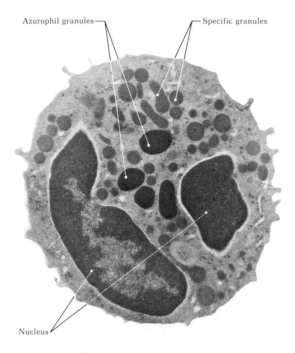

Azurophil granules

Specific granules

Nucleus

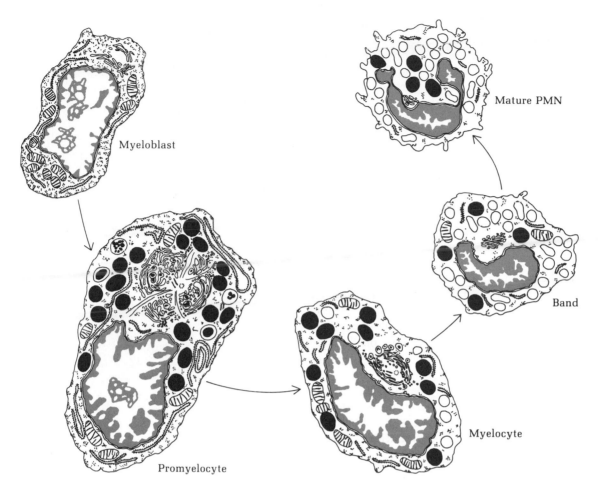

**Figure 11-3.** Stages in the maturation of PMN leukocytes. The myeloblast is a relatively undifferentiated or embryonic cell. The promyelocyte (or progranulocyte) and myelocyte are stages of intense secretory activity associated with the formation of azurophil and specific granules, respectively. The band cell is a nonsecretory, smaller intermediate that is beginning to show changes in the shape of the nucleus. The final product, the mature PMN, has a multilobed nucleus and a cytoplasm containing primarily glycogen and granules. The mature PMN contains 75–90% specific granules and only 10–25% azurophil granules.

(see Chapter 13 for details of antibody structure). Thus, specific antibodies act as a bridge to bring particulate matter into intimate contact with the phagocyte. Attachment, however, is also enhanced by various humoral factors. For example, it seems likely that the alternate pathway for the activation of complement (Chapter 14) provides a major

mechanism for nonspecific attachment. This pathway, also known as the properidin pathway, can be activated by naturally occurring polysaccharides and lipopolysaccharides, as well as by aggregates of IgA, resulting in the splitting of the C3 component of complement to form C3a and C3b. The C3b polypeptide will bind to a wide variety of particulate substances, including lipopolysaccharides, membranes, and cell walls, and also to specific receptor sites on the phagocyte. Thus, like antibodies, C3b acts as a bridge to bring particulate matter into close physical contact with the leukocyte membrane.

Basic amines also act as nonspecific factors that stimulate phagocytosis of infecting microorganisms—probably by binding to the invading microorganism and, like C3b, bringing the bacterium into close physical contact with membrane sites on the leukocyte.

The act of phagocytosis (ingestion) usually rapidly follows attachment of a particle to the leukocyte cell membrane. This is achieved by the formation of a vacuole (called a phagosome) which is formed by the invagination of the phagocyte plasma membrane to surround the attached particle, followed by separation of the phagosome from the newly reconstituted membrane of the phagocyte (see Figure 11-4).

At the time of phagocytosis there is a burst of metabolic activity within the phagocyte in which the stores of glycogen in the cytoplasm of the PMN are metabolized. Part of the resulting glucose is converted to lactic acid via the glycolytic pathway and part of the glucose is metabolized via the hexosemonophosphate shunt. Both pathways result in the formation of reduced coenzymes, that is, NADH from glycolysis and NADPH from the shunt reactions. During the reoxidation of the reduced coenzymes, large amounts of hydrogen peroxide are formed by the PMN in the following manner:

1. $\text{NADH} + \text{H}^+ + \text{O}_2 \xrightarrow{\text{NADH Oxidase}}$
$$\text{NAD} + \text{H}_2\text{O}_2$$

2. $\text{NADPH} + \text{H}^+ + \text{O}_2 \xrightarrow{\text{NADPH Oxidase}}$
$$\text{NADP} + \text{H}_2\text{O}_2$$

Since a major amount of the NADH formed during glycolysis is used in the glycolytic pathway to reduce pyruvic acid to lactic acid, it seems that the hexosemonophosphate

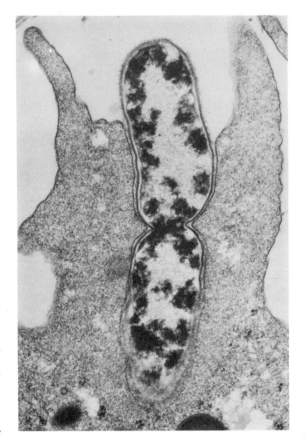

**Figure 11-4.** PMN engulfing a microorganism. When a bacterium is internalized by a PMN, the plasma membrane invaginates to form the wall of a phagosome. Note that the plasma membrane follows precisely the contour of the bacterium. ($\times 35{,}000$)

shunt provides the main source of reduced coenzyme for the formation of $\text{H}_2\text{O}_2$.

## Antimicrobial Systems of the Phagocyte

It is evident that the PMN has several different mechanisms available to kill ingested bacteria; although they usually operate simultaneously, it is possible to look at each system individually.

LYSOSOMES. In 1955 Christian de Duve discovered that many of the small granules within the cytoplasm of animal cells contain hydrolytic enzymes. These granular structures have been named lysosomes because they contain enzymes capable of hydrolyzing the major constituents of living cells, that is proteins, nucleic acids, fats, and carbohydrates. Lysosomes are present in the cytoplasm of essentially all animal cells, and they probably have many roles, including maintenance of our tissue cells by facilitating normal turnover of cell constituents. However, here we shall be concerned with the function of lysosomes in the host's phagocytic cells, where they function to kill bacterial invaders.

Immediately after phagocytosis occurs, lysosomes begin to fuse with the membrane of the phagosome and release their contents into the phagosome. Since the lysosomes exist as small granules within the phagocyte, this process is called degranulation and the resulting phagosome is now referred to as a phagolysosome (see Figure 11-5). Over 60 different enzyme activities have been found within lysosomes. Among these are a number of proteases, lipases, carbohydrases, RNase, DNase, acid phosphatase, and a peroxidase which has been given the name of myeloperoxidase. It appears likely that a number of these enzymes are involved in the killing and digestion of phagocytosed microorganisms, but we shall limit our discussion to several that have been shown to be of primary importance.

MYELOPEROXIDE-HALIDE-PEROXIDE SYSTEM.
The hydrogen peroxide that was produced during the metabolic burst following phagocytosis diffuses from the cytoplasm of the PMN into the phagolysosome. There, in conjunction with myeloperoxidase (MPO)

**Figure 11-5.** After engulfment, lysosomal enzymes from azurophil granules along with enzymes in specific granules enter the phagosome, by fusion of the granule membranes with the phagosome membrane. The ingested bacterium within the phagolysosome is killed and either digested or retained within a residual body, from which it can be excreted by fusion with the plasma membrane of the PMN.

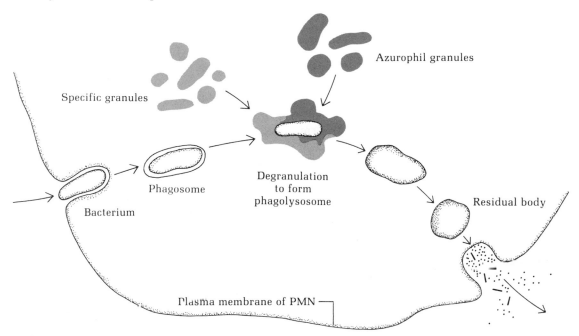

and a halide ion from the PMN, it exerts its bactericidal effect. The biochemical mechanism by which the MPO-halide-$H_2O_2$ system kills the phagocytosed microorganisms is still controversial, but the following two proposals have experimental support:

1. The halide involved in this system is the chloride ion, and the microbicidal (killing) effect results from the formation of hypochlorite (a strong oxidizing agent) according to the following equation:

$$H_2O_2 + Cl^- \xrightarrow{\text{MPO}} ClO^- + H_2O$$

2. The halide involved in this system is the iodide ion, and death results from an iodination of proteins in the microorganisms which is catalyzed by MPO in the presence of $H_2O_2$.

Perhaps both events occur. Certainly, chloride is present in large amounts, and hypochlorite is an effective microbicidal compound. On the other hand, the addition of iodide to the system demonstrates that it is much more active than chloride on a molar basis. The concentration of iodide, however, in the PMN under physiological conditions is extremely low, which would argue against iodine as the usual ion involved in the MPO microbicidal system.

SUPEROXIDE ANION. Experimental evidence supports the conclusion that PMN's form superoxide ($O_2^-$) during their burst of metabolism following phagocytosis. The superoxide ion is by itself extremely toxic (see Chapter 4), and unless scavenged by the enzyme superoxide dismutase, it may well exert a toxic effect on phagocytosed organisms—particularly those anaerobic pathogens that do not possess their own superoxide dismutase. However, another important function of superoxide is to serve as an intermediate in the oxidative production of hydrogen peroxide according to the following equation:

$$O_2^- + O_2^- + 2H^+ \xrightarrow[\text{dismutase}]{\text{superoxide}} O_2 + H_2O_2$$

MYELOPEROXIDASE-INDEPENDENT ANTIMICROBIAL SYSTEMS. A number of additional enzymes are emptied into the phagolysosome during degranulation of the PMN and undoubtedly are involved in the antimicrobial action of the leukocyte. A few of the better understood factors are lysozyme, which hydrolyzes the peptidoglycan cell wall of certain sensitive bacteria; lactoferrin, which can chelate iron present in the phagolysosome and thus prevent growth of the phagocytosed organism; and basic proteins such as phagocytin and leukin, which have been shown to exert antimicrobial activity, although their mechanism of action or contribution to the killing effect is not known. In addition, acid produced by the metabolic activities of the PMN lowers the pH of the phagolysosome to a pH of 3 or 4, which alone may cause the death of many microorganisms.

## OTHER PHAGOCYTIC CELLS

A second phagocytic cell, called a monocyte, also is produced in the bone marrow and released into the blood stream, and after one or two days migrates through the vessel walls into the surrounding tissues. The monocyte then begins to differentiate into one of a number of large phagocytic cells called macrophages or mononuclear phagocytes (see Figure 11-6). These cells are dispersed throughout the body—some fixed primarily along the blood vessels in the liver, spleen, bone marrow, and lymph nodes, while others maintain their motility and are called wandering or tissue macrophages. Fixed phagocytic macrophages usually have been referred to collectively as the reticuloendothelial system. However, since neither reticulum nor endothelial cells are probably involved in the process of particle clearance, it has been suggested that a more acceptable terminology would be the mononuclear phagocyte system.

The details of macrophage action have been less thoroughly studied than those of

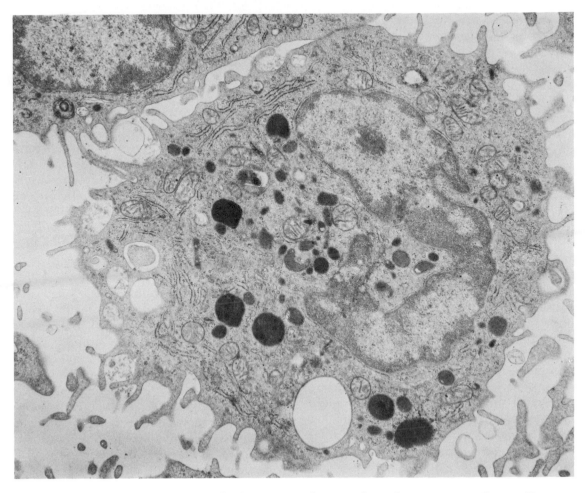

**Figure 11-6.** Electron micrograph of a peritoneal macrophage from a mouse. These cells were obtained from a peritoneal cavity stimulated with a lipid emulsion. Cytoplasmic processes are prominent, some clearly finger-like. Lysosomal dense bodies are numerous— some small and homogeneous, others large and heterogeneous. ($\times$ 12,000)

the polymorphonuclear neutrophils, but the following generalizations can be made:

1. Phagocytosis, including the ability to ingest both foreign particles and antibody-coated bacteria, is analogous to that described for PMN's. Specific receptors for antibody molecules (Fc portion) and complement (C3b) exist on the membranes of macrophages as on PMN membranes

2. Granules in monocytes, like PMN's, contain lysosomal enzymes and in some species

peroxidase. Macrophages also contain stores of lysosomal enzymes packaged in tiny vesicles. Unlike the situation in PMN's, lysosomal enzymes are continuously synthesized during the tissue phase of the macrophage with the result that the mature macrophage possesses many times more lysosomal enzymes than does the monocyte at the time it begins to differentiate into a macrophage.

3. Following the formation of the phagosome, lysosomal granules (in monocytes) or stored lysosomal enzymes in vesicles

(macrophages) fuse with the phagosome to release their hydrolytic enzymes, forming a phagolysosome.

4. The phagocytizing monocyte or macrophage undergoes a burst of metabolic activity which results in the formation of hydrogen peroxide; however, myeloperoxidase is absent from these cells in some species. Thus, even though the MPO system seems to be an important microbicidal event for the PMN's, the mononuclear phagocytes can make efficient use of killing techniques which have yet to be fully elucidated.

In general, the mononuclear phagocytes are considered to be a second line of defense, since PMN's characteristically are first to arrive at a site of inflammation. This probably results from the fact that even though both cell types are attracted by a bacterial infection, PMN's migrate faster and thus appear first. PMN's, however, are short-lived and in the event of a chronic infection are soon replaced by the longer-lived macrophages. In addition, there are certain microorganisms (such as tubercle bacilli, brucellae, and *Toxoplasma* parasites) that preferentially attract macrophages to the site of the infection. Such organisms are phagocytized by the macrophages, but by an as yet unknown mechanism they are able to inhibit the degranulation of the macrophage. Such organisms therefore continue to multiply intracellularly within the macrophage phagosome, usually resulting in a chronic infection. In some cases the macrophages (with their intracellular bacteria) pile up into a type of nodule which becomes surrounded by connective tissue. These walled-off nodules are termed granulomas, or in the case of tuberculosis, tubercles.

Another role played by macrophages appears to be as one of the mediators of the inflammatory response. It has been shown that in addition to their phagocytic and intracellular digestive properties, macrophages can secrete various proteases which may be involved in chronic inflammation and delayed-type hypersensitivity reactions

(see Chapter 17). The most likely candidate of the macrophage-secreted enzymes for inducing an inflammatory reaction is a plasminogen activator that converts the humoral proteolytic enzyme, plasminogen, to its active form, plasmin. Interestingly, the administration of steroids (which are antiinflammatory) appears to inhibit the migration of monocytes from the bone marrow, with a resulting inhibition of inflammation and plasminogen activator secretion. It has been proposed that the normal role of plasminogen activator is to activate plasminogen, which then digests some of the supporting structures of blood vessels to allow the migration of monocytes into the various body compartments.

In addition, macrophages are also the active cells involved in specific cell-mediated immunity (Chapter 17). In this case, however, macrophages are stimulated by lymphokines that are secreted by certain lymphocytes. Lymphokine-stimulated macrophages are considerably more active in phagocytosis and killing than nonstimulated cells, and they have been referred to as angry or activated macrophages.

Last, we shall see that macrophages are necessary for the production of specific humoral antibodies; this role for macrophages will be discussed in Chapter 15.

## DEFECTS IN INTRACELLULAR KILLING

The role of the phagocyte as a major defense against disease became more obvious with the discovery that some individuals produce leukocytes that are defective in their ability to phagocytize and destroy invading microorganisms. Such persons experience repeated episodes of infection in spite of the presence of high levels of circulating specific antibodies. We shall briefly discuss several types of defects in the following sections.

### Chronic Granulomatous Disease

Chronic granulomatous disease (CGD) is a frequently fatal, usually sex-linked, genetic disorder that is characterized by repeated bacterial infections—most commonly with chronically infecting organisms such as *Staphylococcus aureus* or gram-negative rods. These individuals possess PMN's that phagocytize invading bacteria normally but are unable to kill many of the ingested microorganisms, as indicated in Figure 11-7.

**Figure 11-7.** *Staphylococcus aureus* and *Serratia marcescens* were incubated with PMN's from a patient with chronic granulomatous disease and with PMN's from a normal control. The inability of the patient's PMN's to kill either species of bacterium is readily apparent from the number of viable bacteria.

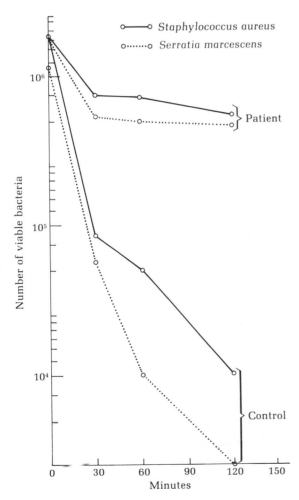

The major defect in the PMN's of these patients has been shown to be related to the inability of the phagocyte to produce hydrogen peroxide. This seems to result from a specific enzymatic defect involving NADH oxidase, the enzyme that catalyzes the major hydrogen peroxide generating reaction. This enzyme appears to be present in near-normal amounts, but it fails to become activated after phagocytosis and thus is not available to aid in $H_2O_2$ production. The defective PMN's also are therefore unable to produce superoxide, another source for $H_2O_2$ production. Interestingly organisms which metabolically generate their own $H_2O_2$, such as streptococci and lactobacilli, are killed normally by CGD PMN's. This suggests a major role for $H_2O_2$ in the usual cidal (killing) mechanism.

**Chediak-Higashi Syndrome**

Individuals with Chediak-Higashi syndrome (CHS) suffer recurrent infections similar to those described for persons with chronic granulomatous disease. However, this defect results from the presence of giant lysosomes formed in the promyelocyte, a precursor stem cell to the PMN (see Figure 11-8). These abnormal lysosomes do not fuse readily with a cytoplasmic phagosome. Such cells also have other defects, including a defective chemotactic response to infection.

**Myeloperoxidase Deficiency**

Individuals whose PMN's completely lack MPO are for the most part well and free from recurrent infections, although a case of recurrent candidiasis from an MPO-deficient patient has been reported. It is clear, therefore, that MPO is not the only cidal pathway. Phagocytes from MPO-deficient individuals produce $H_2O_2$ and possess other cidal mechanisms which involve superoxide, $H_2O_2$-ascorbic acid, lysozyme, and the ability to produce an acid pH within the phagolysosome.

In summary, the primary importance of

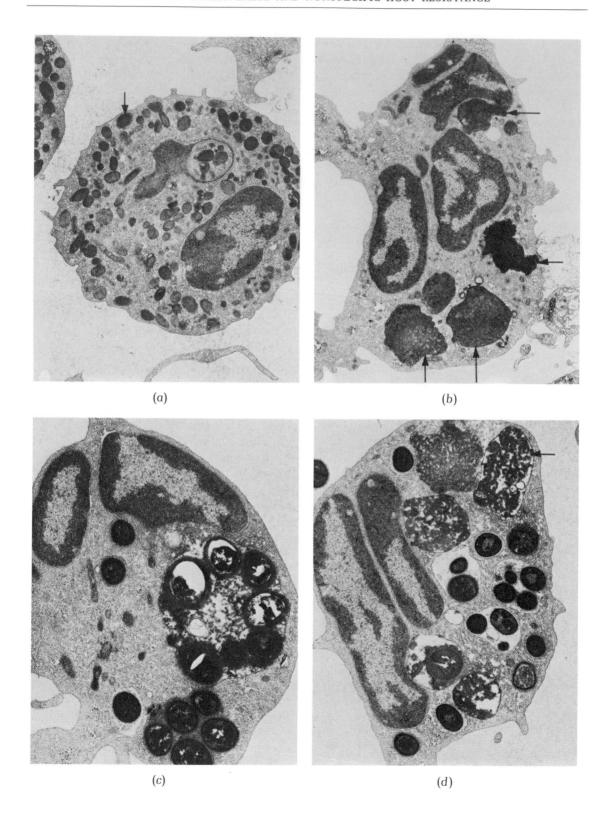

(a)

(b)

(c)

(d)

**Figure 11-8.** Electron micrographs of PMN's from normal controls and from patients with Chediak-Higashi syndrome (CHS). PMN's have been stained histochemically for peroxidase, causing the azurophil lysosomes to appear dark. *a.* Normal PMN with arrow pointing to one of the many small lysosomes. *b.* PMN from patient with CHS. Arrows point to the very few, large lysosomes. *c.* Normal PMN 60 minutes after mixing with staphylococci, showing phagosomal fusion with peroxidase activity in the phagolysosomes and a lack of peroxidase-positive granules in the cytoplasm (compare with *a*). *d.* CHS-PMN 60 minutes after mixing with staphylococci. Note the persistence of structurally intact peroxidase-positive giant lysosomes (arrow).

the phagocytic cell is well established. The release of phagocytes from the bone marrow and their chemotactic response to infection and inflammation are major defenses preventing overt disease. Defects in either phagocyte mobilization or the phagocytosis and killing of invading organisms is manifested by frequent episodes of infectious disease in spite of the presence of high levels of specific circulating antibodies. Much that we know concerning the mechanisms of killing invading bacteria has been learned from studies of individuals with defective phagocytes, and it seems probable that additional defects in certain phagocytic cells will be discovered which will add to our knowledge of their regulation and microbicidal activities.

## REFERENCES

Babior, B. M., R. S. Kipnes, and J. T. Curnutte. 1973. Biological defense mechanisms: The production by leukocytes of superoxide, a potential bactericidal agent. *J. Clin. Invest.* **52**:741–744.

Bellanti, J. A., and D. H. Dayton, eds. 1975. *The Phagocytic Cell in Host Resistance.* Raven Press, New York.

Black, F. L. 1975. Infectious diseases in primitive societies. *Science* **187**:515–518.

Boggs, D. R., and A. Winkelstein. 1975. *White Cell Manual,* 3rd ed. F. A. Davis Co., Philadelphia.

Boxer, L. A., M. Watanabe, M. Rister, H. R. Besch Jr., J. Allen, and R. L. Baehner. 1976. Correction of leukocyte function in Chediak-Higashi syndrome by ascorbate. *New Engl. J. Med.* **295**:1041–1045.

Carr, I. 1973. *The Macrophage: A Review of Ultrastructure and Function.* Academic Press, New York.

Cline, M. J. 1975. *The White Cell.* Harvard Univ. Press, Cambridge, Mass.

Klebanoff, S. J. 1971. Intraleukocytic microbicidal defects. *Annu. Rev. Med.* **22**:39–62.

Klebanoff, S. J., and C. B. Hamon. 1972. Role of myeloperoxidase-mediated antimicrobial systems in intact leukocytes. *J. Reticuloendothel. Soc.* **12**:170–196.

Mandell, G. L. 1974. Bactericidal activity of aerobic and anaerobic polymorphonuclear neutrophils. *Infect. Immun.* **9**:337–343.

Nelson, D. S., ed. 1976. *Immunobiology of the Macrophage.* Academic Press, New York.

Simmons, S. R., and M. L. Karnovsky. 1973. Iodinating ability of various leukocytes and their bactericidal activity. *J. Exp. Med.* **138**:44–63.

Weinberg, E. D. 1975. Metal starvation of pathogens by hosts. *Bioscience* **25**:314–318.

Weiss, L. 1972. *The Cells and Tissues of the Immune System.* Prentice-Hall, Englewood Cliffs, N.J.

Wilkinson, P. C. 1974. *Chemotaxis and Inflammation.* Churchill Livingstone, London.

# 12

# Structure of Antigens
# and Antibodies

In the previous chapter we considered the nonspecific mechanisms by which the body protects itself from infections. However, since everyone occasionally becomes ill, common sense tells us that these mechanisms are insufficient for protecting us against all pathogenic invaders. We are aware that following recovery from many childhood diseases there probably will be no recurrence, and we consider ourselves immune to that particular disease. In other words, we do not anticipate a second attack of mumps, chickenpox, or measles. The state of being highly resistant to a specific pathogenic organism is called immunity, and the type we are concerned with here is referred to as specific and acquired immunity, since it is directed against particular organisms and it occurs as a response to a given stimulus.

What is the nature of this specific acquired immunity? What happens in the body that will prevent a subsequent attack by the same organisms? Acquired immunity is understood best by visualizing a system whereby animals are able to "distinguish" between materials that make up their own bodies and those which are foreign. This system does not normally react against its own cells, but will set into motion a series of complex reactions that aids in the elimination or neutralization of foreign substances such as cells from other animals, bacteria, viruses, and toxins. It is this ability to recognize "self" as opposed to "nonself" that forms the basis for specific acquired immunity.

In order to understand the formation of these protective reactions, it is necessary to know something of the nature of the foreign substances that induce their synthesis.

## Antigens

Foreign materials that gain entrance to the body and induce a specific immune response are called immunogens or antigens, abbreviated simply Ag. The resulting specific immune response may take the form of substances called antibodies (abbreviated Ab) that circulate in the bloodstream (antibody-mediated immunity or AMI), or may

158

take the form of certain cells that have acquired an increased ability to destroy other cells (cell-mediated immunity or CMI), or both. In either case, acquired immunity enables the body to destroy or neutralize invading organisms or toxins.

Chemically, antigens are usually composed of protein, polysaccharide, or combinations such as glycoproteins, nucleoproteins, or glycolipids. Many of the antigens of concern to us occur as components of various membranes or structures surrounding bacteria, viruses, or even cancer cells. Examples of such antigens include bacterial capsules, the cell wall lipopolysaccharides of gram-negative bacteria, specific glycoproteins occurring in cell membranes, or the attachment sites on viruses that interact with specific receptors on mammalian cells. Some antigens are more effective in inducing a specific immune response than are others; or stated another way, there are strong antigens and weak antigens. Some proteins such as diphtheria or tetanus toxoids are strong antigens when injected and induce a good immune response, whereas foreign antigens occurring on the surface of a cancer cell may be weak and elicit a poor immune response or none at all.

## PROPERTIES OF ANTIGENS

An antigen may be a soluble substance such as horse serum proteins or a bacterial toxin, or it may exist on particulate matter such as a red blood cell, a bacterial cell, or a virus. In any case, it must have a molecular configuration with certain consistent characteristics to be able to induce antibody formation. Let us look at some of the properties a molecule must possess to be an effective antigen, or, for that matter, to be any kind of an antigen.

First and foremost, an antigen must be foreign to the host. We can easily see that unless this were true, an animal would produce antibodies against antigens on its own cells and subsequently destroy them. A theory, first proposed by Sir Macfarlane

Burnet, postulated that during the prenatal period the developing lymphoid system learns to distinguish "self" from "nonself." As will be described in Chapter 15, this so-called learning of self may result from the destruction of those cells which have the potential to synthesize antibodies to self. As a result, one develops a permanent self-tolerance to antigens that are normal components of one's own cells. We shall also learn that occasional alterations of normal antigens or other malfunctions can induce the immune system to respond toward antigens which are self, resulting in autoimmune diseases.

The second property a substance must have to be capable of inducing an antibody response is that it must be a reasonably large molecule. It is rare for any compound with a molecular weight of less than 6000 daltons to act alone as an antigen. This seems unusual, because the substances (antibodies) formed in response to the presence of an antigen react with only a small portion of the antigen. The portion of the antigen that specifically combines with antibody is spoken of as its determinant group.

If we could degrade the antigen—that is, chemically break it down and isolate a determinant group (which would probably have a molecular weight varying from 200 to 1000 daltons)—we would find that this isolated portion of the antigen still reacts with the antibodies formed in response to the original antigen but by itself is unable to induce the production of antibodies when injected into an animal. For many macromolecular proteins, however, it would be difficult to isolate the determinant groups of an antigen—particularly in those instances where a determinant group consists of an area of a protein that has folded back and forth to create a specific tertiary structure that is recognized by the antibody.

Considerable insight into the nature of an antigen and the specificity of an antibody to its antigenic determinant evolved from experiments carried out by Karl Landsteiner and his collaborators over 40 years ago. They prepared synthetic antigens by coupling a number of aromatic compounds to carrier proteins, as shown in Figure 12-1 for the coupling of m-aminobenzene sulfonic acid to chicken serum. When this synthetic antigen was injected into a rabbit, antibodies of two major specificities were produced, one which reacted with the chicken serum and another that combined specifically with the m-aminobenzene sulfonic acid. Note that even though m-aminobenzene sulfonic acid could not by itself induce antibody formation, it would react with preformed antibodies that had been induced by the synthetic antigen. These small molecules of known chemical composition that can be chemically attached to large proteins have been given the name of haptens. Thus, by definition, a hapten is a molecule that is too small to induce antibody synthesis; but when conjugated to a large carrier protein, the hapten becomes one of the determinant groups toward which the antibody is directed. It is apparent, therefore, that antibodies can be produced that are specific for small molecules (haptens) provided the haptens are coupled to a large carrier.

The fact that uncoupled hapten binds to its antibody in the absence of a carrier opened a new area of research concerned with the molecular specificity of antibodies. These experiments relied on the observation that when a hapten binds to its specific antibody, it blocks the antibody-combining site from additional reactions with haptenic molecules on a carrier. Slight changes could be made in a hapten to study the effect of such alterations. It was then possible to judge the

**Figure 12-1.** Schematic diagram illustrating the coupling of an aromatic hapten to a carrier protein. The final protein will induce antibody synthesis to both the carrier protein and the aromatic hapten.

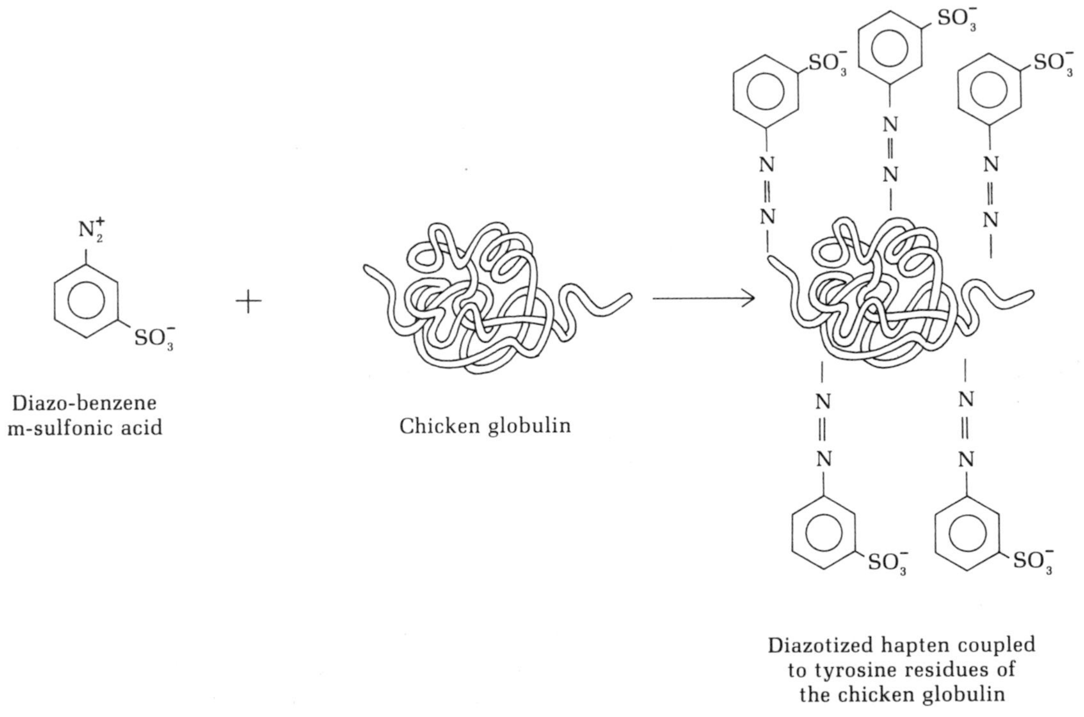

Diazo-benzene
m-sulfonic acid

Chicken globulin

Diazotized hapten coupled
to tyrosine residues of
the chicken globulin

**Table 12-1. Effect of Moving or Altering Side Groups on Aromatic Haptens**

| Antigens made from chicken serum and: | Position of the substituents | | |
|---|---|---|---|
| | NH$_2$ with R* (ortho) | NH$_2$ with R (meta) | NH$_2$ with R (para) |
| Aminobenzene sulfonic acid[a] | $+\pm$[b] | $++\pm$ | tr. |
| | $+\pm$ | $+++$ | $\pm$ |
| Aminophenyl arsenic acid | O | $+$ | O |
| | O | $+$ | O |
| Aminobenzoic acid | O | $\pm$ | O |
| | O | $+$ | O |

*R denotes the groups SO$_3$H, AsO$_3$H$_2$, COOH.

[a] 2 drops of immune serum for m-aminobenzene sulfonic acid were added to 0.2 cc of the antigens, diluted 1 : 500.

[b] Readings were taken after 1 hour at room temperature (first line) and after standing overnight in the ice box (second line).

changed haptenic group's ability to inhibit the reaction of antibody to its specific hapten bound to a carrier molecule. The specificity of antibody for its inducing antigenic determinant was astonishing. As shown in Table 12-1, merely moving the sulfonic acid group from the *meta* to the *ortho* or *para* positions greatly diminished the combining ability of the antibodies induced by the serum-conjugated *m*-aminobenzene sulfonic acid. One can also see that, if the sulfonic acid side group is changed to an arsenic acid or carboxyl group, the *m*-aminobenzene sulfonic acid antibodies lose almost all ability to react with the altered hapten group. Thus, one can conclude that the specificity of an antigen lies primarily in its three-dimensional shape. Moreover, for an antigenic determinant or hapten to induce an antibody response it must be combined with a large carrier molecule.

Finally, in order for a substance to stimulate antibody synthesis, it must possess at least two determinant groups that are foreign to the host. (As we shall see in Chapter 17, this is not necessarily true for the induction of a cell-mediated response.) We

shall discuss the reasons for this two-determinant group requirement in Chapter 15 and, therefore, shall confine our immediate discussion to what is meant by two determinant groups.

If, for example, a rabbit is immunized with the same hapten consisting of *m*-aminobenzene sulfonic acid linked this time to rabbit globulin, one sees no antibody response to either the carrier globulin or the *m*-aminobenzene sulfonic acid. If, however, the *m*-aminobenzene sulfonic acid is linked to guinea pig or chicken globulin, the rabbit can synthesize antibodies to both the globulin and to the *m*-aminobenzene sulfonic acid. Thus, it is clear that the rabbit possesses the ability to make antibodies to *m*-aminobenzene sulfonic acid; but for this to occur, the hapten must be linked to a carrier also foreign to the host. Antibodies might be produced using rabbit globulin in the rabbit if such large quantities of *m*-aminobenzene sulfonic acid were complexed so that the normal tertiary structure of the rabbit globulin was distorted. This would not, however, invalidate our conclusion that an antigen must possess two foreign determinants, since the distorted rabbit globulin would be recognized by the rabbit as a foreign substance.

This is all very good, but in everyday life our immune system is challenged to make antibodies to native proteins composed of amino acids that do not necessarily have aromatic side groups attached. What are the foreign determinants in such cases? The answer to this question requires remembering what is meant by the tertiary structure of a protein. This can be defined rather simply by stating that the ultimate shape of a native protein is determined by its amino acid sequence. As a result of hydrogen bonding, disulfide bonds, hydrophobic forces, and so forth, a polypeptide folds back and forth upon itself to assume a specific and reproducible form.

Using crystalline sperm whale myoglobin (composed of 153 amino acid residues of known sequence), M. Zouhair Atassi has conclusively shown that the antigenic sites of this protein are found in five small regions (6 or 7 amino acids each) which possess different, specific configurations in the native protein. The antigenic determinants in some proteins are highly dependent on the native three-dimensional structure of the protein, and if these conformational structures are destroyed by denaturation of the native antigen, the determinant group is lost. On the other hand, many antigenic determinants consist of a linear sequence of six or seven amino acids (as in whale myoglobin) and denaturation has little effect on their ability to bind to antibody. Such determinants are designated "linear" to distinguish them from the native three-dimensional "conformational" determinants. Figure 12-2 illustrates a schematic drawing of the myoglobin molecule showing its five antigenic sites.

The antigenic determinants of polysaccharides are somewhat variable. Elvin Kabat, using dextran as an antigen, has shown the specific determinants to consist of oligosaccharides containing a maximum of six or seven monosaccharides, illustrating once

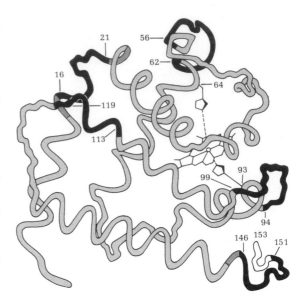

**Figure 12-2.** A schematic diagram showing the mode of folding of sperm whale myoglobin. The five solid black portions represent entire antigenic reactive regions. The dark grey segments, each corresponding to only one amino-acid residue, can be part of the antigenic reactive regions with some antisera. The light grey regions represent parts of the molecule that reside outside of the reactive regions. The numbers identify landmark amino-acid residues.

again that the maximum size for an antigen determinant is in the range of 1000 daltons. It is also of interest that the specificity of antibodies to polysaccharides is dependent not only upon the size of the determinant group but also upon the sugars involved and the linkage between these sugars. Thus, a dextran composed of $\alpha$ 1–3 glucosidic linkages would induce a quite different antibody specificity than a dextran made up of $\alpha$ 1–4 linkages.

We have now covered the three important properties a compound must possess in order to be an antigen: (1) it must be foreign to the host, (2) it usually must be a reasonably large molecule, and (3) it must possess at least two determinant groups foreign to the host.

Antigen

# Antibodies

Unfortunately, we are still on that circuitous route where some definitions must continue to be phrased in unknown terms; eventually we shall travel the entire circle and, hopefully, all will then be clear.

Just as we defined antigens (Ag) in terms of antibody (Ab), the order must be reversed to define Ab as a specific immunoglobulin which is synthesized in response to an antigenic stimulation.

In discussing the properties of antibodies the generalization can be made that all antibodies are proteins containing a small amount of carbohydrate attached to the molecule. Some have a greater tendency to become attached to tissues than others, but all are soluble and can be found in serum.

In the early days of immunology, before the complexity of serum was appreciated,

serum proteins were classified according to their solubility as either albumins or globulins. It was observed that circulating antibodies were found only in globulins and that if one subjected serum to electrophoresis, it would separate into albumin and three major globulin components. These components were designated as alpha, beta, and gamma globulin. Almost all circulating Abs were found in the gamma globulin fraction (see Figure 12-3), and as a result, the term gamma globulin was used for years as a synonym for circulating Abs. However, since there are exceptions, the more proper name, immunoglobulins (abbreviated Ig), is used as a general name of antibodies. Actually, the name immunoglobulin is a generic term that includes antibodies and all proteins that have structural similarities to

**Figure 12-3.** *a.* Electrophoresis scale diagram of rabbit serum containing antibodies to egg albumin. Peaks for alpha, beta, and gamma globulin are shown. *b.* Same diagram after absorption of serum with egg albumin. Note dramatic decrease in size of the gamma globulin peak, demonstrating that the anti-egg albumin antibodies were gamma globulins.

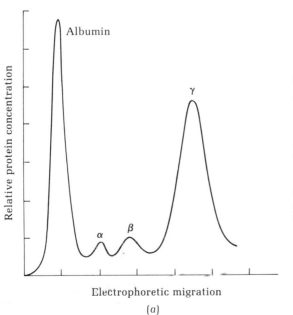

*(a)*

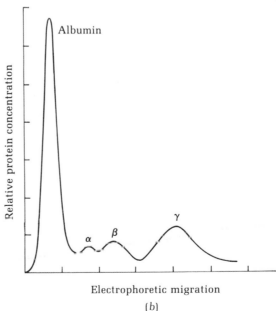

*(b)*

antibodies but for which no specificity is known—for example, myeloma proteins.

## STRUCTURE OF ANTIBODIES

It would probably be safe to say that during the past several decades no group of proteins has received such intense study as has the collection of immunoglobulins. Early investigations beginning around 1950 revealed that most Ab molecules had a molecular weight of about 150,000 daltons and contained 15 to 20 disulfide bonds. Treatment of Ab molecules with sulfhydryl agents to selectively cleave some of these bonds yielded equimolar amounts of two intact peptide chains. One of the resulting peptides possessed a molecular weight of approximately 50,000 daltons and the other a molecular weight of about 25,000 daltons (75,000 total). Since the original intact antibody molecule had a molecular weight of 150,000 daltons, it appeared probable that it was composed of two of the heavy chains (50,000 daltons) and two of the light chains (25,000) which were held together by disulfide bonds.

A major breakthrough came when Rodney Porter demonstrated that digestion of rabbit Ig with the proteolytic enzyme papain cleaved the molecule into two major fractions plus a small amount of short peptides. One fraction (45,000 daltons) still possessed the antigen-binding site and was thus named fragment-antibody binding, or as it is now called, Fab. The other fragment could be crystallized and because of this property was called fragment-crystallized, or Fc (50,000 daltons).

Surprisingly, although Fab still possessed an antigen binding site, it was monovalent (possessed only one reactive site for Ag), and hence could not crosslink antigen molecules. However, when one added up the molecular weights of the isolated Fab and Fc fragments, plus the observation that Fab was monovalent, it appeared that the original antibody molecule contained two Fab fragments and one Fc fragment.

This postulate was soon proven when antibody molecules were treated with the proteolytic enzyme, pepsin. In this case a single large component (100,000 daltons) was obtained, plus a series of small peptides. Moreover, the large component was divalent, possessing the two antigen binding sites of the original antibody molecule. Since the large component had a molecular weight about 10 percent higher than two Fab fragments from a papain digestion of antibody, it was named $F(ab')_2$. Let us try to put the following information together to postulate a model for the basic structure of antibody: (1) it is composed of two heavy chains (50,000 daltons each) and two light chains (25,000 daltons each) which are joined by disulfide bonds; (2) treatment with papain yields two monovalent Fab fragments (45,000 daltons each) and one Fc fragment (50,000 daltons); (3) treatment with pepsin

**Figure 12-4.** Schematic stick model of IgG showing two heavy and two light chains held together by interchain disulfide bonds.

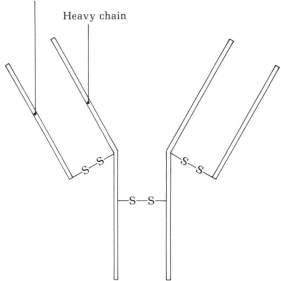

Light chain

Heavy chain

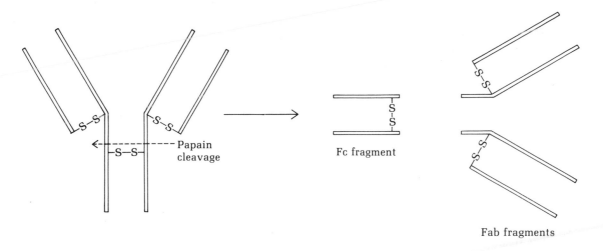

**Figure 12-5.** Schematic illustration of the digestion of IgG with papain to yield one Fc fragment and two Fab fragments.

splits the molecule into one divalent $F(ab')_2$ fragment (100,000 daltons) and some small peptides. Based on this evidence, a much over-simplified "stick" model of antibody was proposed, as shown in Figure 12-4. Here we can see a molecule composed of two heavy chains and two light chains. Depending upon which side of the interchain disulfide bond the heavy chain is cleaved, the reaction will yield two monovalent Fab fragments and an Fc fragment (see Figure 12-5), or one $F(ab')_2$ fragment and some small peptides (see Figure 12-6). It can be seen that the $F(ab')_2$ obtained following pepsin digestion contains a larger portion of heavy chain than does isolated Fab obtained through papain hydrolysis.

Later in this chapter our molecular model

**Figure 12-6.** Schematic illustration of the digestion of IgG with pepsin to yield one $F(ab')_2$ fragment plus small peptides.

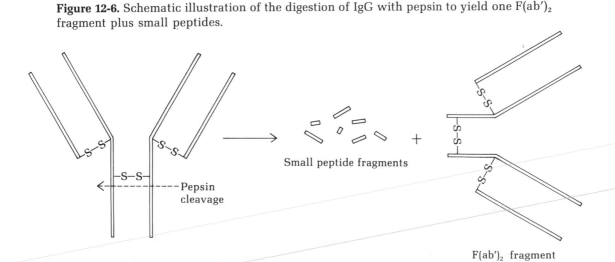

for antibody structure will become considerably more complex, but this simplification will suffice until we can ease into a more comprehensive model to explain the incredible diversity of antibodies.

## CLASSES OF IMMUNOGLOBULINS

In general, most antibodies have a molecular weight of 150,000 daltons and are composed of two heavy and two light chains. When subjected to analytical centrifugation, they possess a sedimentation coefficient of approximately 7 Svedberg units, and are referred to as 7S antibodies. However, if a crude preparation of immunoglobulin is centrifuged in a similar manner, one finds that the sedimentation coefficients can range from 7S to 19S, representing molecular weights varying from 150,000 to 1,000,000 daltons. Zone electrophoresis also demonstrates a large charge heterogeneity of immunoglobulins. Quite obviously, it is not possible to characterize an immunoglobulin molecule at a molecular level unless reasonable quantities of a single species of antibody can be obtained.

A source of such singular immunoglobulin became available when it was recognized that individuals with a malignancy of the lymphoid system called multiple myeloma possess large amounts of immunoglobulin in their serum. Because this malignancy is the result of large numbers of daughter cells that have arisen from a single Ab-forming cell, these cells all synthesize an identical immunoglobulin and the resulting immunoglobulin is, therefore, homogeneous (Chapter 15). Using the different purified immunoglobulins from many different patients with multiple myeloma, it was possible to study the chemical and antigenic characteristics of a series of different immunoglobulins.

Initial studies soon revealed that immunoglobulins could be divided into different classes based on their antigenic properties. In other words, when immunoglobulin (i.e., antibody) is injected into a species of animal different from the one from which it was obtained, the receiving animal will produce antibodies to the foreign immunoglobulin. Using these antibodies to compare the immunoglobulins from a large series of myeloma patients, it was seen that they could be divided into five major classes. Also, it was discovered that the antigenic differences among these five classes exist in their heavy chains. These heavy chains have been designated by the Greek letters alpha ($\alpha$), gamma ($\gamma$), delta ($\delta$), epsilon ($\epsilon$), and mu ($\mu$), and the corresponding classes of immunoglobulin are named IgA, IgG, IgD, IgE, and IgM. It is now known that all normal individuals possess varying amounts of immunoglobulin from each of these five classes.

Similar studies of the antigenicity of light chains revealed that there are two major types, called kappa ($\kappa$) and lambda ($\lambda$). Both $\kappa$ and $\lambda$ light chains, however, are found in all five classes of immunoglobulin. Thus, the five classes of immunoglobulin are distinguished by antigenic differences in their heavy chains. It should be pointed out that any one homogeneous immunoglobulin—such as that produced from a single clone (progeny of a single cell) of antibody-producing cells—will contain only $\kappa$ or $\lambda$ light chains, but not both, and only one type of heavy chain. Thus, a particular single cell produces only a single light chain and a single heavy chain.

### IgG

IgG makes up over 70% of the total human immunoglobulin. We shall characterize its structure before discussing the other four classes. Also, to keep the record straight, our discussion will be confined to human immunoglobulins, even though most major classes of immunoglobulins occur also in other animals.

IgG SUBCLASSES. Based on antigenic differences, IgG can be subdivided into four subclasses. These subclasses have been designated as IgG1, IgG2, IgG3, and IgG4, and studies have shown that the specific antigenic determinants for these IgG subclasses are located in the Fc portion of the antibody molecule. The reason that these antigenic differences are designated as subclasses rather than additional classes of Ig is based on the degree of homology among the various antigenic types of Ig. Thus, if the amino acid sequences of Ig are compared, one sees that the subclasses of IgG possess more than 90% identity among the constant regions of their heavy chains, whereas the same comparison between IgG and IgM reveals only about a 32% homology. Thus, in summary, all IgG molecules have common antigenic determinants on their heavy chains (which make them IgG) plus specific determinants in the Fc portion of the heavy chain which enables one to subdivide them into subclasses. Since the subclasses of IgG differ in the Fc portion of the molecule—the part responsible for complement fixation (Chapter 14), for fixing the IgG to certain cell surfaces, and for passage of human maternal antibody through the placenta to the fetus—it is not surprising that these subclasses differ in those effector functions that are controlled by the Fc fragment. Antiserum that is specific for each subclass of IgG can be prepared by injecting the purified subclass (obtained from patients with multiple myeloma) into rabbits. The resulting anti-IgG rabbit serum can be further purified by absorbing out contaminating antibodies using other purified subclasses of IgG. Using such monospecific antiserum it has been shown that IgG1, 2, 3, and 4 comprise about 59, 30, 8, and 3%, respectively, of the total human IgG. Remember, however, that all of these subclasses are encoded in separate genes, and thus all normal humans possess all four subclasses of IgG just as they possess all classes of immunoglobulin.

IgG ALLOTYPES. In contrast to subclasses, allotypes are minor variations in structure that will vary from one individual to another. In other words, subclass IgG1 from one person may show a minor antigenic difference from the IgG1 obtained from another person. These differences are specified by an allelic locus which is not sex-linked and thus follows typical autosomal Mendelian segregation. As a result they can be used, for example, as evidence in paternity litigation. There are two general types of allotypes based on their position in the IgG molecule, which are designated Gm and Inv.

Gm allotypes occur on the heavy chain ($\gamma$) of IgG molecules. There have been about 25 different Gm allotypes described (designated by numbers), each representing a different allele which codes for about a two-amino-acid difference between one Gm allotype and another. The IgG1 subclass heavy chain may carry markers from two or three different Gm loci (located at different positions in the heavy chain) while the other IgG subclasses carry only a single Gm determinant. Note that each subclass of IgG carries its own Gm genetic allele and each can therefore express a different Gm allotype. Therefore, an individual's Gm allotype could be listed as IgG1, Gm1 and Gm3; IgG2, Gm23; IgG3, Gm15; and IgG4, Gm4a. Unlike many genetic loci in which the maternally or paternally acquired gene may be dominant (such as in eye color), the Gm alleles are codominant. Thus individuals who are heterozygous at an allele will express both the paternal and maternal Gm specificity, although any one antibody-synthesizing cell will express only one of the two allelic genes.

The second allotype, called Inv, is found only on $\kappa$ light chains. There appear to be two different loci that code for a single amino-acid change at positions 153 and 191 on the $\kappa$ chain. Thus far only three Inv types have been described as occurring in IgG, IgA, and IgM. Since IgD and IgE also possess $\kappa$ light chains, it seems probable that the Inv allotype will also be found in these classes of immunoglobulin. Table 12-2 summarizes

**Table 12-2. Properties of Human Immunoglobulins**

| IG | Heavy (H) chain designation | Mol. wt. ($\times 10^{-3}$) | No. of domains in H chain | Mol. wt. of H chain ($\times 10^{-3}$) | Percentage of CHO | Normal serum cone (mg/ml) | Half-life (days) | Fixation of guinea pig complement | Attachment to monocytes |
|---|---|---|---|---|---|---|---|---|---|
| IgG1 | $\gamma_1$ | 146 | 4 | 51 | 2–3 | 9 | $21 \pm 5$ | + | + |
| IgG2 | $\gamma_2$ | 146 | 4 | 51 | 2–3 | 3 | $20 \pm 2$ | ± | − |
| IgG3 | $\gamma_3$ | 165 | 4 | 60 | 2–3 | 1 | $7 \pm 1$ | + | + |
| IgG4 | $\gamma_4$ | 146 | 4 | 51 | 2–3 | 0.5 | $21 \pm 2.5$ | −[a] | − |
| IgM | $\mu$ | 970 | 5 | 72 | 9–12 | 1.5 | 5 | + | − |
| IgA1 | $\alpha_1$ | 160 | 4 | 52–56 | 7–11 | 3 | 6 | −[a] | − |
| A₂m(1) | | | | | | | | | |
| IgA2 | $\alpha_2$ | | | | | | | | |
| A₂m(2) | | 160 | 4 | 55–58 | 7–11 | 0.5 | 6 | −[a] | − |
| SIgA | $\alpha_1$ or $\alpha_2$ | 380–390 | 4 | 52–58 | 7–11 | 0–0.05 | | − | − |
| IgD | $\delta$ | 172–200 | 4 or 5 | 60–69 | 9–11 | 0.03 | 3 | − | − |
| IgE | $\epsilon$ | 188–196 | 5 | 72–76 | 12 | 0.0003 | 2.3–4 | −[a] | − |

[a]Complement can be activated by aggregated molecules via an alternate pathway.

the properties of IgG together with those of the other classes of immunoglobulin.

AMINO-ACID SEQUENCING OF IgG. Using homogeneous IgG preparations from myeloma patients, it has been possible to determine the amino-acid sequence of a number of light and heavy chains. Light chains are particularly easy to obtain because many myeloma patients secrete large amounts of pure homogeneous light chains known as Bence-Jones proteins in their urine.

When the amino-acid sequence from a large number of different $\kappa$ light chains was determined, an astonishing result was obtained. Starting from the amino-terminal end, approximately half of the amino-acid sequence (about 110 amino acid residues) showed extreme variation among different preparations of $\kappa$ chains (although myeloma protein from one patient possessed a single sequence). However, the second half of the light chain possessed a highly constant amino-acid sequence for all $\kappa$ chains. (Variations in the constant region were found only for the Inv allotypes.) Similarly, various $\lambda$ chains possessed a variable amino acid sequence in their amino-terminal half, and a highly constant region in their carboxy-terminal half. These regions were appropriately named Variable$_{Light}$ ($V_L$) and Constant$_{Light}$ ($C_L$).

Amino-acid sequencing of heavy chains from different IgG molecules also showed that approximately 115 residues on the amino-terminal end were highly variable while the remainder of the heavy chain was constant (exceptions were the Gm and subclass differences in the constant region). However, because the heavy chain is twice as long as the light chain, the constant region is approximately three times as long as the constant region of the light chains. Moreover, it was found that the IgG molecule contained at least a dozen intrachain disulfide bonds. Since the amino-acid sequence was known, it was now possible to construct a more detailed model of an IgG molecule showing the variable and constant regions as well as the intrachain and interchain disulfide bonds. Figure 12-7 schematically represents such a model, showing that the light chain is divided into one variable and one constant region ($V_L$ and $C_L$), while the heavy chain exists in four units—one variable and three constant regions—which are designated as $V_H$, $C_{H1}$, $C_{H2}$ and $C_{H3}$. We shall see that the different immunoglobulin classes differ in a number of properties such as the ability to fix complement, to cross the placenta from mother to fetus, to bind to phagocytes, skin, or lympocytes, and to bind to mast cells. Each of these biological properties appears to be associated with a specific region in the immunoglobulin molecule and, as a result, each of the variable and constant regions is referred to as a domain.

## SITE OF ANTIBODY DIVERSITY

It is now well established that the specificity of antibody is a function of the tertiary structure of the variable regions of its light and heavy chains. This, in turn, is a function of the amino-acid sequence that exists in the variable regions. Moreover, if the amino-acid sequences from a large number of different immunoglobulins are compared, one can categorize them into families based on similarities of their variable regions. In other words, immunoglobulins within a specific family will possess similar stretches of amino acids in their variable region. Since it is estimated that the human may be able to synthesize thousands of different antibodies, how is it possible to generate this degree of diversity from a small number of immunoglobulin families? The answer may lie in "hot spots" of variability where amino-acid substitutions, deletions, or insertions occur within specific areas of the variable regions. Thus, a comparison of the variable regions from immunoglobulins of the same family shows that the major variations and gaps occur at approximately the same positions in each chain, as shown in Figure 12-8. Most of these hot spots of variability have

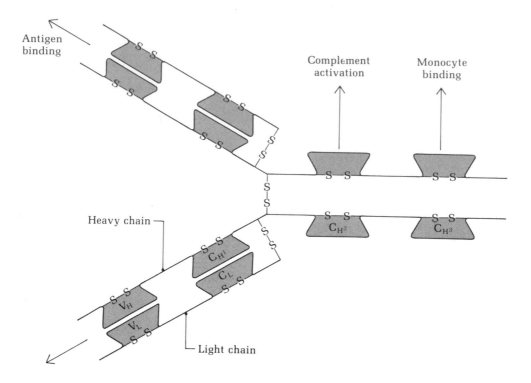

**Figure 12-7.** Schematic illustration of IgG showing both intra- and interchain disulfide bonds. Each loop in the peptide formed by an intrachain disulfide bond represents a single domain (grey areas labeled $V_H$, $C_{H^1}$, etc.). The $C_{H^2}$ is involved in complement fixation while the $C_{H^3}$ possesses sites that can bind to monocytes. Another effector function somewhere in the $C_{H^2}$ or $C_{H^3}$ domains is the capacity for transplacental transfer.

been shown to be a part of the contact binding area of antibody with its antigen. The somatic mutation theory proposes that the variations occurring in these hot spots are the result of mutations that occurred in the cell after fertilization. This is in contrast to a germ-line theory for antibody diversity, which suggests that all of the variable regions of antibody specificities occurred during evolution, are coded on separate genes, and are inherited as such. This latter concept argues that each antibody-producing cell originally possesses the genetic potential to respond to many antigens, but the final outcome perhaps depends upon a random selection of which immunoglobulin it synthesizes and carries on its surface. Still another pro-

posal suggests that the variable hot spots are encoded in a large variety of episomes (extra-chromosomal DNA). This concept proposes that these episomes become inserted into specific locations in the chromosomal DNA and specify those regions of high variability occurring in the antibody molecule. There are strong and weak points for all theories, and it may be possible that the truth lies somewhere in between these proposals.

IDIOTYPES.  If antibodies from an animal are injected into a second animal of the same allotype or even into a genetically identical animal, one might not expect the second animal to recognize these antibodies as foreign. However, some recipients unexpectedly do recognize these immunoglobulins as foreign. This can be explained by the fact that the site of variation in such antibodies occurs within the variable regions of the molecule and reflects the fact that any one clone of antibody-forming cells may synthesize antibodies possessing a unique structure in their variable region. These variants, called idiotypes, are expressed as antigenic differences among antibodies that are induced by the same antigen within a single individual or single species. In other words, antibodies from two different animals of the same allotype, induced by the same antigen, may possess sufficiently different structures in their variable region that rabbit A would recognize antibodies from rabbit B as foreign, and vice versa. Also, if the antibodies induced by injecting this antigen into a single rabbit were used to immunize a goat, the goat anti-rabbit serum might show a series of different antibodies directed against the antigen. The anti-idiotype may be directed against the antibody-combining site and

**Figure 12-8.** Variability at different amino acid positions for the variable region of the light chains. Variability is equal to the number of different amino acids at a given position divided by the frequency of the most common amino acid at that position. One can see that the variability is concentrated in three regions of the molecule (hot spots): 24–34, 50–56 and 89–97. Variations in length (caused by insertions at positions marked GAP) have been found in the first and third of these regions. It has been proposed that positions 24–34 and 89–97 contain the complementarity-determining residues of the light chain, those which make contact with the antigenic determinant. The heavy chain also has similar regions of very high variability.

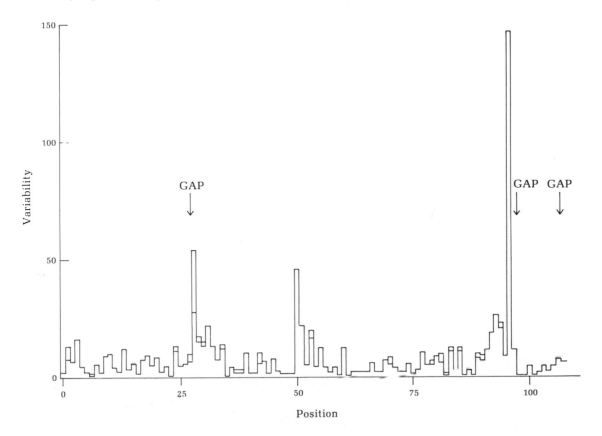

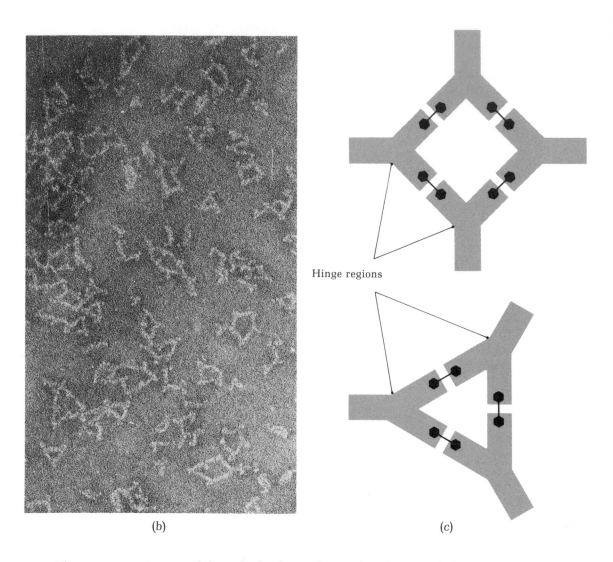

**Figure 12-9.** *a.* Structural formula for bis-N-dinitrophenyl-octamethylene-diamine, the hapten used to bind IgG to form polymers such as those diagrammed in Figure 12-9c. *b.* Electron micrograph of polymers produced by reaction of rabbit anti-DNP IgG with an equivalent amount of a divalent hapten (bis-N-dinitrophenyl-octamethylene-diamine). The antibody molecules are centered at the corners of the polygonal shapes. The Fc fragments project from the corners and the Fab fragments form the edges of the polygons. Note how the polymers consist of dimers, trimers, tetramers, and pentamers. (×260,000) *c.* Schematic illustration of a trimer and tetramer made of IgG monomers as shown in *b.* Note how the arms of the Fab portion must open wider for the tetramer than for the trimer.

hence be site specific, or it may be determined by other areas of the variable region, in which case one can only conclude that the variable portion of an antibody can vary among antibodies possessing the same specificity. The fact that a single myeloma protein (which arises from the malignant growth of a single antibody-producing cell) is of one idiotype supports the conclusion that each idiotype originates from a separate clone of antibody-producing cells.

ELECTRON MICROSCOPY OF IgG. Several important concepts concerning antibody reactions were observed by Robert Valentine and Michael Green from the electron microscopy of purified and specific IgG directed against dinitrophenol, when it was reacted with the synthetic dihapten, bis-N-dinitrophenyl-octamethylene-diamine (see Figure 12-9a). As can be seen in Figure 12-9b, antibody was able to form dimers, tetramers, and pentamers with this synthetic hapten (depending upon the number of haptens and Ab molecules in a given complex.) These combinations are schematically illustrated in Figure 12-9c. The antigen-reacting site is located between the L and H chains at the N-terminal end of the Fab portion of the molecule. Moreover, careful examination of the electron micrographs of IgG treated with pepsin to remove the Fc fragment shows that this treatment had no effect on the ability of the antibody to bind to the hapten and form dimers, trimers, and larger configurations. Finally, examination of the schematic drawing (Figure 12-9c) clearly shows that the angle between the Fab arms of the molecule must be variable— it can open or close depending upon the size of the antigen, or, as in this case, to fit the various multiples of hapten bound by the antibody.

Amino-acid sequences have shown that this area of bending possesses (1) a high proline content and (2) interchain disulfide bonds between the heavy chains. It is believed that these properties make this region flexible, allowing for considerable spreading of the Fab arms of the molecule; and, therefore, this part of the heavy chain is called the hinge region. Additional detailed information concerning the three-dimensional structure of immunoglobulin has been derived by X-ray diffraction studies, and current models are based in large part on the X-ray data. We shall turn to the other four classes of immunoglobulin, comparing their structures and functions with that of IgG.

## IgM

IgM was so named because it is a macroglobulin, at least five times larger than IgG. It has a sedimentation coefficient of 19S and a molecular weight of approximately 900,000 daltons. Considerable information concerning its structure has accumulated from the study of IgM isolated from patients with Waldenstrom's macroglobulinemia. These individuals have a malfunction in their lymphoid system that results in the synthesis of copious amounts of IgM.

If one gently breaks the interchain disulfide groups with sulfhydryl agents, the IgM molecule will dissociate into five 7S subunits, each having a molecular weight of about 180,000 daltons. Each of these 7S subunits is composed of two light chains (either $\kappa$ or $\lambda$) and two heavy chains designated $\mu$ chains. Interestingly, although the $\lambda$ and $\kappa$ light chains appear to be identical to those found in all classes of immunoglobulins, the $\mu$ chain is about 20,000 daltons larger than the $\gamma$ heavy chain of IgG. As a result, $\mu$ chains contain one variable region plus four (rather than three) constant regions. In addition, IgM also contains approximately 12% by weight of carbohydrate, linked at five positions in the $\mu$ chain.

Thus, each IgM molecule is actually composed of five monomeric 7S units, and the general formula for IgM can be written as either $(\mu_2\lambda_2)_5$ or $(\mu_2\kappa_2)_5$. Dissociation of an IgM molecule into its monomeric units also releases a 20,000 dalton peptide which has been designated as the J chain. It is not

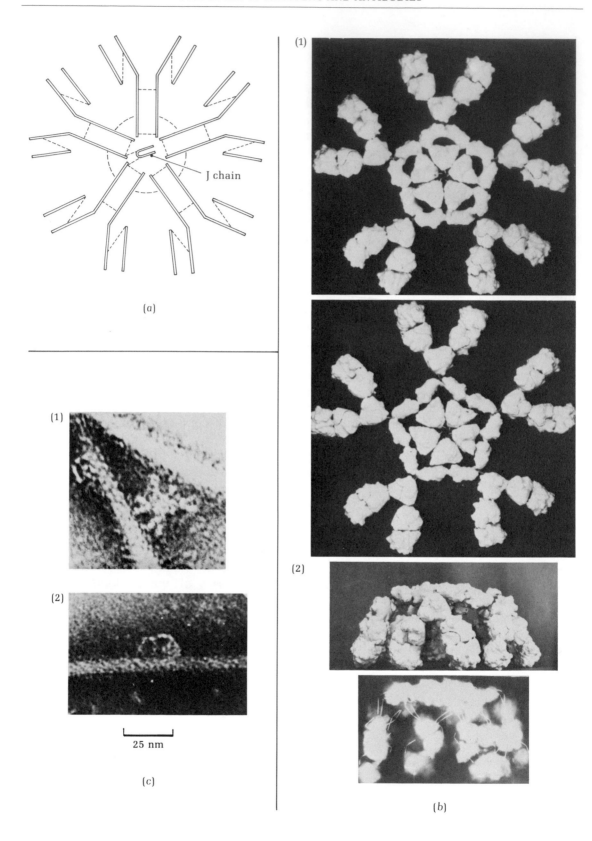

J chain

(a)

(1)

(2)

25 nm

(c)

(1)

(2)

(b)

known just where this J chain fits into the IgM molecule, but it is believed to be bound to one or perhaps two of the $\mu$ chains. Figure 12-10 gives a schematic representation of an IgM molecule; since IgM also possesses a hinge region in its heavy chain, it is not surprising that electron microscopy has shown that its shape can vary when reacting with an antigen, as shown by the models and micrographs in Figure 12-10b and c.

Because IgM contains ten Fab fragments, one would predict that it possesses ten antigen-combining sites. Such has not always been found to be the case. It appears many antigens are too large to fit physically into each of the ten potential antigen binding sites. Thus, one frequently finds that IgM is capable of binding only five molecules of antigen—apparently because large antigens may sterically block half of the potential binding sites.

As will be amplified in Chapters 14 and 15, IgM is usually the first antibody to appear following induction by an antigen. However, IgM synthesis is not prolonged, and IgG antibodies soon become the most prevalent class. IgM is, however, much more efficient than IgG in its ability to fix complement (Chapter 14), resulting in the lysis and death of most gram-negative bacteria. This increased efficiency appears to be due to the close proximity of the complement-binding sites on each of the Fc regions of the 7S subunits.

## IgA

The basic structure of IgA is similar to that described for IgG; it contains two light chains (either $\kappa$ or $\lambda$) and two heavy poly-peptides that have been designated as $\alpha$ chains. Of course, the antigenic properties of the $\alpha$ chains set IgA aside as a separate class of immunoglobulins, but IgA possesses an additional property that has led some immunologists to call it our first line of defense; namely, in addition to occurring in the serum as a 7S monomer, it is also found externally in almost all the body secretions. Thus, secreted IgA is present in the mucus of the lungs and gastrointestinal tract, as well as in saliva, tears, seminal fluid, urine, and colostrum (Table 12-3). Curiously, the secreted IgA occurs primarily as dimers of the monomeric unit (370,000 daltons with a sedimentation value of 11S), and a small amount is also found in higher multiples with sedimentation values from 16 to 20S. Secreted IgA antibodies possess a J chain (molecular weight 15,000 to 15,500 daltons), as was described for the multimeric IgM molecule, and, in addition, are linked to a second polypeptide (60,000 daltons) which has been designated as the secretory piece. It is not known just when and where these two additional polypeptides are added to the IgA molecule. It is possible that the J chain is involved in linking the monomeric units to form dimers and higher multiples, and it appears to be synthesized by plasma cells in the sub-epithelial tissue, as are heavy and light chains of IgA. The monomers are thought to be dimerized as they are secreted; otherwise, random dimerization in serum or secretions might yield rather inefficient dimers of mixed specificity. The secretory piece appears to be synthesized by the epithelial cells and added to the IgA molecules as they are transported into the external secretions. Its function is not known,

**Figure 12-10.** a. Schematic stick model of IgM. The dashed lines represent interchain disulfide bonds. It is not certain whether the J chain is linked to one or two $\mu$ chains. b. (1) IgM models made from cast domains, showing all five $F(ab')_2$ arms with alternative arrangements of $C\mu 3$ and $C\mu 4$ domains. (2) 'Table' form of the IgM model corresponding to the 'staple' in electron micrographs and X-ray photograph of this model (compare with c). c. Electron microscopy of IgM antibodies. The bar represents 25 nm. (1) IgM cross-linking two bacterial flagella. (2) IgM, seen in profile as a 'staple,' bound to a single flagellum.

**Table 12-3. Concentrations of Immunoglobulins and Relative Counts of Cells Producing the Different Classes of Immunoglobulins**

| Organ or Secretion | Conc. of immunoglobulins mgm % | | | Concentration ratio | Cell count ratio[a] |
|---|---|---|---|---|---|
| | IgG | IgA | IgM | IgG/IgA | IgG/IgA |
| Serum | 1000 | 160 | 110 | 6 | |
| Colostrum[b] | 30 | 600 | 0.50 | 0.05 | |
| Parotid saliva | 0–tr | 10 | 0–tr | <0.1 | |
| Nasal | 10 | 20 | 0–tr | 0.5 | 1 : 6 |
| Tears | 0–tr | 20 | — | <0.1 | |
| Bronchial | | | | | 1 : 5 |
| Gastric | | | | | 1 : 16 |
| Intestinal | 140 | 150 | — | 0.9 | 1 : 22 |
| Colon | | | | | 1 : 23 |
| Rectum | | | | | 1 : 16 |
| Appendix | | | | | 1 : 1 |
| Bile (gall bladder) | 143 | 160 | — | 0.9 | — |

[a]Quantitative cell counts using fluorescent antibody technique.
[b]Average values in first three days. Concentration of all immunoglobulins falls progressively as lactation proceeds.

but it may be involved in the transport of IgA to an external environment, or it may protect the secreted IgA from proteolytic digestion by extracellular proteases that are present in gastrointestinal and other secretions. Figure 12-11 depicts a schematic stick model of an IgA dimer.

SUBCLASSES OF IgA. Based on minor antigenic differences in their $\alpha$ chains, IgA can be divided into two subclasses, which have been designated as IgA1 and IgA2. These subclasses are found in all normal individuals; however, IgA2 can be additionally divided into two heritable allotypes (analogous to the Gm allotypes described for IgG) which are called $A_2m(1)$ and $A_2m(2)$. Transfusion of blood containing one of these allotypes into an allotype-negative individual can stimulate anti-$A_2m(1)$ or anti-$A_2m(2)$ antibody formation, possibly causing a transfusion reaction in subsequent transfusions.

## IgD

This class of immunoglobulins is present in the serum at a level of only about 0.2% of the concentration of IgG. In fact, were it not for a patient with multiple myeloma who was synthesizing abnormal amounts of IgD, it might still not have been found as a circulating antibody class.

IgD molecules have a molecular weight of approximately 180,000 daltons and, like other monomeric antibodies, are composed of two light and two heavy chains. The heavy chains, designated $\delta$ chains, contain about 12% carbohydrate and, as in the other cases, contain the antigenic determinants that define this class of immunoglobulins.

Because of the very low concentration of IgD in the serum and the unusual lability of the molecule during purification, it has been difficult to assign specific functions to this class of immunoglobulins. Only recently has a preliminary concept of its role in the immune system been proposed, namely as

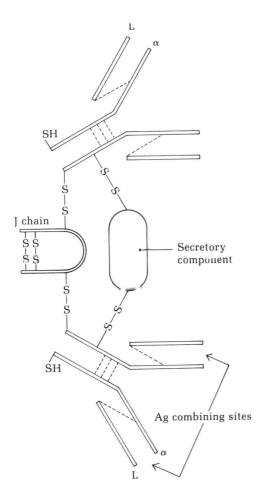

**Figure 12-11.** Schematic structural model of secretory IgA. It is uncertain whether the J chain is linked to one or two α chains.

a regulator for the synthesis of the other classes of immunoglobulins. At this point, the following paradox seems to exist: (1) B type lymphocytes, which are destined to differentiate into antibody-producing plasma cells, have a considerable amount of immunoglobulin on their cell surface; (2) it is generally believed that it is the reaction of antigen with the specific surface immunoglobulin which sets into motion the series of events which leads to cell differentiation and antibody synthesis; (3) although the major serum immunoglobulin is IgG and the major extracellular immunoglobulin is

IgA, these classes are not found on the cell surfaces of B lymphocytes (or, at most, rarely); and (4) IgD occurs in very low concentrations in the serum, but is found on the surface of the majority of B lymphocytes. It is, therefore, proposed that the function of IgD is to act as a cell surface receptor for antigen and to regulate the differentiation of B lymphocytes into antibody-producing cells that synthesize the other classes of immunoglobulins. This role will be amplified in Chapter 15 when we discuss the overall synthesis of immunoglobulins.

## IgE

Although this class of immunoglobulin is present in serum in minute concentrations, we have more definitive information concerning its function than we have for IgD, as shown in Table 12-2.

First of all, IgE immunoglobulins are responsible for the countless allergies with which certain individuals suffer: food, ragweed and other pollens, dust, and almost any other material imaginable. Although structurally similar to IgG, the heavy chains, called ε, are about 20,000 daltons larger than the IgG γ chains and as a result possess an additional domain in the Fc portion of the molecule, which provides IgE with a rather unusual property. IgE may exist in the allergic individual in considerably higher concentrations than in the nonallergic person; however, if IgE is injected into the skin of a normal individual, it will remain localized for weeks or months, whereas skin-fixing IgG will persist for a much shorter period. Thus, when a specific antigen (such as ragweed pollen) comes into contact with IgE antibody fixed to the surface of a mast cell, the reaction results in the release of pharmacologically active substances such as histamine and serotonin which dilate capillaries, alter permeability, and cause bronchial constrictions characteristic of an allergic rhinitis (such as hay fever). Apparently the major differences between IgE and the other classes of immunoglobulins reside in the Fc portion of the IgE molecule, because it is this part of the antibody that fixes so tightly to mast cell membranes.

It would seem unusual that an antibody possessing such destructive properties should have persisted so long during the evolution of the human race. However, circumstantial evidence suggests that IgE may also function as a protective antibody. This postulate arises from the observation that individuals in tropical areas may possess 20 times as much IgE as those from more northern areas. It has also been observed that IgE levels may rise following infection with certain parasites—especially helminths (see Chapter 44). Together these two observations suggest the possibility that the normal physiological function of IgE is to destroy invading parasites by reacting with antigens on their surfaces while its Fc fragment is still bound to a mast cell. This would result in the release of histamine and the possible destruction of the parasite. In the event that this is the major physiological function of IgE, those individuals living in northern climates but endowed with the genetic ability to mount an IgE response to environmental antigens may find some small comfort during their wheezing and sneezing by realizing that IgE may be a useful antibody for those who live in the tropics.

## REFERENCES

Atassi, M. Z. 1975. Antigenic structure of myoglobin: The complete immunochemical anatomy of a protein and conclusions relating to antigenic structures of proteins. *Immunochemistry* 12:423–438.

Capra, J. D., and J. M. Kehoe. 1975. Hypervariable regions, idiotypy and the antibody combining site. *Adv. in Immunol.* 20:1–40.

Cooper, M. D., and A. R. Lawton, III. 1974. The development of the immune system. *Sci. American* 231:58–72.

Davies, D. R., E. A. Padlan, and D. M. Segal. 1975. Three-dimensional structure of immunoglobulins. *Annu. Rev. Biochem.* 44:639–667.

Day, E. D. 1972. *Advanced Immunochemistry.* Williams and Wilkins, Baltimore.

Givol, D. 1973. Structural analysis of the antibody combining site. *Cont. Topics in Molec. Immunol.* 2:27–50.

Heidelberger, M., and F. E. Kendall. 1935. A quantitative theory of the precipitin reaction. *J. Exp. Med.* 62:697–720.

Kabat, E. A. 1968. *Structural Concepts in Immunology and Immunochemistry.* Holt, Rinehart and Winston, New York.

Kabat, E. A. 1960. The upper limit for the size of human antidextran combining sites. *J. Immunol.* 84:82–85.

Kochland, M. E. 1975. Structure and function of the J chain. *Adv. in Immunol.* 20:41–70.

Landsteiner, K., and J. van der Scheer. 1936. On cross reactions of immune sera to azoproteins. *J. Exp. Med.* 63:325–339.

Moss, A. J., Jr., G. V. Dalrymple, and C. M. Boyd. 1976. *Practical Radioimmunoassay.* C. V. Mosby, St. Louis.

Nisonoff, A., J. E. Hopper, and S. B. Spring. 1975. *The Antibody Molecule.* Academic Press, New York.

Porter, R. R. 1972. The antigen-binding sites of immunoglobulins. *Cont. Topics in Molec. Immunol.* 1:165–180.

Sela, M., B. Schechter, I. Schechter, and F. Borek. 1967. Antibodies to sequential and conformational determinants. *Cold Spring Harbor Symp. Quant. Biol.* 32:537–545.

Spiegelberg, H. L. 1972. γD Immunoglobulin. *Cont. Topics in Molec. Immunol.* 1:165–180.

Tiselius, A., and E. A. Kabat. 1939. An electrophoretic study of immune sera and purified antibody preparations. *J. Exp. Med.* 69:119–131.

Valentine, R. C., and N. M. Green. 1967. Electron microscopy of an antibody-hapten complex. *J. Molec. Biol.* 27:615–617.

Walker, L. J., and H. Taub. 1976. *Fundamental Skills in Serology.* Charles C. Thomas, Springfield, Ill.

Wu, T. T., and Kabat, E. A. 1970. An analysis of the sequences of the variable regions of Bence Jones proteins and myeloma light chains and their implication for antibody complementarity. *J. Exp. Med.* 132:211–250.

# 13

## Antigen-Antibody Reactions

It has been said that there are more experimental methods for studying antigen-antibody reactions than there are ways of cooking potatoes. In some minds, this chapter may prove the validity of that statement. But first some basic concepts that will help to understand the various systems to be described need to be established.

The study of antigen-antibody reactions in the laboratory is called serology, reflecting the fact that it is a measure of antibodies or antigens found in the serum (the amber-colored fluid that exudes from coagulated blood). Using standard serological tests, a known antigen (Ag) can be tested with an individual's serum in a search for its specific antibody (Ab), or conversely, a serum containing known Abs may be reacted with organisms isolated from a patient to confirm or to assist in the identification of the organism. Serologic techniques are also used for typing blood in blood banks, for typing tissue before transplant operations, for typing immunoglobulins, and for many other clinical tests.

A number of methods can be used to determine the presence or the amount of a specific Ab in an individual's serum. The particular method used depends in part

upon the sensitivity desired but mostly upon the physical state of the Ag, in other words whether it is on the surface of a cell, a soluble toxin or protein, a virus, or an encapsulated organism. Because most Abs have two or more identical antigen-combining sites and most naturally occurring Ags possess multiple, different reactive sites, a reaction between Ab and Ag can form a lattice-work of many Ag and Ab molecules. If the Ag is on the surface of particulate material such as a bacterium or a red blood cell, the end result is a clumping of the cells or agglutination. A soluble Ag may form an Ag-Ab complex that becomes too large to stay in solution, and the result is a precipitation, or a precipitin reaction. Other reactions merely measure the gain or loss of a property of the Ag. An example of this is a reaction with a bacterial toxin to neutralize it; the Ab neutralizing the toxin is given the general name antitoxin. In still other reactions Ab neutralizes viruses so that they cannot infect susceptible cells (neutralizing Ab), or Abs called opsonins may react with bacterial cells to make them more easily phagocytized by leukocytes.

The multiplicity of Ab names does not, however, indicate different types of anti-

bodies for each reaction; it merely denotes
the type of reaction being measured. Thus,
if sufficient antitoxin is mixed with a soluble
toxin, it will produce a precipitin reaction, or
if this soluble toxin is adsorbed to particles
such as styrene beads, the same specific
antibody will agglutinate the beads, or enhance their phagocytosis. Therefore, specific
Ab names such as precipitin, agglutinin,
antitoxin, and others are used only to indicate the physical state of the Ag or the type
of Ag-Ab reaction being measured. With this
in mind, we now may consider some specific
techniques for measuring Ag-Ab reactions.

## THE PRECIPITIN REACTION

The precipitin reaction yields a visible
precipitate of Ag and Ab. Thus, if one mixes
a clear sample of a dilution of serum containing Abs with a solution of the correct
Ag, the mixture will become opalescent
within minutes to hours and a flocculent
precipitate will appear in what had been a
clear solution. Such reactions are usually
carried out by adding a constant amount of
Ab (antiserum) to each of a series of 10 or 12
tubes that contain increasing amounts of
Ag—in other words, tube 1 contains the least
Ag and tube 12 the most. During an incubation time of 2 to 24 hours, a reaction occurs
between the Ag and its specific Ab, which
results in a visible precipitate in those tubes
in which the Ab and the Ag are in correct
proportion to each other so that they can
form an insoluble lattice. If one wishes to
make this a quantitative test, it is a relatively simple matter to collect the resulting
precipitate and determine the amount of Ag
and Ab in each precipitate—especially if the
Ag is a non-nitrogen-containing polysaccharide. Figure 13-1 shows a typical precipitin curve obtained by plotting the amount
of Ab in the precipitate against the amount of
Ag added to each tube. Remembering that
each tube receives an identical quantity of
Ab, it can be seen that only a small amount
of precipitate is formed in the first few tubes,
which contain relatively little antigen and,

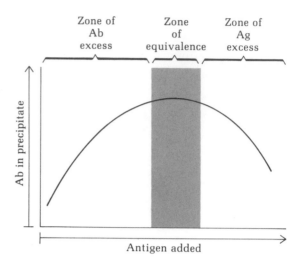

**Figure 13-1.** Precipitin curve illustrating
the effect of Ag concentration on the total
amount of antibody precipitated as insoluble complexes of Ab and Ag.

hence, an excess of Ab. In the tubes containing more Ag, the amount of precipitate increases up to a point, after which it decreases as a result of smaller complexes
being formed in the zone of Ag excess.
Assays of the supernatant solution will
show that those tubes containing too little
Ag still contain free Ab, whereas in those
with high concentrations of Ag, no free Ab can
be detected in the supernatant solution in
spite of the fact that little or no precipitation occurred in those tubes. Only in tubes
of maximum precipitation is all Ag and all
Ab removed from solution. These zones, as
shown in Figure 13-1, are designated as the
zone of Ab excess, the equivalence zone,
and the zone of Ag excess. In the zone of Ab
excess, all Ag has reacted with Ab and has
been precipitated. Conversely, in the zone of
Ag excess, all of the Ab has reacted with Ag,
but in those tubes of high Ag concentration,
the complexes remain soluble because the
large excess of Ag binds Ab into small complexes which do not crosslink to form large
insoluble aggregates. Figure 13-2 is a schematic illustration of the type of complexes
formed in each zone.

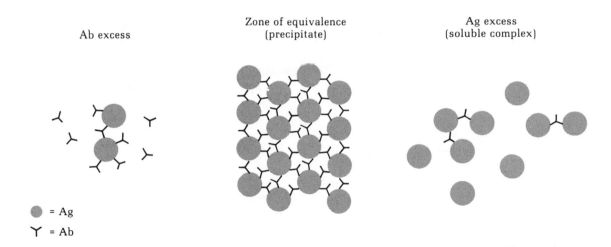

**Figure 13-2.** Schematic illustration of the complexes formed as a function of Ag-to-Ab ratios.

Beyond the fact that the precipitin curve demonstrates that Ab and Ag must be present in optimal proportions for maximum precipitation to occur, it also shows that Ab and Ag can react with each other in multiple proportions. Thus, unlike a chemical reaction in which, for example, one mole of $Na_2SO_4$ reacts with one mole of $BaCl_2$ to form one mole of $BaSO_4$ and two moles of NaCl, Ag-Ab precipitates may contain variable proportions of reactants. This is illustrated in Table 13-1, where it can be seen that the ratio of Ab to Ag in the precipitate varied from 21.5 in Ab excess to 6.6 in a tube containing Ag excess. Moreover, this table shows that even in the equivalence

**Table 13-1. Addition of Egg Albumin (Ea) to a Constant Quantity of Antibody (Anti-Egg-Albumin)**

| Ea N added (mg) | Ea N pptd. (mg) | Total N pptd. (mg) | Antibody N by difference (mg) | Ratio Antibody N:EaN in ppt. | Tests on supernatant |
|---|---|---|---|---|---|
| 0.029 | Total | 0.665 | 0.635 | 21.5 | Excess Ab |
| 0.049 | Total | 1.005 | 0.956 | 19.5 | Excess Ab |
| 0.079 | Total | 1.320 | 1.241 | 15.7 | Traces Ab and Ea (?) |
| 0.082 | Total | 1.370 | 1.288 | 15.7 | Excess Ab |
| 0.088 | Total | 1.422 | 1.334 | 15.2 | Slight excess Ab |
| 0.098 | Total | 1.468 | 1.370 | 14.0 | No Ab or Ea |
| 0.122 | Total | 1.570 | 1.448 | 11.9 | No Ab or Ea |
| 0.140 | Total | 1.502 | 1.452 | 10.4 | No Ab or Ea |
| 0.157 | Total | 1.606 | 1.449 | 9.2 | No Ab or Ea |
| 0.195 | 0.194 | 1.650 | 1.456 | 7.5 | Excess Ea |
| 0.234 | 0.202 | 1.542 | 1.340 | 6.6 | Excess Ea |
| 0.296 | | 1.025 | | | |

zone, where all Ab and all Ag had been precipitated, the ratio of Ab to Ag could vary from 14.0 to 9.2.

### Modifications of the Precipitin Reaction

A number of modifications of the classical precipitin reaction have been developed. Most such changes are designed either to increase the sensitivity of the reaction or to identify specific Ag–Ab reactions occurring in a system containing multiple Ags and Abs.

DOUBLE DIFFUSION (OUCTERLONY TECHNIQUE). When soluble Ag and soluble Ab are placed in separate small wells punched into agar that has solidified on a slide or glass plate, the Ag and the Ab will diffuse through the agar. The holes are located only a few millimeters apart and Ab and Ag will interact in the area in which they are in optimal proportions to form a line of precipitate. Because different Ags will diffuse at different rates and since different Ags may require different concentrations of Ab for optimal precipitation, the position of the precipitin band will usually vary for each Ag. Figure 13-3 is a schematic illustration of double diffusion in which there are several identical and nonidentical Ags. Thus, you can see that this technique can in some cases determine the number of Ags present in a solution. Figure 13-4 is an example of actual double-diffusions showing similarities, partial identities, and nonidentities.

SINGLE DIFFUSION (OUDIN TECHNIQUE). The Oudin technique is seldom used, but it will also separate some Ag-Ab precipitates. The antiserum (containing the Abs) is mixed with melted agar, poured into a small tube and allowed to solidify. The Ag solution is then layered on top of the solidified agar. As in the case of double diffusion, different Ags will diffuse at variable rates and will require different proportions of Ag to Ab for precipitation to occur. As the Ags diffuse through the agar gel, a line of precipitate will form when Ag and Ab are in optimal proportions (see Figure 13-5). As the process continues, the precipitin lines appear to move further down the tube, becoming more separated from each other. However, the actual pre-

**Figure 13-3.** Schematic illustration of double diffusion with various combinations of identical and nonidentical Ags. In each case well number 1 contains crude Ab; all other wells contain Ags. The conclusions are shown under each slide.

Well **1** contains crude Ab; all other wells contain Ag.

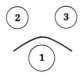 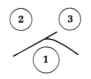 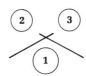

(a) **2** and **3** are identical.

(b) **2** and **3** contain one identical Ag, but **2** has one Ag not present in **3** (partial identity).

(c) **2** and **3** contain non-identical Ags.

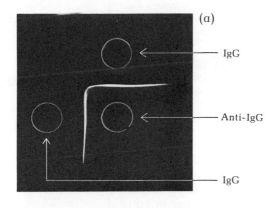

(a)

— IgG

— Anti-IgG

— IgG

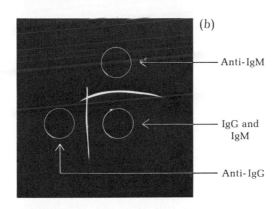

(b)

— Anti-IgM

— IgG and IgM

— Anti-IgG

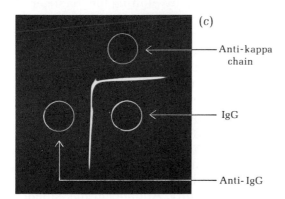

(c)

— Anti-kappa chain

— IgG

— Anti-IgG

**Figure 13-4.** Double diffusion; a. Identity: human IgG in both antigen wells and anti-human IgG in the antibody well. b. Nonidentity: mixture of IgG and IgM in one antibody well and anti-IgG in one antibody well and anti-IgM in the other antibody well. c. Partial identity: IgG in the antigen well and anti-IgG in one antibody well and anti-kappa chain in the other antibody well.

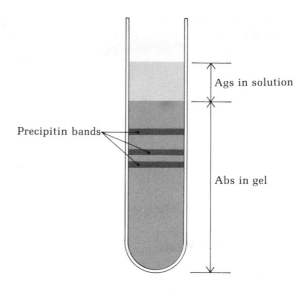

Ags in solution

Precipitin bands

Abs in gel

**Figure 13-5.** Single diffusion of Ags downward through Abs immobilized in a gel.

cipitate doesn't move. What occurs is that as more Ag diffuses through the agar, the precipitated line becomes an area of Ag excess. Since Ag-Ab reactions are reversible, this results in the solubilization of the precipitate and its reformation at a position further down the tube where optimal proportions of Ag and Ab exist. Different Ags can, however, diffuse together to form a single precipitin line. Therefore, if either this technique or double diffusion is used to show the purity of a specific Ag, it must be supported by additional evidence.

IMMUNOELECTROPHORESIS. This procedure combines electrophoresis and double diffusion for the separation of Ag-Ab reactions in gels. In essence, one places a small drop of solution containing the Ags (usually proteins) into a small hole punched out of solidified agar on a slide. The slide is then placed in an electric field to allow for the electrophoretic migration of the Ags. Different Ags will migrate at different rates or even in different directions, depending upon their size and charge. After the completion of the electrophoresis, a trough is removed from the agar along one or both sides of the slide

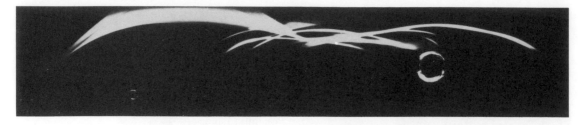

**Figure 13-6.** Immunoelectrophoresis: whole human serum was placed in the well (circle) and subjected to electrophoresis. After two hours, the electric current was turned off and anti-whole human serum was placed in a trough along the length of the slide. The precipitin lines are formed where the antibodies and the antigens (separated components of whole human serum) diffuse together in optimal proportions.

and the appropriate antiserum is placed into the troughs. As before, the Abs and the Ags diffuse toward each other, resulting in the formation of precipitin bands whenever they are both in zones of optimal proportions. Since diffusion is a function of molecular weight, immunoelectrophoresis adds a second parameter for separating antigens, that is, the charge of the antigen. Thus immunoelectrophoresis is more likely to separate similar high molecular weight antigens than is simple diffusion alone. As shown in Figure 13-6, this procedure can be used to separate many antigens as well as to indicate the potential purity of an antigen.

RADIAL IMMUNODIFFUSION. This procedure is used only to quantitate the amount of a specific Ag present in a sample and can be used for many Ags. One diagnostic application of this procedure is to measure the amount of a specific immunoglobulin class present in a patient's serum.

The assay is carried out by incorporating monospecific antiserum (antiserum containing only Ab to the Ag for which you are assaying) into melted agar and allowing the agar to solidify on a glass plate in a thin layer. Holes are then punched into the agar and different dilutions of the Ag are placed into the various holes. As the Ag diffuses from the hole, a ring of precipitate will form at that position where Ag and Ab are in optimal proportions (see Figure 13-7). However, if the Ag solution is concentrated, the area near the hole will contain Ag excess and, therefore, the Ag must diffuse further before it will be present in optimal concentration. Thus, the diameter of the precipitated ring is a quantitative function of Ag concentration. Using known concentrations of the Ag in question, one can prepare a standard curve by plotting the diameter of the precipitin ring versus Ag concentration. Once a standard plot is obtained, one need only to measure the diameter of the precipitin ring to calculate the concentration of Ag in the unknown solution.

Radial immunodiffusion is used routinely for the laboratory diagnosis of multiple myeloma or agammaglobulinemia. In either case, antibody to the various classes of immunoglobulins (IgG, IgA, IgM, IgD, or IgE) is incorporated into the agar before allowing the agar to solidify. Aliquots of the patient's serum are then added to the holes punched in the agar. By noting the diameter of the resulting precipitin ring it is possible to quantitate the amount of any class of immunoglobulin present in the patient's serum.

RADIOIMMUNOASSAYS. This is one of the newest, most sensitive, and most versatile techniques available for determining trace

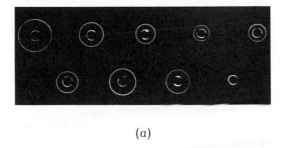

(a)

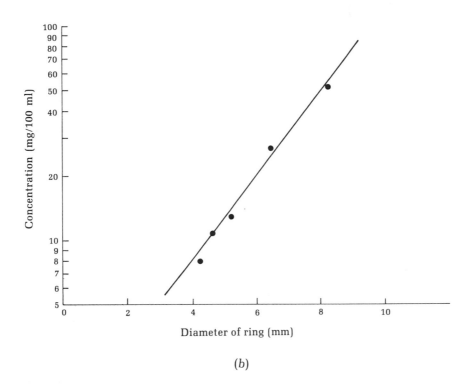

(b)

**Figure 13-7.** Radial immunodiffusion. *a.* Anti-IgA is incorporated into the agar and small wells are punched out, into which the patient's serum is placed. The top row consists of standards containing 52, 28, 13, 8 and 10.2 mg per 100 ml of standard IgA. The wells in the bottom row received serum from four different patients. *b.* A curve is drawn by plotting the diameter of the precipitin rings in the top row against the logarithm of the concentration of IgA. The concentration of IgA in each patient's serum can then be read from the curve after measuring the diameter of each precipitin ring in the bottom row; in these cases concentrations are 17, 30, 22 and less than 1 mg of IgA per 100 ml of serum.

amounts of haptens or Ags. The entire procedure is based on competition for the reactive sites on the specific Ab between a known amount of a highly radioactive Ag and an unknown amount of the same, but nonradioactive Ag. If no unlabeled Ag is present, the Ag-Ab complex will be highly radioactive. If equimolar amounts of radioactive and nonradioactive Ag are present, the complexes would contain only half as much radioactivity, and if there were a huge excess of unlabeled Ag, the complexes would contain very little radioactivity. One can, therefore, prepare a standard curve for a specific system by adding increasing amounts of nonradioactive Ag and measuring the decrease in radioactivity occurring in the Ag-Ab complexes. This curve will allow the quantitation of Ag present by merely counting the radioactivity present in the Ag-Ab complexes.

But, here is the tricky part of this assay. The reaction is usually carried out with Ag excess, and the concentrations of Ab and Ag used are so small that precipitation does not occur. Thus, one must separate the soluble Ag-Ab complexes from any residual soluble radioactive Ag before counting. This may be accomplished by any one of several techniques. For example, using albumin as an Ag, R. S. Farr showed in 1958 that soluble Ag-Ab complexes could be precipitated by adding ammonium sulfate to a final concentration of 40% saturation. This Farr technique is now used to precipitate the radioactive Ag-Ab complexes formed during the radioimmunoassay, but it is of value only if free Ag remains soluble in 40% ammonium sulfate.

Another procedure for precipitating Ag-Ab complexes out of solution is the double Ab technique. This method is based on the fact that Abs are antigenic if injected into a foreign host. Thus, the injection of human immunoglobulin into a goat will induce goat Abs that will react with and precipitate human Abs. Therefore, if our radioimmunoassay utilizes human Abs, one can merely add goat antiserum containing anti-human immunoglobulins to the solution containing the Ag-Ab complexes. This will form yet larger complexes, resulting in the precipitation of the soluble Ag-Ab complexes formed during the radioimmunoassay. The precipitate can then be counted for incorporated radioactivity. A schematic diagram of the radioimmunoassay is shown in Figure 13-8.

Taking advantage of its extreme sensitivity (measuring picograms of Ag per ml) the radioimmunoassay is used to measure the concentration of certain hormones such as insulin, testosterone, growth hormone, and glucagon. It is also used to determine the presence of the hepatitis B Ag (see Chapter 36), which may be present in the serum of asymptomatic blood donors.

## AGGLUTINATION REACTIONS

When Ag is present on the surface of a cell or particle, the addition of Ab will cause a clumping or agglutination of the cells. This reaction is analogous to the precipitin reaction in that antibody merely acts as a bridge to form a lattice network of Ab and cells. Of course, since cells are so much larger than a soluble Ag, the result is more visible when the cells aggregate into clumps.

The usual agglutination test is actually only a semi-quantitative measure of Ab since, unlike the precipitin test, one cannot normally determine the milligrams or moles of antibody that are attached to a clump of bacterial cells. Instead, serial dilutions of the serum are made, as shown schematically in Figure 13-9. When the dilutions of antiserum are completed, a constant amount of cells is added to each tube and, following several hours of incubation at 37°, clumping is recorded by visual inspection. The titer of the antiserum is given as the reciprocal of the highest dilution that causes clumping. Thus, an antiserum which agglutinated at a dilution of 1 to 128 (but not at 1 to 256) would be reported to have a titer of 128. Note that

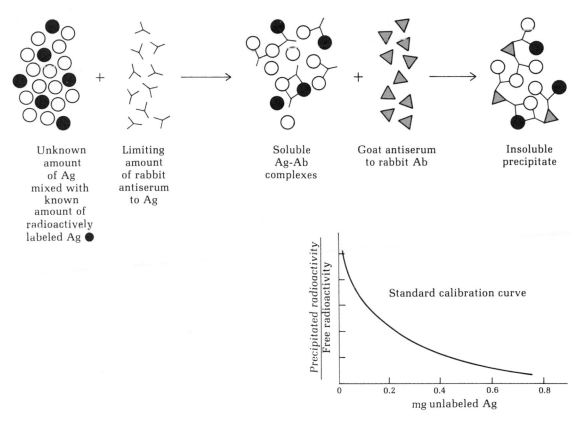

**Figure 13-8.** Radioimmunoassay used to quantitate trace amounts of an Ag such as human growth hormone. The ratio of precipitated to free radioactivity is measured after the process. The amount of unlabeled Ag present can then be determined from a calibration curve. The standard curve is prepared in a similar manner, using a constant amount of radioactively labeled Ag with varying known amounts of unlabeled Ag.

**Figure 13-9.** Double dilutions of Ab carried out in an agglutination reaction. Each tube contained one ml of saline before beginning the double dilutions with antiserum. The numbers under each tube represent the dilution of serum in that tube.

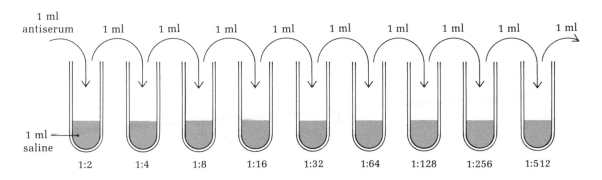

this is not an absolute value but rather expresses a relative concentration of a specific antibody present in the serum.

Since a cell has many antigenic determinants on its surface, one does not normally see zones of Ab excess as described for the precipitin reaction. Occasionally antibodies are formed, however, that will react with the antigenic determinants on a cell but will not cause agglutination (for example, anti-Rh and anti-*Brucella* Ab). Such Abs have been named blocking Abs because they are unable to agglutinate the cells. At one time blocking Abs were thought to be monovalent (possessing only one Ag binding site) and thus unable to form a lattice; however, since they can be made to cause agglutination under special conditions, this concept no longer has credence. A more likely explanation is that whole cells carry a net negative charge making them subject to an electrostatic repulsion which cannot be overcome by 7S Ab. This would result in having both Ab reactive sites from a single Ab molecule binding to adjacent determinants on the same cell, failing, therefore, to crosslink them to form an aggregated mass of cells. Their presence is suspected when one sees agglutination occurring at high dilutions of antiserum but not in the lower dilutions containing a more concentrated antiserum. As the serum is diluted, the concentration of blocking Ab falls to the point that it is no longer inhibitory.

## ISOANTIBODIES

Early in the practice of blood tranfusion, it was observed that the recipient had to be compatible with the donor if a serious transfusion reaction was to be avoided. It was soon learned that the basis of incompatibility was immunological in nature and that some individuals possessed naturally occurring antibodies in their serum that would lyse other types of red blood cells. This led to the discovery of the ABO system of classification for red blood cells.

It was observed by Karl Landsteiner that if serum from a number of individuals was mixed with red blood cells (RBC's) obtained from these persons in all possible combinations, the RBC's were agglutinated in some instances. On the basis of these findings, he determined that RBC's could be classified into four major types which were designated as A, B, O, and AB. This classification is based on the presence (or absence) of two antigens A and B which may be present together, singly, or not at all on RBC's. These RBC antigens have been termed isoantigens (or alloantigens).

Unexpectedly, Landsteiner found that each individual's serum contained isoantibodies (subsequently shown to be of the IgM-type) against those A and B isoantigens that were not present on the person's RBC's. Thus, as shown in Table 13-2, type A persons possess Ab to type B Ag on RBC's; type B individuals possess Ab to type A Ag on RBC's; type O persons have both anti-A and anti-B Abs, while type AB individuals have neither of these Abs. The origin of the isoantigens is a heritable trait but the origin of the isoantibodies is not known. It has been postulated that they arise as a result of an antibody response to antigens in the intestinal flora which are structurally similar to the A and B isoantigens. The occurrence of structurally similar Ag from widely diverse sources is not unusual. One such Ag has been named the Forssman Ag. This Ag, which stimulates the formation of anti-

**Table 13-2. Isoantigens and Isoantibodies Associated with the ABO Classification of Red Blood Cells**

| Blood type | Isoantigen on RBC | Isoantibody in Serum |
|---|---|---|
| A | A | B |
| B | B | A |
| AB | AB | None |
| O | None | AB |

bodies capable of lysing red blood cells of sheep (in the presence of complement—see Chapter 14), is found in many animal and bacterial sources. Antibodies to Forssman Ag are referred to as heterophile Ab and their presence in humans is used as a diagnostic aid for infectious mononucleosis.

A sometimes fatal transfusion reaction with fever, prostration, and renal insufficiency may occur if a patient receives blood from a different blood group; this results from the hemolysis of the transfused cells by the patient's own isoantibodies and serum complement. Careful tests to identify the blood group in both the recipient and donor, as well as compatibility tests to ascertain possible agglutination of donor cells (crossmatching), must be carried out before transfusion to avoid this hazard.

## Rh Factor

The Rh factor (so-called because it also occurs on the RBC's of *Rhesus* monkeys) present in about 85 percent of the population is an antigen found on red blood cells but not related to the A and B antigens. Unlike the ABO system, isoantibodies to Rh antigen do not occur. If, however, an Rh negative individual receives Rh positive red blood cells, that person will respond by making Ab to the Rh factor.

This is particularly dangerous when a mother is Rh negative and the father is Rh positive because, if the fetus is genetically Rh positive, any fetal blood that enters the mother's circulation will induce the formation of Abs that are directed against the Rh factor in the red blood cells of the fetus. Since these antibodies will be of the IgG type, they can cross the placenta to react with the red blood cells of the fetus. This results in a hemolytic disease known as erythroblastosis fetalis.

Since exposure of an Rh negative mother to the Rh positive cells of her baby does not normally occur in sufficient concentrations to induce a primary response until the time of delivery, a first child is usually not in danger. However, if the mother makes a primary response to the Rh Ag at the time of delivery, a secondary response (anamnestic response) can be induced at a later date with much smaller amounts of Rh Ag. Thus, a subsequent Rh positive fetus might trigger the mother to form anti-Rh antibodies that would then cross the placenta and destroy the fetal RBC's. To avoid this, we can take advantage of the fact that an excess of injected antibody to the Rh positive RBC's will react with and destroy such cells, preventing the mother from making a primary response to the Rh factor. This procedure is now routinely done at the time of delivery to Rh negative mothers with Rh positive babies. Fortunately, even though there are 27 known Rh specificities, only Ag D appears to be a sufficiently strong Ag to stimulate the synthesis of destructive, hemolytic antibodies, and hence it is anti-D (Rhogam) that is used in these cases.

COOMBS ANTI-GLOBULIN TEST.  Anti-Rh antibodies are of the IgG type, but they will not normally agglutinate Rh positive red blood cells. The best explanation for this observation is that there are insufficient Rh factor sites to permit 7S anti-Rh Ab to overcome the normal electrostatic repulsion that exists among RBC's. A clever way to measure these nonagglutinating Abs was described by Coombs. He reasoned that if red blood cells were coated with anti-Rh Abs, the addition of antibodies to the Rh Abs would cause the erythrocytes to agglutinate. Thus, he injected human immunoglobulin into rabbits to stimulate them to make anti-human immunoglobulin (also known as Coombs reagent). The anti-globulin test for Rh Abs could then be accomplished as follows: (1) react Rh positive red blood cells with the serum to be tested; (2) after a short incubation, add anti-human immunoglobulin; if the serum contained Rh Abs, the red blood cells would then agglutinate as shown schematically in Figure 13-10.

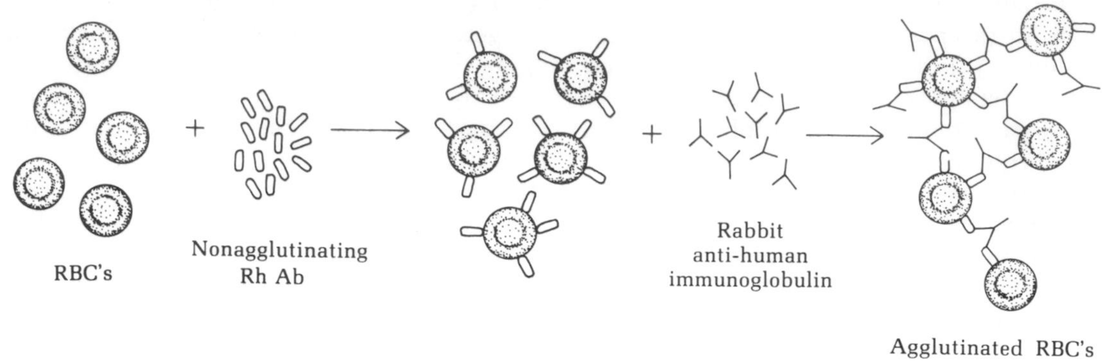

RBC's     +     Nonagglutinating Rh Ab     →         +     Rabbit anti-human immunoglobulin     →

Agglutinated RBC's

**Figure 13-10.** Coombs anti-globulin test used to detect nonagglutinating Rh Abs.

### Passive Agglutination Reactions

Because the difference between a precipitin reaction and an agglutination reaction is based on whether the Ag is soluble or particulate, a precipitin reaction can be measured as an agglutination reaction by adsorbing a soluble Ag to the surface of a cell or particle. One may use synthetic particles such as polystyrene beads, but since red blood cells can be made to readily adsorb many soluble Ags, they are frequently used for this purpose.

Most polysaccharides or lipopolysaccharides will spontaneously adsorb to the surface of red blood cells. Proteins do not adsorb well unless the erythrocytes are first treated with tannic acid. These "tanned" cells are then mixed with a soluble protein Ag prior to their use in passive hemagglutination.

Such tests are frequently carried out in plastic agglutination trays in which two-fold dilutions of antiserum can be accomplished using a standardized loop. The addition of the tanned red blood cells possessing the adsorbed Ag to the Ab-containing wells results in agglutination patterns, as shown in Figure 13-11.

### SPECIAL SEROLOGIC TESTS

There are a number of serologic tests that are highly specialized and sometimes

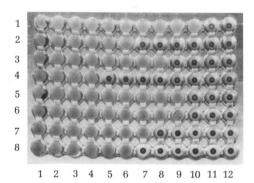

**Figure 13-11.** Hemagglutination patterns. The wells in each horizontal row contain double dilutions of antiserum (0.05 ml) to which 0.05 ml of appropriate red blood cells are added. Horizontal rows 1 through 4 contain sheep's red blood cells (SRBC) and serum from rabbits immunized with SRBC. Rows 5 through 8 contain SRBC that have been coated with human gamma globulin (HGG) and serum from rabbits immunized with HGG. Positive hemagglutination is seen as diffuse clumping of the red blood cells, while a negative reaction appears as a small button of red blood cells that have settled to the bottom of the well, as in the right-hand wells here.

difficult to process. An example of these would include the *Treponema pallidum* immobilization test (TPI) for syphilis. It is based on the fact that the live organisms become immobilized if mixed with serum containing specific antisyphilitic antibodies. Complement fixation is also a specialized technique for the determination of specific antibodies. However, because of the complexity of the complement system, it will be discussed separately in Chapter 14.

The hemagglutination inhibition test (red cell agglutination inhibition) is used to identify certain viruses that by themselves routinely cause the agglutination of red blood cells. If, however, specific antibodies to the virus are mixed with the virus before the red blood cells are added, agglutination is inhibited. Thus, by using known antiserum, one can identify an unknown virus or quantitate a known virus.

Another specialized procedure is the chemical attachment of a fluorescent dye to an Ab. If cells are then treated with this fluorescent Ab, the Ab combines with its specific Ag and the entire complex becomes visible when viewed with a special fluorescence microscope.

The fluorescent antibody technique can also be used in an indirect method in the following manner. Antihuman immunoglobulin is prepared (as described for the Coombs anti-globulin test) and made fluorescent by the attachment of fluorescent dye. These Abs are then used to provide a rapid detection of a specific human Ab. For example, let us suppose we want to check a patient's serum for the presence of Abs to the organism that causes typhoid fever, *Salmonella typhi.* We would mix a dilution of the patient's serum with the *S. typhi* organisms and, after a few minutes, wash off the excess serum and add fluorescently labeled anti-human immunoglobulin. If the patient's serum contained Ab to *S. typhi,* these Abs would have reacted with the Ags on the surface of the bacterial cells. The fluorescently labeled anti-human immunoglobulin subsequently added would then react with the

human immunoglobulin on the *S. typhi,* causing cells to fluoresce. On the other hand, if the patient's serum did not contain specific Abs to *S. typhi,* no human immunoglobulin would react with the bacterial cells and the subsequent addition of the fluorescently labeled anti-human immunoglobulin would not result in the presence of fluorescent cells. This same technique can be and is, indeed, used for many different types of Ab reactions, since the fluorescent anti-human immunoglobulin will react with all human antibodies. This method is frequently referred to as the indirect fluorescent Ab technique or the fluorescent sandwich technique. Using an antiserum known to be specific for a particular organism, this same technique can also be used for the rapid identification of an unknown bacterium.

An essentially identical technique in which the antibody is labeled with ferritin (a protein that contains a high concentration of iron) is also useful. Such Ab is electron dense and, when viewed with the electron microscope, will appear as dark bodies.

This chapter has been largely concerned with techniques that detect and measure Abs and Ags. The techniques described, however, are artificial laboratory procedures that do not reflect the natural role of immunoglobulins. The remainder of this unit will emphasize the *in vivo* role of immunoglobulins and the immune response in combating disease.

## REFERENCES

Davis, N. C., and M. Ho. 1976. Quantitation of immunoglobulins, in N. R. Rose and H. Friedman, eds. *Manual of Clinical Immunol.* Amer. Soc. Microbiol., Washington, D.C. 4–16.

Froese, A., and A. H. Sehon. 1975. Kinetics of antibody-hapten reactions. *Cont. Topics in Molec. Immunol.* **4**:23–54.

Gehle, W. D., and K. O. Smith. 1976. Detection of soluble immune complexes by ultracentrifugation. *J. Immunol. Methods* **10**:289–291.

Gill, T. J., III. 1976. Principles of radioimmunoassay, in N. R. Rose and H. Friedman, eds. *Manual of Clinical Immunol.* Amer. Soc. Microbiol., Washington, D.C. 169–171.

Jerne, N. K. 1973. The immune system. *Sci. American* **229**:52–60.

Kochwa, S. 1976. Immunoelectrophoresis (including zone electrophoresis), in N. R. Rose and H. Friedman, eds. *Manual of Clinical Immunol.* Amer. Soc. Microbiol., Washington, D.C. 17–35.

Macario, A. J. L., and E. C. de Macario. 1975. Antigen-binding properties of antibody molecules: Time-course dynamics and biological significance. *Current Topics in Microbiol. and Immunol.* **71**:125–170.

Morris, D. A. N., M. D. Smith, and J. Greyson. 1976. Surface immune precipitation: A new method for rapid quantitative antigen analysis. *J. Immunol. Methods* **9**:363–372.

Simons, M. J., and A. A. Benedict. 1974. Radioelectrocomplexing: A general radioimmune assay procedure for the detection of primary binding of antigen by antibody. *Cont. Topics in Molec. Immunol.* **3**:205–254.

# 14

# Complement and Complement Fixation

Around the beginning of the twentieth century it was observed that antiserum could exert two entirely different effects on gram-negative bacteria or red blood cells. In one case, when fresh specific antiserum was used, such cells were lysed. On the other hand, if the antiserum was heated to 56°C for 30 minutes or aged a week or so, it could no longer cause lysis, but would instead agglutinate the bacteria or red blood cells. However, when fresh normal serum, such as guinea pig serum, was added to the heated or aged antiserum, it regained its ability to cause cell lysis. It was thus apparent that the lytic effect required two factors: (1) specific antibody, and (2) a labile component present in normal serum. This latter substance has been given the name complement. Subsequent research has revealed that complement is an incredibly complex multicomponent system which is composed of at least twelve different proteins.

Before outlining the details of complement activation, however, it would be worthwhile to consider the biological purpose of the complement system. This can be best emphasized by noting that once antibody has reacted with its antigen, it can do no more. In other words, antibody might precipitate an antigen or, if cellular, might cause agglutination; but, with the exception of the neutralization of toxins or of virus infectivity by steric hindrances, antibody alone is a rather ineffective means of protection. Thus, practically, the major function of a specific antibody is to recognize a foreign antigen and bind to it. By doing so, it provides a site for the initiation of the reactions of the complement system. It is the activation of this system that (1) leads to the lysis of foreign cells, (2) enhances phagocytosis of invading microorganisms, and (3) causes a local inflammation, stimulating the chemotactic activity of the host's leukocytes. The following sections of this chapter will be concerned with a step-by-step dissection of the component parts and reactions of the complement system and the role that this system plays in the destruction of foreign cells.

## CLASSICAL PATHWAY OF COMPLEMENT ACTIVATION

As will become apparent, the operation of the complement system consists of a number of reactions, each of which activates the next reaction in the series. A primary event must occur, however, to initiate the reactions that eventually involve the many com-

**Table 14-1. Proteins of the Classical Human Complement System**

| Protein | Serum concentration ($\mu g/ml$) | Sedimentation coefficient (S) | Molecular weight | Relative electrophoretic mobility | Number of chains |
|---------|---------|---------|---------|---------|---------|
| C1q | 180 | 11.1 | 400,000 | $\gamma_2$ | 18 |
| C1r | — | 7.5 | 180,000 | $\beta$ | 2 |
| C1s | 110 | 4.5 | 86,000 | $\alpha$ | 1 |
| C1t | — | 10.0 | — | — | — |
| C2 | 25 | 4.5 | 117,000 | $\beta_1$ | — |
| C3 | 1600 | 9.5 | 180,000 | $\beta_2$ | 2 |
| C4 | 640 | 10.0 | 206,000 | $\beta_1$ | 3 |
| C5 | 80 | 8.7 | 180,000 | $\beta_1$ | 2 |
| C6 | 75 | 5.5 | 95,000 | $\beta_2$ | 1 |
| C7 | 55 | 6.0 | 110,000 | $\beta_2$ | 1 |
| C8 | 80 | 8.0 | 163,000 | $\gamma_1$ | 3 |
| C9 | 230 | 4.5 | 79,000 | $\alpha$ | — |

**Table 14-2. The Cytolytic Complement Reaction: Functional Units and Membrane Sites.**

*First site: Activation of recognition unit*

$$C1 + \boxed{Ab} \longrightarrow \boxed{Ab \begin{smallmatrix} \diagup C1q - C1t \\ \diagdown C1r - C1s \end{smallmatrix}} \longrightarrow C\overline{1s}$$

*Second site: Assembly of activation unit*

$$C4 \xrightarrow{C\overline{1s}} C4a + C4b^*$$

$$C2 \xrightarrow{C\overline{1s}} C2a^* + C2b$$

$$C4b^* + C2a^* \longrightarrow \boxed{C\overline{4b2a}}$$

$$\boxed{C\overline{4b2a}} + C3 \longrightarrow C3a + C3b^*$$

$$\boxed{C\overline{4b2a}} + C3b^* \longrightarrow \boxed{C\overline{4b2a3b}}$$

*Third site:*
*Assembly of membrane attack mechanism*

$$C5 + \boxed{C\overline{4b2a3b}} \longrightarrow C5a + C5b^*$$

$$C5b^* + C6 + C7 + C8 + C9 \longrightarrow \boxed{C5b\text{-}9}$$

Notes:
1. All components enclosed in boxes are bound to a site on the cell membrane.
2. Bars denote activated enzymes.
3. Asterisks denote enzymatically activated binding sites.

ponents of the complement system (see Table 14-1). In the case of the classical pathway, the initiating event occurs when the first component of complement reacts with antigen-antibody complexes in which the antibody is either IgM or IgG. Neither IgA, IgD, nor IgE is effective in activating complement in this way.

Once initiated, the activation of the complement system may have a varied effect, depending upon the type of foreign cell involved in the antigen-antibody reaction. In the case of a gram-negative bacterium or a red blood cell, the integrity of the cell membrane is destroyed, resulting in the lysis and death of the cell. Gram-positive organisms, however, are not lysed, but the activation of complement by a gram-positive cell and specific antibody will result in the release of fragments of complement components which aid in phagocytosis by binding to the Ag, forming a bridge between it and a host leukocyte. The complex reactions that produce all of these effects can be divided into three series of reactions involving the complement system: (1) the recognition unit, (2) the assembly of the activation unit, and (3) the assembly of the attack unit. Table 14-2

**Figure 14-1.** Pictorial representation of the three-site model of complement transfer from solution to the solid phase of the target cell surface. The C1 complex is reversibly bound to antibody molecules (Site I) through its C1q and C1r subunits. An internal reaction leads to activation of C1s. C$\overline{1s}$ activates labile sites in C2 and C4 by enzymatic removal of activation peptides. The C$\overline{4b,2a}$ enzyme (C3 convertase) is thereby enabled to assemble at membrane Site II topologically distinct from Site I. C$\overline{4b,2a}$ converts itself to C$\overline{4b,2a,3b}$ (C5 convertase) by cleavage of C3 and assimilation of C3b. Many monomeric C3b fragments are bound in the process within the microenvironment of a C$\overline{4b,2a}$ complex. These clusters of C3b bound at a fourth category of membrane sites (not indicated in the drawing) are responsible for the immune adherence reaction. C$\overline{4b,2a,3b}$ in cleaving C5 initiates the self assembly of the C5b-9 complex which attacks the membrane at a third, topologically distinct site (Site III). The membrane lesion at Site III is caused, in all probability, by the insertion into the membrane of a small specialized portion of one of the subunits of the complex. C3a and C5a are activation peptides with anaphylatoxin activity.

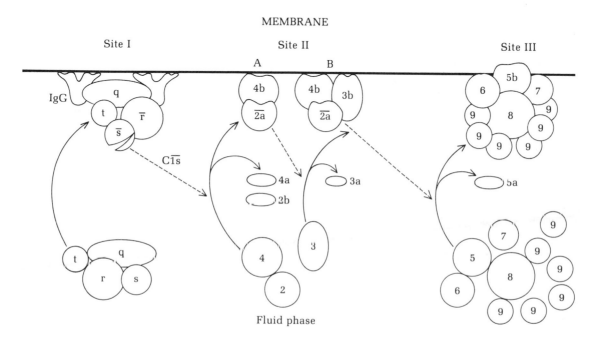

summarizes the reactions of complement leading to the formation of the attack complex, and Figure 14-1 gives a schematic model of the series of reactions leading to the formation of the attack complex.

### The Recognition Unit

Of the nine known components of complement, only the first component, C1, is involved in the recognition unit. This component, as indicated in Table 14-1, is actually composed of four different proteins, C1q, C1r, C1s, and C1t, which interact with each other on an antigen-antibody complex. The precise mechanism through which this interaction occurs is still somewhat obscure, but the over-all function of the recognition unit is to convert the C1s subunit of C1 into an enzyme which starts the assembly of the activation unit.

The reaction begins when both C1q and C1r bind to the Fc fragment of the antigen-antibody complexes. The binding site of C1q is located in the fourth domain ($C_{H4}$) of IgM, and on the second domain ($C_{H2}$) of IgG. (Subclass IgG4 will bind C1q but, for unexplained reasons, it does not cause the activation of the complement system.) The exact site of binding for the C1r subunit is not known, but it binds to the Fc fragment at a site that is distinct from that of C1q.

C1q is a rather unusual protein made up of six subunits, each of which possesses its own binding site for the Fc fragment of IgG or IgM. For the complement system to be activated, the proteins comprising the first component of complement must crosslink at least two molecules of IgG, presumably by C1q. This means that a minimum of two IgG molecules must be bound very closely together on the cell membrane to be an effective activator; on the other hand, a single molecule of IgM will initiate the sequence. This occurs because IgM is a pentameric molecule possessing a multimeric Fc fragment able to bind to several of the "arms" of the C1q. Thus, one IgM molecule on the surface of a RBC is sufficient to cause complement-mediated lysis; a RBC must bind an average of 700 molecules of IgG antibody to ensure that two molecules are close enough to be cross-linked by C1q. IgM is obviously more efficient in complement-mediated reactions than IgG.

The sequence of events that occur after the binding of C1q and C1r to the antigen-antibody complex is not completely known. It is thought, however, that C1s binds to C1r and that the C1t binds through a $Ca^{++}$ dependent linkage to C1q to form a bridge between C1q and C1s. In general, the binding of C1r to the antibody is thought to result in a conformational change in the C1r molecule that exposes an enzymatically active site able to cleave C1s to form $\overline{C1s}$. (Complement components which have been modified to become enzymatically active are written with a bar over the complement designation, as in $\overline{C1s}$.) It is thought that the activation of C1s requires a rigid complex that is provided when C1q links several IgG molecules together. The specific role of C1t is not known, but it appears to interact with both C1q and C1s to aid in producing the conformational change required to reveal the active site of C1r. Thus, the recognition unit consists of the binding of C1q and C1r to the Ag-Ab complex and the sequential activation of C1r and C1s. Activated $\overline{C1s}$ initiates the assembly of the activation unit.

### Assembly of the Activation Unit

The assembly of the activation unit occurs in the following steps: (1) $\overline{C1s}$ cleaves C4 into C4a and C4b. This exposes a hydrophobic binding site on C4b which binds to a site on the cell membrane (different from the formation of the recognition unit); (2) $\overline{C1s}$ also cleaves C2 into C2a and C2b; (3) C2a combines with C4b to form the active enzyme $\overline{C4b,2a}$ or, as it is also called, C3 convertase. Immediately after being formed the $\overline{C4b,2a}$ cleaves C3 into two fragments, C3a and C3b. The C3b binds to the $\overline{C4b,2a}$ to form another enzyme, $\overline{C4b,2a,3b}$, named C5 convertase. This $\overline{C4b,2a,3b}$ is the activation unit of complement, and at this point in the series of reactions it is bound to the cell membrane. Note, however, that this enzyme is not bound at the Ag-Ab reaction site, and it may not even be on the same cell.

## Assembly of the Membrane Attack Complex

The only enzymatic step in this final series of reactions is the cleavage of C5 by the C5 convertase into C5a and C5b. The other reactions are nonenzymatic and occur spontaneously as follows: (1) C5b reacts with one molecule each of C6 and C7; (2) this complex is then able to bind one molecule of C8 to form C5b,6,7,8; (3) six molecules of C9 then join to this tetramolecule to form a C5b-9 complex consisting of ten molecules of the complement system (see Figure 14-2) with a total molecular weight of approximately one million daltons. The C5b-9 complex is the actual attack complex, and it binds to a site on the cell membrane causing membrane destruction and lysis of the cell. Table 14-2 summarizes the reactions occurring in the classical pathway of complement activation.

## Mechanism of Complement Lysis

Early theories of membrane damage by the attack complex of complement postulated that perhaps the damage was the result of a lipase activity in the C5b-9 complex. However, no enzymatic degradation products can be found in synthetic lipid bilayers which have been damaged by complement, and it is now generally believed that the C5b-9 complex becomes inserted into the outer leaflet of the membrane. Current ideas suggest that one peptide chain of the C8 component may extend through both leaflets of the cell membrane. By a mechanism that is still poorly understood, this results in the formation of a hydrophilic channel which can be seen by electron microscopy to exist as a small donut-shaped hole in the membrane (see Figure 14-3). It should be noted

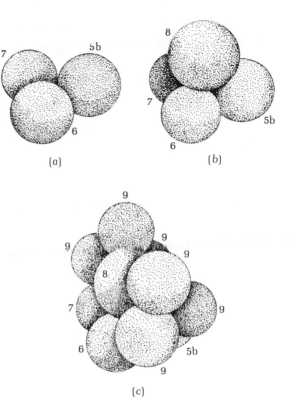

(a)   (b)

(c)

**Figure 14-2.** Model of the C5b-9 decamolecular membrane attack mechanism of complement showing three stages of its assembly. The relative sizes are roughly proportional to the molecular weights of the proteins. The numerals refer to the corresponding complement components. a. Model of the membrane-bound C5b,6,7 trimolecular complex, displaying triangular geometry and constituting the proposed binding site for C8. b. Model of the tetramolecular complex C5b,6,7,8 having the geometry of a tetrahedron. c. Model of the fully-assembled decamolecular C5b-9 complex, exhibiting two C9 trimers bound in triangular arrangement to the C8 portion of the tetrahedron.

that one $\overline{C1s}$ molecule can result in the formation of many $\overline{C4b,2a}$ complexes, which after combination with C3b can generate many attack complexes. Thus, once the recognition event occurs, there is a cascade of reactions that may result in gross membrane damage.

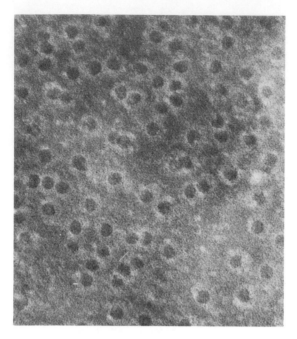

**Figure 14-3.** Sheep erythrocyte membrane treated with antibody and human complement. Subsequent treatment with trypsin was used to remove other protein but did not affect the round lesions caused by complement. (×320,000)

## ALTERNATE PATHWAY OF COMPLEMENT ACTIVATION

The alternate pathway of complement activation (also called the properdin pathway) does not require the presence of specific antibodies for initiation and, as a result, provides a mechanism of nonspecific resistance to infection. Moreover, this pathway does not utilize C1, C4, or C2, which are the early reactants in the classical pathway of complement activation. Keep in mind, however, that the over-all result of this pathway is the same as that of the classical pathway: C3 is split into C3a and C3b, and C5 is cleaved to form C5a and C5b, thus permitting the spontaneous formation of the C5b-9 membrane attack complex. The enzymes catalyzing these conversions are entirely different from the C3 and C5 convertases described for the classical pathway of complement activation.

## Recognition and Assembly via the Alternate Pathway

There are still unknown factors involved in the alternate pathway, and the terminology of the reactants can be mind-shattering to the novice; however, note that this pathway bypasses both the recognition unit and the assembly of the activation unit as described for the classical pathway. Instead there are at least three normal serum proteins that, when activated, form a functional C3 convertase and a C5 convertase. These are initiating factor (IF), C3 proactivator convertase (D), and C3 proactivator (B). In addition, properdin, which is also a normal component of serum, enters the pathway as an accessory component to protect the C3 and C5 convertase from inactivation by C3b inactivator. In brief, the activation of the complement system by way of the alternative pathway is as follows:

1. Particles (usually foreign cells) containing polysaccharides, lipopolysaccharides, zymosan (a yeast cell wall polysaccharide) or aggregated IgA act on an initiation factor, IF, (molecular weight of 170,000 daltons) present in serum, converting it to an active form, $\overline{\text{IF}}$. IF, therefore, is the recognition unit for the alternate pathway.

2. $\overline{\text{IF}}$ then reacts with C3, Factor B (C3 proactivator) and Factor D (C3 proactivator convertase) to form an initial C3 convertase as shown below:

$$\overline{\text{IF}} + \text{C3} + \text{B} + \text{D} \xrightarrow{\text{Mg}^{++}} \text{C}\overline{\text{3,B,IF}}$$

It is not known whether Factor D is an integral part of this enzyme.

3. The initial C3 convertase ($\text{C}\overline{\text{3,B,IF}}$) splits C3 to form C3a and C3b. The C3b is deposited on the surface of the activating particle (which would normally be a cell membrane).

4. C3b binds Factor B, forming the transient intermediate C3b,B, which is then subject to cleavage by the activated C3 proactivator convertase, $\overline{\text{D}}$, to form $\text{C}\overline{\text{3b,Bb}}$. This is the

active C3 convertase of the alternate pathway.

5. As more C3b is generated by $\overline{C3b,Bb}$, it continues to attach to the membrane. When a critical density of C3b becomes bound to the $\overline{C3b,Bb}$ (thought to be at least three molecules), the specificity of the convertase is shifted from a C3 to a C5 convertase (designated $\overline{C3b_n,Bb}$).

6. Properdin (molecular weight of 212,000 daltons) enters the reaction sequence and binds to both the C3 and C5 convertase to protect the complex from the action of C3b inactivator (a normal component of serum). Properdin interaction, therefore, is the terminal event in the assembly of the activation unit for this pathway.

7. Once the C5 convertase is formed, C5 is cleaved to form C5a and C5b and the spontaneous formation of the attack complex (C5b-9) quickly follows.

### The C3b Cascade

It can be seen that the major regulating component for either the classical or alternative pathway is the presence of C3b. Once C3b becomes available from either pathway, C5 convertase is formed and the membrane attack complex can be assembled. It is not surprising, therefore, that normal serum contains a C3b inactivator which dampens this reaction by destroying C3b. In the absence of C3b inactivator, any C3b would continue to act as a feedback amplifier, converting all of the C3 component of complement to C3a and C3b.

### ADDITIONAL COMPLEMENT-MEDIATED REACTIONS

During the formation of the membrane attack complex, C3 and C5 are cleaved into the peptides C3a, C3b, C5a, and C5b respectively. The importance of these reactions can be seen by the fact that the formation of one recognition unit ($\overline{C1s}$) may eventually activate many molecules of C3 and C5, and that the cleavage of both of these components is further amplified by the presence of C3b. As discussed earlier in this chapter, C5b reacts spontaneously with the subsequent components of complement to form the attack complex. The other products of these reactions—C3a, C3b, and C5a—are, however, involved in events other than the lysis of the target cell.

### Anaphylatoxins

C3a and C5a will bind to the membranes of mast cells and platelets, causing the release of pharmacologically active mediators such as histamine and serotonin. The role of these mediators in immediate-type hypersensitivity is discussed in detail in Chapter 16; suffice it to say here that their major effect is to increase capillary permeability and to cause the constriction of smooth muscle. Large concentrations of C3a and C5a in the bloodstream would result in fatal shock similar to the anaphylactic shock described in Chapter 16 (hence the name anaphylatoxins), but the release of small amounts of histamine from mast cells and platelets has probable benefit, by increasing capillary permeability at the site of inflammation. This permits a much more rapid movement of leukocytes through the capillary wall to an infected area.

It is evident, however, that while small amounts of histamine at the site of inflammation may be helpful, large amounts could be disastrous. Fortunately, serum also contains an inactivator which very rapidly destroys both C3a and C5a. The inactivator is actually a carboxypeptidase B that cleaves the carboxyterminal arginine from each of these anaphylatoxins, resulting in their complete inactivation.

### Chemotaxis

Any material that attracts leukocytes to an area of inflammation is a chemotactic agent. Both C5a and C5b,6,7 (the partially formed attack complex) are chemotactic. We can, therefore, see that the activation of complement by either the classic or the alternate pathway will result in an increased infiltration of leukocytes into an area of inflammation.

### Immune Adherence

Excess C3b will bind to Ag-Ab complexes (for example, Ab bound to an Ag on the surface of a bacterium). Since leukocytes also possess specific receptor sites on their membranes for C3b, this immune adherence of C3b greatly facilitates the phagocytosis of the C3b-coated cell.

### GENETIC DEFECTS RESULTING IN COMPLEMENT DEFICIENCIES

Both animals and humans have been found to possess genetic defects that result in either a deficiency of some complement component or in a deficient regulatory system for the control of the activated components of complement. For the most part, those individuals unable to synthesize C2 or C4 because of genetic makeup do not appear to suffer from frequent infections—probably because they can still utilize the alternate pathway of complement activation.

Defects at the C3 level have been observed in individuals who are unable to synthesize C3, as well as in persons who lack the C3b inactivator to destroy the C3b component. These latter persons will, therefore, be subjected to C3b amplification (as described for the alternate pathway) with the result that essentially all of the normal C3 will be split to C3a and C3b. This causes abnormally low serum levels of C3. In cases of inability to synthesize C3 or lack of the C3b inactivator, persons are subject to recurrent infections, apparently because they can neither form the attack complex, mount an effective chemotactic response, nor stimulate phagocytosis.

A regulatory deficiency has been described in which the inhibitor that inactivates C1s is lacking. As one might guess, unless there is some way to turn off the recognition unit, the cascade of reactions involving the complement series will result in consider-

able damage to the host. Normal serum contains a glycoprotein that rapidly inactivates C1s. Those individuals lacking this inactivator suffer from occasional local accumulations of fluid which, particularly if localized in the larnyx, can be fatal. The precise mechanism of the edema (hereditary angioneurotic edema) is not readily apparent.

### COMPLEMENT FIXATION

As was described earlier in this chapter, complement reacts with antigen-antibody reactions involving IgM and IgG. As a result, complement undergoes a series of complex reactions and is depleted, or fixed. The measurement of complement fixation *in vitro* thus provides a sensitive technique for the determination of antigen-antibody reactions. A complement fixation test can be used to determine the presence or absence of an antigen-antibody reaction in the following manner.

First, because we wish to add a known amount of complement to the system, serum from an individual is heated to 56°C for 30 minutes to inactivate any complement present. Then, since we are trying to assess the level of a specific antibody in the serum, we make a series of double dilutions of the serum, following which known amounts of complement (usually in the form of fresh guinea pig serum or freshly dissolved lyophilized guinea pig serum) and antigen are added to each tube of diluted antiserum. The assay is incubated overnight to allow complement to fix and any C5b-9 complexes to decay. Since these assays comprise very small amounts of antibody and antigen, no visible reaction will occur, and the only way to ascertain if a reaction occurred is to determine whether the added complement was fixed. To do this, an indicator system must be added to the reaction tubes.

The indicator system consists of sheep's red blood cells and specific antibody to sheep's red blood cells which cause lysis only in the presence of complement. If no complement is present, there will be no lysis. Therefore, if we now look at our test system, we will see that if antibodies are present in the individual's serum, complement will have been fixed, and our subsequently added indicator system does not undergo lysis. On the other hand, if the person's serum does not contain the antibodies for which we are testing, complement will still be available for the lysis of our indicator system. The amount of RBC lysis that occurs can be determined by centrifuging down any unlysed RBC's and measuring with a spectrophotometer the amount of hemoglobin that has been released into the supernatant solution. One may plot the percent of RBC's lysed against the dilution of antibody present in the test system, but in actual practice, the antibody titer is usually reported as the reciprocal of the serum dilution that resulted in the lysis of half of the added red blood cells. It must be stressed, however, that because of the complexity of the complement system, any complement fixation test must include controls to ascertain that neither the antigen nor the antiserum alone could inactivate complement and that in the absence of both antigen and antiserum the added complement was effective for the lysis of the red blood cells.

Complement fixation tests may be used as an aid for the diagnosis of syphilis (Wasserman test), pertussis, gonorrhea, histoplasmosis, and a number of other diseases.

## REFERENCES

Assimeh, S. N., and R. H. Painter. 1975. The identification of a previously unrecognized subcomponent of the first component of complement. J. Immunol. 115:482–487.

Assimeh, S. N., and R. H. Painter. 1975. The macromolecular structure of the first component of complement. J. Immunol. 115:488–494.

Bitter-Suermann, D., U. Hadding, H-U. Schorlemmer, M. Limbert, M. Dierich, and P. Dukor. 1975. Activation of alternate pathway by some T-independent antigens. J. Immunol. 115:425–430.

Colten, H. R. 1976. Biosynthesis of complement. Adv. in Immunol. 22:67–118.

Cooper, N. R. 1973. Activation of the complement system. Cont. Topics in Molec. Immunol. 2:155–183.

Fearon, D. T., and K. F. Austen. 1975. Initiation of C3 cleavage in the alternate pathway. J. Immunol. 115:1357–1361.

Gewurz, H., and L. A. Suyehira. 1976. Complement, in N. R. Rose and H. Friedman, eds. Manual of Clinical Immunol. Amer. Soc. Microbiol., Washington, D.C. 36–47.

Humphries, G. M. K., and H. M. McConnell. 1975. Antigen mobility in membranes and complement mediated immune attack. Proc. Nat. Acad. Sci. USA 72:2483–2487.

Kolb, W. P., and H. J. Muller-Eberhard. 1975. The membrane attack mechanism of complement. J. Exp. Med. 141:724–735.

Mayer, M. M. 1973. The complement system. Sci. American 229:54–66.

Medicus, R. G., O. Gotze, and H. J. Muller-Eberhard. 1976. Alternative pathway of complement: Recruitment of precursor properdin by the labile C3/C5 convertase and the potentiation of the pathway. J. Exp. Med. 144:1076–1093.

Muller-Eberhard, H. J. 1975. Complement. Annu. Rev. Biochem. 44:697–724.

Muller-Eberhard, H. J. 1972. The molecular basis of the biologic activities of complement. The Harvey Lectures 1970–71. Academic Press, New York, 75–104.

Pillemer, L., L. Blum, I. H. Lepow, O. A. Ross, E. W. Todd, and A. C. Wardlaw. 1954. The properdin system and immunity. I. Demonstration and isolation of a new serum protein, and its role in immune phenomena. Science 120: 279–285.

Podack, E. R., W. P. Kolb, and H. J. Muller-Eberhard. 1976. The C5b-9 Complex: Subunit composition of the classical and alternative pathway-generated complex. J. Immunol. 116:1431–1434.

Reid, K. B. M., and Porter, R. R. 1975. The structure and mechanism of activation of the first component of complement. Cont. Topics in Molec. Immunol. 4:1–22.

Schreiber, R. D., O. Gotze, and H. J. Muller-Eberhard. 1976. Alternative pathway of complement: Demonstration and characterization of initiating factor and its properdin-independent function. J. Exp. Med. 144:1062–1075.

# 15

## Antibody Synthesis and Immunological Unresponsiveness

Having defined antigens as molecular structures that induce the synthesis of antibodies, we are now ready to look at the sequence of events occurring when the antibody-forming system is confronted with a foreign antigen.

As far back as 1900, Paul Ehrlich proposed a theory for antibody formation in which he visualized that certain cells of the body possessed surface receptors for antigens. Then, when a foreign antigen such as a toxin or a virus combined with the surface receptor, the entire complex was released from the cells. This in turn, stimulated the cell to make more receptor—some of which was released to become circulating antibody (see Figure 15-1). As we shall see, Ehrlich's concept is not too far from present theories of antibody synthesis, but it was generally disregarded for many years because immunologists could not imagine that an animal could possess cells with surface receptors to such an incredibly large array of antigens, including artificially synthesized compounds in which the antigenic determinant groups were aromatic phenols. In contrast, an instructional theory for antibody formation was advanced by Linus Pauling and others, in which it was proposed that antigen acted as a template around which the newly synthesized anti-

**Figure 15-1.** Ehrlich's selection hypothesis proposed that the combination of Ag with a cell receptor (Ab) stimulated the cell to synthesize and shed additional receptors (Abs).

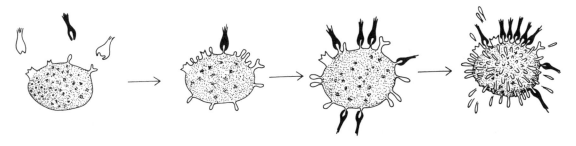

body could wrap itself to form a specific tertiary structure that would in turn bind more antigen (see Figure 15-2). This concept remained in vogue until it was realized that the tertiary structure of a protein was dependent upon its amino-acid sequence, and thus antibody specificity could not result from instruction by the antigen.

This brought us back to a variation of Ehrlich's original concept of antibody formation. In simple terms, the clonal selection hypothesis, as advanced by Sir Macfarlane Burnet, proposed that antigen reacted with a surface receptor on a cell and that this reaction induced the cell to divide into more cells and to secrete antibody that would react with the stimulating antigen (see Figure 15-3). Burnet also postulated that if such cells reacted with antigen during fetal development, the cell was destroyed. Accordingly, by the time of birth all cells that could react with self would have been eliminated. It should be emphasized that all is not as simple as implied in this brief introduction. The fact that antigen stimulates the proliferation of the antibody-producing cells has been amply demonstrated; however, the mechanism through which the animal recognizes self versus nonself is not fully known and may be more complex than proposed in the original hypothesis. We shall have occasion to return to this problem later in this chapter.

## CELLS INVOLVED IN ANTIBODY SYNTHESIS

It is beyond the scope of this text to review all the experimental data that implicated the small lymphocyte as a precursor to the antibody-producing cell (the plasma cell) and showed secondary lymphoid tissue (spleen and lymph nodes) to be the major centers of antibody synthesis. Suffice it to say that rats depleted of their lymphocytes by continual drainage from the thoracic duct are unable to respond to an antigenic challenge by producing antibody. Replacement of the lymphocytes restores the ability to mount a primary antibody response. Other experiments have

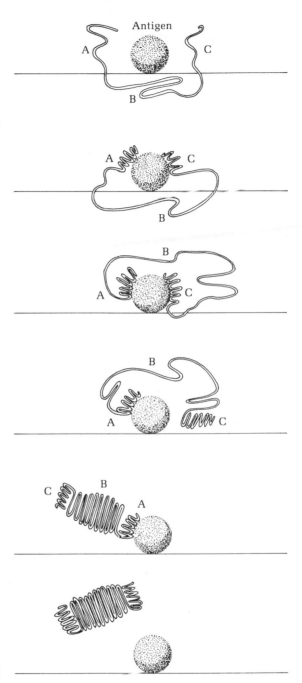

**Figure 15-2.** Pauling's Ag template theory proposed that Ag reacted with a nascent antibody chain causing the chain to fold around the antigen in such a manner as to acquire specific reaction sites complementary to the Ag.

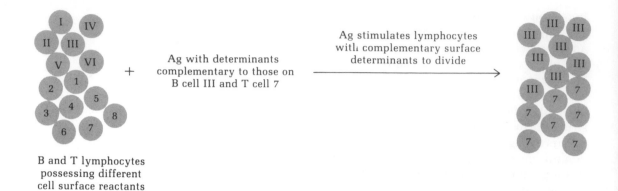

**Figure 15-3.** Burnet's clonal selection theory, similar to Ehrlich's hypothesis, proposes the reaction of Ag with a few specific cells, causing these cells to proliferate into clones of antibody-producing cells.

shown that the injection of small lymphocytes into an animal whose own lymphocytes had been destroyed by heavy irradiation restores the ability to synthesize antibodies. It is now well established that small lymphocytes are either directly or indirectly responsible for antibody production.

### Thymus and Bursa

The duality of the immune system was suggested when it was discovered that sensitivity to some bacteria and fungi could not be transferred from one animal to another with antiserum but could be transferred using living white cells. It therefore appeared that the body possessed two immune systems, one mediated by circulating antibodies and the other mediated only by intact living cells. This concept was soon borne out by case reports of children who suffered from excessive bacterial infections and were found to be unable to form circulating antibodies. These same individuals, however, were not subject to recurrent viral or fungal infections, and it was observed that they did possess a system of cell-mediated immunity (see Chapter 17). Other reports of children who were unable to mount a cell-mediated immune response but formed some circulating antibodies soon followed. An insight into the origins of these

two immune systems arose out of experiments with chickens and mice.

A chicken has a lymphoid organ called the bursa of Fabricius, a small pouch of lymphoid cells located in the lower gut (see Figure 15-4). Removal of the bursa from newly hatched chickens destroys their ability to produce circulating antibodies but does not affect their cell-mediated immune system. Removal of the thymus, however, suppresses all cell-mediated immunity and partially inhibits the chicken's ability to form circulating antibodies. This latter experiment was also done with newborn mice, where it was demonstrated that removal of the thymus completely eliminated cell-mediated immunity even though the mouse could still produce antibodies to some antigens. Since mammals do not possess a bursa, the reverse experiment was not possible with mice.

Thus, it appears that the thymus is necessary for the development of cell-mediated immunity, and in the chicken the bursa of Fabricius is necessary for the development of antibody-producing cells.

### T Cells and B Cells

It seems appropriate to digress for a moment to consider the origin and distribution of lymphoid tissue since it is the cells of this tissue that eventually differentiate to form the immune system.

All circulating cells (red cells, white cells and platelets) are believed to arise from the same stem cell. In the normal course of events a circulating stem cell (which originated in the fetal liver or adult bone marrow) becomes committed to differentiate through one of a series of specific pathways to form the final mature circulating cell. This is shown schematically in Figure 15-5, where one can see that after the stem cell becomes a committed progenitor cell, it is sequestered in some organ of the body and undergoes a specific cellular differentiation to form the final mature end cell.

**Figure 15-4.** The location of the bursa of Fabricius and thymus in the chicken. The multi-lobed thymus is the origin of T lymphocytes, while the bursa (found only in birds) is the organ from which B lymphocytes originate. After leaving the thymus or the bursa, the lymphocytes may colonize the spleen or bone marrow.

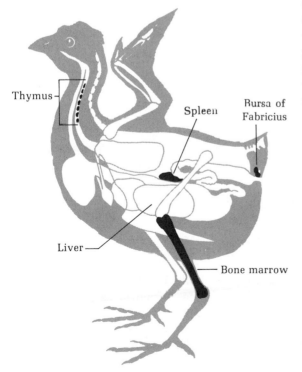

The eventual role of the end cell is known to be influenced by the organ in which cell differentiation occurred. Thus, a progenitor cell that enters the thymus differentiates into a small lymphocyte (called a thymocyte) and eventually emerges as a mature T cell to seed secondary lymph organs such as the spleen and lymph nodes. Similarly, progenitor cells entering the bursa of chickens (or its currently unknown equivalent in mammals) differentiate into small lymphocytes called B cells, which seed the same secondary lymph organs as T cells. Thus, although we do not yet know the primary lymphoid organ in mammals that is analogous to the bursa of Fabricius, we do know that it exists and that all vertebrates possess thymus-derived small lymphocytes (T cells) and bursa-equivalent-derived small lymphocytes (B cells).

### Cooperative Effect of T and B Cells in Producing Antibody

As was discussed earlier in this section, removal of the thymus from neonatal mice eliminates their cellular immune system and limits their capacity to produce antibodies to many antigens. The injection of mouse thymus cells into such animals restores both their cell-mediated immunity and their normal antibody-producing ability. Surprisingly, repopulation of lethally irradiated non-thymectomized mice with thymus cells does not result in their ability to form antibody. If, however, both thymus cells and bone marrow lymphocytes are injected into lethally irradiated mice, their antibody-producing system is restored to normal. The additional observation that bone marrow cells alone are ineffective for most antigens indicates that two different cell types are required for antibody synthesis, lymphocytes from the thymus and lymphocytes from the bone marrow. It is now recognized that the thymus lymphocytes develop into T cells and that the bone marrow contains the B lymphocytes.

The next question one might ask is whether it is the B cells, or T cells, or both, that develop into the actual antibody-synthesizing cells. There have been a number of complicated

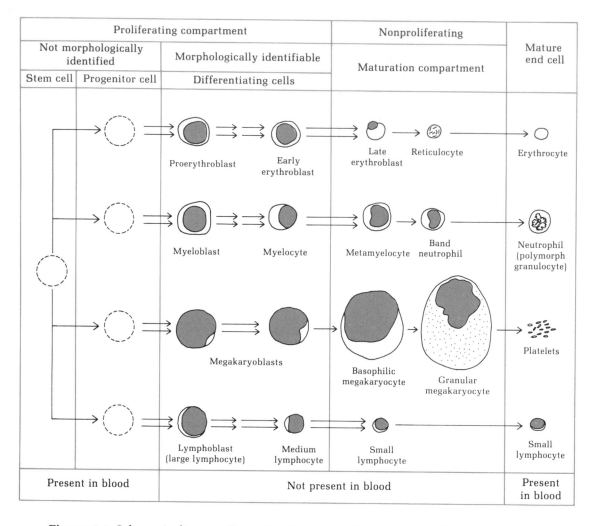

**Figure 15-5.** Schematic diagram illustrating the nomenclature and morphology of various blood cells as they differentiate from stem cells to mature end cells.

experiments designed to answer this question, but we shall point out here only the observation that if bone marrow and thymus cells are obtained from animals possessing different immunoglobulin allotypes (see Chapter 12) and injected into irradiated mice, the resulting immunoglobulin is always the same allotype as the bone marrow donor. These data, along with other experiments, have firmly established that the actual antibody-producing cells arise only from the B cells and that even though T cells are required for the synthesis of most antibodies, they

neither make antibody nor differentiate into antibody-producing cells. Thus, the role of the T cell in antibody synthesis is that of a helper cell.

### The Role of the Macrophage in Antibody Synthesis

The fact that both B cells and T cells are required for antibody synthesis seems about as complicated as it ought to be. However, experimental data have conclusively shown that the macrophage is also a participant in this complex business of antibody formation.

Macrophages are large mononuclear phagocytes that wander through tissues by squeezing between cells, although many are fixed in the endothelial lining of spleen, liver, and lymph nodes to make up the mononuclear phagocyte system (also called the reticuloendothelial system). They are active phagocytic cells and ingest and degrade foreign particulate matter—particularly bacteria and viruses.

Their role in antibody synthesis became apparent when Donald Mosier found that mouse spleen cells could be separated into two groups based on their adherence to a plastic surface. In short, he placed spleen cells (obtained from mice that had been immunized with sheep's red blood cells) in a plastic dish for 30 minutes and then very gently washed free the cells that did not stick to the plastic. After enriching or purifying the nonadhering cell types by allowing them to stick to a plastic dish several more times, he observed that the nonadhering cells were almost all lymphocytes, whereas those cells that stuck to the plastic were primarily macrophages (see Figure 15-6).

He then used each population of these cells in an *in vitro* Jerne plaque assay to determine the number of cells that could produce antibodies to sheep red blood cells (SRBC). This is carried out by suspending the adhering or nonadhering spleen cells in agar containing SRBC and complement. As you can see, any cell that produces antibodies to SRBC will, in the presence of complement, cause their lysis. One need only count the clear plaques of lysis to determine the number of antibody-producing cells (see Figure 15-7). Mosier's results are shown in Table 15-1, where it can be seen that macrophage-rich (MR) cells did not form anti-SRBC antibodies, nor did the lymphocyte-rich (LR) fractions. However, when these cell lines were mixed together, many antibody-producing plaques were seen.

Subsequent data has confirmed the observation that the macrophage is indeed involved in some way with antibody produc-

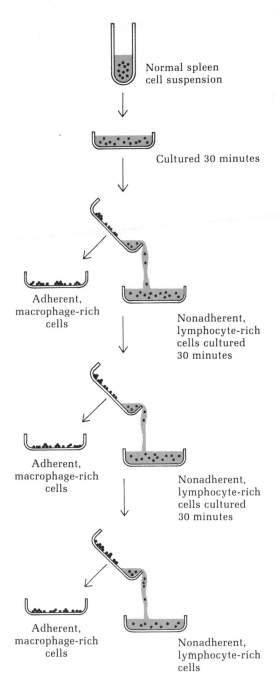

**Figure 15-6.** Method of culturing mouse spleen cells to obtain adherent (macrophage-rich) and nonadherent (lymphocyte-rich) populations.

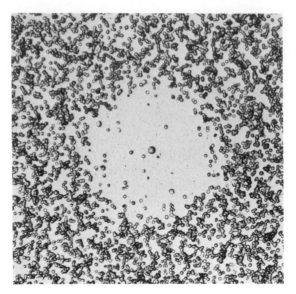

**Figure 15-7.** Jerne plaque showing an antibody-producing cell from the spleen of a mouse immunized with sheep red blood cells (SRBC). Note the clear area where the antibody (in the presence of complement) lysed the surrounding SRBC as it diffused away from the antibody-producing cell. ($\times$70)

**Table 15-1. Plaque-Forming Cell Response *In Vitro* of Various Cell Populations**

| Cell populations | Plaque-forming cells, day-4 response |
|---|---|
| Normal spleen cells | 1 |
| Normal spleen cells + SRBC | 191 |
| MR + SRBC + Normal spleen cells | 127 |
| MR + SRBC + LR | 68 |
| MR + SRBC | 0 |
| LR + SRBC | 1 |

Notes:
1. Figures are averages of three separate experiments.
2. SRBC denotes $10^7$ sheep red blood cells.
3. MR denotes a macrophage-rich population.
4. LR denotes a lymphocyte-rich population.

tion, even though it is well established that the macrophage does not itself synthesize antibodies. Its precise role has yet to be elucidated, although it is in all likelihood involved with presenting the antigen on the macrophage surface in a manner in which it can interact with those T cells that specifically recognize the antigen. The macrophage might do this through phagocytosis followed by partial degradation of the antigen, resulting in a more effective presentation to the T cell of the antigenic determinants, or it may act by merely providing a sticky surface for the antigen, thus bringing T cells into intimate contact with the macrophage.

### Differences Between B and T Cells

Morphological examination of B and T cells using light microscopy shows essentially no differences between these two cell lines. Both are small lymphocytes approximately 8 $\mu$m in diameter and both are nonphagocytic, motile cells. Early observations of lymphocytes with the scanning electron microscope indicated that the cell surface of the B cell was covered with spiny protrusions while that of the T cells was relatively smooth. This, however, is now known to be an artifact and there is currently no known morphological difference between B and T cells.

Antigenically, however, considerable differences have been observed. For example, if one stains these cells with fluorescently labeled anti-human immunoglobulin, the B cells will become strongly fluorescent while the T cells do not react with the anti-Ig. One can, therefore, conclude that B cells have considerable amounts of immunoglobulin on their cell surface whereas T cells either do not possess immunoglobulins or, if they do, the amount is too small to be seen with fluorescently labeled anti-Ig.

The search for other antigenic differences between B and T cells calls for the injection of T cells from one animal into another animal and then, after an antibody response, the adsorption of the antiserum with cells from the donor (which should not, of course, contain T cells). The adsorbed serum is then tested to see if it contains antibodies which are specific for T cells. Such experiments are difficult to carry out in humans, but it has been clearly demonstrated that T cells from mice do indeed possess alloantigens (antigens present in some individuals of a species, but absent in others) that are not known to exist in B cells.

The first thoroughly studied T-cell alloantigen in mice has been designated as Thy 1 (old terminology, theta Ag). Thus far, two mouse allotypes have been described, Thy 1.1 and Thy 1.2. By using the proper cells to adsorb the antisera, it is possible to obtain pure monospecific Thy 1.1 or 1.2 antisera. Treatment with anti-Thy 1 and complement results in the selective destruction of the corresponding T cells. It is, therefore, possible to determine the percentage of T cells present in the various lymphoid organs by reacting the lymphocytes with anti Thy 1 and complement and noting the number of lymphocytes killed by this treatment. Table 15-2 shows the results from such an experiment.

Several other alloantigens such as Ly and Tla antigens also occur on mouse T cells. The significance of Tla is unknown; the Ly Ags will be discussed in Chapter 17 under functional subclasses of T cells.

Antigens other than immunoglobulins have also been reported to be present on B cells and not on T cells; the importance or function of these antigens is not known and little can be said about them at this time. There are, however, two receptors present on B cells that do not occur on T cells, namely, the Fc receptor and the complement receptor.

FC RECEPTOR. This receptor will specifically bind to the Fc portion of antigen-antibody

Table 15-2. Percentage of Thymus-Derived Lymphocytes in Various Tissues from Two Inbred Strains of Mice (Balb/c and CBA)

| | Killed with anti-Thy 1 (%)[a] (A) | Killed with normal mouse serum (%)[a] (B) | Cytotoxic index (%)[b] | Number of experiments |
|---|---|---|---|---|
| I. BALB/C MICE | | | | |
| Blood lymphocytes | 73 (72–76) | 9 (6–13) | 70 | 4 |
| Lymph node | 67 (64–71) | 11 (6–14) | 63 | 5 |
| Spleen | 40 (37–46) | 10 (9–12) | 33 | 4 |
| Peritoneal lymphocytes | 37 (32–46) | 4 (1–6) | 34 | 3 |
| Peyer's patches | 29 (27–30) | 11 (5–15) | 20 | 3 |
| II. CBA MICE | | | | |
| Blood lymphocytes | 71 (61–80) | 5 (2–8) | 70 | 15 |
| Lymph node | 75 (72–78) | 9 (2–13) | 72 | 3 |
| Spleen | 38 (35–42) | 9 (7–13) | 32 | 3 |
| Peritoneal lymphocytes | 36 (25–46) | 6 (5–7) | 32 | 3 |
| Peyer's patches | 34 (28–38) | 11 (9–13) | 25 | 3 |

a) Expressed as mean (range in parenthesis).
b) This cytotoxic index [(A − B/100 − B) × 100] is based on the assumption that both Thy 1-bearing and non-Thy 1-bearing cells are proportionally represented among the dead cells in the control tubes with normal mouse serum.

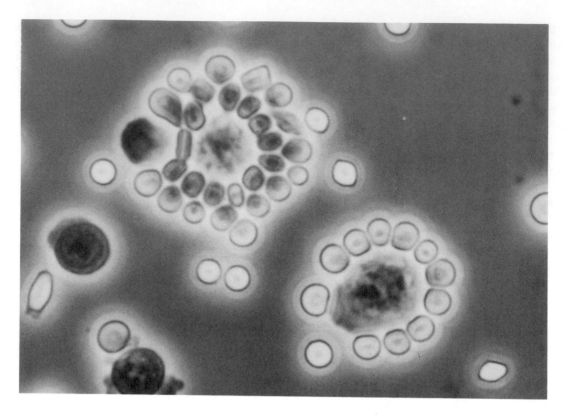

**Figure 15-8.** Rosettes consisting of erythrocytes binding to the surface of lymphocytes. It is not possible to know whether the lymphocytes are B or T cells, but since B cells characteristically bind greater numbers of erythrocytes, one could speculate that one rosette contains a B cell while the other consists of erythrocytes surrounding a T cell. (×2000)

complexes or aggregated IgA. It can be demonstrated by coating red blood cells with antibody and mixing them with B lymphocytes. The Fc portion of the antibody that projects from the surface of the red blood cell will bind to receptors on the B cells resulting in the formation of rosettes of erythrocytes surrounding each B cell. T cells, on the other hand, will form rosettes with RBC's in the absence of Ab (see Figure 15-8).

COMPLEMENT RECEPTOR. B cells also possess a receptor that will bind to complement, but only if the complement has first reacted with an antigen-antibody complex. The reason for this is that the receptor is specific for the C3b portion of complement, which would be readily available only after binding to an antigen-antibody complex.

## MODEL FOR ANTIBODY SYNTHESIS

Some antigens are spoken of as T-cell independent, since they can induce antibody formation in the absence of T cells. Such antigens are characteristically large molecules made up of a repeating sequence of monosaccharides such as dextrans, lipopolysaccharides, or capsular antigens. It should also be noted that T-independent antigens stimulate only IgM synthesis and that 7S antibody is produced only as a result of T-cell cooperation. However, for most antigens it is now conclusively established that antibody production requires the interaction of three different cell types: B cells, T cells, and macrophages. Moreover, the clonal selection theory of Burnet, the generally accepted model for the origin of antibody-producing cells, proposes that each individual possesses B cells and T cells that can interact with as many as a million different antigenic determinants. Thus, in the presence of an antigen the lymphocytes possessing specific receptors for the antigen will react and, as a result, are selected out to divide, differentiate, and produce antibody.

We shall now dissect this complicated affair so that we can better understand the role of each of the various components involved in antibody formation.

## KINETICS OF ANTIBODY FORMATION

As one might expect, the rate and extent of antibody production is influenced by several external factors. For example, antibody levels generally increase with increasing amounts of antigen, but this is not proportional after a certain concentration of antigen is reached. Also, the physical condition of the antigen will influence the rate of antibody production, and it is generally true that particulate antigens stimulate a more rapid antibody synthesis than do soluble protein antigens.

Adjuvants may also be used to enhance the immunogenicity of soluble antigens. Most adjuvants are designed to interact with the antigen and then release it slowly over a prolonged period; alum-precipitated toxoids have been used extensively in human immunizations, and water and oil emulsions of antigen containing killed tubercle bacilli have been widely used in animal immunizations. This latter mixture, called Freund's complete adjuvant, causes a fairly intense inflammatory response and is used in experimental animals for the stimulation of antibody directed against T-cell dependent antigens. Since Freund's adjuvant appears to

stimulate T cells, it is ineffective when used with T-cell independent antigens.

To define the basic terminology of the kinetics of antibody formation, we shall for the moment confine ourselves to the appearance of antibody following the injection of antigen into an animal. We shall not be concerned with either the mechanism of antibody synthesis or the class of antibody that is produced.

### Primary Response

The appearance of antibodies in the blood serum following an initial exposure to antigen is known as the primary antibody response. As already pointed out, both the rate and the extent of the primary response are dependent upon the nature of the antigen, size of dose administered, route of administration, and the sensitivity of the serologic technique used to quantitate the antibody. Figure 15-9 depicts a typical primary response curve. In a usual case measurable antibody appears after about five days and reaches a peak in two to three weeks. The duration of antibody in the serum is dependent upon a continued stimulation of antibody production by antigen and upon the

**Figure 15-9.** Antibody response curves. Because of the large variability for different Ags, time is shown as arbitrary units. However, a maximum primary response might require 10 to 20 days, whereas a secondary response occurs in 1 to 3 days.

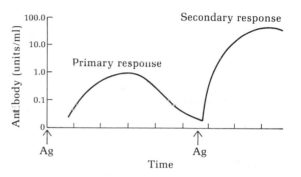

rate of antibody turnover, which varies for each class of immunoglobulin. (Under average conditions, the half life of IgG is estimated to be approximately 23 days.)

## Secondary Response

As also shown in Figure 15-9, a second exposure to an antigen, months or even years after the primary response, results in an almost immediate appearance of antibodies (within one to three days) reaching levels that may be 10 to 15 times higher than that occurring during the primary response. This may happen even if there was no measurable antibody level at the time of the second injection of antigen. Since the antibody-secreting cells are short-lived, this type of response cannot be attributed to a reactivation of dormant plasma cells, but rather to an activation of memory cells as described in the following sections.

## Role of the B Cells in Antibody Formation

After the injection of an antigen, there is a lag time of variable duration followed by an exponential rise in circulating antibody. One can determine the number of antibody-forming cells in the spleen using the Jerne plaque technique. As with antibody levels, one sees an exponential rise. The fact that the increase in antibody level is the result of proliferation of antibody-producing cells can also be confirmed by showing that tritiated thymidine (thymidine is a component of DNA) is incorporated into antibody-producing cells during the primary response.

It appears then that antigen reacts with those B cells that possess a complementary immunoglobulin on their cell surface. This interaction (along with T-cell helper function) induces B-cell transformation into lymphoblasts which go on to form plasma cells and memory cells. Not much is known about memory cells, but there seems little doubt that they are long-lived lymphocytes which,

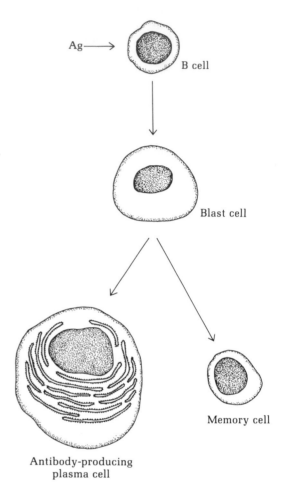

**Figure 15-10.** Antigen reacts with B cells with complementary immunoglobulin to stimulate the formation of plasma cells and memory cells.

in the case of B memory cells, are precommitted to differentiate into plasma cells following stimulation by their respective antigen. This is supported by the fact that the mature plasma cell lives only a few days and there would be no secondary response in the absence of memory cells. As we shall discuss later, T cells also form memory cells, and these memory cells are also necessary for a secondary antibody response to occur. Figure 15-10 illustrates a schematic concept for the formation of plasma cells and memory cells following Ag stimulation.

## Immunoglobulin Classes

If one determines the class of antibody synthesized during the usual primary response, it is seen that IgM (19S Ig) appears early, is short-lived, and is followed by the appearance of 7S Ig (usually IgG), as shown in Figure 15-11. This can be readily demonstrated in the laboratory by treating antiserum with reducing agents such as mercaptoethanol that will cause the IgM to dissociate into 7S Ig subunits that no longer form antigen-antibody crosslinks. Such treatment has no effect on the usual 7S immunoglobulins such as IgG and IgA.

Although the detailed mechanism of this shift is not known, there is substantial data that the change in antibody class actually involves a shift within the cell, whereby the same variable light ($V_L$) and variable heavy ($V_H$) chains are shifted from association with genes producing $\mu$ heavy chains to those producing the $\gamma$ chains for IgG. The fact that a single cell can do this is exemplified by a myeloma cell line that simultaneously produces both IgM and IgG. These two classes of immunoglobulin can be assumed to be synthesized by the same cell line, for both Ig classes possessed the same idiotype and an identical amino-acid sequence in their variable regions.

The regulation of this shift is a little vague, but data by Ellen Vitetta and Jonathan Uhr have prompted the theory that the switch is controlled by the class of immunoglobulin existing on the surface of the B cell. In brief, they showed the following: (1) B cells in newborn mice have only IgM on their surfaces; (2) by adulthood 60–70% of the B cells in the spleen and 85–95% of those that populate the Peyer's patches in the gut possess IgD on their cell surface; and (3) B cells do not possess IgG or IgA on their surface.

From these data they have postulated that IgD is the triggering receptor for the replication and differentiation of B lymphocytes. Moreover, they suggest that those cells bearing IgD are the precursors of plasma cells which, if present in Peyer's patches, will become IgA-secreting cells and, if present in the lymph nodes, will become IgG producers. They also postulate that some cells bear both IgD and IgM on their surface and that following exposure to antigen such cells will either secrete IgM or will become IgM memory cells.

They propose that since isolated IgD is extremely susceptible to proteolytic cleavage, it is protected while on the surface of the B cell. After binding to antigen, a reactive site on the IgD may be exposed to a proteolytic enzyme, causing the triggering of the B cell.

Much of this theory is based on somewhat abstract reasoning, but it is certainly tempting to postulate some regulating role for IgD, since it is present on such a high percentage of B lymphocytes in adults and yet is hardly measurable as a circulating antibody class. These data also support the postulate that a

**Figure 15-11.** Classes of Ab produced during the primary response. Note that IgM comes up first but only reaches low titers and soon disappears. IgG appears later than IgM, but reaches much higher levels for a longer time.

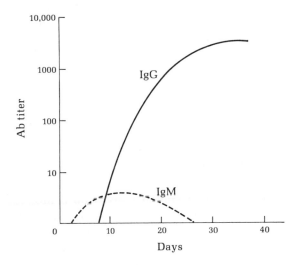

cell can switch from IgM synthesis to IgD synthesis and finally to IgG, IgA, and probably IgE production.

### Changes in Antibody Affinity

Antibody affinity represents the strength of the binding between antibody and antigen. To put it another way, a high affinity antibody has a close physical fit between its combining site and the antigen; one with low affinity does not. It can be observed that antibody arising early in the immune response possesses lower affinity than late antibody. Also, antibody synthesized as a result of a large antigenic stimulus possesses lower affinity than antibody induced by a smaller amount of antigen. This has been explained by the fact that large amounts of antigen will stimulate a heterogeneous population of B cells possessing immunoglobulin receptors that react with both "good" and "poor-fitting" antigens. On the other hand, when only small amounts of antigen are used, B cells with high-affinity immunoglobulin can successfully compete with those possessing low-affinity receptors. This, of course, results in the synthesis of high-affinity antibody.

### Role of T Cells in Antibody Formation

The requirement for T cell cooperation for 7S antibody synthesis is now well established, but the mechanism of this interaction is still somewhat obscure. It appears that T cells do not possess immunoglobulins on their cell surfaces; they do, however, specifically bind to antigenic determinants. This can be shown by allowing T cells to interact with a very highly radioactive antigen. Only those T cells reacting with the antigen are destroyed by the radioactivity (antigen suicide) while T cells that recognize other antigens are unharmed.

### Carrier Effect

It is also established that a helper T cell interacts with one antigenic determinant while a B cell combines with a second one to initiate antibody synthesis. If we combine a hapten

such as dinitrophenol (DNP) to a carrier protein, antibodies are produced which will react with both the carrier and the hapten. We would now like to ask whether T cells also proliferate to produce memory cells specific for the carrier.

To answer this question N. A. Mitchison immunized mice with a hapten-carrier conjugate consisting of 4-hydroxy-3-iodo-5-nitrophenacetyl azide conjugated to chicken gamma globulin (NIP-CGG). After 10–20 weeks, the mice were given booster injections of either: (1) NIP-CGG, (2) NIP-bovine gamma globulin (NIP-BGG), or (3) NIP-ovalbumin (NIP-OA). Only those boosted with NIP-CGG responded with a secondary Ab response to NIP, even though all of the mice had shown a primary response to NIP. (If 1000- to 10,000-fold larger booster injections were used, the mice would show an antibody response to conjugates such as NIP-BSA or NIP-OA; however, at these levels of conjugate injection it is difficult to distinguish between a primary and a secondary response.) Clearly, then, unless tremendously large doses of carrier conjugate were given, the mice responded with a secondary Ab response only when the NIP was presented on the same carrier that had been used to elicit the primary response.

An additional insight into this phenomenon was obtained from Mitchison's experiments in which spleen cells from primed mice, those that had undergone a primary response to a particular carrier-hapten conjugate, were collected and injected into lethally irradiated nonprimed mice. Results from these experiments confirmed the observation that a secondary response to a hapten did not occur unless it was complexed to the same carrier that induced the primary response. It was shown, however, that one could stimulate a secondary antibody response from a conjugate such as NIP-BSA if the irradiated mouse received spleen cells from a mouse that had mounted a primary response to NIP-OA and spleen cells from a different mouse that had received only BSA. Thus, the added presence of spleen cells that had been primed only with carrier protein (BSA) is sufficient to allow a secondary response to the NIP-BSA. If, however, the BSA-primed spleen cells are treated with anti-Thy 1 antibodies and complement, the T cells are destroyed and the BSA spleen cells are then ineffective in the above experiment. It thus appears clear that T cells, like B cells, form specific memory cells that must be present before a secondary antibody response can occur.

**Nature of the T-Cell Receptor and Signal**

In all this messy business of antibody synthesis, one of the more frustrating aspects has been to determine the specific nature of the T-cell receptor and the T-cell signal that turns the B cell on to proliferate and differentiate into a plasma cell. It is established that T cells possess specific receptors for antigenic determinants, but the detailed chemistry of these receptors is far from clear. Unlike B cells, treatment with labeled anti-immunoglobulin does not result in the appearance of fluorescently labeled T cells.

An insight into the nature of the T-cell receptor and the signal to the B cell has come from the work of A. J. Munro and M. J. Taussig, who extracted a specific soluble T-cell factor which could substitute for intact T cells in the activation of B cells. In essence, these investigators injected T cells and antigen into a lethally irradiated mouse to induce a specific "primary response" of the T cells to the antigen. After seven days, the "educated" T cells were isolated and incubated in a test tube with the specific antigen. Six to eight hours later the T cells were removed; the soluble supernatant solution along with B cells and antigen were injected into a second irradiated mouse. After twelve days, the mouse was sacrificed and a Jerne plaque assay was carried out to determine how many spleen cells were producing antibody to the specific antigen. The experimental procedure along with the results is depicted schematically in Figure 15-12, where it can be seen that not only did this system induce an antigenic response but the response was specific for

the antigen with which the T cell had been educated.

A partial characterization of this T-cell factor has shown that it is a protein with a molecular weight of approximately 50,000 daltons. It will not react with anti-immunoglobulins and appears, therefore, not to be an immunoglobulin. Munro and Taussig have demonstrated, however, that the T-cell factor possesses a specific antigen binding site by showing that it is absorbed when passed through a column containing the specific immobilized antigen.

These results seem to invalidate an older concept that T-cell function requires a cell-to-cell interaction with the B cell. Figure 15-13 is a schematic diagram illustrating a possible relationship between T-cell factor and B cells in a cell cooperation for antibody synthesis.

More recently H. Binz and H. Wigzell from Uppsala University in Sweden presented evidence at the XLI Cold Spring Harbor Symposium on Quantitative Biology that one receptor on T cells is a new class of immunoglobulin heavy (H) chain which has tentatively been named "tau" ($\tau$). These investigators concluded from their experiments that the antigen receptor on the T cell exists in the variable region of the $\tau$ heavy chain. Tau is a polypeptide of approximately 75,000 daltons which does not react with conventional anti-immunoglobulin antibodies.

One can only speculate about the actual function of the T-cell factor. However, if we digress for a moment to list a few facts that we do know about antibody synthesis, perhaps a plausible model will evolve. (1) Any substance that induces the proliferation of a cell is called a mitogen; such a stimulation is called a mitogenic effect. (2) Antibody synthesis requires the proliferation of both B and T cells, and thus antigen acts either directly or indirectly as a mitogen. (3) T-cell independent antigens such as lipopolysaccharides are directly mitogenic for B cells. Our model would then propose that most antigens are ineffective as mitogens for B cells but can interact with specific T cells to

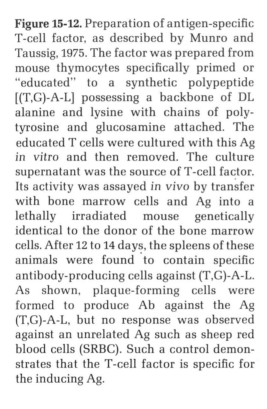

**Figure 15-12.** Preparation of antigen-specific T-cell factor, as described by Munro and Taussig, 1975. The factor was prepared from mouse thymocytes specifically primed or "educated" to a synthetic polypeptide [(T,G)-A-L] possessing a backbone of DL alanine and lysine with chains of polytyrosine and glucosamine attached. The educated T cells were cultured with this Ag *in vitro* and then removed. The culture supernatant was the source of T-cell factor. Its activity was assayed *in vivo* by transfer with bone marrow cells and Ag into a lethally irradiated mouse genetically identical to the donor of the bone marrow cells. After 12 to 14 days, the spleens of these animals were found to contain specific antibody-producing cells against (T,G)-A-L. As shown, plaque-forming cells were formed to produce Ab against the Ag (T,G)-A-L, but no response was observed against an unrelated Ag such as sheep red blood cells (SRBC). Such a control demonstrates that the T-cell factor is specific for the inducing Ag.

After 12-14 days of antigen and bone marrow cells in second mouse:

| Ag | Plaque-forming cells in spleen |
|---|---|
| None | None |
| SRBC | None |
| (T,G)-A-L | 10,000 |

induce both proliferation and the release of antigen bound to T-cell factor. It is tempting to propose that it is this latter complex which acts as a mitogen when it is bound to the cell surface of its specific B cell.

## CONTROL OF THE IMMUNE RESPONSE

It has been known for a long time that the immune response is subject to genetic control. Inbred strains of laboratory mice and guinea pigs designated as low responders and high responders have been studied. Crossbreeding experiments with such animals show that the genes controlling the immune response are located in an area designated as the major histocompatibility complex (MHC). The importance of this group of genes for the control of both cellular and humoral immunity is now known to be so great that no discussion of the immune response can ignore them. On the other hand, a detailed discussion of the complexity of the major histocompatibility gene complex would go far beyond the scope of this text. In brief, (and we shall return to this gene complex in Chapter 17) the major histocompatibility complex consists of a series of genes which control a large number of immunological responses. These genes are linked to a segment of a mouse's chromosome number 17 and are called the H-2 complex in the mouse or the HLA region for the human counterpart.

The MHC of the mouse can be divided into four regions—*K, I, S,* and *D*—and several of these regions can be associated with multiple effects on the immune system. The I region, however, appears to control the humoral immune response. In fact, there is now considerable evidence to support the proposal that the *Ir* genes (a subregion of *I*) code for at least two functions associated with antibody production: (1) T-cell recognition of antigen which is required for cell cooperation, and (2) B-cell response to T-cell mediators. A brief survey of the evidence for these conclusions follows:

Using lethally irradiated mice as walking test tubes for antibody production, A. J. Munro and M. J. Taussig injected these mice with soluble T-cell factor and B cells obtained from strains of mice that responded with high antibody titers following the injection of a synthetic Ag (high responders) and strains that showed very little Ab response under identical conditions (low responders). These investigators found that some low responders lacked B cells that could be turned on by Ag and T-cell factor from high responders but possessed T cells that were as effective as T cells from high-responder strains. Other low-responder strains lacked both B and T cells that could interact with the Ag, and one low-responder strain possessed normal B cells and was defective only in its T-cell population. They concluded from crossbreeding among these low- and high-responder strains that there are two genes in

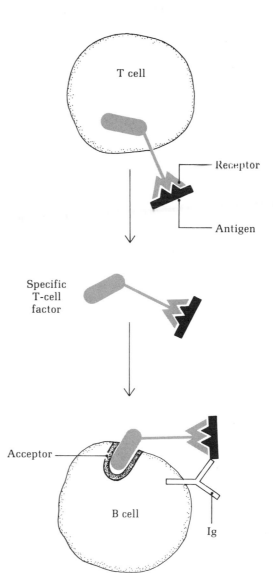

**Figure 15-13.** Model showing a possible relationship between T-cell receptor, specific T-cell factor, and B-cell acceptor in cell cooperation and a mechanism of B-cell triggering. The immune-response genes are believed to code for the T-cell receptor, the T-cell factor, and the B-cell acceptor.

the immune response region (Ir genes) that code for T and B-cell cooperation: (1) one codes for a T-cell-specific factor that interacts with Ag, and (2) the other controls the B-cell acceptor function for the T-cell factor and Ag.

It therefore appears that T cells possess two independent receptor molecules: (1) a heavy chain ($\tau$) that specifically binds to the antigen, and (2) a receptor that recognizes self through antigens coded by the Ir genes. This concept explains the observation that T cells respond optimally only when they see antigens in association with their own MHC antigens, i.e., on macrophages that are genetically histocompatible. One can thus visualize a model for T-cell proliferation as follows: (1) antigen binds to the surface of the macrophage; (2) T cells possessing the correct $\tau$ chain then bind to the antigen on the macrophage surface; (3) an interaction between the macrophage immune-region-associated antigens and T-cell receptor results in a mitogenic effect upon the T-cell; and (4) T-cell factors are released, causing B-cell proliferation and differentiation into antibody-producing plasma cells.

## IMMUNOLOGICAL UNRESPONSIVENESS

In this section, we shall be primarily concerned with the suppression of the immune response, and will construct a model that attempts to explain why an individual cannot make antibodies to antigens that are present on that animal's own cells. Quite obviously, this lack of response is through no defect in their antigenicity because such cells will readily stimulate antibody production if they are implanted into another person. Recall that this recognition of "self" versus "nonself" was proposed by Burnet to occur during fetal life by a mechanism in which those cells capable of making antibody to self were destroyed. Thus, by the time the fetal immune system had matured sufficiently to make an immune response, all of the B and T cells that could react with self had been eliminated.

This concept still provides an over-all working model for tolerance to self, but we can now supply some of the details involved.

### Neonatal Tolerance

During the first several weeks after birth the neonatal mouse is unable to produce antibodies to most antigens. This immune system may be used to determine which components are missing or nonfunctional.

Neonatal spleen cells contain normal adult numbers of Thy 1-bearing T cells and immunoglobulin coated B cells. Also, if one stimulates such cells with a B-cell mitogen like bacterial lipopolysaccharide, some antibody is produced. Thus, it would appear that neonatal spleen cells contain functional B cells but lack functional helper T cells. To test this hypothesis, adult T cells were added to two-week-old spleen cells and stimulated with sheep's red blood cells to form anti-SRBC. Surprisingly, no antibody was produced. If, however, the pre-existing neonatal T cells were first removed with anti-Thy 1 and complement, the neonatal system was easily reconstructed by the addition of adult T cells. Thus, it appears that the neonatal T cells are able to suppress antibody formation even in the presence of all of the necessary components of the antibody-producing system. We now know that this is, in fact, the case and that neonatal spleen and thymus cells contain a separate class of T cells that can nonspecifically suppress the differentiation of B cells to plasma cells. Moreover, as the mouse (or perhaps any animal) grows older, the number of its nonspecific suppressor cells decreases. After the following section, we will hypothesize how these nonspecific suppressor T cells may be involved in tolerance to self.

### Adult Tolerance

Adult tolerance can be defined as the inability to make an immune response as a result of a previous exposure as an adult to a specific antigen. Based on Burnet's theory of tolerance to self, the most obvious question is whether one can induce a permanent tolerance by exposure of an immunologically immature neonate to any foreign antigen, and, if so, could tolerance also be established in the immunologically mature adult? Sir Peter Medawar and his collaborators showed in 1953 that newborn mice could be rendered permanently and specifically tolerant to foreign antigens by injecting those antigens into the immunologically immature animal. One would expect that this tolerance develops by a mechanism not unlike that which occurs for tolerance to self.

The development of tolerance in the adult is not quite as easy to establish as it is in the neonate; however, using the proper conditions, one can induce tolerance to almost any antigen. In general, tolerance in the adult requires the presence of more antigen than in the neonate, perhaps so as to overload the immune system. Also, the closer the relationship that the tolerogen (the Ag to which tolerance is being induced) is to self, the easier it is to induce tolerance. This is probably a function of the number of determinants that differ between donor and recipient. In any event, we would now like to ask whether adult tolerance is a function of T cells, B cells, or both.

It has been reported that mice cannot be made tolerant to SRBC if they are first deprived of their T cells but will develop tolerance if the T cells are replaced. Moreover, tolerant mice do not produce antibody to SRBC even when given spleen cells from nontolerant animals; and if spleen cells from tolerant mice are injected into nontolerant mice, the recipients become tolerant. Thus, it appears that at some point T cells are required for an animal to express tolerance. Satisfactory explanations for these observations are still in a state of flux; but, since adult tolerance results from exposure to a specific tolerogen, it would seem that these suppressor T cells must exert a specific suppressor effect against only the inducing tolerogen, even if only to eliminate a specific B-cell population.

If sufficient tolerogen is used, B cells also appear to become tolerant, or to at least lose their ability to form antibodies to the tolerogen. This can be demonstrated by the injection of normal T cells and tolerant B cells into an irradiated mouse followed by challenge with the tolerogen. The production of B-cell tolerance, however, requires the use of considerably larger amounts of tolerogen than are required to induce T-cell tolerance. It also requires the continued presence of higher amounts of tolerogen than does T-cell tolerance. Thus, B-cell tolerance is lost much sooner than T-cell tolerance.

## Proposed Model for Immunological Unresponsiveness

With the concept that tolerance may result from the presence of suppressor T cells to the tolerogen, we are now ready to suggest a cellular model for tolerance. This model, as suggested by David Benjamin (1977, personal communication) is based in part on the model for antibody synthesis reported by Ellen Vitetta and Jonathan Uhr (1975) in which they proposed that B cells coated with a mixture of IgM and IgD produced IgM, and that IgG, IgA, or IgE were synthesized by B cells possessing only IgD on their surface. They also proposed that the reaction of antigen with B cells possessing only surface IgM would result in tolerance for that antigen. Our model supposes that since B cells may have either IgM or IgD on their surface, each of these immunoglobulins must serve a different function. Thus, since IgM-coated B cells occur at a time when tolerance is easiest to produce, it seems reasonable to suggest that such cells may even be eliminated by reaction with antigen. Second, since IgM is the first antibody synthesized, it might well be synthesized by a cell that is intermediate in its transition from an IgM to an IgD coated cell. Finally, since most B cells possess IgD, one could postulate that they produce the more abundant classes of antibody, namely 7S antibodies such as IgG, IgA, and IgE, or that they differentiate into short-lived IgG, IgA, and IgE-bearing cells that produce the corresponding antibodies.

Benjamin's over-all explanation for both neonatal and adult-type tolerance is schematically shown in Figure 15-14. Here we can see that a stem cell first differentiates into an IgM-coated B cell which migrates to the spleen. In the spleen nonspecific suppressor T cells prevent its differentiation into a mixed IgD-IgM B cell capable of producing IgM antibody. Thus, during a neonatal period, all antigens would result in tolerance, possibly by clonal elimination. The next step in the maturation of the immune response would be the loss of

nonspecific suppressor T cells as the animal grows older, which would then permit the differentiation of the IgM-bearing cell into first a mixed IgM-IgD coated cell and later a cell bearing only IgD. At this point, one could induce tolerance by stimulating the formation of specific suppressor T cells which would either block helper T-cell function or block maturation of helper cells to activated helper T cells. As depicted in Figure 15-14, this would not necessarily prevent the formation of IgM antibodies by the tolerant animal. This has, in some cases, been found to be true; in other words, animals tolerant to certain antigens may produce specific IgM but not 7S

**Figure 15-14.** Possible model for B-cell differentiation and for the T-cell suppression of the immune response. Antigen reacting with a B cell possessing only IgM receptors eliminates the B cell, resulting in tolerance to the Ag. During fetal and early life nonspecific suppressor T cells prevent B-cell differentiation. Adult tolerance could result from specific suppressor cells that arise later in life, acting at both of the two sites shown to prevent Ab synthesis.

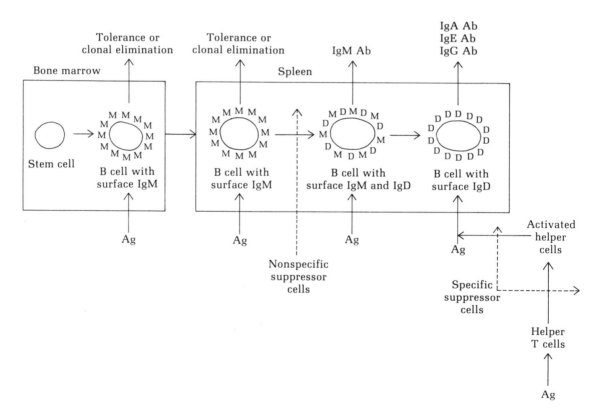

antibodies. Moreover, this model explains adult B-cell tolerance, since large amounts of antigen may cause the clonal elimination of IgM-coated cells as well as induce the formation of specific suppressor T cells. As antigen levels fall, however, new IgM-coated cells would be formed from stem cells and specific suppressor cells would disappear.

Admittedly, this model requires additional experimentation before it can be confirmed (and indeed it may not be entirely correct); but it is experimentally testable and might explain for the first time laboratory results obtained from both neonatal and adult tolerant animals.

## Immunosuppressive Drugs

Thus far, we have been concerned with mechanisms of suppressing specific parts of the immune system without suppressing the entire adult response. With organ transplants becoming more commonplace, however, there are occasions when the entire immune system must be suppressed to prevent transplant rejection. This may be accomplished by one or more of the following ways: (1) irradiation to destroy lymphocytes, especially T cells, (2) use of anti-lymphocytic serum (ALS) to destroy T cells, or (3) the use of immunosuppressive drugs, some of which may prevent lymphocyte proliferation while others such as the corticosteroids destroy the lymphocytes. In any event, all of these techniques are dangerous because of the toxicity of the agents and because they leave the individual without protection to a number of infectious diseases and neoplastic disorders that are normally controlled by the immune system. Examples will be discussed later in this text.

## REFERENCES

Asherson, G. L., and M. Zembala. 1975. Inhibitory T cells. *Current Topics in Microbiol. and Immunol.* **72**:55–100.

Bennich, H., and S. G. O. Johansson. 1971. Structure and function of human immunoglobulin E. *Adv. in Immunol.* **13**:1–55.

Claman, H. N., and E. A. Chaperon. 1969. Immunologic complementation between thymus and marrow cells—A model for the two-cell theory of immunocompetence. *Transplantation Rev.* **1**:93–113.

Cooper, M. D., and A. R. Lawton, III. 1974. The development of the immune system. *Sci. American* **231**:58–72.

Hopper, J. E., and A. Nisonoff. 1971. Individual antigenic specificity of immunoglobulins. *Adv. in Immunol.* **13**:57–99.

Jandinski, J., H. Cantor, T. Tadakuma, D. L. Peavy, and C. W. Pearce. 1976. Separation of helper T cells from suppressor T cells expressing different Ly components. I. Polyclonal activation: suppressor and helper activities are inherent properties of distinct T-cell subclasses. *J. Exp. Med.* **143**:1382–1390.

Katz, D. H., and D. Armerding. 1976. The role of histocompatibility gene products in lymphocyte triggering and differentiation. *Fed. Proc.* **35**:2053–2060.

Katz, D. H., and B. Benacerraf, eds. 1974. *Immunological Tolerance: Mechanisms and Potential Therapeutic Applications.* Academic Press, New York.

Kehoe, J. M., and J. D. Capra. 1974. Phylogenetic aspects of immunoglobulin variable region diversity. *Cont. Topics in Molec. Immunol.* **3**:143–159.

Lerner, R. A., and F. J. Dixon. 1973. The human lymphocyte as an experimental animal. *Sci. American* **228**:82–91.

Marchalonis, J. J. 1975. Lymphocyte surface immunoglobulins. *Science* **190**:20–29.

Metcalf, D., and M. A. S. Moore. 1971. *Haemopoietic Cells.* North-Holland, Amsterdam.

Miller, J. F. A. P., and G. F. Mitchell. 1969. Thymus and antigen-reactive cells. *Transplantation Rev.* **1**:3–42.

Mitchison, N. A. 1971. The carrier effect in the secondary response to hapten-protein conjugates. *Eur. J. Immunol.* **1**:10–27.

Mosier, D. E. 1967. A requirement for two cell types for antibody formation *in vitro. Science* **158**:1573–1575.

Munro, A. J., and M. J. Taussig. 1975. Two genes in the major histocompatibility complex control immune response. *Nature* **256**:103–106.

Raff, M. 1976. T-cell recognition at Cold Spring Harbor. *Nature* **263**:10–11.

Rosenthal, A. S., ed. 1975. *Immune Recognition.* Academic Press, New York.

Shevach, E. M. 1976. The role of the macrophage in genetic control of the immune response. *Fed. Proc.* **35**:2048–2052.

Taussig, M. J., and A. J. Munro. 1976. Antigen specific T-cell factor in cell cooperation and genetic control of the immune response. *Fed. Proc.* **35**:2061–2066.

Taussig, M. J., E. Mozes, and R. Isac. 1974. Antigen-specific thymus cell factors in the genetic control of the immune response to poly (tyrosyl, glutamyl)-poly-D, L-alanyl-poly-lysyl. *J. Exp. Med.* **140**:301–312.

Taylor, R. B., and A. Basten. 1976. Suppressor cells in humoral immunity and tolerance. *Brit. Med. Bull.* **32**:152–157.

Tomasi, T. B., Jr. 1970. Structure and function of mucosal antibodies. *Annu. Rev. Med.* **21**:281–298.

Vitetta, E. S., and J. W. Uhr. 1975. Immunoglobulin-receptors revisited. *Science* **189**:964–969.

Weiss, L. 1972. *The Cells and Tissues of the Immune System.* Prentice-Hall, Englewood Cliffs, N.J.

Williamson, A. R. 1976. Biological origin of antibody diversity. *Annu. Rev. Biochem.* **45**:467–500.

# 16

# Immediate-Type Hypersensitivity

Our study of immunology has, thus far, been primarily concerned with the protective aspects of our immune system. For at least a century, however, it has been known that a second injection of an antigen into an experimental animal occasionally results in a violent and often fatal reaction. Such results were unexpected since the antigen itself was innocuous and induced no reaction in other control animals.

Around the turn of the century the Austrian physician Clemens von Pirquet coined the term "allergy" (Greek, "altered reaction") to describe a previously-exposed person's ability to react to an agent in a manner different from that of another individual who had not yet been in contact with such a substance. Over the years, the term "hypersensitivity" has also been used to describe those immunological reactions that are damaging to the host. At the present time the terms allergy and hypersensitivity are used synonymously. Paradoxically, immunity and hypersensitivity employ similar mechanisms but are differentiated in that the latter reactions result in damage, rather than protection, to the host.

## IMMEDIATE AND DELAYED-TYPE HYPERSENSITIVITY

Early studies of hypersensitivity reactions revealed that some occurred within minutes after a second exposure to an antigen, while others required 24 to 48 hours to attain a maximum reaction. As a result, the former type was referred to as immediate hypersensitivity and the latter as delayed hypersensitivity. However, the division was really not that clear, since the lag time between challenge and maximum reaction time was actually more of a continuum, making the labels "immediate" or "delayed" rather arbitrary.

A much better criterion for this classification was discovered when it was observed that some types of hypersensitivity could be passively transferred with serum from an allergic individual, while others required the transfer of intact lymphocytes. In other words, some hypersensitivities are initiated by soluble antibodies, while others occur only as a cell-mediated response. Current terminology has designated all hypersensitivities that are mediated by soluble anti-

223

bodies as immediate-type, whereas those associated only with intact cells are referred to as delayed-type. In this chapter we shall be concerned only with the immediate type; the following chapter will discuss delayed-type reactions and cell-mediated immunity.

## TYPES OF ALLERGIC REACTIONS

Before an allergic reaction can occur, an individual must be sensitized to the antigen involved. This sensitization normally follows contact with the antigen in question (frequently called the allergen), but it can also be passively induced by the injection of preformed antibody to the allergen. In either case, subsequent contact with the allergen causes the destruction of certain host cells, resulting in the release of pharmacologically active mediators whose major effect is to cause smooth muscle contraction and to dilate capillaries. Table 16-1 divides the immediate-type hypersensitivities into three major groups on the basis of the class of antibody involved, the requirement for complement, and the type of cell destruction that

releases the pharmacological mediators. The first of these to be discussed is anaphylaxis.

## ANAPHYLAXIS

Depending primarily upon the route by which antigen enters the body of a sensitized individual, an anaphylactic reaction may vary from a severe and frequently fatal systemic reaction to a local manifestation such as a food allergy, hay fever, asthma, or cutaneous anaphylaxis. Early studies of these allergies were hampered by the lack of an *in vitro* assay for antibodies to a specific allergen. In fact, it was originally believed that the antibodies causing such allergic reactions were monovalent, although it is now known that the inability to detect them was merely a function of their extremely low serum concentration (approximately 0.5 to 1.0 $\mu$g per ml) and the insensitivity of the available *in vitro* serological tests. Fortunately, an *in vivo* technique for their detection became available when it was shown that such allergic responses could be passively transferred to a nonallergic individual. This was demon-

### Table 16-1. Immediate-Type Hypersensitivities

| Group | Ab involved | Complement involved | Examples | Mediator cells |
|-------|-------------|---------------------|----------|----------------|
| Anaphylaxis | IgE | No | Anaphylactic shock<br>Cutaneous anaphylaxis<br>Hives<br>Asthma<br>Hay fever<br>Drug allergies | Primarily mast cells but may also include basophils |
| Immune complex syndromes | Any class, but primarily IgG or IgM | Yes | Serum sickness<br>Arthus reaction<br>Glomerulonephritis<br>Rheumatoid Arthritis<br>Systemic lupus erythematosis | Primarily neutrophils and platelets |
| Autoimmune reactions | Any class, but primarily IgG | Yes | Transfusion reactions<br>Rh incompatibility<br>Hemolytic anemia | None |

strated by the German scientist Carl Prausnitz in the following manner: he injected serum from an associate named Heinz Küstner (who was highly allergic to fish) into his own skin and one day later a minute amount of fish extract was injected into the same site. Within minutes a pale, elevated area arose which was surrounded by an area of redness. This same reaction, designated as a wheal and flare or a wheal and erythema, also occurs in an allergic individual when small amounts of allergen are injected into the skin. The skin-sensitizing antibodies responsible for this reaction have been referred to for many years as Prausnitz-Küstner (P-K) antibodies, or as reagins.

Subsequent studies of reagins showed that they possess a number of properties that differentiate them from the other classes of circulating antibodies; namely, they are destroyed by heating at 56°C for 1 to 4 hours and they possess an unusual tendency to bind to skin cells. Moreover, to carry out a P-K antibody transfer as described above, one must allow a latent period of approximately 24 hours between the intradermal injection of the antiserum and the allergen. Thus, it appears that the injected antibody must first be fixed to certain cells before a wheal and flare response could be elicited. The discovery of two myeloma patients who produced large amounts of a hitherto undescribed class of immunoglobulin made it possible to produce specific antibodies to these myeloma proteins. Such antibodies were found to react with κ and λ light chains but did not react with the heavy chains of known immunoglobulins. These antibodies did, however, react with reagins. It was concluded that reagins constitute a fifth class of immunoglobulin, now designated as IgE.

## Properties of Human IgE

Normal individuals possess less than 1 μg per ml of serum IgE, although highly allergic persons may have concentrations 30 times as high. Because IgE normally occurs in such minute amounts, the physical and chemical characteristics of this class of immunoglobulin have been determined using IgE isolated from myeloma patients.

Like the other immunoglobulins, IgE contains two light chains, either κ or λ, and two heavy chains, which have been designated as ε chains. The ε chains, however, contain 550 amino residues as compared to 440 residues for γ chains. Thus, IgE appears to possess an additional domain in its Fc portion, which, as we shall see, endows this molecule with an unusual property. IgE also possesses approximately four times more carbohydrate on its ε chain than does the γ chain of IgG.

AFFINITY OF IgE FOR SKIN AND MAST CELLS. Early studies revealed that if one injected reaginic antibodies into the skin, they would remain localized for as long as two months. It now appears probable that the additional domain in the ε chain is responsible for this ability, since attachment can be competitively inhibited by prior injection of the Fc portion from IgE myeloma protein but not by the corresponding Fab fragments. IgE is found primarily bound to mast cells, which line the capillaries in connective tissues, and on leukocytes known as basophils. Immunoglobulins that bind to cells are called cytotropic antibodies. Those that bind only to cells obtained from the same species of animal are called homocytotropic, whereas those that bind to cells of other species (but not their own cells) are referred to as heterocytotropic. It is probably fortunate that IgE can neither cross the placenta nor initiate the classical complement activation pathway. Table 16-2 summarizes the properties of IgE as compared to IgG antibodies.

MEASUREMENT OF IgE. Until recently, reaginic antibody could be measured only by an *in vivo* assay in which an allergen was injected into the skin and the site observed for the appearance of a wheal and flare. In fact, hay fever and asthma patients are frequently injected intradermally with minute amounts

Table 16-2. Comparison of IgE and IgG Antibodies

| Property | IgE | IgG |
|---|---|---|
| Heat stability (56°C for 4 hours) | Labile | Stable |
| Ability to fix in skin | ~2 months | ~2 days |
| Ability to cross placenta | No | Yes |
| In vitro assay | Radio-immunoassay | Many serologic reactions |
| Molecular weight | 188,000 | 150,000 |
| Sedimentation coefficient | 8.2 S | 6.6 S |
| Carbohydrate content | 12% | 3% |

of extracted pollens, dust, food, and other substances to determine the nature of the allergen responsible for their discomfort.

The availability of myeloma IgE made it possible to prepare purified anti-IgE antibodies. Using these antibodies and known radioactivity labeled ($^{125}$I) IgE, several radio-immunoassays have been developed that will detect as little as 1 ng of IgE (see Figure 16-1a). One can also carry out an in vitro assay for IgE antibodies to a specific allergen by adsorbing the allergen to sephadex particles which are then mixed with the serum to be tested. After an appropriate incubation period, the particles are washed and allowed to react with radioactively-labeled anti-IgE. The amount of radioactivity binding to the beads is a measure of the IgE which had bound to the specific allergen (see Figure 16-1b).

## Effect of Cytotropic IgE-Antigen Reactions

Immediate-type hypersensitivity reactions have been described as antibody-adherent, antigen-adherent, or aggregate. Although any of these types can be produced experimentally, under normal conditions anaphylactic reactions are antibody-adherent reactions involving cytotropic antibody and its specific allergen. In other words, the initiating event of an anaphylactic reaction is typically the binding of antigen with IgE antibodies that exist on the surface of mast cells. These cells are characterized by the possession of large cytoplasmic granules that contain a number of pharmacologically active substances, particularly histamine. The binding of antigen results in the cross-linking and aggregation of the surface IgE molecules, and this in turn causes degranulation (expulsion of the cytoplasmic granules) of the mast cells. The actual symptoms of the various forms of anaphylaxis are the direct result of the release of histamine and other mediators from the IgE-coated mast cells. Experimental evidence strongly suggests that the aggregation of the IgE on the cell surface initiates the degranulation of the mast cell. Thus, the use of anti-IgE or aggregated Fc fragments from IgE will also produce a wheal and flare reaction when injected intradermally, inasmuch as anti-IgE will cause aggregation of existing IgE on mast cells, and aggregated Fc fragments from IgE will bind to mast cells as an aggregate, causing their degranulation.

MEDIATORS RELEASED BY MAST CELLS. There seems little doubt that the release of histamine by the mast cell accounts for most of the symptoms occurring in human anaphylaxis. Plasma histamine rises during anaphylaxis, and the injection of histamine into a guinea pig will induce most of the acute symptoms of anaphylaxis. Histamine acts by causing an increase in tissue permeability, capillary dilation, and smooth muscle contraction. Antihistamines, therefore, will alleviate many of the symptoms of anaphylaxis such as difficulty in breathing due to bronchial constriction and shock due to increased vascular permeability.

Serotonin (5-hydroxytryptophan) is released by the degranulation of mast cells and is also released from platelets. Like histamine it causes smooth muscle contraction, capillary dilation, and increased capillary permeability. Certain animals, particularly rats and mice, are extremely sensitive to serotonin, and in these animals its release is a major contributor to the pathology of anaphylaxis. Humans, however, are not particularly sensitive to serotonin, and its release is not believed to play a major role in human anaphylaxis.

Slow-reacting substance of anaphylaxis (SRS-A) appears to be a low-molecular-weight acidic lipid that is released by the degranulation of mast cells. SRS-A causes constriction of human bronchioles, and it is thought to be synthesized or activated at the time of the antigen-antibody reaction. Very little is known about its chemical structure, but its action is not blocked by antihistamines. It is thought to be involved in the symptoms of human asthma and hay fevers.

There are also several kinins whose plasma concentration increases during anaphylaxis.

**Figure 16-1.** Schematic illustration of a radioimmunoassay. *a.* Assay to determine the amount of IgE present in a patient's serum. *b.* Assay to quantitate a specific IgE.

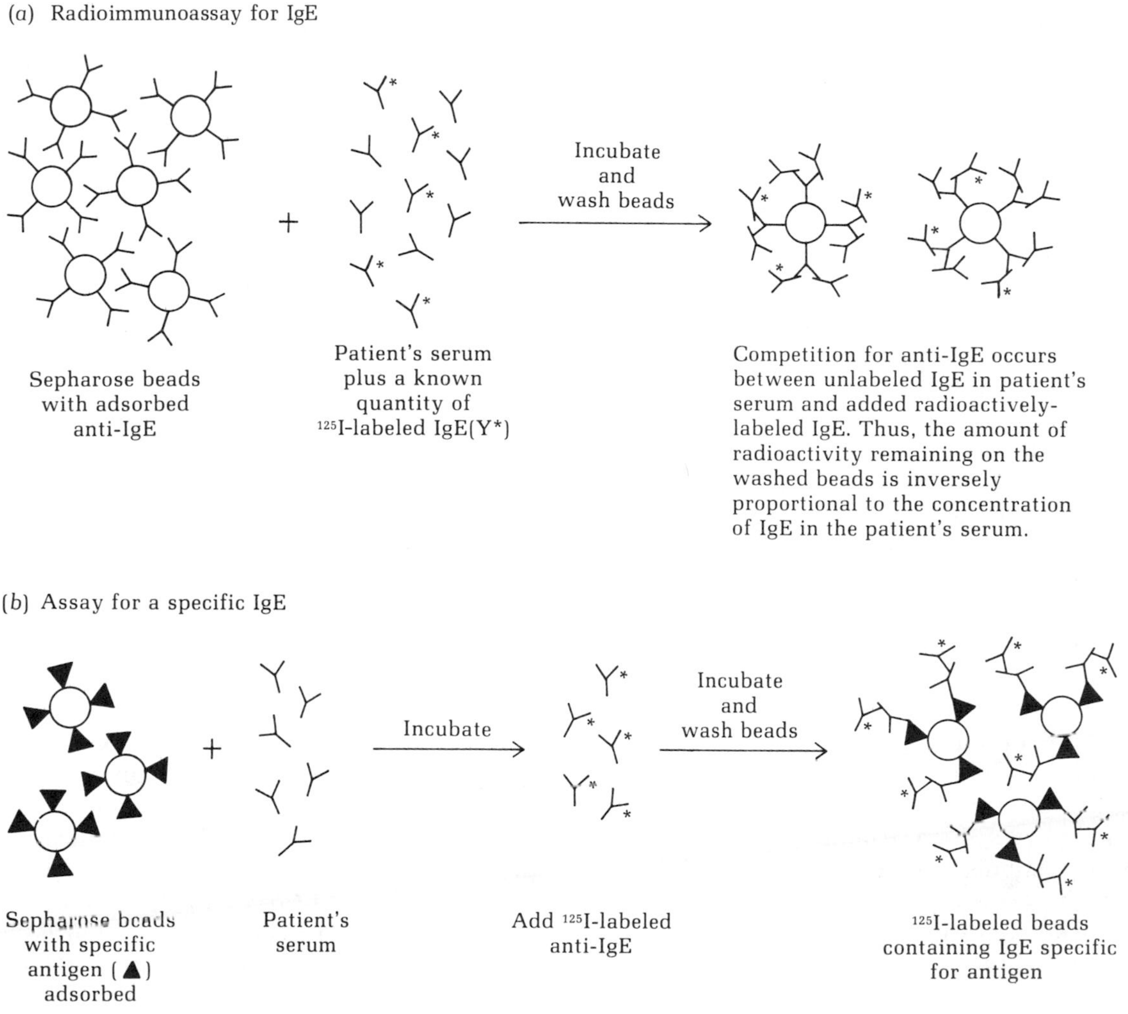
(a) Radioimmunoassay for IgE
Incubate and wash beads
Sepharose beads with adsorbed anti-IgE
Patient's serum plus a known quantity of 125I-labeled IgE(Y*)
Competition for anti-IgE occurs between unlabeled IgE in patient's serum and added radioactively-labeled IgE. Thus, the amount of radioactivity remaining on the washed beads is inversely proportional to the concentration of IgE in the patient's serum.
(b) Assay for a specific IgE
Incubate
Incubate and wash beads
Sepharose beads with specific antigen (▲) adsorbed
Patient's serum
Add 125I-labeled anti-IgE
125I-labeled beads containing IgE specific for antigen

These substances, of which bradykinin is the best-studied, arise as degradative peptides from normal serum proteins. When injected into animals, they cause increased capillary permeability and smooth muscle contraction, thereby mimicking symptoms of anaphylaxis.

## Types of Anaphylaxis

We have now established that anaphylactic reactions occur as a result of pharmacologically active mediators released when an antigen binds to cytotropic antibody, usually on the surface of a mast cell. It is not surprising that the availability of antigen will influence the rate of release of these mediators and, hence, the type and severity of the anaphylactic symptoms. Since antigen availability is usually dependent upon the route by which antigen enters the immune system, we can use this criterion to divide anaphylaxis into various subtypes.

SYSTEMIC ANAPHYLAXIS. This extremely severe reaction frequently results in death within minutes after the antigen is injected into a susceptible person or animal. Prior to the availability of antibiotics, most cases of human anaphylaxis were caused by the injection of heterologous (foreign) antiserum into a highly sensitive individual. Now, however, antibiotic therapy has greatly reduced the use of foreign antisera for the treatment of disease. Unfortunately, antibiotic therapy itself has become an important cause of human systemic anaphylaxis. For example, even though penicillin is chemically quite innocuous to the animal body, many persons become remarkably hypersensitive to this antibiotic. The injection of penicillin into such individuals results in an IgE-antigen reaction with the rapid release of histamine into the circulatory system. Another common example of systemic anaphylaxis is an individual highly sensitive to bee or wasp stings.

The major effect of histamine in systemic anaphylaxis is the contraction of smooth muscle; however, the organ affected varies among animals. Fatal anaphylaxis in humans results from respiratory failure caused by constriction of the smooth muscles in the bronchi.

LOCAL ANAPHYLAXIS. These allergies, sometimes called atopic allergies, occur spontaneously in about 10% of the population. The antigens involved are common environmental allergens such as the pollens of grass and ragweed, dander, house dust, and various foods. Symptoms depend upon the route of entry of the allergen; for example, pollens and dander that are usually inhaled cause asthma or hay fever. On the other hand, ingested allergens such as foods produce symptoms of gastrointestinal upset or hives.

The symptoms of atopic allergies result from the reaction of homocytotropic IgE antibodies with allergen and the subsequent release of histamine and SRS-A. Thus, they are caused by an antibody-adherent reaction, which is actually a manifestation of localized anaphylaxis.

CUTANEOUS ANAPHYLAXIS. As was described earlier in this chapter, the injection of minute amounts of allergen into the skin of a sensitive individual results in the rapid development of a wheal and flare. Such a reaction is another manifestation of localized anaphylaxis, since the inflammation is caused by cell mediators (primarily histamine) released by the reaction of IgE with allergen.

Certain subclasses of human IgG are heterocytotropic in that they will fix to cells of a phylogenetically distant species, such as a guinea pig, but not to human cells. It is possible to demonstrate extremely minute amounts of such antibody by a procedure known as passive cutaneous anaphylaxis (PCA). This is usually accomplished by injecting 0.1 ml of a highly diluted antiserum into the skin of a guinea pig (representing as little as 0.1 $\mu$g/ml of protein). After allowing 3 to 6 hours for the heterocytotropic antibody to fix to skin cells, antigen mixed with a dye such as Evans blue is injected intravenously. The reaction of the antigen with the cell-fixed antibody releases mediators, resulting in increased capillary dilation and permeability allowing the dye to enter the inflamed area. It is visualized by the staining of the skin (with the Evans blue) at the site of inflammation.

**Desensitization and Blocking Antibodies**

It should now be evident that anaphylaxis—whether systemic or localized—results from antigen reacting with cytotropic antibody and the subsequent release of pharmacologically active mediators. Under normal circumstances this hypersensitivity is caused by homocytotropic antibodies (such as IgE in humans), so one might rightly guess that the presence of noncytotropic antibody might compete with cytotropic antibody in binding the allergen. It follows that desensitization to an allergen such as ragweed pollen can be accomplished by the repeated injection of minute amounts of the pollen to stimulate the formation of IgG antibodies. IgG antibodies are not cytotropic in the human and can, therefore, act as blocking antibodies to intercept the allergen before it can bind to the cytotropic IgE antibodies. Obviously, this type of desensitization can be dangerous, and very small amounts of antigen must be used in a hypersensitive person to avoid inducing a systemic anaphylactic shock.

**Treatment of Anaphylactic Reactions**

Successful treatment of anaphylactic-type hypersensitivities is based on either (1) inactivation of released cell mediators, or (2) inhibition of their release. In the first case, antihistamines can be used to block the effect of histamine; however, these agents will not completely prevent the symptoms of anaphylaxis because they do not inhibit the action of the other pharmacological mediators. Also, there is considerable variation in sensitivity to histamine among various species of ani-

mals; humans and guinea pigs are exquisitely sensitive whereas rats and mice are relatively insensitive.

The release of mediators following reaction of allergen with cytotropic antibody can be prevented by 3'5'-cyclic AMP (cAMP). Hence, drugs such as epinephrine and isoproterenol which stimulate the synthesis of cAMP or the methylxanthines which inhibit its degradation have been used for many years to control the symptoms of anaphylaxis. In fact, it is not unusual for individuals highly sensitive to insect stings to carry a syringe containing epinephrine, for injection into themselves in the event of a sting.

**Genetics of IgE Production**

Although the details concerning the genetic control of IgE antibody production are unknown, there is little doubt that atopic allergies are heritable traits. This is confirmed by the observation that more than half of such patients have a family history of atopic diseases. Experimentally, it has been shown that some mouse strains are unable to produce IgE antibodies but can produce normal concentrations of the other immunoglobulin classes. In crosses between these strains and high IgE producers, the ability to mount an IgE response is dominant.

Interestingly, the major difference between atopic and nonatopic humans appears to be in the ability of atopic persons to respond to trace amounts of allergen normally available in the environment for sensitization, since most persons will form cytotropic antibodies if they are sensitized with an unusually and sufficiently large dose of allergen.

**IMMUNE COMPLEX SYNDROMES**

There are a number of clinical syndromes in which the symptoms and pathology of the disorder are initiated by the deposition of immune complexes composed of antibody and antigen in various tissues of the body. Based on the route and amount of antigen available and in some cases on the nature of the antigen itself, the immune complex destruction of tissue may occur locally or as a widely disseminated inflammation.

## Arthus Reaction

Early in the twentieth century, Maurice Arthus, a French physiologist, found that after receiving several weekly injections of horse serum, rabbits acquired the ability to respond with a marked local inflammation to later intradermal injections of the same antigen. This reaction, subsequently known as the Arthus reaction, requires the presence of large amounts of precipitating antibody and is thus mediated by either IgG or IgM classes of immunoglobulins. The series of events leading to the inflammation characteristic of the Arthus reaction appears to occur as follows: (1) Intradermally injected antigen reacts with precipitating antibody (IgG or IgM) to form an immune precipitate that penetrates the local blood vessel walls. (2) These complexes fix complement, resulting in the formation of the active chemotactic factors, C5a and C5b,6,7 (see Chapter 14). The attracted polymorphonuclear leukocytes ingest the immune precipitates, causing the release of lysosomal enzymes. (3) The lysosomal enzymes catalyze the necrosis of adjacent cells, resulting in more inflammation.

Platelets and mast cells appear to be involved in the early stages of the Arthus reaction, and it appears that the release of vasoactive amines from these cells causes an increased permeability, permitting the immune complexes to penetrate into the capillary walls. However, these cells do not seem to be of primary importance as mediators of inflammation, since antihistamines do not inhibit the course of the Arthus reaction.

The time course of the Arthus reaction is considerably slower than that described for reaginic antibodies. Slight swelling and edema may begin within one to two hours, and the usual reaction will reach a maximum in approximately four hours. Since the intensity of the inflammation is a function of the amount of antibody-antigen complexes, the rate of healing may depend on the severity of the local necrosis.

Clinically, Arthus reactions characterized by localized lung lesions have been described in individuals who inhale spores from a thermophilic *Aspergillus* (whose normal habitat is decaying vegetation) or in those who inhale mold spores used in the manufacture of certain cheeses.

## Serum Sickness Syndrome

Serum sickness gets its name from the type of reaction that may follow the injection of a foreign antiserum, such as tetanus antitoxin from a horse. Since the horse serum contains foreign proteins, the patient begins to synthesize antibodies to the antigens in the horse serum. After about a week, antibodies are rapidly being synthesized and immediately react with the circulating foreign serum. Because the synthesized antibody binds to antigen as fast as it is being synthesized, the products of the reaction are soluble immune complexes containing an excess of antigen (see precipitin reaction, Chapter 13).

As the soluble immune complexes fix complement, platelets become clumped and lysed —possibly because of the formation of a C5b-9 attack complex (see Chapter 14) or as a result of cytotropic antibody on basophils, causing their lysis and the liberation of a platelet-activating factor. The released histamine and other pharmacologically-active mediators cause an increase in the permeability of the vascular endothelium which, in turn, permits the soluble immune complexes to penetrate the blood vessel walls. The subsequent fixation of complement causes a polymorphonuclear response followed by phagocytosis of the immune complexes and the release of lysosomal enzymes. The over-all pathology of serum sickness is not unlike a disseminated Arthus reaction in which the immune complexes have been deposited in the blood vessel walls, kidneys, and tissues throughout the body. The major symptoms include fever, joint pain, rash, and an enlarged spleen and lymph nodes. The leukocytic destruction of the immune complexes results in the immune clearance of the foreign serum, and recovery usually occurs in a few days.

One can also experimentally induce a serum sickness syndrome by the infusion of preformed immune complexes. However, to be effective they must be soluble complexes that can penetrate the vascular epithelium and can fix complement. This property is found only in a condition of slight antigen excess; complement is not fixed by complexes containing large antigen excess, and near the equivalence point the immune precipitate is cleared before it can penetrate the blood vessel walls.

The reactions described for serum sickness can occur as a result of other foreign substances. Many persons develop allergies of this type to antibiotics. In these cases, it is believed that the low-molecular-weight antibiotic becomes attached to proteins in the host and, as a result, becomes large enough to be antigenic.

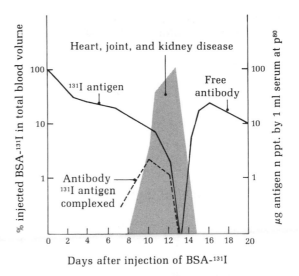

Days after injection of BSA-$^{131}$I

**Figure 16-2.** Elimination of radioactively labeled bovine serum albumin (BSA-$^{131}$I) antigen from the circulation of a rabbit. The antigen is slowly cleared until antibodies are formed. Antigen then complexes with antibody to form soluble complexes that are deposited in the heart, joints, and kidneys. Grey area illustrates occurrence of lesions resulting from deposition of immune complexes. After antigen is cleared, free antibody is found in the serum.

## Experimental Immune Complex Diseases

Using serum sickness as a model for immune complex disease, one might correctly surmise that situations can be produced in which large amounts of antigen may be presented to the immune system to bring about the formation of soluble immune complexes. This has been studied experimentally in rabbits following the injection of bovine serum albumin (BSA). If the disappearance of the BSA is followed, one sees a slow catabolism during the first eight days, occurring at about the same rate as that of the rabbit's own albumin. Once antibody synthesis is under way, there is a rapid immune clearance of the BSA, as shown in Figure 16-2. During this period of immune clearance, soluble antibody-antigen complexes are deposited in the arteries, glomeruli, joints, and heart, resulting in inflam-

mation such as described for the Arthus reaction.

A chronic immune complex disease can also be induced and maintained by the daily injection of an antigen such as BSA into a rabbit. In this case, the amount of antigen injected is critical, since it must be just sufficient to produce a temporary state of antigen excess after each injection.

The most common lesion formed in immune complex diseases occurs in the basement membrane of the kidney, causing a chronic or acute glomerulonephritis (inflammation of the kidney glomeruli). This is readily manifested clinically by an increase of protein in the urine (proteinurea) and elevated levels of cholesterol and urea in the blood. If one maintains this chronic state by the continued injection of antigen, the subsequent glomerulonephritis invariably leads to death.

Arteritis (inflammation of an artery), resulting from the deposition of these complexes in the blood vessels and heart, is seen more frequently during an acute episode of the disease than when one maintains a chronic state by frequent injections of antigen. Damage of the arteries appears to be due to the fixation of complement, resulting in the attraction and subsequent degranulation of neutrophils. The mechanism of kidney damage is not as clearly understood, since depletion of either neutrophils or the third component of complement (C3) has been reported not to alter the extent of kidney injury. In either case, it appears probable that the release of vasoactive amines from circulating platelets is a necessary prerequisite for the increased permeability permitting the entrance of the immune complexes into the vessel wall. It is currently believed that these amines are released from the platelets by the mechanisms described for serum sickness.

### Naturally-Occurring Immune Complex Diseases in Animals

We have established that immune complex disease occurs whenever there is sufficient antigen in the circulation to form soluble immune complexes with precipitating antibody. It would not be surprising, therefore, that immune complex diseases can occur naturally. A mutation occurring in ranch mink, which resulted in a desirable change in coat color, was described in 1941. These mutants, known as Aleutian mink, were found to develop an illness pathologically similar to the serum sickness syndrome already described, i.e., glomerulonephritis and widespread arteritis. Subsequent studies have shown that this disease is caused by Aleutian disease virus (ADV), but unlike most viruses, ADV infectivity is not neutralized by circulating antibody. Thus, in this disease a constant supply of antigen is being

supplied to the immune system to provide the major components of an immune complex disease.

Certain strains of mice that are infected with lymphocytic choriomeningitis virus *in utero* become life-long carriers of the virus (see Chapter 40). It was long believed that this carrier state was the result of an acquired tolerance to the virus; however, such carriers do develop pathological changes consistent with immune complex disease. The reason these carrier mice are unable to neutralize the virus is unclear, but it has been proposed that it may represent a quantitative phenomenon in which the carrier mice are deficient in their ability to make a sufficiently strong immune response to eliminate the virus.

### Naturally-Occurring Immune Complex Diseases in Humans

Quite a number of human maladies readily fit the description of immune complex diseases. For the most part, however, the antigen that initiates these diseases is not known; our discussion will, therefore, be limited to only a few human disorders in which the symptoms of the disease appear to be related to an immunological response.

SYSTEMIC LUPUS ERYTHEMATOSIS. This disease closely resembles serum sickness as manifested by the pathologic changes seen in the kidney and the blood vessels. The antibodies found in systemic lupus erythematosis (SLE) are directed against a variety of host cellular antigens, but the most important ones appear to be a heterologous population of antibodies directed against DNA. The series of events that releases the antigen and induces the formation of antinuclear antibodies is not known, although the presence of a persistent viral infection has long been suspected. Thus, a virus that could integrate its DNA into the host genome could code for the presence of foreign antigens on the cell surface. Immune destruction of such cells could supply the nuclear antigens that initiate SLE. This is still conjecture, however, and results from additional research are necessary to learn the specific inducing events that lead to SLE.

GLOMERULONEPHRITIS. As already discussed, most immune complex diseases result in kidney damage. There are only a few cases, however, in which the infectious agents that initiate this syndrome have been identified.

Group A streptococcal infections, particularly those caused by type 12, have long been known to cause an acute glomerulonephritis (Chapter 18). The specific nature of the streptococcal antigen involved in this immune complex disease is not known, but several laboratories have demonstrated the presence of IgG, complement, and streptococcal antigens in the granular deposits along the glomerular capillary walls.

Chronic glomerulonephritis has been reported to be associated with malaria (Chapter 43) and with hepatitis B infections (Chapter 36). In both cases, it seems likely that the immune system is presented with large amounts of antigen over an extended period of time, resulting in the occurrence of immune complex disease.

RHEUMATOID ARTHRITIS. This disease is characterized by a chronic inflammation of the joints in which there are high levels of immunoglobulins, complement, and complement-fixing aggregates of immunoglobulins. The resulting inflammation may well result from a reaction such as described for the Arthus reaction, in which the major damage results from the release of lysosomal enzymes following the phagocytosis of the immune complexes. The greatest mystery concerning rheumatoid arthritis is the nature of the antigen involved. There is, however, circumstantial evidence that aggregated IgG might function as the inducing antigen.

## AUTOIMMUNE REACTIONS

Autoimmune reactions are defined here as immunological reactions against self that occur in the absence of cell mediators. For the most part, these disorders are diseases in which autoantibodies are formed against antigens on the cells of a specific organ such as the kidney or against antigens on one's own platelets and red cells.

What happens to induce individuals to synthesize antibodies to their own tissues? In some cases, it seems that target tissues or cells are normally sequestered from the immune system, and only if conditions allow their release into the circulatory system can antibody formation occur. This appears to be true in the case of spermatozoa and brain tissue, since the injection of these tissues into the circulatory system may result in male infertility or allergic encephalitis, respectively. This does not, however, explain other autoimmune diseases such as hemolytic anemia that seem to occur as a result of antibody synthesis to a readily available autoantigen (see Table 16-3). One concept proposes that

**Table 16-3. Autoimmune Diseases Occurring in Humans**

| Disease | Autoantigen |
|---------|-------------|
| Hashimoto's thyroiditis | Thyroid cell surface |
| Hemolytic anemia | Red blood cell surface |
| Pernicious anemia | Intrinsic factor (necessary for vitamin $B_{12}$ absorption) |
| Allergic encephalitis | Brain cell surface |
| Systemic lupus erythematosis | DNA of many cells |
| Thrombocytopenic purpura | Platelet surface |
| Rheumatoid arthritis | ? IgG in synovial membrane |
| Myasthenia gravis | Receptor for acetylcholine |
| ? Rheumatic fever | Heart |
| ? Subacute glomerulonephritis | Kidney |

specific suppressor T cells normally prevent the production of autoantibodies; thus, the loss of specific suppressor T cells alone could result in autoantibody production. Or if a minor modification in the antigen occurs (such as that which could result from lysosomal hydrolysis), a new T-cell determinant might be created that could stimulate existing T cells to cooperate with functional B cells to produce destructive autoantibodies. This same principle could apply to cross-reacting antigens found in microorganisms. Thus, Group A streptococci (Chapter 18) may in some cases be able to present a new T-cell determinant on an antigen that cross-reacts with heart tissue, resulting in the occurrence of rheumatic fever. It also seems possible that cellular antigens might be altered by microorganisms to provide new T-cell determinants, or even that microorganisms might themselves act as adjuvants to bypass the T-cell requirement.

In any event, there seems to be a familial tendency for autoimmune diseases to occur, and persons with one autoimmune disease are much more likely to have a second autoimmune disease. Any complete explanation will probably also include genetic defects inherent in the suppressor T-cell population.

## REFERENCES

Bazaral, M., H. A. Orgel, and R. N. Hamburger. 1974. Genetics of IgE and allergy: Serum IgE levels in twins. *J. Allergy and Clin. Immunol.* **54:**288–304.

Bazaral, M., H. A. Orgel, and R. N. Hamburger. 1971. IgE levels in normal infants and mothers and an inheritance hypothesis. *J. Immunol.* **107:**794–801.

Becker, E. 1971. Nature and classification of immediate-type allergic reactions. *Adv. in Immunol.* **13:**267–313.

Burnet, F. M. 1972. *Auto-Immunity and Auto-Immune Disease.* F. A. Davis, Philadelphia.

Cochrane, C. G., and D. Koffler. 1973. Immune complex disease in experimental animals and man. *Adv. in Immunol.* **16:**185–264.

Flick, J. 1972. Human reagins: Appraisal of the properties of the antibody of immediate-type hypersensitivity. *Bacteriol. Rev.* **36:**311–360.

Grundbacher, F. J. 1975. Causes of variations in serum IgE levels in normal populations. *J. Allergy and Clin. Immunol.* **56:**104–111.

Henderson, L. L., J. B. Larson, and G. J. Gleich. 1975. Maximal rise in IgE antibody following ragweed pollination season. *J. Allergy and Clin. Immunol.* **55:**10–15.

Hoffman, D. R., and Z. H. Haddad. 1974. Diagnosis of IgE-mediated reactions to food antigens by radioimmunoassay. *J. Allergy and Clin. Immunol.* **54:**165–173.

Johansson, S. G. O., H. H. Bennich, and T. Berg. 1972. The clinical significance of IgE. *Progr. Clin. Immunol.* **1:**157–181.

Lockey, R. F. 1974. Systemic reactions to stinging ants. *J. Allergy and Clin. Immunol.* **54:**132–146.

Weigle, W. O. 1971. Recent observations and concepts in immunological unresponsiveness and autoimmunity. *Clin. Exp. Immunol.* **9:**437–447.

# 17

# Cellular Immunity

Each normal vertebrate animal possesses two immune systems, a humoral one composed of soluble immunoglobulins and a cellular system that depends on the action of living cells that have become sensitized to a specific antigen. These two systems of immunity are separate entities, but they are not mutually exclusive. Thus, the same antigen may and frequently does induce both specific antibody synthesis and a specific cellular response.

Although unaware of the nature of the inflammatory response, Robert Koch first described cellular hypersensitivity in 1891. He observed that if tubercle bacilli were injected into the skin of a guinea pig previously infected with tubercle bacilli, an intense area of inflammation would develop in one to two days at the site of the infection. This response did not occur in noninfected control animals. Koch later found that he could use a concentrate of the broth culture in which the tubercle bacilli had grown and obtain a similar inflammatory response in an animal that had been previously infected with tubercle bacilli (see tuberculin in Chapter 25). Since it required 24–48 hours for this inflammation to reach a peak, he referred to it as delayed

hypersensitivity; later, when similar systems were described, they were called tuberculin-type or delayed-type hypersensitivities. It was also observed that the intravenous injection of tuberculin into a sensitized guinea pig could cause a systemic shock; however, unlike systemic anaphylaxis, fatal tuberculin shock required a comparatively large amount of tuberculin and even then it did not occur until 6 to 24 hours after challenge.

The most puzzling aspect of this reaction was that, unlike the Arthus-type sensitivity, it could not be passively transferred using serum from a sensitized animal. Moreover, the cutaneous reaction differed histologically from the Arthus reaction in that it contained primarily monocytic leukocytes rather than polymorphonuclear cells. The first major breakthrough in our understanding of this type of hypersensitivity came in 1942 when Karl Landsteiner and Merrill Chase showed that tuberculin hypersensitivity could be passively transferred from a sensitized to a nonsensitized guinea pig using washed, intact, viable, white cells. This observation clearly showed that delayed-type hypersensitivity was mediated by cells and could function in the absence of humoral antibody.

**Table 17-1. Differences in Delayed and Immediate-Type Hypersensitivity**

| Property | Delayed-Type | Immediate-Type |
|---|---|---|
| Mediators | Cells | Antibodies |
| Time for skin reactions to reach maximum | 24–48 hours | Minutes to several hours |
| Type of cells involved | Lymphocytes and macrophages | Mostly polymorphonuclear leukocytes |
| Passively transferred with: | T cells | Soluble antibodies |

Considerable efforts have since been expended to determine whether cellular hypersensitivity (as seen in a delayed-type skin reaction) was actually synonymous with cell-mediated immunity. It now seems likely that the hypersensitivity and cellular immunity represent the same phenomenon and, as a result, the terms are used interchangeably. Some of the major properties that differentiate delayed-type hypersensitivity from immediate-type hypersensitivity are listed in Table 17-1.

## NATURE OF INDUCING ANTIGENS

It is well established that a single antigen may induce both humoral antibody synthesis and specific cellular immunity. However, in the case of cellular immunity, it appears that the lower limits of antigen size are usually larger than that required for the induction of immunoglobulin synthesis. And, somewhat surprisingly, the parameters of specificity seem to be more rigid for the cellular reaction than is generally seen in an antibody response. For example, if one experimentally immunizes an animal with dinitrophenol that has been complexed to guinea pig albumin (DNP-GPA), one can induce antibody formation to DNP-GPA as well as a delayed-type hypersensitivity to the complexed DNP. As was discussed in Chapter 15, the humoral antibodies produced will also bind to DNP if it is complexed to a large number of different and unrelated carrier proteins. Delayed hyper-

sensitivity, however, shows a higher degree of conjugate specificity, and minor changes in the carrier protein may result in little or no delayed-type skin reaction when injected into a host sensitized with DNP-GPA. Therefore, it seems that the recognition system for delayed-type hypersensitivity must distinguish both the hapten and the carrier before a reaction will occur.

Most of us, however, do not come into contact with such novel antigens as DNP-GPA and would ask what kind of natural antigens would sensitize our cellular immune system. This question cannot be answered with a single, concise reply; however, cellular immunity is, for the most part, directed against antigens occurring on whole cells or on many kinds of viruses. The perplexing aspect is that although we can list some generalities concerning what types of organisms are most likely to evoke a strong cellular immune response, we cannot always predict which immune system will actually provide protection against reinfection. For example, cellular immunity appears to be responsible for providing essentially all of our protection against mycotic infections (Chapter 29), as well as for providing immunity to reinfection by bacteria causing tuberculosis, leprosy, brucellosis, and listeriosis. Infections caused by clostridia, shigellae, and pseudomonads are probably held in check more by our humoral immune system than by our cell-mediated immune reactions. In general, it seems that humoral antibodies have little effect on those bacteria that are able to survive and multiply within host macrophages, and, as we shall discuss in the next section, a cell-mediated immune response provides our major protection against such bacteria.

Since viruses all reproduce as intracellular agents, it is a little more difficult to assign a reason for the variation in the type of immune response to these agents. A cellular response, however, appears to control virus infections such as mumps, vaccinia, herpes, and tumor viruses, but may be of little value in the prevention of such diseases as polio, common colds, or yellow fever.

A delayed-type skin response known as allergic contact dermatitis provides an exception to the generalization that cellular immunity is usually induced by antigens on whole cells. The allergens in these cases are generally low-molecular-weight chemicals such as the catechols of poison ivy, cosmetics, drugs, or antibiotics. Sensitization occurs when these substances combine with skin proteins to form the large antigens necessary to induce a delayed-type hypersensitivity. Once an individual is sensitized, subsequent skin contact with the allergen, resulting in the formation of the same carrier-conjugate, will induce a delayed-type reaction that reaches maximum intensity in about 24 to 48 hours and is characterized by the presence of large numbers of mononuclear cells in the deep layer of the skin. This sequence of events is depicted schematically in Figure 17-1 Superficially, vesicles also form which may coalesce to form blisters.

It is obvious that we cannot accurately predict which antigens are likely to stimulate which immune system. It is generally accepted that the cell-mediated response is

**Figure 17-1.** Schematic illustration showing the acquisition of allergic contact dermatitis to poison ivy. Dermatitis would not normally occur as a result of a primary sensitization because the inducing Ag would be gone before sufficient T cells became available. On secondary contact, however, T memory cells are rapidly converted to activated T cells.

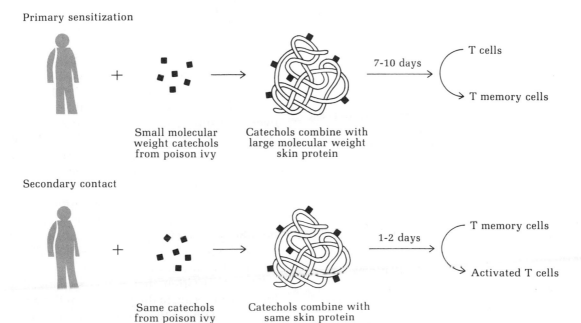

phylogenetically older than the humoral one, and some investigators believe the body responds to all antigens with at least a "weak" cell-mediated immune response. We also know that for many antigens such a response can be very weak and unimportant, while for others it provides the only protection to the body. Usually the administration of an antigen in adjuvant (see Freund's adjuvant, Chapter 13), and an intradermal rather than an intravenous injection favors the induction of a delayed-type response.

## CELLULAR BASIS OF IMMUNITY

In vivo measurements of cell-mediated hypersensitivity have helped in the retrospective diagnosis of some fungal, bacterial, and viral infections. Their value is based on the observation that cell-mediated inflammation to many infectious agents can be invoked by either the intradermal injection of a small amount of microbial products (as shown in Table 17-2) or by a test in which these products are applied to a patch that is allowed to remain in contact with the skin for approximately 24 hours. One must remember, however, that cell-mediated hypersensitivity may last for years after clinical recovery from a disease. A single positive skin test can therefore be interpreted only as evidence of a past or present infection that may be either clinical or subclinical. However, if a conversion from negative to positive is observed and if this occurs in association with clinical symptoms, the test is quite useful. In spite of the use of such skin reactions for more than half a century, it was not until techniques became available for in vitro measurements of cell-mediated hypersensitivity that an insight into the molecular mechanism of these reactions came to light.

### Cell Types in Cellular Immunity

One of the early techniques for the in vitro determination of cell-mediated hypersensitivity measured the inhibition of migration of white cells in the presence of a specific sensitizing antigen. This procedure is generally carried out by placing peripheral white blood cells or peritoneal exudate cells from a sensitized animal into a capillary tube. Under normal conditions, these cells migrate out of the open end of the capillary tube when placed into a tissue culture medium. If, however, the antigen to which the animal had been sensitized is added to the culture, the migration is inhibited, as shown in Figure 17-2. This inhibition is highly specific for the antigen to which the cells have been sensitized. If one obtains macrophages from a nonsensitized animal and mixes them with lymphocytes from a sensitized animal, migration of these macrophages are also inhibited in the presence of the specific antigen to which the lymphocytes are sensitized. Moreover, it requires only about one sensitized lymphocyte for each 99 macrophages to demonstrate this inhibition of migration, and the addition of either anti-lymphocytic serum or anti-Thy 1 serum completely abolishes the inhibition of macrophage migration. Thus, cellular immunity is not only mediated by lymphocytes but is a primary property of the T lymphocyte, since only the T cell would be affected by antiserum to the Thy 1 antigen.

The observation that a few sensitized T lymphocytes can, in the presence of their specific sensitizing antigen, inhibit the migration

**Table 17-2. Some Microbial Products Used to Elicit Delayed-Type Hypersensitivity Reactions in Sensitive Individuals**

| Product | Disease |
| --- | --- |
| Tuberculin | Tuberculosis |
| Brucellergin | Brucellosis |
| Lepromin | Leprosy |
| Histoplasmin | Histoplasmosis |
| Blastomycin | Blastomycosis |
| Coccidioidin | Coccidioidomycosis |
| Killed mump virus | Mumps |

|  | No antigen | Ovalbumin | Toxoid |
|---|---|---|---|

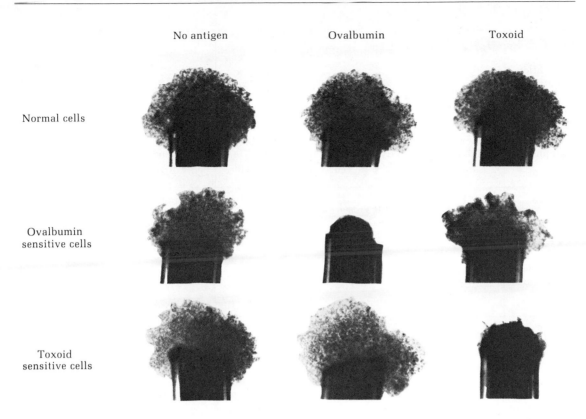

Normal cells

Ovalbumin sensitive cells

Toxoid sensitive cells

**Figure 17-2.** Effect of ovalbumin and diphtheria toxoid on the migration of peritoneal cells obtained from guinea pigs exhibiting delayed-type hypersensitivity to ovalbumin or diphtheria toxoid. Photographs were taken after 24 hours incubation of each cell type with the respective antigen. Migration was inhibited only by the antigen to which the guinea pig exhibited a delayed-type hypersensitivity.

of normal macrophages indicates that there must be a soluble factor produced by the sensitized lymphocyte that mediates the inhibition. This has been found to be the case, and the responsible soluble substance, called migratory inhibition factor (MIF), has been shown to be a glycoprotein synthesized by the sensitized T cell following contact with its specific antigen. Paradoxically, if T lymphocytes are treated with the antigen to which they have been sensitized in the absense of any macrophages, no soluble mediators are released. Furthermore, if purified macrophages are treated with antigen, they stimulate T cells to produce MIF, even though the macrophages are washed free of antigen

before mixing with T cells. Neither the culture supernatant nor homogenates of these macrophages can stimulate purified immune T cells. There is no ready explanation for these results (shown in Figure 17-3), but it has been demonstrated that for macrophages to be effective in stimulating T cells, they must be antigenically similar; they must share at least one major antigen with the T cell. These observations indicate that the stimulation of T cells to synthesize MIF requires close contact between macrophage and lymphocyte. Moreover, they show that even though the specificity of cell-mediated immunity lies in the T lymphocyte, the activation of the macrophage is a circuitous route:

| | (a) | (b) | (c) | (d) | (e) |
|---|---|---|---|---|---|
| Migration pattern | 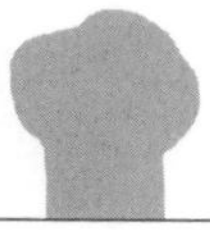 | | 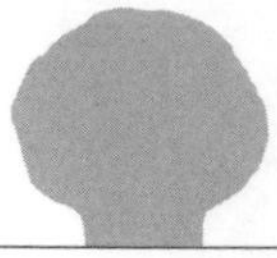 | | 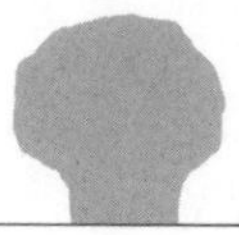 |
| Lymphocyte | Non-purified lymph node cell 2 x 10⁷ cells | Purified lymphocyte 2 x 10⁷ cells | Purified lymphocyte 2 x 10⁷ cells | Purified lymphocyte 2 x 10⁷ cells | None |
| Stimulation | PPD 25 μg/ml | PPD 25 μg/ml | Non-pulsed purified macrophage 0.1 x 10⁷ cells | PPD-pulsed purified macrophage 0.1 x 10⁷ cells | PPD-pulsed purified macrophage 0.5 x 10⁷ cells |
| Migration index (%) | 52 | 105 | 100 | 36 | 77 |

**Figure 17-3.** Migration patterns obtained by stimulation of lymphocytes sensitized to PPD (purified protein derivative extracted from tubercle bacilli): (a) crude leukocyte preparation containing both lymphocytes and macrophages, (b) in the absence of macrophages, (c) containing both lymphocytes and macrophages but not pulsed (treated) with PPD, (d) macrophages pulsed with PPD prior to mixing them with sensitized lymphocytes, and (e) PPD plus macrophages but no lymphocytes. The macrophages here are the adherent cells of peritoneal exudate cells.

antigen must first bind to compatible macrophages, which only then can induce the T cell to synthesize MIF and other soluble mediators as described in the following sections.

## Macrophage Stimulation by Lymphocyte Mediators

Although the liberation of MIF from the stimulated lymphocyte keeps the macrophage localized in the area of inflammation, the macrophage expresses the actual acquired immunity by inhibiting the intracellular multiplication of the infectious agent. This increase in macrophage activity appears to be stimulated by various products released from the sensitized lymphocyte. Soluble mediators, such as MIF, that are released from antigen-stimulated lymphocytes have been given the general name of lymphokines. Many of them have yet to be characterized

and are assigned specific names that describe only their effects on other cells.

CHEMOTACTIC FACTOR FOR MACROPHAGES. Observations of cell types found at the sites of delayed-type skin reactions have shown the major type of cell present to be a rapidly dividing monocyte which eventually differentiates into a mature macrophage. The assumption that antigen-induced lymphocytes release a factor that attracts monocytes has been proven by *in vitro* experiments using chambers separated by a micropore filter. Monocytes were placed into one chamber and lymphocytes plus antigen into the other chamber. Chemotactic activity was evaluated by counting the number of monocytes that migrated through the filter into the lymphocyte chamber. The results clearly demonstrated that a chemotactic factor is released when lymphocytes react with antigen and, futhermore, that the reaction is specific for the antigen to which the lymphocytes are sensitized. A partial characterization of this chemotactic factor for macrophages indicates that it is a protein capable of being separated from MIF on gel electrophoresis.

MACROPHAGE ACTIVATING FACTOR.   Acquired immunity to diseases such as tuberculosis and brucellosis has been clearly shown to require activation of macrophages. Observations to support this conclusion have repeatedly demonstrated that macrophages from immunized animals have acquired an enhanced bacteriostatic or bactericidal activity not seen in control macrophages obtained from nonimmune animals. The changes that take place are spoken of as macrophage activation and, in general, include: (1) increased phagocytic activity, (2) increased metabolic activity, and (3) increased numbers of lysosomes and lysosomal enzymes. (In fact, because of the increased activity of such stimulated macrophages, some investigators have referred to them as "enraged or activated macrophages.")

The molecular events culminating in the enhancement of macrophage function are not known. *In vitro* experiments have shown that the supernatant solution from a mixture of stimulated lymphocytes and macrophages will mediate this activity. Attempts to purify the macrophage activating factor indicate that it is a glycoprotein similar to the same mediator that inhibits the migration of macrophages (MIF), but it may or may not be identical to MIF.

It should be emphasized that the stimulation of the lymphocyte is a specific event which under normal circumstances occurs only when the sensitized lymphocyte interacts directly or indirectly with its antigen. An exception is seen with various plant proteins, collectively referred to as plant lectins, that are able to nonspecifically mimic the antigen stimulation of lymphocytes. Once the macrophage is activated, however, its action is nonspecific. For example, macrophages activated by tuberculin-sensitive lymphocytes will also show an enhanced activity toward any organism present.

CELL-MEDIATED IMMUNITY IN VIRAL INFECTIONS.   One can eliminate immunity to many virus infections by treatment with anti-lymphocytic or anti-Thy 1 serum, both of which destroy T cells. Thus, there is little doubt that cell-mediated responses are involved in many types of viral immunity. The mechanism of viral destruction is not known, although it also appears to be associated with the accumulation of monocytes.

### Transfer Factor

In the beginning of this chapter, cell-mediated immunity was defined as a response that could be passively transferred only with intact living lymphocytes. The one exception to this definition appears to occur only in humans. H. S. Lawrence reported that cell-mediated responses to streptococcal antigens could be passively transferred in humans using soluble extracts of sensitized lymphocytes. The active component, called transfer factor, is a low-molecular-weight molecule, resistant to treatment with trypsin, RNase, and DNase. Little is known about the chemistry or the mode of action of this material and it is currently the subject of much research and debate.

## DIRECT CYTOTOXICITY OF LYMPHOCYTES

Lymphocytes are also capable of directly killing target cells to which they have been sensitized. The effector lymphocytes are completely inhibited by anti-Thy 1 serum and are, therefore, solely comprised of T cells. Essentially any type of tissue cell may serve as a target cell. This direct cytotoxicity requires cell-to-cell contact and will not function if a membrane is placed between the effector and target cells. Furthermore, it is specific only for the target cell to which the effector is sensitized; third-party cells within the mixture are not harmed.

The mechanism of this direct cytotoxicity is not known; it is known that the effector lymphocyte must be living and metabolically active. The target cell can be seen to undergo morphological damage after 12 to 20 hours of contact, and by 48 to 72 hours the destruction is massive. It appears that the effector T lymphocyte is not damaged during the cytotoxic attack on the target cell and remains capable of attacking additional target cells; data such as shown in Figure 17-4 however, would support a one-hit phenomenon between lymphocyte and target cell, within a 48-hour time period.

Neither humoral antibodies nor complement are involved in this process; however, since the cytotoxic effect requires such close contact between the effector and target cells, antibody to either cell may sterically block the cytotoxic reaction.

## CYTOTOXICITY OF SOLUBLE MEDIATORS RELEASED BY LYMPHOCYTES

We have discussed the antigen-mediated release of lymphokines that influence the behavior of macrophages. Also included in the catalog of substances released by antigen-stimulated lymphocytes are soluble media-

**Figure 17-4.** Relationship between the number of lymph node cells and surviving target cells after being cultured together for 48 hours. Target cells in this case were Lewis tumor cells, and sensitized lymph node cells were obtained from rats immunized against Lewis histocompatibility antigen. *a.* Note that only sensitized lymph node cells are cytotoxic for the target cells. *b.* The fact that there is a straight-line exponential relationship between the dose of lymphocytes and the percentage of target cells surviving supports the concept of a single-hit event for the cytocidal activity of the lymphocyte.

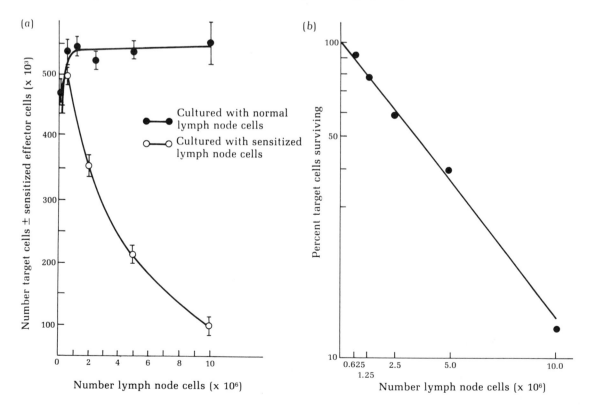

tors that kill target cells. The term lymphotoxin (LT) has been used to describe one such mediator.

The antigen-cell interaction is specific, although various plant lectins such as phytohemagglutinin or concanavilin A will also induce the release of LT. Since LT will act on a large variety of normal and neoplastic cells, "innocent bystander" cells may also be killed when sensitized T cells are stimulated by antigen to synthesize and release LT. Lymphotoxin appears to be a moderately stable protein that acts on the plasma membrane of target cells.

A variety of other cytotoxic mediators are released by the action of antigen with its sensitized T cell. Most of these have not been well characterized, and they have been assigned names descriptive of their action on target cells—for example, cloning inhibitory factor, skin reactive factor, proliferation inhibition factor, chemotactic factor, and blastogenic factor. The relationship of these mediators to each other or to the other mediators reported to be released by sensitized lymphocytes is at this time unknown. It is also not currently known whether a single population of T lymphocytes is responsible for both direct cytotoxicity and the release of mediators.

## CELLULAR ASPECTS OF TRANSPLANTATION REJECTION

It has been known for hundreds of years that only under very restricted circumstances can one successfully transplant skin or organs from one individual to another. When such transplants are made, the foreign tissue is usually killed and rejected approximately 10 to 14 days after transplantation. If a second transplant from the same donor is applied, it is rejected much sooner than was the first transplant. A second transplant from a different, unrelated donor, however, requires essentially the same time period for rejection as did the first transplant. These observations clearly establish the following facts: (1) rejection is the result of an immunological reaction; (2) a second transplant from the same donor calls forth an anamnestic response which results in a more rapid rejection; and (3) rejection is directed at specific tissue antigens which, in most cases, differ from one individual to another.

### Tissue Transplant Terminology

Since graft rejection is the result of an immunological reaction, tissue that is antigenically identical to that of the recipient would not be expected to be rejected. Thus, autografts, which are transplants from one area to another in the same person, or isografts, which are transplants between genetically identical persons (identical twins), would not be rejected. This is also observed in strains of mice and guinea pigs that have been inbred so that all offspring are genetically identical.

Allografts (older terminology: homografts) are transplants between genetically nonidentical animals of the same species, such as human to human or mouse to mouse. Xenografts are grafts that cross species lines. Since the intensity of a rejection is a function of the degree of antigenic difference between donor and recipient, one might correctly expect that xenografts are vigorously rejected, whereas the rejection of an allograft depends upon the relatedness between the donor and the recipient. This terminology is summarized in Table 17-3.

**Table 17-3. Types and Examples of Tissue Grafts**

| Type | Example |
|------|---------|
| Autografts | From one area of an individual's body to another area |
| Isografts | Between genetically identical animals, such as identical twins or inbred strains of animals |
| Allografts | Between members of the same species, such as human to human |
| Xenografts | From one species to another, such as monkey to human |

## CELL-MEDIATED VERSUS HUMORAL REJECTION

Allograft destruction is histologically characterized by the infiltration of lymphocytes into the foreign tissue. In fact, the transfer of lymphoid cells from an animal that has rejected an allograft will confer upon the recipient the ability to respond with an accelerated rejection of tissue from the same allograft donor, indicating that immunological memory resides in the lymphocytes. Moreover, neonatally thymectomized mice are frequently unable to reject allografts, but will acquire this ability if given lymphocytes from a syngeneic (genetically identical) animal. It therefore seems to be established that allograft rejection is a function of lymphocyte-mediated immunity.

The passive transfer of serum, even though it contains antibodies to the foreign tissue, does not normally result in an accelerated allograft rejection. One seeming contradiction to this statement is seen if skin is transferred to an individual who possesses a high titer of humoral antibody to the transplanted skin. Such grafts are rejected very quickly—even before they can vascularize—and therefore they are called white grafts. In such cases, the graft does not even begin to "heal-in," and it is really a matter of semantics as to whether it ever truly existed as a graft.

## HISTOCOMPATIBILITY

### Histocompatibility or Transplantation Antigens

Since allograft rejection is caused by a cell-mediated immune response, it is reasonable to conclude that transplanted cells possess surface determinants that are recognized as foreign by genetically nonidentical animals or persons. These determinants, termed histocompatibility or transplantation antigens, have been extensively studied in the mouse and to a lesser extent in other animals, including humans. They have been shown to be glycoproteins (45,000 daltons) associated with a second small protein (11,000 daltons) known as $\beta_2$-microglobulin. An unusual characteristic of the histocompatibility antigens is that the $\beta_2$-microglobulin part of these antigens possesses a similar molecular weight and considerable amino acid homology with the constant domain of the light chain of the IgG molecule.

### Histocompatibility Genes

There are a number of gene loci that code for cellular antigens involved in allograft rejection. For example, about 40 such genes have been detected in the mouse, and it would appear likely that humans are no less complex. In at least ten different animals ranging from amphibians to humans, the histocompatibility antigens evoking the strongest response (that is, the ones most responsible for allograft rejection) have been shown to be coded in a single chromosomal segment, termed the major histocompatibility complex (MHC). This same complex also controls a number of other immunological reactions such as (1) the ability to respond to a specific antigen, and (2) the recognition of incompatibility that leads to a proliferative response (blast formation) when lymphocytes of different allotypes are mixed together in vitro.

The MHC of the mouse, the H-2 complex, has been subjected to a more thorough genetic study than that of any other animal, because of the availability of so many inbred strains. Figure 17-5 is a chromosome map of the H-2 complex, including some of the known traits that are controlled by the MHC.

Although there is still much to be learned about the H-2 complex, it seems established that the major histocompatibility antigens are controlled by two loci, termed H-2K and H-2D, and that there are multiple alleles within a population for each of these loci. Each allele of these loci can code for one histocompatibility antigen (mol. wt. approx. 45,000 daltons) and each of these antigens will contain one determinant that is specific for a given nonrecombinant haplo-

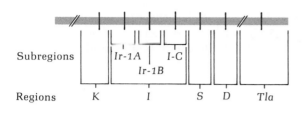

| Subregions | | | | | | |
|---|---|---|---|---|---|---|
| | | Ir-1A | I-C | | | |
| | | Ir-1B | | | | |
| Regions | K | I | | S | D | Tla |

| Genetically variant traits controlled by the H-2-Tla complex | |
|---|---|
| Trait | Controlling region |
| Serologically detected alloantigen | K,D |
| Transplanted antigens | K,D,Tla,I |
| Cell-mediated lympholysis target antigens | K,D |
| Thymus-leukemia cellular alloantigens | Tla |
| Tumor virus susceptibility | K or I |
| Immune responses | I |
| Mixed-leukocyte reaction | K,I,D |
| Graft-versus-host reaction | K,I,D |
| I-region lymphocyte antigens | I |
| T-cell-B-cell interactions | I |
| Complement levels | S |

**Figure 17-5.** Genetic fine structure map of the H-2-Tla gene complex of mouse chromosome 17, showing regions and subregions. Note that although the Tla region is not part of the H-2 complex, it is closely related and controls traits similar to those of the H-2 complex.

type (termed a private specificity) plus additional determinants that may be shared with other haplotypes (termed public specificities). (A haplotype is a single combination of alleles at the loci comprising the H-2 complex; it is defined by the immunologic response that follows a challenge with a tissue graft from a nonidentical animal. Moreover, each individual has two MHC haplotypes, one inherited from each parent.) There are data also, however, which show that some histocompatibility loci (which are also of moderate strength in inducing allograft rejection) exist in the Tla region (which is linked to the MHC) and in the I region of the MHC.

## Cell-Mediated Lympholysis

When lymphocytes are mixed with target cells that possess different histocompatibility antigens, the target cells are lysed. This cell-mediated lympholysis (CML) is a function of specific histocompatibility differences between killer and target cells and is, therefore, controlled by the K and D regions of the H-2 complex. It can be measured by labeling target cells with $^{51}$Cr and determining the release of chromium from the lysed cells.

## Immune Response Genes

Different H-2 haplotypes also show different patterns of high or low antibody responses to various antigens. These responses are under the control of the I region of the H-2 complex. In fact, susceptibility to certain leukemia-producing viruses has been shown to be influenced by a single gene in the I region, and it is postulated that the genetic constitution of this region may play an important role in the disease resistance of natural populations. Recent data have suggested that the I region gene products may function by coding for a T-cell factor necessary for its interaction with a B lymphocyte.

MIXED LYMPHOCYTE REACTION. When allogenic lymphocytes (those possessing different alloantigens) are mixed together in vitro they undergo blast formation, enlarging, becoming more basophilic, and synthesizing DNA at a faster rate than normal (see Figure 17-6). In laboratory practice, the extent of this mixed lymphocyte reaction (MLR) is measured by determining the amount of tritiated thymidine incorporated into DNA after incubating the lymphocytes together for several days. It is usually made unidirectional by treating the donor's lymphocytes with X-irradiation or mitomycin C (to prevent DNA replication), so that only the recipient's lymphocytes can undergo blast formation.

The extent to which a recipient's lymphocytes incorporate tritiated thymidine is

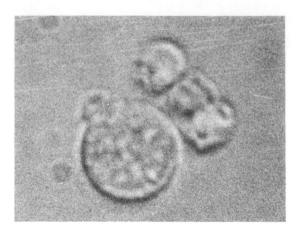

**Figure 17-6.** Blast formation. Mouse thymocytes were incubated in the presence of concanavalin A for 48 hours. Note one large lymphocyte that has undergone blast formation adjacent to three smaller unstimulated lymphocytes. Antigen-induced blast formation is morphologically identical.

directly correlated with the degree of antigenic differences between the two allogenic lymphocytes and, hence, can be used to predict allograft compatibility. It was believed for years that the blast formation seen in the MLR was due to differences in the histocompatibility antigens. It is now known, however, that the major stimulatory factors are controlled by genes termed lymphocyte activating determinants (Lad), which exist in the immune response region (I region) of the H-2 complex. However, weak stimulation is also associated with the K and D regions that control the structure of the histocompatibility antigens.

GRAFT VERSUS HOST REACTIONS. If spleen or bone marrow cells are injected into an immunologically unresponsive host—a newborn animal or an X-irradiated adult—the injected lymphocytes recognize the host tissue as foreign and will initiate a graft versus host reaction (GVHR). In the newborn mouse the GVHR causes a loss in weight, skin lesions, diarrhea, and eventually, death. As a result,

it has been called the runting syndrome. A GVHR would also occur if allogenic (immunologically foreign) lymphocytes were injected into a normal adult. In such cases, however, the tremendous numbers of host lymphocytes are able to destroy the injected lymphocytes before any of the symptoms of a GVHR can occur.

Genetic evidence indicates that the GVHR is actually an *in vivo* equivalent of the MLR, showing that it is also under major control of the I region of the H-2 complex.

## HUMAN HISTOCOMPATIBILITY GENES

The genetic control of histocompatibility antigens in the human is very much like that described for the mouse. The human major histocompatibility complex, called the HLA complex, controls the structure of the major human histocompatibility antigens as well as the functions associated with the immune response genes.

Because of the obvious impossibility of controlled human mating experiments, the determination of histocompatibility specificities and mapping of the HLA complex cannot be accomplished as in the mouse. Sera have been collected from thousands of individuals and tested for antibodies capable of agglutinating lymphocytes obtained from donors. A complement-mediated cytotoxicity test is now used in which the antiserum is mixed with the lymphocytes or platelets to be tested in the presence of complement. Killing of the cells is determined by the addition of a dye such as trypan blue. Living cells will not take up the dye; membrane-damaged cells become stained. Individuals from whom antisera were taken included those who would be most likely to have received allogenic lymphocytes, such as persons who had received multiple blood transfusions, those who had rejected organ grafts, mothers who had given birth to multiple children and had as a result become immunized against those fetal antigens of paternal specificity, and individuals who were purposefully immunized with skin grafts or leukocyte injections.

The distribution of antigens in family pedigrees show that the HLA complex contains at least four regions. A World Health Organization nomenclature committee, which met in Denmark during 1975, has recommended the following names be given to the HLA regions: (1) HLA-A (formerly the LA locus), (2) HLA-B (formerly the FOUR locus), (3) HLA-C (formerly the AJ locus), and (4) HLA-D (for the locus controlling the determinants identified by MLR typing). The probable order of these four loci on the chromosome is D, B, C, A. The HLA complex contains three loci that code for histocompatibility antigens. Using the serological tests described on the cells obtained from thousands of individuals, 18 antigens have been described for the A locus, 24 for the B locus, and 5 for the C locus. Each of these antigens has been numbered, and monospecific serum that will react with them has been isolated. It is therefore possible to specifically type the major histocompatibility antigens of both a donor and a recipient to partially evaluate the probability of allograft compatibility.

The MLR in humans, as in the mouse, appears to be under the control of the immune response genes of the HLA complex. It is well established that incompatibilities as measured by the MLR may lead to transplant rejection in spite of compatibility at the A, B, and C loci. It is particularly important for bone marrow transplants given to individuals with aplastic anemia or severe combined deficiency diseases that there be MLR compatibility between donor and recipient, since the same genetic factors apparently control both the MLR and GVHR. This, in fact, has been shown to be the case, since patients receiving bone marrow transplants from mismatched MLR donors often die from a GVHR, while grafts between nonidentical HLA and MLR matched individuals (mostly siblings) are usually manageable.

One major technical problem is that there is no serological method to determine the antigens involved in the MLR, and current procedures for the MLR require several days to obtain either a positive or negative result.

## TOLERANCE OF ALLOGRAFTS

The method for inducing tolerance to a cell-mediated function is essentially the same as was described in Chapter 15 for the induction of antibody-associated tolerance to foreign antigens, but the mechanism by which such tolerance is maintained is not fully understood.

In essence, one can inject cells from mouse strain A into neonatal mouse strain B. Strain B will become permanently tolerant to cells of strain A and even as an adult will accept allografts from strain A. Inducing tolerance with living cells is, however, a little different from merely injecting a protein such as bovine serum albumin. In both cases, the immunologically immature animal is unable to react to the tolerogen, but in the latter situation, the injected antigen is eventually metabolized and no longer present. Injected living cells, however, grow and provide a continued source of tolerogen and, hence, may act by sheer amount to prevent the neonatal animal from ever forming cells that will react with the foreign tissue.

Interestingly, a strain B mouse that has been made tolerant to strain A cells will reject those strain A cells if the adult animal is injected with sufficient lymphocytes from a normal adult strain B mouse. These injected lymphocytes are not tolerant and see the strain A cells as foreign, as shown schematically in Figure 17-7.

A somewhat paradoxical situation is seen when one induces antibody formation to the allogenic cells before implanting the graft. An enhancement of graft survival appears to occur as a result of blockage of the histocompatibility antigens by noncytotoxic antibodies. This prevents either the induction of cell-mediated immunity or the action of killer cells on the implanted graft.

## CELLULAR ASPECTS OF TUMOR IMMUNITY

It has been known since early in the twentieth century that lymphocytes and mononuclear

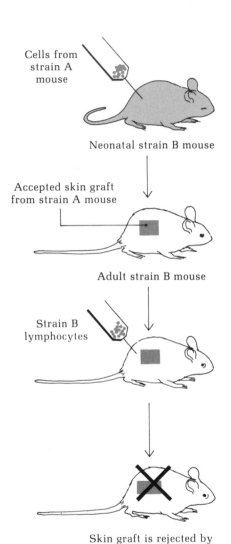

Cells from
strain A
mouse

Neonatal strain B mouse

Accepted skin graft
from strain A mouse

Adult strain B mouse

Strain B
lymphocytes

Skin graft is rejected by
injected strain B lymphocytes

**Figure 17-7.** Schematic diagram showing the induction of tolerance by the injection of "foreign" lymphocytes into a neonatal mouse and the breaking of this tolerance by the subsequent injection of genetically identical lymphocytes from a nontolerant inbred mouse.

cells were involved in tumor destruction; it has not been until the last several decades that technical advances allowed some insight into the immunological mechanism of tumor destruction.

### Immune Surveillance

Although it has been difficult to obtain unequivocable proof, it is generally accepted that immune forces provide our major defense against malignant tumors. In other words, it seems likely that there are frequent genetic changes in our somatic cells that could result in a clinical malignancy were it not for a mechanism for eliminating these cells. This concept is based in large part on the following observations: (1) most malignancies occur at an age (very old or neonatal) when immunological functions are partly inactive, and (2) any procedure that decreases the cell-mediated immune response (thymectomy, anti-lymphocytic serum, immunosuppressive drugs) increases the likelihood that a tumor will develop. Thus the concepts have evolved that immune surveillance is a normal function of our immune system and that the elimination of a newly developed tumor cell is analogous to allograft rejection.

### Nature of Tumor Antigens

Immune surveillance could not function unless tumor cells acquired antigens capable of being recognized as foreign to the immune system. The observation that tumor cells do possess unique antigens has been clearly demonstrated. As will be discussed in a later chapter, all tumors that are caused by viruses acquire a tumor antigen specific for the inducing virus. For example, all tumors produced by a polyoma virus will have the same tumor antigens, and any tumor induced by a herpesvirus will acquire antigens that are specified by that herpesvirus. Carcinogen-induced tumors also possess antigens not present on the normal cell; however, the origin of these antigens is unknown. Even when multiple tumors are induced in an animal by a single chemical carcinogen, each tumor will possess separate, specific antigens. Some tumors possess antigens that are present normally only during fetal development. Such antigens are undoubtedly expressed by a normal gene that is derepressed in some manner in the malignant cell; since these fetal antigens normally disappear before the maturation of the immune system, they are recognized as foreign. The significance of such antigens is not known, but the appearance of antibodies to fetal antigens could provide an early screening method for the detection of certain malignancies.

**Mechanism of Tumor Destruction**

In many malignancies one can demonstrate both humoral antibodies and a delayed-type hypersensitivity directed against the tumor cells, and there has been tremendous effort expended to determine which immune system is actually responsible for tumor immunity. The over-all consensus is that even though serum antibodies plus complement can destroy the malignant lymphocytes involved in leukemia or lymphosarcoma, tumor immunity is cellular rather than humoral in nature. This is supported by the passive transfer of tumor immunity with intact cells and by *in vitro* techniques showing that lymphocytes will undergo blast formation when incubated with autologous tumor cells. Also, inhibition of macrophage migration as well as lymphocyte-mediated cytotoxicity can frequently be demonstrated by appropriate *in vitro* techniques.

Recent evidence in guinea pigs and mice has led to the conclusion that the immune response genes present in the major histocompatibility complex control an animal's potential to respond to a specific antigenic stimulus. This has received some support from recent correlations between certain HLA types and the frequency of certain malignancies and autoimmune diseases. Some investigators have reported that any stimulation of cell-mediated immunity can be beneficial for the immune rejection of

tumors. As a result, some cancer patients have been given an avirulent mycobacterium (BCG) which induces a cell-mediated immunity to tuberculosis. Drugs such as levamisole have also been used to nonspecifically stimulate the cellular immune system in patients who have a defective cellular response. Results, however, have been equivocal and there is certainly no general consensus that such measures are beneficial. The future will undoubtedly provide greater insight into these questions as well as into genetic control of our immune responses.

**CELL-MEDIATED AUTOIMMUNITY**

As discussed in the preceding chapter, autoimmune diseases are invariably associated with the presence of humoral antibodies against the concerned cells or organs. As a result, it has usually been assumed that these antibodies were the cause of the autoimmune disease. It is becoming increasingly apparent, however, that cell-mediated responses may be the causal event in some autoimmune diseases. For example, experimental allergic encephalitis is accompanied by a humoral antibody response to the myelin-containing tissues; but the disorder is passively transferred with intact lymphoid cells and not with serum. Similarly, the serum from patients with thyroiditis (Hashimoto's disease) contains high titers of humoral antibody to thyroglobulin and to cell membranes obtained from the thyroid. The experimental disease in rats and mice, however, appears to be a cell-mediated response.

It therefore seems probable that some autoimmune diseases, such as the hemolytic anemias, may be strictly antibody-mediated, while others may be cell-mediated or result from the combined effect of the two immune systems.

**FUNCTIONAL SUBCLASSES OF T CELLS**

We have discussed the fact that T lymphocytes are involved in a number of different immunological functions; they can (1) act as helpers in the synthesis of humoral Ab; (2) act as suppressors of Ab synthesis and cell-mediated functions; (3) initiate graft versus host reactions; (4) carry out direct cytotoxic reactions on target cells; and (5) release lymphokines that can kill cells directly or stimulate macrophages. One might ask if this diversity of function results from the antigenic stimulation of a single T-cell clone that subsequently differentiates to cause this myriad of heterogeneous functions or if there exist subclasses of T cells that are preprogrammed and require only the proper antigenic stimulation to carry out a specific function.

This enigma has been partially solved. It has been determined that mouse T lymphocytes possess at least four antigen systems, designated Ly antigens. Each system is comprised of two alleles which specify a cell-surface alloantigen. Since these are genetically determined, inbred mice will express only one allele for each Ly antigen, and it is, therefore, possible to obtain antiserum against specific Ly alleles. For example, if T cells from a mouse strain of Ly phenotype 1.2, 2.2, 3.2, and 4.2 were injected into another strain that was phenotypically 1.1, 2.2, 3.2 and 4.2, the antibodies formed would be directed against the alloantigen, Ly 1.2. In the presence of complement, such antisera would destroy all T cells possessing alloantigen Ly 1.2. Thus, using a series of monospecific anti-Ly antisera it is possible to eliminate specific populations of T cells.

This research is still incomplete, but it demonstrates that there are subpopulations of T cells. In one case, cells depleted of Ly 1 T lymphocytes were unable to display appreciable helper activity for antibody synthesis but were unimpaired in their ability to generate a cytotoxic response. On the other hand, cells depleted of Ly 2 and 3 T lymphocytes showed effective helper response but possessed greatly diminished cytotoxic ability. Another investigation has revealed that T helper cells can be distinguished from T suppressor cells on the basis of differences in their Ly antigen. These preliminary experiments show more than one subpopulation of T lymphocytes, and since subpopulations are genetically determined, they obviously exist prior to antigenic stimulation. It seems probable that future research will discover additional subpopulations of T cells.

## IMMUNODEFICIENCY DISEASES

There are a number of diseases in which an individual is unable to respond to an antigenic stimulation. Defects in antibody production go by various names such as antibody deficiency syndrome, hypogammaglobulinemia, or agammaglobulinemia. Many of these disorders are heritable defects. Only during the last few decades has it been possible to keep such individuals alive long enough to determine the nature of the clinical syndrome. However, we can now broadly categorize immunodeficiency diseases as defects in B cells, T cells, or both. There are several B-cell disorders which range from almost complete agammaglobulinemia to specific deficiencies in the production of IgA or both IgA and IgG. Agammaglobulinemia is the most severe form of this disease, and it is usually acquired as an X-chromosome-linked genetic defect characterized by the inability of the stem cell to differentiate into a B cell. As a result such persons form very little humoral antibody and suffer from recurrent infections. They do, however, produce normal T cells and appear to develop a normal cellular immune system. Therefore, they can normally handle viral, fungal, and some bacterial infections.

A different situation was reported in 1974 by Thomas Waldmann and his collaborators who investigated a number of patients that were unable to make adequate amounts of immunoglobulins and, as a result, suffered from frequent recurrent infections. Their results showed that lymphocytes from some of these patients inhibited antibody formation by lymphocytes from normal individuals. Thus, what appeared at first to be a type of B-cell deficiency is now postulated to result from a defect in the production of suppressor T cells, in which too many nonspecific suppressor cells are made.

A disease caused by T-cell deficiency, DiGeorge's syndrome, is manifested by the almost total lack of a thymus. The disease does not appear to be familial and probably occurs because of a failure in fetal cell differentiation. Afflicted persons respond poorly to T-cell dependent antigens and possess a severely defective cellular immune system. Grafts of fetal thymus have in some cases produced dramatic improvement.

Undoubtedly the most severe of the immunodeficiency diseases is the combination of B and T-cell deficiency. It occurs as a heritable disorder that may be transmitted as either an autosomal or X-linked recessive trait. It is characterized by the lack of bone marrow lymphocytes and may well result from a defect in the stem cell's ability to differentiate into mature B and T cells. Bone marrow grafts from compatible siblings can provide effective B and T-cell functions.

A disorder known as secretory component deficiency is characterized by inability to synthesize the secretory piece necessary for the secretion of IgA. Such an individual possesses normal serum levels of all classes of immunoglobulin, including IgA, but no IgA can be found in the patient's saliva, jejunal fluid, or at the intestinal-mucosal sites. Clinically, this deficiency is accompanied by a constant low-grade diarrhea with occasional severe diarrheal exacerbations. Stool cultures show the presence of large numbers of the yeast *Candida albicans*. The existence of this deficiency emphasizes the importance of secretory IgA in the control of intestinal microorganisms.

Figure 17-8 provides a summary of the various blocks which can lead to immune deficiency diseases.

## SUPPRESSION OF CELL-MEDIATED IMMUNITY

With the advent of organ transplants has come the necessity to suppress cell-mediated reactions in order to prevent allograft rejection. Ideally, one would like to create a state of permanent tolerance to the allogenic cells given to the recipient. Unless tolerance to the specific donor's cells was acquired neonatally, however, the prospect of developing

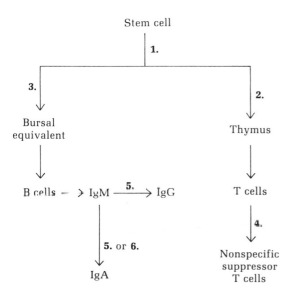

**Figure 17-8.** Schematic illustration depicting the various points that the immune system may be blocked, resulting in an immunodeficiency disease.

1. Genetic defect in which stem cell cannot differentiate into either a T cell or a B cell (combined deficiency)

2. Failure to develop a functional thymus, resulting in T cell deficiency

3. Inability of stem cell to differentiate into a B cell— usually acquired as an X-linked genetic defect

4. Increased production of nonspecific suppressor T cells

5. Inability to differentiate into a 7S Ab-producing plasma cell

6. Inability to produce secretory piece, resulting in normal levels of serum IgA, but no secreted IgA

true tolerance in the adult is dim. If, however, donor cells are closely matched with recipient's cells in the major histocompatibility complex loci, the possibility of suppressing the cell-mediated response sufficiently to allow acceptance of the allograft is good. This can be accomplished in several ways.

The administration of anti-lymphocytic serum (ALS) will preferentially remove the majority of sensitized T cells, permitting the survival of the foreign tissue. But since ALS is usually made in horses, it will contain foreign proteins, and its continued use can result in the occurrence of an immune-complex disease. In addition, since T cells are removed, individuals receiving ALS show only a poor humoral antibody response.

Drugs most commonly used to effect immunosuppression include the corticosteroids (such as prednisone) which nonspecifically block cell-mediated responses. In a usual kidney transplant case, the recipient is given ALS in the beginning and then treated with prednisone and perhaps an analog of purine such as imuran.

While these measures are essential for the survival of an allograft, they are not without danger. Not only is the patient more susceptible to infection but the very system responsible for immune surveillance of malignant cells is seriously suppressed.

## REFERENCES

Alexander, P. 1976. The functions of the macrophage in malignant disease. *Annu. Rev. Med.* **27**:207–224.

Asherson, G. L., and M. Zembala. 1976. Suppressor T cells in cell-mediated immunity. *Brit. Med. Bull.* **32**:158–164.

Bach, F. H. 1976. Genetics of transplantation: The major histocompatibility complex. *Annu. Rev. Genetics* **10**:319–339.

Burnet, F. M. 1974. Transfer factor—a theoretical discussion. *J. Allergy and Clin. Immunol.* **54**:1–13.

Campbell, P. A. 1976. Immunocompetent cells in resistance to bacterial infections. *Bacteriol. Rev.* **40**:284–313.

Cantor, H., and E. A. Boyse. 1975. Functional subclasses of T lymphocytes bearing different Ly antigens. *J. Exp. Med.* **141**:1376–1389.

Claman, H. N. 1975. How corticosteroids work. *J. Allergy and Clin. Immunol.* **55**:145–151.

Collins, F. M. 1974. Vaccines and cell-mediated immunity. *Bacteriol. Rev.* **38**:371–402.

Crowle, A. J. 1975. Delayed hypersensitivity in the mouse. *Adv. in Immunol.* **20**:197–264.

Granger, G. A., R. A. Daynes, P. E. Runge, A. M. Prieur, and E. W. B. Jeffes, III. 1975. Lymphocyte effector molecules and cell-mediated immune reactions. *Cont. Topics in Molec. Immunol.* **4**:205–241.

Grebe, S. C., and J. W. Streilein. 1976. Graft-versus-host reactions: A review. *Adv. in Immunol.* **22**:120–221.

Kirkpatrick, C. H. 1975. Properties and activities of transfer factor. *J. Allergy and Clin. Immunol.* **55**:411–421.

McCluskey, R. T., and S. Cohen, eds. 1974. *Mechanisms of Cell-Mediated Immunity*. John Wiley and Sons, New York.

Nossal, G. J. V. 1974. Lymphocyte differentiation and immune surveillance against cancer, in T. J. King, ed. *Developmental Aspects of Carcinogenesis and Immunity*. Academic Press, New York.

Ohiski, M., and K. Onoue. 1975. Functional activation of immune lymphocytes by antigenic stimulation in cell-mediated immunity. *Cellular Immunol.* **18**:220–232.

Old, L. J. 1977. Cancer immunology. *Sci. American* **236**:62–79.

Perlmann, P., and G. Holm. 1969. Cytotoxic effects of lymphoid cells *in vitro*. *Adv. in Immunol.* **11**:117–193.

Pollack, S. 1974. Serum factors and cell-mediated destruction of tumor cells, in T. J. King, ed., *Developmental Aspects of Carcinogenesis and Immunity*. Academic Press, New York.

Poulik, M. D., and R. A. Reisfeld. 1975. $\beta_2$-Microglobulins. *Cont. Topics in Molec. Immunol.* **4**:157–204.

Reisfeld, R. A., and B. D. Kahan. 1972. Markers of biological individuality. *Sci. American* **226:** 28–37.

Shreffler, D. C., and C. S. David. 1975. The H-2 major histocompatibility complex and the I immune response region: Genetic variation, function and organization. *Adv. in Immunol.* **20:**125–195.

Waldmann, T. A., S. Broder, R. M. Blaese, M. Durm, M. Blackman, and W. Strober. 1974. Role of suppressor T cells in pathogenesis of common variable hypogammaglobulinemia. *Lancet* **2:** 609–613.

Watanabe, N., S. Kojima, and Z. Ovary. 1976. Suppression of IgE antibody production in SJL mice. I. Nonspecific suppressor T cells. *J. Exp. Med.* **143:**833–845.

Woodruff, J. F. 1975. T Lymphocyte interactions with viruses and virus-infected tissues. *Progr. in Med. Virol.* **19:**121–161.

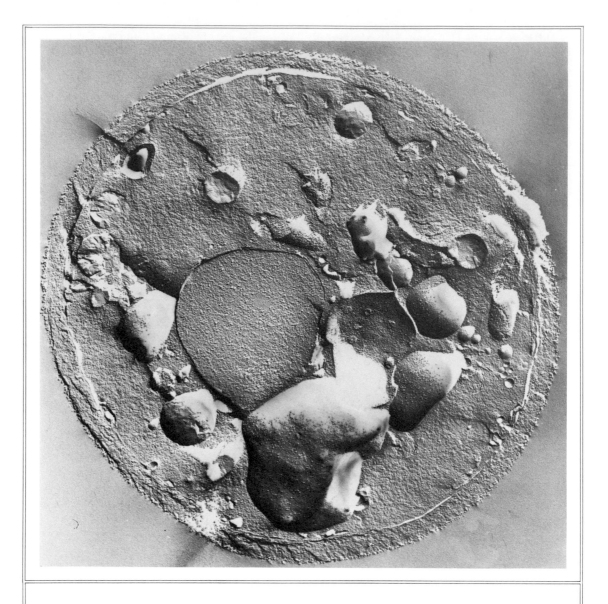

# UNIT THREE

# Bacteria and Fungi

IT has been just over 100 years since the germ theory of disease was accepted by scientists. Since then, the relationship between humans and pathogenic microorganisms has changed drastically, mostly in our favor, but, as we shall see, the conquest of one problem has frequently resulted in the appearance of new challenges in the control of infectious organisms. Though our hospitals are no longer the death traps of the nineteenth century, new life-saving techniques have resulted in types of infections unheard of several decades ago.

During the past century we first learned that microorganisms cause diseases such as smallpox, bubonic plague, cholera, and typhoid fever; such microorganisms were found to require a mechanism to be transmitted from an infected person or animal to a noninfected host. This concept gave rise to the science of epidemiology, and the epidemiologist learned where to break the link in the chain of transmission. Thus, better sanitation of drinking water drastically curtailed typhoid fever and dysentery; control of mosquitoes eliminated urban yellow fever; and scrubbing and disinfectants reduced surgical infections.

Second, during this century of rapidly developing knowledge, the science of immunology began with the discovery that individuals could be protected from many diseases caused by microorganisms by artificially inducing a specific immunity. By the middle of the twentieth century, diseases such as smallpox, diphtheria, tetanus, and whooping cough could be prevented, and during the past quarter century effective vaccines have become available for many other infectious diseases.

The third era in the conquest of infectious diseases began in the 1930's and '40's when chemotherapeutic drugs and antibiotics appeared, apparently destined to eliminate bacterial infections. We soon learned that many microorganisms can mutate to antibiotic-resistant forms, so the microbiologist battles constantly to develop new antibiotics to replace those which are no longer effective.

So, where do we stand now? Many dreaded organisms have been curtailed to the point where they no longer cause important disease —particularly in the Western World. But recent medical knowledge and techniques have led indirectly to the occurrence of many previously rare or unknown infections caused either by organisms considered as normal flora or by organisms previously thought of as nonpathogens. These infections result when host resistance is reduced to the degree that "normal flora" or "nonpathogens" are able to grow and flourish in areas where they otherwise could not penetrate, or, if they did invade, would be killed by our immune mechanisms. A few situations leading to this type of infection include: (1) the use of immunosuppressants to prevent the rejection of organ transplants; (2) the use of kidney dialysis machines and heart pumps; (3) the frequent use of urethral catheters; and (4) the use of antibiotics that destroy part of our normal flora. In fact, any procedure which destroys the protection offered by an intact skin and mucosa, interferes with the immune system or cough reflexes, or changes the normal flora is conducive to serious infections by "harmless" organisms. Thus, to fully understand the numerous problems in the diagnosis and prevention of infections, it is vital that we know about those organisms that have a permanent home in some area of the human body, that is, our normal flora.

We can categorize our normal flora as helpful (symbionts), harmless (commensals), and potentially harmful (opportunists). However, it must be kept in mind that these groups are not mutually exclusive and that given the opportunity, even a symbiont may become a pathogen. Therefore, these categories are of value only in describing the normal role of the organism in relation to the human body. Most of the organisms comprising the normal flora of the body are considered to be commensals; under normal circumstances they give no evidence of benefit or harm to the host. In general, commensals may be extremely important because they provide an environment unfavorable for the growth of many potentially pathogenic organisms.

Some organisms are not really "normal flora," but may be present in a large percentage of the members of a population without causing disease. For example, *Staphylococcus aureus* can be carried on the skin and in the noses of 20% of the members of a population without appearing to cause any illness. However, if a person should have a respiratory infection, such as measles or influenza, in which the ciliated epithelial cells are destroyed, the staphylococcus can cause a severe and frequently fatal pneumonia. Another example is *Streptococcus pneumoniae* (the pneumococcus), which occasionally may be harbored by 10–50% of normal people and yet is a major cause of lobar pneumonia in humans who are stressed by a defect in either a nonspecific or a specific immune mechanism.

So, let us survey several major areas of the human body and see what one may expect to find as normal flora.

SKIN. The pH of the skin is usually about 5.6 as a result of the presence of acids, especially propionic acid produced by the predominant deep-seated flora of *Corynebacterium* and *Propionibacterium*. However, as one might guess, the skin is subject to a considerable transient population of microorganisms, which routinely includes staphylococci, sarcinae, nonpathogenic mycobacteria, spore-forming bacilli from the soil, alpha-hemolytic streptococci, and contaminating organisms normally found in the intestinal tract (such as the gram-negative enterics, the enterococci, and potentially pathogenic yeasts such as *Candida albicans*).

MOUTH AND RESPIRATORY TRACT. The alpha-hemolytic streptococci appear to be the major organisms isolated from the mouth and upper respiratory tract. However, many obligately anaerobic organisms, such as spi-

rochetes, fusiform bacteria, and *Bacteroides*, also reside in crypts around the teeth but (because of the difficulty of laboratory cultivation) are not isolated routinely.

Other bacteria occasionally found in the upper respiratory tract of healthy individuals include *Corynebacterium pseudodiphtheriae*, *Streptococcus pneumoniae*, *Haemophilus influenzae*, beta-hemolytic streptococci, *Neisseria meningitidis*, and *Klebsiella pneumoniae*. In addition, staphylococci and other species of *Neisseria* are frequently present. Many of these organisms are not "normal" flora in the strict sense of the word, since they are really potential pathogens for both the individual who harbors them as well as for close contacts.

INTESTINAL TRACT. Although food contains many microorganisms, the stomach has no normal flora, and because of the acidity, few organisms exist for long in the stomach. Normally, organisms begin to appear in the jejunum and the ileum (the second and third segments of the small intestine), but it is not until near the lower end of the ileum that large numbers of bacteria occur.

In the upper intestinal tract, the major organisms found are enterococci, staphylococci, lactobacilli, and occasionally *Escherichia coli*.

Over 95% of the flora of the lower intestinal tract consists of obligately anaerobic bacteria —mainly *Bacteroides*, but also *Bifidobacterium*, *Clostridium*, anaerobic streptococci, plus many obligately anaerobic gram-negative bacteria. Because of the difficulty in growing these obligate anaerobes, the facultatively anaerobic enterics, such as *Escherichia*, *Enterobacter*, and *Pseudomonas*, which actually comprise only 3–4% of the intestinal flora, were at one time believed to be the major intestinal flora.

GENITOURINARY TRACT. The urinary tract, except for the urethra of the male, is normally sterile. In the male, staphylococci, diphtheroids, and short gram-negative rods frequently can be isolated from the exterior part of the urethra; nonpathogenic cocci may be present in the urethra of the female. In addition, mycoplasmas have been isolated from the urethras of both males and females, and *Mycobacterium smegmatis,* a rapidly growing acid-fast bacillus, is present on the external genitalia of both sexes.

Between puberty and menopause, the vaginal area has an acid pH, while prior to puberty and after menopause the secretions are neutral to alkaline. This change in pH results in changes in the normal flora of the vagina; under neutral to alkaline conditions, coliforms, diphtheroids, micrococci and streptococci predominate. In an acid environment, lactobacilli constitute the major organisms, but diphtheroids, yeast, alpha-hemolytic streptococci, and anaerobic cocci are found in lesser numbers.

EYE. It is surprising that the eye is so seldom infected, since one might initially think of it as being particularly susceptible to disease. However, the normal flora is meager; *Corynebacterium xerosis, Staph. aureus, Staph. epidermidis,* and diptheroids may be frequently found, and other organisms may be transient contaminants of the conjunctiva.

This very brief survey should reinforce the point that today's student of medical microbiology must learn not only the characteristics and epidemiology of the organisms routinely considered as pathogens, but must also be alerted to a new brand of infections, called nosocomial infections, acquired as a result of hospital procedures and frequently caused by "normal flora."

Unit Three is designed to differentiate between those organisms that are considered to be commensals and those that are regarded as pathogens. This unit will emphasize, however, that given an opportunity, many of the organisms making up our normal flora can cause serious and sometimes fatal infections.

## GENERAL REFERENCES

Briody, B. A. and R. E. Gillis, eds. 1974. *Microbiology and Infectious Disease.* McGraw Hill, New York.

Burrows, W. 1973. *Textbook of Microbiology,* 20th ed. W. B. Saunders Co., Philadelphia.

Davis, B. D., R. Dulbecco, H. N. Eisen, H. S. Ginsberg, W. B. Wood, and M. McCarty. 1973. *Microbiology,* 2nd ed. Harper and Row, New York.

Frobisher, M., and R. Fuerst. 1973. *Microbiology in Health and Disease,* 13th ed. W. B. Saunders, Philadelphia.

Gillies, R. R. 1975. *Lecture Notes on Medical Microbiology.* Blackwell Scientific Pub., London.

vonGraevenitz, A., and T. Sall. 1973. *Pathogenic Microorganisms from Atypical Clinical Sources.* Marcel Dekker, New York.

Joklik, W. K., and H. P. Willett, eds. 1976. *Zinsser Microbiology,* 16th ed. Appleton Century Crofts, New York.

Lennette, E. H., E. H. Spaulding, and J. P. Truant, eds. 1974. *Manual of Clinical Microbiology,* 2nd ed. American Society for Microbiology, Washington, D.C.

Moffet, H. L. 1975. *Clinical Microbiology.* J. B. Lippincott, Philadelphia.

Myrvik, Q. N., N. N. Pearsall, and R. S. Weiser. 1974. *Fundamentals of Medical Bacteriology and Mycology.* Lea and Febiger, Philadelphia.

Smith, L. DS. 1975. *The Pathogenic Anaerobic Bacteria,* 2nd ed. Charles C. Thomas, Springfield, Ill.

# 18

---

# The Gram-Positive Pyogenic Cocci

Those invasive cocci which are frequently involved in purulent (pus-forming) lesions are usually referred to as the pyogenic cocci. Many secrete toxic substances, undoubtedly responsible for the pathology of the lesions they produce, but the major property permitting them to cause disease is their ability to resist phagocytosis in the absence of specific antibodies. Thus, we shall see that one's major defense against the pyogenic cocci is the production of humoral antibodies (opsonins) which stimulates their phagocytosis and destruction. We shall see also that some infections caused by the pyogenic cocci can be acute, and, without antibiotic therapy, an antibody response may not be sufficiently rapid to overcome the infection.

## Streptococci

Streptococci are important pathogens both because of the many severe infections they produce and because of the complications (sequelae) that may occur after recovery from the acute infection.

The bacteria classified in the genus *Streptococcus* share certain morphological and biochemical characteristics, of which the most noticeable is their appearance. They are spherical cells that divide in only one direction, but rather than separating into individual cocci, the daughter cells tend to remain together forming pairs or chains of cocci (see Figure 18-1). The length of chain likely to be observed when stained specimens are examined depends to some extent on the species of streptococcus (*Strept. pneumoniae* has a tendency to remain in pairs), whether the organisms were grown on solid or liquid medium, and how roughly they were handled in the process of making a smear. The streptococci are all gram-positive and nonmotile.

### METABOLISM OF THE STREPTOCOCCI

Nutritionally, the streptococci are very demanding in their growth requirements, having lost the ability to synthesize many required nutrients. For example, some streptococci require as many as 15 different amino acids, all of the known B vitamins, and some purines or pyrimidines for growth. Obviously, such a complex synthetic medium would be used only in a research laboratory. For routine culturing of streptococci, a complex undefined medium containing peptones, meat infusion, salts, glucose, and agar for solidification is used. To this is added 5% sterile defibrinated blood before the medium is poured into petri dishes. The resulting plates are usually referred to as blood agar plates, valuable both for growing and for identifying the streptococci.

Most streptococci are considered facultative anaerobes, although obligately anaerobic streptococci exist and are normal inhabitants of the female genital tract. But even the term facultative anaerobe is somewhat misleading because the streptococci obtain all of their energy requirements from the fermentation of sugars to lactic acid, whether they are growing aerobically or anaerobically. They have no aerobic metabolism, and, since they are unable to synthesize heme, a necessary prosthetic group of the cytochromes, they have no mechanism for an aerobic metabolism requiring the transport of electrons through a cytochrome system to molecular oxygen. Their growth in the presence of air is also limited because of the spontaneous aerobic oxidation of reduced pyridine nucleotides (NADH or NADPH). In the absence of cytochromes, this results in a two-electron transfer to oxygen to form $H_2O_2$. Most bacteria can protect themselves from the killing effect of $H_2O_2$ because they synthesize the enzyme catalase, which quickly converts $H_2O_2$ to $H_2O$ and $O_2$. However, the streptococci are unable to synthesize this enzyme, since catalase also contains a heme prosthetic group, and, as a result, may form lethal amounts of $H_2O_2$ during aerobic growth. In laboratory practice, the streptococci are grown on blood agar plates, and red blood cells provide a good source of catalase for the destruction of any $H_2O_2$ formed during aerobic metabolism.

**Figure 18-1.** Chains of *Streptococcus mutans* ($\times$ 5,000). As discussed later in the chapter, this streptococcus utilizes sucrose to produce an acid capable of eroding tooth enamel.

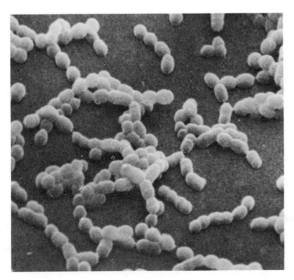

## HEMOLYSINS

As streptococci grow, they secrete a large number of toxins and enzymes. We do not know the exact role of many of these products in the production of disease, but some of them are used for the identification of the streptococci and in some cases for the diagnosis of a recent streptococcal infection. Among these secreted products may be one or more hemolysins that cause the lysis of red blood cells in the medium. Although there is no evidence that hemolysin plays any part in the disease syndrome, the streptococci are divided into three groups based on the presence or absence of hemolysis and on the type of red cell destruction caused by the hemolysin.

The alpha-hemolytic streptococci produce an incomplete hemolysis of the red blood cells resulting in a greenish-brown discoloration surrounding the colony. The partially opaque area contains unlysed red blood cells and a green unidentified reduced product of hemoglobin. The streptococci producing alpha-hemolysis are also called viridans streptococci, or occasionally they are referred to as the green streptococci after the green zone of discoloration around the colony.

The beta-hemolytic streptococci cause a hemolysis of red blood cells surrounding the colony, resulting in a completely clear zone in which no color remains. This beta-hemolysis occurs as the result of the secretion of two different hemolysins by the streptococci—designated streptolysin S and streptolysin O. Streptolysin S was so named because early work with this hemolysin showed that it could be extracted from the cells with serum. However, because it is stable in the presence of atmospheric oxygen (streptolysin O is not), the S could represent "stable" as well as "serum" extractable. Since streptolysin O is reversibly inactivated in the presence of oxygen, the beta-hemolysis one sees on the surface of a blood agar plate is primarily the result of streptolysin S rather than streptolysin O. If, however, the streptococci are grown anaerobically, both hemolysins produce beta-hemolysis.

The third major group of streptococci produces no hemolysins, and hence has no effect on blood cells in an agar medium. Members of this group of streptococci sometimes are called the gamma-hemolytic streptococci, although the term is really a misnomer because they are not at all hemolytic.

## CLASSIFICATION OF THE STREPTOCOCCI

Until the 1930's the classification of the streptococci was confused. Many streptococci were considered specific for the disease entity from which they were isolated and were given names based on that type of infection. Examples were such names as *Streptococcus erysipelatos* for an organism isolated from the skin infection, erysipelas, and *Strepto-*

**Table 18-1. Major Criteria Used in Sherman's Biochemical Classification of the Streptococci**

| Group | Characteristics |
|---|---|
| Pyogenic (all Lancefield groups except D and N) | Mostly beta-hemolytic |
| | Will not grow at 45° C or in the presence of 6.5% NaCl |
| Viridans (not classifiable in Lancefield's classification) | alpha-hemolytic |
| | Will grow at 45° C but not in the presence of 6.5% NaCl |
| Lactic (Lancefield's Group N) | Nonhemolytic |
| | Will not grow at 45° C or in the presence of 6.5% NaCl |
| | Will grow at 10° C in the presence of 0.1% methylene blue in milk |
| Enterococcus (Lancefield's Group D) | Usually not hemolytic |
| | Will grow at 45° C in the presence of 6.5% NaCl |
| | Will grow at pH 9.6 |

*coccus scarlatinae* for one isolated from scarlet fever. A biochemical classification proposed by J. M. Sherman (see Table 18-1) proved valuable in the overall classification of this genus, but since essentially all acute infections were caused by organisms in Sherman's pyogenic group, this classification was of little value to the medical epidemiologist. The present classification of the streptococci still uses the criteria proposed by Sherman, but, in addition, uses antigenic properties to subdivide most of the streptococci into groups and types. This latter classification was originally proposed by Rebecca Lancefield in 1933, and it became obvious as a result of her classification that a single streptococcal species could be responsible for a variety of disease entities.

Rebecca Lancefield found that if streptococci are placed in dilute acid (pH 2) and heated at 100°C for 10 minutes, a soluble carbohydrate antigen is extracted from their cell walls. This carbohydrate, which she called C carbohydrate, can also be extracted with formamide by heating the cells at 150°C for 15 minutes. All streptococci, except the viridans group (see Table 18-1) possess a C carbohydrate, and when the C carbohydrate from many different streptococcal isolates was categorized using antibodies obtained by immunizing rabbits with the streptococci, it was found that there were 13 different antigenic C carbohydrates. Based on these antigenic differences in their C carbohydrate, Lancefield divided the streptococci into groups designated by letters, as shown in Table 18-2. Thus, the organisms in group A all possess the same antigenic C carbohydrate, and the organisms in group B all possess another C carbohydrate. The C carbohydrate from group A has been shown to consist of a long polymer of rhamnose to which are attached residues of N-acetylglucosamine (see Figure 18-2). Furthermore, it soon became apparent that each group had a specific habitat, that is, group A were primarily human pathogens, group B primarily cattle pathogens, and so on (see Table 18-2).

**Table 18-2. Lancefield's Group Classification and Normal Habitat of Streptococci**

| Group | Normal Habitat |
|-------|----------------|
| A | Humans |
| B | Cattle |
| C | Wide variety of animals and humans |
| D | Intestinal tract of humans and animals (enterococci) |
| E | Swine |
| F | Humans |
| G | Humans and dogs |
| H | Humans |
| K | Humans |
| L | Dogs |
| M | Dogs |
| N | Dairy products (never hemolytic on blood agar) |
| O | Humans |

**Figure 18-2.** Diagrammatic representation of the streptococcal group A carbohydrate.

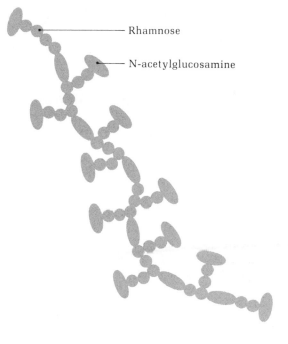

Rhamnose

N-acetylglucosamine

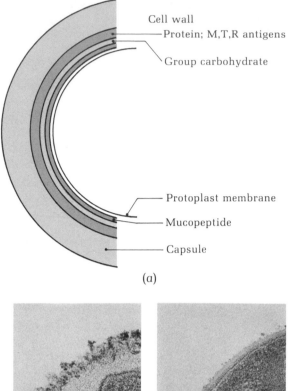

(a)

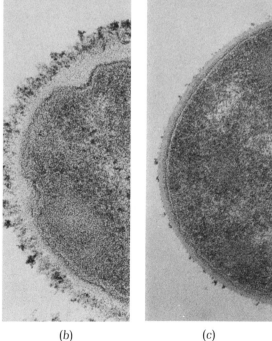

(b)          (c)

**Figure 18-3.** *a.* Layers of the cell wall and capsule of a group A streptococcus. *b.* Section through a streptococcal cell showing fimbriae of M protein (× 100,000). *c.* Section through a type of streptococcal cell without M protein (× 80,000; compare with *b*).

Though common, these habitats are not rigid.

In addition to the carbohydrate used to classify the streptococci into groups, other antigens are present in each group. Some of these antigens are not involved in the virulence of the streptococci nor of value in a specific classification, and so will not be discussed. However, each Lancefield group does contain a type-specific substance which allows a further subdivision of the group into specific types. The type-specific antigen in some groups is a carbohydrate (different from the C carbohydrate), whereas in group A, containing the major human pathogens, it is a cell wall protein called the M protein. Figure 18-3*a* shows a schematic representation of a typical group A *Streptococcus* cell; Figure 18-3*b* shows a section through a cell and M protein.

## GROUP A BETA-HEMOLYTIC STREPTOCOCCI

Although human infection may be caused by organisms from several Lancefield groups, group A contains most of the streptococci known to produce acute disease, and members of group A may lead to late nonsupporative (non-pus-forming) complications such as rheumatic fever, acute glomerulonephritis, and erythema nodosum. These organisms are all beta-hemolytic. On the basis of antigenic differences in the M protein, the group is subdivided into over 50 types designated by numbers. The M protein is also important in the virulence of group A streptococci for two reasons: first, it is antiphagocytic, and, as a result, organisms possessing M protein are able to maintain an infection in the absence of specific antibodies because they resist phagocytosis; second, the M protein is the antigen which induces type-specific immunity. Thus, even though antibodies are formed against a number of streptococcal antigens, including the C carbohydrate, only the type-specific anti-M protein antibodies provide immunity, since these antibodies act as opsonins to allow the virulent organisms to be phagocytosed.

Many group A streptococci also possess a capsule of hyaluronic acid, but as hyaluronic acid is a normal component of connective tissue, anti-capsular antibodies are not formed. The capsule does provide additional antiphagocytic protection, but since the M protein actually extends through the capsule as fine fimbrae, the presence of the capsule does not protect the cell from the opsonic effect of anti-M antibodies.

Group A streptococci also posses an additional type-specific antigen named the T protein. Unlike the M protein, the T antigens are not involved in the virulence of the organisms, nor are they related to type-specific immunity. It is not customary, therefore, to determine the T-antigenic specificity of a streptococcus unless the isolate is one of those rare group A streptococci that does not possess an M protein.

The group A streptococci excrete a number of enzymes and toxins, most of which appear to have some role in the production of disease but no one of which provides a clear-cut answer to the disease-producing potential of these virulent organisms. The enzyme streptokinase promotes the lysis of fibrin blood clots and is thought by some to be at least partially responsible for the rapid spread of streptococcal infections by preventing the formation of a fibrin barrier around the infected site. However, antibodies to streptokinase do not seem to influence the infection, and its role is vague. Streptokinase was originally thought to be a proteolytic enzyme and, as such, was named fibrinolysin. Subsequently, it was shown to act by catalyzing the conversion of an inactive plasma component, plasminogen, into the active proteolytic enzyme, plasmin.

Streptodornase is a general name given to the streptococcal enzymes that degrade DNA, the DNases. They are capable of degrading the viscous DNA resulting from the disintegration of the host's leukocytes and may contribute to the more rapid spread of the infection. Preparations of streptodornase and streptokinase have in the past

been used therapeutically to thin thick exudates of pus or necrotic tissue.

Hyaluronidase depolymerizes hyaluronic acid, and it seems almost paradoxical that some streptococci produce hyaluronic acid capsules as well as an enzyme that destroys it. Hyaluronidase is believed to play a role in the spread of streptococci through tissues by hydrolyzing the host's hyaluronic acid and has therefore been called spreading factor.

NADase cleaves the nicotinamide portion from the coenzyme nicotinamide adenine dinucleotide (NAD), but no data suggest that this enzyme is involved in the disease-producing potential of the streptococci.

Streptolysin O is an oxygen-labile hemolysin which binds to cholesterol in the cell membrane and causes the lysis of erythrocytes. However, since anemia is not a usual result of streptococcal infections, it is not this function which contributes to the virulence of the organisms; it is the ability of streptolysin O to penetrate the host's leukocytes and cause a release of the enzymes in the cell's lysosomes, resulting in degranulation and death of the leukocyte (see Chapter 11). The release of these hydrolytic enzymes may also destroy adjacent tissue and contribute further to the streptococcal infection. Furthermore, streptolysin O is capable of suppressing chemotaxis and leukocyte mobility. The fact that streptolysin O is antigenic and that anti-streptolysin O (ASO) will prevent the hemolysis of erythrocytes provides a very important tool for determining a recent group A streptococcal infection. Such information is an important aid in the diagnosis of the late complications of streptococcal infections which usually occur after the organisms have been eliminated from the host.

Streptolysin S is a small polypeptide of about 28 amino-acid residues, active only when bound to a nonspecific carrier such as RNA or streptococcal cell wall. In addition to causing beta-hemolysis, it is able to inhibit chemotaxis and phagocytosis as well as to exert a cytotoxic effect on various types of eucaryotic cells. It is believed to act by binding to phospholipid in the target cell membrane, and it has been shown that mere external contact of group A streptococci with leukocytes was sufficient to kill the phagocytic cells. It seems clear, therefore, that this hemolysin is an important factor of group A streptococcal infections. Unlike its O counterpart, streptolysin S is not antigenic—probably because of its small size.

## PATHOGENICITY OF BETA-HEMOLYTIC STREPTOCOCCI

### Streptococcal Pharyngitis

Streptococcal pharyngitis is the most frequent manifestation of group A infections. This condition may be very acute—in which case the mucous membranes of the tonsils and pharynx are red and edematous (filled with fluid) with a purulent exudate; cervical lymph nodes may be enlarged, and the temperature is usually high. Complications include spread of the organisms to the middle ear or, rarely, to the meninges. Pneumonia is not usual but might occur in conjunction with a viral respiratory infection such as influenza or measles. Epidemics of streptococcal pharyngitis are usually the result of personal contact with either infected persons or healthy carriers. Epidemiological studies have shown that commonly a school child brings the infections home and spreads them in the family.

### Scarlet Fever

Scarlet fever may be caused by any type of group A streptococcus that produces an erythrogenic toxin. Not all group A organisms make this exotoxin, since its synthesis is restricted to organisms that are lysogenic, i.e., that carry a prophage in which the information for toxin production is encoded in the prophage DNA. Scarlet fever, therefore, is generally the result of a streptococcal sore throat caused by an erythrogenic toxin-producing organism; although the bacteria may remain localized in the throat, the dissemination of the toxin causes the appearance of a diffuse skin rash.

Immunity to scarlet fever results from the presence of antitoxin to the erythrogenic toxin; however, since there are three antigenically distinct erythrogenic toxins, it is possible to have the disease more than once. It is important to note that although immunity to scarlet fever is directed against the toxin, immunity to a streptococcal infection is type-specific and directed against the M protein. Thus, it is possible for an individual who has antitoxic immunity to become infected with a group A erythrogenic toxin-producing streptococcus of a type for which anti-M protein immunity has not been acquired. Such an individual would not show the rash because of antitoxic immunity, but would act as a source of scarlet fever.

Susceptibility to scarlet fever can be determined by the intradermal injection of a minute quantity of the diluted toxin, a procedure known as the Dick test. If antitoxins are present, the toxin is neutralized, and there is no skin reaction. If there are no antitoxins in the blood, an area of inflammation develops around the site of the injection within 24 hours. However, because of the known multiple etiology of scarlet fever, the Dick test has little significance.

The Schultz-Charlton reaction is used as a diagnostic procedure in which a small amount of polyvalent antitoxin is injected intradermally into the rash area. If the rash is the result of scarlet fever, there will be a blanching of the skin at this point within a few hours. Such a procedure can be of value in differentiating the rash of scarlet fever from similar rashes.

### Other Beta-Hemolytic Streptococcal Infections

Puerperal sepsis is a postpartum infection of the uterus which has claimed the lives of many women following childbirth. Modern aseptic techniques and antibiotics have eliminated much of this type of infection from developed countries.

Impetigo or cellulitis can result from group A streptococcal infections of the skin, and, if organisms infect the lymphatics of the skin, the infection is called erysipelas.

Wound infections as well as postpartum infections may be caused by the obligately anaerobic streptococci which are part of the normal flora of the intestinal tract and female genital tract. Such infections usually occur in conjunction with some of the other obligately anaerobic organisms from these areas, for example *Bacteroides*.

## LATE NONSUPPORATIVE COMPLICATIONS

Complications of group A streptococcal infections are rheumatic fever involving the heart and joints, acute glomerulonephritis involving the kidney, and perhaps erythema nodosum involving the skin.

### Rheumatic Fever

Rheumatic fever occurs in a small percentage of individuals two to three weeks after the onset of an untreated pharyngeal infection caused by a beta-hemolytic group A streptococcus. The disease may occur as a sequela of infection by any of the types of group A streptococci; however, there is, at present, no evidence that those which cause rheumatic fever (directly or indirectly) are any different from those that do not. Recovery from rheumatic fever occurs without residual injury to the joints, but the involvement of the heart is important, since permanent damage may occur there. The mechanism by which streptococci produce rheumatic fever is still obscure, but a great deal of circumstantial evidence indicates that it is the result of an immunological reaction. Various theories have postulated that streptococcal antigens, such as the M protein, might be deposited in the joints and heart. In addition, there have been reports that a common cross-reacting antigen exists in some (or all) group A streptococci and the heart. In this case antibodies synthesized in response to the streptococcal infection could react with antigens in the heart causing cellular destruction and permanent damage. The theory that rheumatic fever is the result of an immunological reaction is also supported by postmortem studies which showed large deposits of immunoglobulins and the C3 component of complement within the heart. Thus, even though there are gaps in our knowledge concerning the specific antigen involved, the reaction of an antibody induced by the streptococcus, either directly with heart tissue or with an antigen deposited in the heart, would activate complement resulting in the formation of anaphylatoxins (C3a and C5a) that cause localized tissue damage.

### Glomerulonephritis

Acute glomerulonephritis, an inflammation of the glomeruli in the kidney, is less frequently a consequence of streptococcal infection than is rheumatic fever. Most cases of glomerulonephritis occur about a week after group A, type 12 pharyngeal or skin infections, but a few have been reported to follow types 4, 18, 25, 49, 52, and 55. In this condition, bloody urine (hematuria) is the predominant symptom and is often accompanied by hypertension.

Glomerulonephritis is also believed to be an immunological disease, in which either the streptococci possess or synthesize an antigen which cross-reacts with glomerular basement membranes of the kidney, or they deposit streptococcal antigen-antibody complexes on the basement membranes. In either case, the activation of the C3 and C5 components of complement would lead to tissue destruction.

### Erythema Nodosum

Erythema nodosum are skin lesions that may follow diseases such as tuberculosis or coccidioidomycosis (a fungal infection discussed in Chapter 29), as well as occasional group A streptococcal infections. An explanation for this syndrome is even more vague than that for the other post-streptococcal complications, but it has been proposed that the streptococcal cell wall might be the toxic agent.

## LABORATORY DIAGNOSIS OF BETA-HEMOLYTIC STREPTOCOCCAL INFECTIONS

To prevent late nonsupporative complications, it is essential that beta-hemolytic streptococcal infections be diagnosed promptly and treated adequately. The only positive way to make a diagnosis is to isolate and serologically identify the causative organism. To accomplish this, material from the patient (usually a throat swab) is streaked on a blood agar plate. After approximately 24 hours incubation at 37°C the plate is examined for

**Figure 18-4.** Streptococcal growth in the presence of discs containing bacitracin. Upper left: growth right up to the edge of the disc indicates resistance and, thus, a streptococcus not of group A. Upper right: zone of inhibition around disc indicates sensitivity to bacitracin by a group A streptococcus.

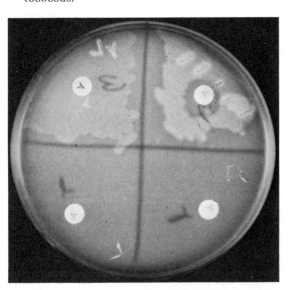

the presence of beta-hemolytic streptococci, indicated by tiny, compact, dull colonies surrounded by areas of clear hemolysis. If a Gram stain of such a colony reveals gram-positive cocci occurring in chains, a tentative diagnosis is made. Serologic identification of the M protein is not routinely done.

Since group A streptococci are more sensitive to the antibiotic bacitracin, presumptive evidence that a beta-hemolytic streptococcus belongs to group A can be obtained by using discs containing a calibrated amount of bacitracin, which will inhibit the growth of group A streptococci but not other groups of streptococci (see Figure 18-4). Fluorescently-labeled antibody against the C substance of group A may also be used for a definitive identification of these organisms.

Immunological procedures are useful in the diagnosis of the late, nonsupporative complications which usually occur when it is no longer possible to isolate the infecting streptococcus. Here, one can determine the amount of antibody present against streptolysin O. If the antistreptolysin O (ASO) titer is high, it indicates a recent infection by beta-hemolytic streptococci.

## TREATMENT OF BETA-HEMOLYTIC STREPTOCOCCAL INFECTIONS

Fortunately, all streptococci, except some enterococci, are sensitive to a wide variety of therapeutic drugs. The sulfonamides suppress their growth but do not prevent the occurrence of the late, nonsupporative complications. Penicillin, which is bactericidal, is the antibiotic of choice, and most experts agree that therapeutic levels of penicillin should be maintained for at least eight to ten days to ensure complete eradication of the organisms. It is extremely important to remember that adequate treatment during the acute infection will prevent the complications of rheumatic fever.

Those individuals who have recovered from rheumatic fever are particularly vulnerable to a recurrence if they again become infected with a group A streptococcus. They are usually kept on low levels of oral penicillin for many years to prevent such an infection. Persons who have recovered from glomerulonephritis are usually not given prophylactic penicillin, since the chances of reinfection with a nephritogenic strain (capable of inducing kidney inflammation) are quite low.

It is next to impossible to control the spread of streptococci because there are so many asymptomatic carriers of beta-hemolytic strains. Depending upon the season, anywhere from 5–30% of apparently healthy persons may carry these potentially pathogenic organisms.

## OTHER STREPTOCOCCAL INFECTIONS

### Subacute Bacterial Endocarditis

The alpha-hemolytic streptococci include a number of species which are normal flora in the throat and the nasopharynx of humans, and the enterococci (Lancefield group D streptococci) which are normal inhabitants of the large intestine. Neither produces acute infections, but they can act as secondary invaders.

The one infection in which these streptococci are unquestionably involved is subacute bacterial endocarditis. This infection may be caused by a number of different bacteria, but the viridans streptococci and the enterococci are the most common etiologic agents. It occurs in those individuals who already have an injured heart valve. Upon reaching the damaged valve, the organisms multiply, causing further changes and frequently releasing a shower of emboli (foreign particulate matter) from the valve. The characteristic findings in such infections are fever, heart murmurs, enlarged spleen, and anemia. Once the disease is suspected, the diagnosis is made by obtaining blood cultures from which the bacteria are isolated. Left untreated, this condition is almost invariably fatal.

Subacute bacterial endocarditis can be difficult to treat because the bacteria are enmeshed in vegetative growths on the heart valve. However, the viridans streptococci are sensitive to penicillin, and usually an intensive course of penicillin therapy for two weeks is effective. When the enterococcus (which is identified by its ability to grow at 45°C in a medium containing 6.5% NaCl) is the infecting organism, a combination of penicillin and streptomycin is usually used.

### Dental Caries

The observation that dental caries are the result of a bacterial infection is now well established. In all likelihood, several organisms are involved, but one candidate is an organism named *Streptococcus mutans*.

*Streptococcus mutans* secretes an extracellular glucosyl transferase, also called dextransucrase, which specifically forms a large insoluble polymer of glucose, i.e., a glucan, according to the following equation:

$$n \text{ sucrose} \xrightarrow{\text{dextransucrase}} (\text{glucan})_n + n \text{ fructose}$$

The glucan adheres tightly to the surface of the tooth and bacterium, bringing viable streptococci into very close association with tooth enamel. As the streptococci in the glucan plaques ferment the fructose cleaved from the sucrose, lactic acid is formed, which as a result of its close contact with the tooth, causes decalcification and decay.

Since this enzyme functions only on sucrose, the avoidance of candies and foods rich in sucrose is effective in reducing tooth decay.

Experimental immunization of monkeys by the injection of *Strept. mutans* cells and cell products into the vicinity of the salivary and parotid glands has been reported to cause the formation of IgA antibody, resulting in fewer plaques on the teeth of immunized animals than in control animals; however, until a better method of inducing IgA antibody is developed, it seems unlikely that this will become a popular procedure.

## GROUP B STREPTOCOCCI

Group B streptococci are the etiologic agents of bovine mastitis, and until recently were not believed to cause serious human disease. However, it is now established that group B streptococci are present in the vaginal flora of approximately 25% of all women, and, although it is extremely rare that these organisms cause overt disease in adults, cases of bacteremia (bacteria in the blood) and meningitis (infection of the membranes surrounding the brain and spinal cord) have occurred in diabetics and in individuals on immunosuppressive drugs.

It is in the newborn that serious infections more commonly occur. About 1% of those children born to mothers infected with group B streptococci will develop bacteremia and pneumonia within the first five days of life, and such infections carry a mortaility rate of 50–70%. Meningitis also occurs, with about a 15% mortality rate, but this complication is usually seen between the tenth and sixtieth day of life. All five serotypes of group B streptococci are equally involved in the early infections. However, type III is more frequently associated with the later meningeal infections of neonates. These infants come from mothers without type III antibody, suggesting that the mother is not the source of the infection. It has been suggested that group B meningitis could be prevented by immunizing expectant mothers to the type III streptococci, thus providing the newborn with protective maternal antibodies.

## STREPTOCOCCUS PNEUMONIAE

*Streptococcus pneumoniae*, formerly named *Diplococcus pneumoniae* but commonly called the pneumococcus, was isolated in 1881 by Pasteur and later shown to be the major cause of lobar pneumonia in humans (infecting one or more lobes of the lung). Perhaps no other bacterium was as important to the early development of immunology and molecular genetics. Studies of pneumo-coccal pneumonia initiated specific serum therapy, which was the major treatment for a variety of infectious diseases until the discovery of antibiotics. Research work with pneumococcal transformation provided the initial proof that DNA alone was the carrier of genetic information.

### Morphology and Metabolism of Pneumococci

Pneumococci are lancet-shaped organisms which are usually arranged in pairs, although short chains may also be seen (see Figure 18-5). They are gram-positive, nonmotile, and non-spore-forming, but virulent organisms are encapsulated. They are particularly sensitive to lysis by an autolytic enzyme which cleaves the bond linking the L-alanine peptide to the muramic acid of the peptidoglycan cell wall. This enzyme, L-alanine-muramyl amidase, routinely becomes activated after the culture enters the stationary phase of growth and will in time cause lysis of the entire culture. The enzyme can also be activated by a number of surface active agents (including detergents), but since bile salts such as sodium taurocholate were originally used, the pneumococci are spoken of as bile soluble, a term that is a misnomer.

Pneumococci require choline for growth, and the choline becomes a constituent of teichoic acid in the cell wall. If ethanolamine is substituted for choline, the pneumococci will grow, but they are then no longer sensitive to lysis, nor can they be genetically transformed. Apparently, the incorporation of ethanolamine in place of choline causes steric differences that result in major changes in cell properties.

Nutritionally, the pneumococci need an enriched medium for growth, and, like other streptococci, lack both cytochromes and catalase. All pneumococci produce alpha-hemolysis when growing on a blood agar medium, and, therefore, closely resemble the viridans streptococci in colonial appearance and morphology.

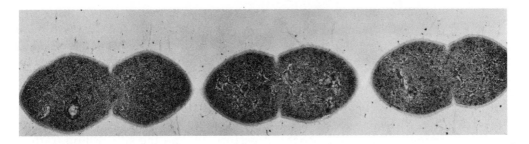

**Figure 18-5.** *Streptococcus pneumoniae* (about × 46,000). Note the diploid arrangement of cells and the lancet shape of individual cells. Capsules are not visible in this electron micrograph.

## Antigenic Structure of the Pneumococci

The pneumococci can be subdivided into over 80 types on the basis of antigenic differences in their polysaccharide capsule. (The ability to transform one type of *Streptococcus pneumoniae* to a new type using purified DNA was discussed in Chapter 7.) They also contain a C carbohydrate analogous to that used by Lancefield to group the streptococci and a type-specific M protein. Unlike the group A streptococci, however, pneumococcal M protein is not antiphagocytic, nor are antibodies to the M protein protective.

## Pneumococcal Pathogenesis

Although the pneumococci excrete a hemolysin called pneumolysin and a neuraminidase, there is no evidence that either substance is involved in their pathogenesis. It appears that the pneumococcus can survive and produce disease in the host primarily because of its capsule. Once a strain loses its capsule, it can be readily phagocytosed and destroyed. Thus, immunity is the result of humoral antibody directed against the capsule, and is, therefore, type specific.

Pneumococcal pneumonia is an acute lung inflammation which may be lobar, that is, involving the tissues in one or more lobes of the lungs, or it may cause a more restricted broncho-pneumonia. The disease is usually sudden in onset and is characterized by chills, fever, and pleural pain (in the area surrounding the lung). The alveoli fill with exudate, and, in about 25% of cases, bacteremia is found early in the course of the disease.

Pneumococci may also invade other tissues, particularly the sinuses, the middle ear, and the meninges. Other secondary complications include septicemia, endocarditis (inflammation of the heart and valves), pericarditis (inflammation of the pericardium, the membrane surrounding the heart), and empyema (an infection of the pleural cavity).

Interestingly, *Streptococcus pneumoniae* is carried as part of the normal flora of the respiratory tract in many healthy individuals. We do not understand why carriers do not suffer from pneumonia, but it appears that the normal lung is quite resistant to infection and that pneumococcal pneumonia occurs most frequently in conjunction with viral infections of the upper respiratory tract. The disease also occurs in persons whose respiratory drainage is impaired, i.e., bedridden patients, heavy smokers, and persons who have inhaled toxic irritants.

## Laboratory Diagnosis

Direct smears of sputum can be stained and observed for gram-positive encapsulated pneumococci. Also, one can perform a quellung test either directly on sputum samples or on the cultured organisms. This test utilizes the fact that if encapsulated bacteria are mixed with type-specific antibodies, the capsule swells to a size considerably larger than normal (see Figure 11-1). The capsular swelling is diagnostic; before the advent of penicillin therapy, it was always necessary to specifically determine which pneumococcal type was causing the infection to ascertain which specific antiserum should be administered. In current practice the quellung test is rarely used for specific typing, but the use of an omni antiserum, which contains antibodies against all types, is of value in providing a definite identification of pneumococci in the sputum.

Because a bile solubility test requires prior growth of the organisms, this determination has been supplanted by a much simpler method: commercially available optochin discs (impregnated with ethylhydrocupreine hydrochloride) are laid down on the surface of an agar plate that has been inoculated with the unknown organism. The pneumococci are exceedingly sensitive to this compound and will fail to grow in the proximity of the disc. The alpha-hemolytic viridans streptococci are insensitive to optochin and will grow adjacent to the implanted disc.

Also, one may inject sputum or spinal fluid intraperitoneally into a white mouse; since mice are very sensitive to pneumococci (as contrasted with other streptococci) the injec-tion of only a few organisms will result in the death of the mouse—usually within one to two days. The organisms can then readily be seen and cultured from the blood drawn from the heart.

In cases of suspected pneumococcal meningitis, essentially the same diagnostic procedures are followed except that a spinal tap is performed, and the spinal fluid (rather than the sputum) is observed. Also, it is routine to withdraw and culture blood from a patient suspected of either pneumonia or meningitis to provide another means of isolating the organism for a definite diagnosis.

### Treatment and Prevention of Pneumococcal Infections

The most effective treatment of pneumococcal infections is the administration of penicillin, since pneumococci have not developed a resistance to this antibiotic. For individuals sensitive to penicillin, erythromycin, lincomycin, or tetracyclines may be used, although pneumococcal resistance to the latter antibiotic has been observed. Prevention of pneumococcal infections appears impractical because the organisms are so widely distributed in the human population. Immunization with pneumococcal polysaccharides is, however, effective, and a vaccine employing the most frequently found types has been successfully employed in large-scale trials.

# Staphylococci

Members of the genus *Staphylococcus* are hearty organisms that cause a tremendous number of infections ranging from localized furuncles (boils) and carbuncles (deeper and larger than a boil—discharging pus from multiple points), to food poisoning, pneumonia, and meningitis. Control of these organisms is particularly difficult since virulent strains are carried asymptomatically in the nasopharynx of 10–50% of normal adults.

### MORPHOLOGY AND METABOLISM OF THE STAPHYLOCOCCI

Members of the genus *Staphylococcus* are spherical cells, approximately 1 $\mu$m in diame-

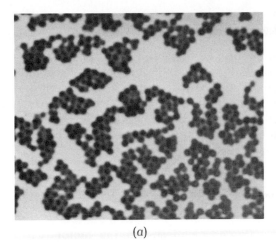

(a)

**Figure 18-6.** a. Clusters of gram-stained *Staphylococcus aureus* (about × 4500). b. Electron micrograph of cells of *Staph. aureus* (× 49,000).

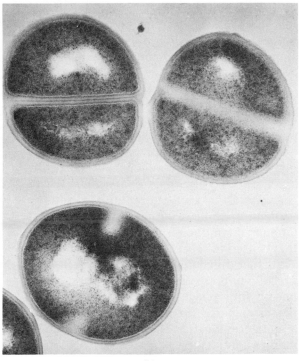

(b)

ter, that in stained smears appear singly, occasionally in pairs, but most frequently as irregular, grape-like clusters (see Figure 18-6). They are gram-positive, nonmotile, non-spore-forming, facultative anaerobes. Their appearance on a gram-stained smear is usually sufficient to distinguish them from the streptococci, since the streptococci are much more prone to form chains of cells (compare with Figures 18-1 and 18-5). If there is doubt, these two genera can be easily separated on the basis of the enzyme catalase. Catalase will break down hydrogen peroxide to form water and oxygen, and if one mixes a loopful of staphylococci on a slide with a drop of 3% hydrogen peroxide, bubbles of oxygen will be visible to the naked eye. Since streptococci do not form catalase, no bubbles will be visible. Also, staphylococcal colonies are considerably larger than those formed by the streptococci.

Staphylococci are facultative anaerobes and ferment a wide variety of sugars to form acid, but no gas. This property permits a differentiation from the large number of avirulent but morphologically similar members of the genus *Micrococcus*. All micrococci are obligate aerobes, and, although they oxidize many sugars, acid is not produced.

Staphylococci grow well on most meat-infusion laboratory media—with or without added sugar; however, synthetic media capable of supporting their growth must contain at least fourteen amino acids and two B vitamins: thiamine and nicotinic acid.

## CLASSIFICATION OF THE STAPHYLOCOCCI

Under present classification, there are two species of staphylococci associated with humans: *Staph. aureus* and *Staph. epidermidis*. Of these, the pathogens are all found in the species *Staph. aureus*, although *Staph. epi-*

*dermidis* (which is part of the normal flora of the skin) may cause occasional small skin abscesses. *Staph. epidermidis* also may occasionally colonize and infect prosthetic cardiac heart valves.

*Staphylococcus aureus* normally produces a light golden pigment; *Staph. epidermidis* colonies are white. In addition, *Staph. aureus* possesses a ribitol teichoic acid (polysaccharide A) in its cell wall that is antigenically distinct from the glycerol teichoic acid (polysaccharide B) of *Staph. epidermidis*. However, it is the ability of *Staph. aureus* to ferment mannitol and to produce coagulase (an enzyme inducing the clotting of plasma) that is used to separate these two species.

Further division of *Staph. aureus* employs phage typing to assign an unknown strain to one of four phage groups. In practice, one places a small drop of each phage group onto a plate previously seeded with the unknown strain of *Staph. aureus*. After overnight incubation, clear plaques of lysis allow one to rank the unknown strain in one of the phage groups shown in Table 18-3. Additional breakdown can be accomplished through the use of individual phages within the assigned group.

The serological typing of *Staph. aureus* into subtypes is difficult, and ordinarily only large diagnostic centers, such as the Center for Disease Control (CDC) in Atlanta, Georgia, are set up for this procedure.

## EXTRACELLULAR TOXINS AND ENZYMES OF THE STAPHYLOCOCCI

The ability of the staphylococci to produce disease depends on their resistance to phagocytosis and their production of extracellular toxins and enzymes. The role of some of the following products is obvious, while others do not appear to be involved in the production of disease.

### Coagulase

Coagulase is an extracellular enzyme that activates a coagulase-reacting factor (CRF) normally present in plasma (possibly prothrombin) causing the plasma to clot by the conversion of fibrinogen to fibrin. All coagulase-producing staphylococci are, by definition, *Staph. aureus*, and, as a result, coagulase production is considered the best laboratory evidence for the potential pathogenicity of a staphylococcus. Seven antigenically different extracellular coagulases have been identified from various staphylococci, but the only pathogenic role suggested for the enzyme is the coating of the organisms with fibrin to inhibit their phagocytosis.

In addition to extracellular coagulase, *Staph. aureus* also possesses a bound coagulase that causes the organisms to clump when mixed with plasma. Bound coagulase can convert fibrinogen directly to fibrin and does not require the presence of CRF for activity.

### Staphylococcal Hemolysins

Hemolysins produced by the staphylococci all give a beta-type hemolysis. There are four hemolysins, alpha, beta, gamma, and delta. These can be differentiated from each other by antigenic distinctions and, as shown in Table 18-4, by the type of erythrocytes which they preferentially will lyse. All four hemolysins possess properties which result in varying degrees of toxicity for leukocytes and tissue cells. In addition, some (particularly

**Table 18-3. Lytic Phage Groups of *Staphylococcus aureus***

| Group | Phage Numbers |
|-------|---------------|
| I | 29, 52, 52A, 79, 80 |
| II | 3A, 3C, 55, 71 |
| III | 6, 42E, 47, 53, 54, 75, 77, 83A, 84, 85 |
| IV | 42D |
| Not grouped | 81, 187 |

**Table 18-4. Classification of Hemolysins by Type of Erythrocyte Lysed**

| Type of Hemolysis | Red Blood Cell Lysed | Usual Source |
|---|---|---|
| alpha | Calf, rabbit, sheep | Human |
| beta | Human, ox, sheep (effective only as hot-cold lysis, i.e., 37°C for 1–2 hrs followed by overnight in refrigerator) | Animal |
| gamma | Guinea pig, horse, human, ox, rabbit, rat, sheep | Human |
| delta | Guinea pig, horse, human, rabbit, rat, sheep | Human |

alpha-hemolysin) are dermonecrotic (kill skin cells) and lethal if injected into mice and rabbits.

## Leukocidin

Leukocidin activity, which is separable from the hemolysins, can be demonstrated in many pathogenic staphylococci. The factor appears to combine with membrane phospholipid, resulting in increased permeability and death of the cell. It may also result in a degranulation of the polymorphonuclear leukocytes similar to that described for streptolysin O.

## Exfoliatin

Exfoliatin is an exotoxin, coded by a plasmid, that causes an acute exfoliative dermatitis called staphylococcal scalded skin syndrome. Staphylococci from phage group II are more frequently involved than other phage groups, and the syndrome may be caused by either or both of two serotypes of exfoliatin. It is characterized by a wrinkling

and peeling of the epidermis, resulting in considerable fluid loss from the denuded skin (see Figure 18-7). Since the epidermal sloughing is caused by a diffusable exotoxin, the infecting staphylococci may or may not be present at the dermal site. This disease is seen most commonly in newborn infants, but it has occurred in adults receiving immunosuppressive therapy. In fact the rarity of this syndrome is surprising since approximately 5% of randomly isolated strains of *Staphylococcus aureus* are reported to produce exfoliatin.

## Staphylococcal Enterotoxins

Enterotoxin, which is an exotoxin, causes a food poisoning (intoxication) which is characterized by severe diarrhea and vomiting. It is excreted by most coagulase-positive staphylococci. Six antigenically distinct enterotoxins, designated A, B, C1, C2, D, and E, have been described, which in some (if not all) cases are coded for by a lysogenic phage. The usual incubation period ranges from two to six hours after the ingestion of food in which the staphylococci have grown and produced enterotoxin. The duration of the acute symptoms is usually less than 24 hours, but an individual may feel debilitated for

**Figure 18-7.** Neonatal mouse injected 24 hours earlier with $1 \times 10^9$ staphylococci from phage group II. The staphylococci were obtained from a patient with scalded skin syndrome.

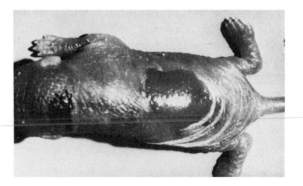

several days. The illness is rarely fatal but patients may be hospitalized for reception of intravenous fluids to replace the fluids lost through diarrhea and vomiting.

## Other Staphylococcal Products

Staphylococci may also excrete enzymes such as penicillinase (which destroys penicillin), hyaluronidase (spreading factor), lipases, and a staphylokinase which causes the lysis of fibrin clots in a manner analogous to that of streptokinase. In addition, *Staph. aureus* possesses a surface component, protein A, which inhibits phagocytosis of the organisms. Protein A binds to the Fc portion of IgG and it has been suggested that this property imparts antiphagocytic activity by competing with leukocytes for the Fc portion of specific opsonins.

## PATHOGENESIS OF STAPHYLOCOCCAL INFECTIONS

In spite of the fact that most persons are either carriers or are exposed frequently to coagulase-positive staphylococci, overt disease (with the exception of staphylococcal food poisoning) in a healthy individual is not a frequent event. Persons most susceptible to serious staphylococcal infections include those whose ability to phagocytose and destroy the staphylococci is not completely developed, or is significantly inhibited. Such persons may include the newborn, surgical or burn patients, persons receiving immunosuppressive drugs, or those with immune deficiency diseases such as chronic granulomatous disease (see Chapter 11). Individuals with lower respiratory viral infections such as influenza or measles and diabetic patients are also more susceptible to staphylococcal infections.

## Skin Infections of Staphylococcal Origin

Infection of a hair follicle by staphylococci resulting in a localized superficial abscess or boil is undoubtedly the most frequent manifestation of staphylococcal disease. These lesions usually heal spontaneously, but, particularly if irritated, may spread to the subcutaneous layers of the skin to produce a furuncle. Such lesions may continue to spread to include multiple contiguous lesions, which are then referred to as carbuncles. The lesions are painful and may require surgical draining before healing.

## Staphylococcal Pneumonia

Staphylococcal pneumonia is rarely a primary event in an otherwise healthy individual. Infection with influenza virus, however, predisposes one to a serious, and frequently fatal, pulmonary infection by staphylococci. Persons with cystic fibrosis are also particularly susceptible to staphylococcal pneumonia.

## Staphylococcal Osteomyelitis

An infection of the bones, staphylococcal osteomyelitis occurs most frequently in boys under the age of 12, and, if untreated, may have a mortality rate of 25%. The source of such infections may be adjacent tissue infections, or it may be spread through the blood stream.

## Wound Infections Involving Staphylococci

Staphylococcal wound infections are less common now than they were in the preantibiotic era, but they are still the single most common hospital-acquired surgical or wound infection. Such infections most often appear to arise from endogenous strains carried by the patient but can also be transmitted by medical personnel or contaminated bedding or equipment.

## Staphylococcal Enteritis

Staphylococcal enteritis is a severe infection of the small or large intestine which may follow gastrointestinal surgery or may occur after intensive antibiotic therapy which destroys much of the normal intestinal flora. The necrotic lesions in the intestinal wall are believed to result from the secretion of enterotoxin by the invading staphylococcus.

Other manifestations of *Staph. aureus* infections include acute bacterial endocarditis, meningitis, impetigo, and the scalded skin syndrome caused by the staphylococcal exotoxin, exfoliatin.

## LABORATORY DIAGNOSIS OF STAPHYLOCOCCAL INFECTIONS

Since staphylococci are so frequently found on the skin and in the nasopharynx, diagnosis may be complicated by the fact that one may not always be certain whether one is dealing with the true etiologic agent of the disease or with a contaminating parasitic staphylococcus. Exudates or blood specimens should be streaked on blood agar plates and, after growth, observed for pigment production and hemolysis. Isolated cultures must also be assayed for the production of coagulase, since it is this property that is most consistently correlated with pathogenicity.

Animal inoculation is not usually of value, but the subcutaneous or intraperitoneal injection of an exfoliatin-producing staphylococcus into a newborn mouse will result in a diffuse sloughing of the epidermis.

## TREATMENT AND CONTROL OF STAPHYLOCOCCI

*Staphylococcus aureus* appears to be consistently adaptable in becoming resistant to drug therapy, and, as a result, many antibiotics soon become ineffective for the treatment of staphylococcal infections. Many strains of staphylococci producing penicillinase can be successfully treated with the penicillinase-resistant semisynthetic penicillin, methicillin (see Chapter 10), but strains resistant to this antibiotic are now being found more frequently. Hence, any isolated staphylococcus must be assayed for antibi-

otic sensitivity as soon as possible, even though therapy should usually commence before such results are available. Once therapy has begun, it should be intensive, so as to kill all organisms before mutation to a slightly higher level of drug resistance can occur.

Control is directed primarily at those individuals who are most susceptible to staphylococcal infections. Thus, the newborn nursery of hospitals and surgical operating rooms are particularly dangerous areas where rigid aseptic procedures must be followed. In the event of a hospital outbreak, the etiologic staphylococcus should be phage-typed and all attending personnel cultured to locate the possible source of the organism.

## REFERENCES

Anthony, B. F., and N. F. Concepçion. 1975. Group B *Streptococcus,*in a general hospital. *J. Infect. Dis.* **132**:561–567.

Baldwin, D. S., and R. G. Schacht. 1976. Late sequelae of poststreptococcal glomerulonephritis. *Annu. Rev. Med.* **27**:49–55.

Bukovic, J. A., and H. M. Johnson. 1975. Staphylococcal enterotoxin C: Solid phase radioimmune assay. *J. Appl. Microbiol.* **30**:700–701.

Fox, E. N. 1974. M-Proteins of group A streptococci. *Bacteriol. Rev.* **38**:57–86.

Genigeorgis, C., and J. K. Kuo. 1976. Recovery of staphylococcal enterotoxin from foods by affinity chromatography. *J. Appl. Microbiol.* **31**:274–279.

Gwaltney, J. M. Jr., M. A. Sande, R. Austrian, and J. O. Hendley. 1975. Spread of *Streptococcus pneumoniae* in families. II. Relation of transfer of *S. pneumoniae* to incidence of colds and serum antibody. *J. Infect. Dis.* **132**:62–68.

Katenstein, A., C. Davis, and A. Braude. 1976. Pulmonary changes in neonatal sepsis due to group B β-hemolytic *Streptococcus*: Relation to hyaline membrane disease. *J. Infect. Dis.* **133**:430–435.

Kloos, W. E., R. J. Zimmerman, and R. F. Smith. 1976. Preliminary studies on the characterization and distribution of *Staphylococcus* and *Micrococcus* on animal skin. *J. Appl. Microbiol.* **31**:53–59.

Kondo, I., S. Sakurai, and Y. Sarai. 1974. New type of exfoliatin obtained from staphylococcal strains belonging to phage groups other than group II, isolated from patients with impetigo and Ritter's disease. *Infect. Immun.* **10:**851–861.

Lacey, R. W. 1975. Antibiotic resistance plasmids of *Staphylococcus aureus* and their clinical importance. *Bacteriol. Rev.* **39:**1–32.

McCarty, M. 1969–1970. *The Streptococcal Cell Wall.* The Harvey Lectures **65:**73–96. Academic Press, New York.

Michalek, S., J. R. McGhee, J. Mestecky, R. R. Arnold, and L. Bozzo. 1976. Ingestion of *Streptococcus mutans* induces secretory immunoglobulin A and caries immunity. *Science* **192:** 1238–1240.

Rogolsky, M., B. B. Wiley, and L. A. Glasgow. 1976. Phage group II staphylococcal strains with chromosomal and extrachromosomal genes for exfoliative toxin production. *Infect. Immun.* **13:**44–52.

Talbot, H. W. Jr., and J. R. Parisi. 1976. Phage typing of *Staphylococcus epidermidis. J. Clin. Microbiol.* **3:**519–523.

Wiseman, G. M. 1975. The hemolysins of *Staphylococcus aureus. Bacteriol. Rev.* **39:**317–344.

Yotis, W. W., ed. 1974. Recent advances in staphylococcal research. *Ann. New York Acad. Sci.* **236.**

# 19

# Neisseriaceae

The gram-negative pyogenic cocci, like their gram-positive counterparts, are able to cause disease because of their ability to resist phagocytosis. However, unlike many of the gram-positive pyogenic cocci, none of the *Neisseria* appear to produce extracellular products that could aid in disease production.

Two species of gram-negative cocci cause serious disease in humans: (1) *Neisseria meningitidis,* the etiologic agent of epidemic meningitis; and (2) *Neisseria gonorrhoeae,* the cause of the venereal disease gonorrhea. Members of other genera of this family that are either normal flora or may on occasion cause disease in humans are found among *Branhamella, Acinetobacter,* and *Moraxella.*

## MORPHOLOGY AND NUTRITION OF THE *NEISSERIA*

Bacteria in the genus *Neisseria* are nonmotile, gram-negative diplococci whose cells are characteristically kidney-shaped with their concave sides adjacent to each other. As a result, the pairs of diplococci sometimes look like small doughnuts (see Figure 19-1).

The nonpathogenic *Neisseria* (part of the normal flora of the nasopharynx) are slightly larger and considerably easier to grow than the pathogenic species; they are able to multiply at 22°C on ordinary laboratory media such as nutrient broth, while the pathogens do not grow well below 37°C and not at all at 22°C. Furthermore, the pathogens are extremely sensitive to fatty acids and trace metals present in peptones and agar. This inhibitory effect can be eliminated by the addition of serum or blood to the growth medium. Moreover, if the blood is heated to 80°C for 10 minutes, it is even more effective. This procedure turns the agar medium a dark brown, and the resulting medium is commonly called chocolate blood agar. The pathogens also require a higher concentration of $CO_2$ for optimal growth than is present in the atmosphere. It is customary, therefore, to culture newly-isolated pathogenic *Neisseria* either in a special incubator containing excess $CO_2$ or in a jar in which a candle has been lit before it is closed. The candle uses about half of the oxygen and releases $CO_2$, resulting in a final concentration of about 10% $CO_2$.

The pathogenic *Neisseria* are fragile organisms and will readily autolyse unless their autolytic enzymes are destroyed by heating

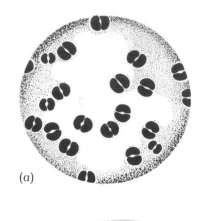

(a)

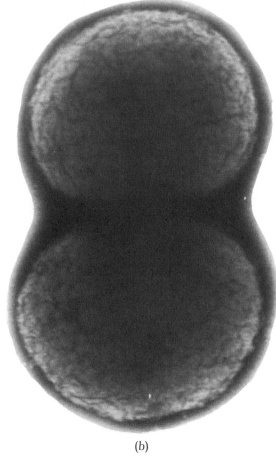

(b)

**Figure 19-1.** *a.* Drawing of "doughnut-shaped" diplococci of *Neisseria gonorrhoeae* as they sometimes appear under the microscope. *b.* Electron micrograph of a negatively-stained pair of *N. gonorrhoeae* cells (× 49,140).

at 65°C for 30 minutes or by the addition of formalin. These techniques are used to preserve cell suspensions for serologic tests.

All *Neisseria,* including the nonpathogens, are oxidase positive, that is, they are able to oxidize dimethyl- and tetramethylparaphenylene diamine. This property can be used to distinguish colonies of *Neisseria* from colonies of other bacteria growing on the same plate. The oxidase test may be carried out by spraying either dimethyl- or tetramethylparaphenylene diamine onto the colonies and observing color changes. Colonies that are oxidase positive turn pink, then dark red, and finally black (see Figure 19-2); oxidase negative colonies are unchanged. The reagent eventually kills the cells, but if the colony is restreaked on fresh media before it turns dark, it can be grown again. The reagent can also be placed on a piece of filter paper, and part of a suspected bacterial colony smeared on the wet filter paper. A positive reaction will be indicated by the development of a dark purple color within 10 to 15 seconds. It should be noted that although the oxidase test is an aid in the isolation and identification of *Neisseria,* any organism that possesses cytochrome C in its respiratory chain will be oxidase positive.

## NEISSERIA MENINGITIDIS

*Neisseria meningitidis,* commonly called the meningococcus, was first described in 1887 as occurring in the spinal fluid of patients with meningitis. Subsequently, it has been shown to be the major etiologic agent for meningitis in humans and also to cause a fulminating, frequently fatal, septicemia resulting in lesions, primarily in the skin, bones, and adrenal glands.

### Antigenic Classification of the Meningococci

Meningococci can be classified into a number of groups based on common antigens. Current serogroups are designated A, B, C, D, X,

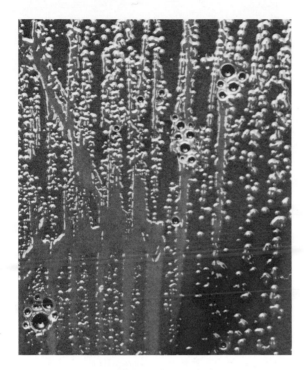

**Figure 19-2.** Black colonies of *Neisseria meningitidis* on chocolate agar indicate a positive oxidase test.

antigen has not been completely characterized, but it appears to be a lipoprotein-lipopolysaccharide complex existing in the outer membrane of these organisms.

## Epidemiology and Pathogenesis of Meningococcal Infections

The meningococcus is a strict parasite of humans and can be routinely cultured from the nasopharynx of asymptomatic carriers. In periods between epidemics, civilian carrier rates range from 2–8%, depending on the season, while in a closed society such as a military camp, the average carrier rate has been reported to exceed 40%, with over 90% of the personnel becoming carriers at some time during 10 weeks of observation.

It therefore is obvious that the organism is spread from person to person via the respiratory route, and that even in a situation where a majority of individuals are carrying the virulent organisms in their nasopharynx, very few ordinarily get sick. However, if we follow the fate of the infecting organism, meningococcal infections can be categorized into three stages.

First occurs the nasopharyngeal infection, which is usually asymptomatic but might result in a minor inflammation. This state may last for days to months and will induce the formation of protective antibodies within a week, even though the infection remains asymptomatic.

Second, in a small percentage of cases the meningococci may enter the blood stream from the posterior nasopharynx—probably via the cervical lymph nodes. This stage, called meningococcemia, may be explosive, resulting in death within 6 to 8 hours, or may begin more gradually with fever, malaise, and a petechial (minute, rounded skin hemorrhages) rash, the lesions of which contain the cocci. The organisms may also cause lesions in the joints and lungs, and, rarely, may cause massive hemorrhages in the adrenals (Waterhouse-Friderichsen syndrome). For unknown reasons, this stage may become chronic on

Y, and Z. Members of groups X and Y have been isolated from cases of meningitis, but X, Y, and Z are frequently found in carriers and have not been involved in large epidemics of meningitis. Interestingly, group Y meningococci have become the predominant meningococcal serogroup causing disease in Air Force personnel in the USA, but the major disease caused by these organisms is pneumonia and not meningitis. Group D strains have not been seen for many years, and it is possible that they no longer exist. Thus, it is groups A, B, and C that are the causes of epidemics of meningitis.

The group-specific antigen for both groups A and C is a polysaccharide capsule surrounding the organisms. In group A it is composed of a polymer of N-acetyl-O-acetyl mannosamine phosphate, and for group C, it consists of a polymer of N-acetyl neuraminic acid which is partially O-acetylated. Group B

rare occasions causing mild symptoms of rash, arthritis, or endocarditis over a long period of time.

The hemorrhagic lesions occurring in both the skin and internal organs, particularly the adrenals, are believed to be due to the release of endotoxin. Electron micrographs show that the meningococcus possesses pili, which probably allows intimate contact with host cells, and that the organisms appear to release blebs of endotoxin (see Figure 19-3). Thus, very close contact by an organism, which in the absence of specific antibody can resist phagocytosis, appears to account for the hemorrhagic lesions characteristic of meningococcal infections.

In the third stage of meningococcal infections the organisms may cross the blood-brain barrier and infect the meninges, causing the major symptoms of severe headache, stiff neck, and vomiting accompanied by delerium and confusion.

Surprisingly, meningococci are also occasionally isolated from areas of the body which are usually considered to be the

**Figure 19-3.** Negatively-stained cell of *Neisseria meningitidis* group B, showing pili and surface blebs of cell-wall lipopolysaccharide, or endotoxin ($\times$ 39,000).

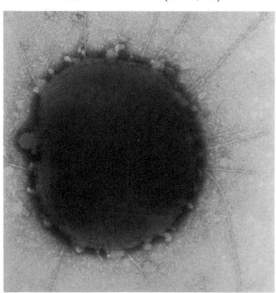

domain of gonococci. Such infections as acute urethritis (inflammation of the urethra), epididymytis (inflammation of the epididymis), vulvovaginitis (inflammation of the vulva and vagina), or cervicitis (inflammation of the cervix of the uterus) would be labeled as gonococcal infections in the absence of a complete laboratory identification of the etiological agent.

### Laboratory Diagnosis of Meningococcal Infections

Spinal fluid, blood, and nasopharyngeal swabs, as well as smears and cultures from skin lesions, may be sources of meningococci. Nasopharyngeal swabs are most effective if done with a cotton swab on a bent wire so that the posterior nasopharynx can be reached without contamination by the normal flora of the mouth.

Frequently, the gram-negative diplococci can be directly observed in white cells sedimented from freshly obtained spinal fluid.

Final identification requires both sugar fermentation tests (Table 19-1) and serological tests using specific group antisera. Since groups A and C possess a capsule, a quellung reaction can result in their identification, and agglutination with specific antiserum can be used for all isolates. In addition, latex particles to which group-specific polysaccharide has been adsorbed can be used in an agglutination procedure to detect antibody to groups A or C meningococci.

Throat swabs are usually streaked on blood or chocolate blood agar, but the selective Thayer-Martin medium is frequently used since it contains polymyxin, vancomycin, and nystatin. These inhibit the growth of many bacteria and yeast contaminants while allowing the growth of the pathogenic *Neisseria*.

### Treatment and Prevention of Meningococcal Infections

Until the early 1960's, the sulfonamides were the drug of choice for treatment of infections

**Table 19.1 Growth Characteristics and Sugar Fermentations by Neisseria and Morphologically Similar Human Parasites**

| Organism | Growth in the Absence of Blood | Glucose | Maltose | Sucrose |
|---|---|---|---|---|
| Neisseria meningitidis | − | + | + | − |
| Neisseria gonorrhoeae | − | + | − | − |
| Neisseria flavescens | + | − | − | − |
| Neisseria sicca | + | + | + | + |
| Branhamella catarrhalis | + | − | − | − |

caused by Neisseria meningitidis, since they readily penetrated the blood-brain barrier. However, the incidence of organisms resistant to sulfonamides has now increased to the point where this treatment is rarely used for meningococcal infections. Fortunately, penicillin is effective and is now considered the drug of choice. Erythromycin or chloramphenicol are also effective and can be used in individuals hypersensitive to penicillin.

Prevention of meningococcal infections has been approached in two different ways: the elimination of carriers and the use of vaccines.

During World War II, entire military camps of thousands of men were given sulfonamides as an effective method of eliminating meningococci from carriers and stopping epidemics. Now that many strains are sulfonamide-resistant, this would probably be of little value. Treatment of the close personal contacts of a patient with a meningococcal infection should be carried out as soon as possible. An antibiotic named minocycline has been extensively used, but because of the frequent side effects of dizziness, nausea, and vomiting (see Table 19-2), it is now recommended that such contacts be treated with 600 mg of rifampin every 12 hours for two days. But occasional rifampin-resistant mutants are now being found, and it may be necessary to use other antibiotics.

Vaccines for groups A and C are commercially available, and they were used in an attempt to stop a major epidemic in Sao Paulo, Brazil, where over 20,000 cases and 3,000 deaths caused by both group A and group C meningococci occurred during 1974. The efficacy of these polysaccharide vaccines has been demonstrated with military recruits, and it seems highly probable that if enough vaccine were available, an epidemic could be stopped early in its evolution.

Unfortunately, group B antigen is not a capsular polysaccharide, and an effective vaccine for group B organisms is not yet available.

## NEISSERIA GONORRHOEAE

No other disease in the United States has grown to the epidemic proportion of gonorrhea during the past decade. Approximately one million cases are reported annually in this country, and these undoubtedly represent only a portion of the total number occurring each year.

### Antigenic Classification of Neisseria gonorrhoeae

Neisseria gonorrhoeae, routinely called the gonococcus, appears to consist of an antigenically heterogenous group of organisms, and no successful immunological classification is available. The organisms are divided into four types based on their colonial appearance (see Figure 19-4), but these morpho-

**Table 19-2. Vestibular Reactions to Minocycline Prophylaxis by Exposure Group and Sex**

| Sex / Exposure Group | No. Treated | No. with Symptoms | Attack Rate % |
|---|---|---|---|
| MALE | | | |
| Hospital | 10 | 9 | 90 |
| College | 6 | 3 | 50 |
| Family and Acquaintances | 15 | 9 | 60 |
| Total | 31 | 21 | 68 |
| FEMALE | | | |
| Hospital | 28 | 28 | 100 |
| College | 7 | 7 | 100 |
| Family and Acquaintances | 17 | 9 | 53 |
| Total | 52 | 44 | 85 |

logical variations are a result of mutations occurring within a single strain. Thus, types 1 and 2 are pathogenic for humans, but after growing on laboratory media overnight, at least half of any culture will show the colonial morphology of types 3 or 4, and after more prolonged cultivation all organisms will appear as the avirulent types 3 and 4.

On a microscopic level, the only obvious difference between the various colonial types is that the virulent types 1 and 2 possess pili while the avirulent types 3 and 4 do not (see Figure 19-5). Since it is well established that pili are involved in the attachment of microorganisms to cells, it appears quite probable that the gonococcus requires close attachment to produce disease. Furthermore, the pili are antiphagocytic, perhaps in part because the organisms are so intimately attached to host cells. Removal of pili from virulent cells by treatment with trypsin results in their phagocytosis and destruction.

Recent reports indicate that virulent gonococci also possess a capsule analogous to that occurring on the meningococci (see Figure 19-6). The role of this capsular material in

**Figure 19-4.** Colony types of *Neisseria gonorrhoeae* (all about × 180). *a.* Type 1 (T1). *b.* Type 2 (T2). *c.* Type 3 (T3). *d.* Type 4 (T4).

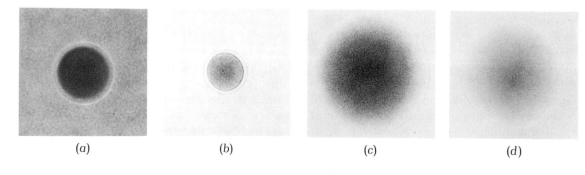

(a)                    (b)                    (c)                    (d)

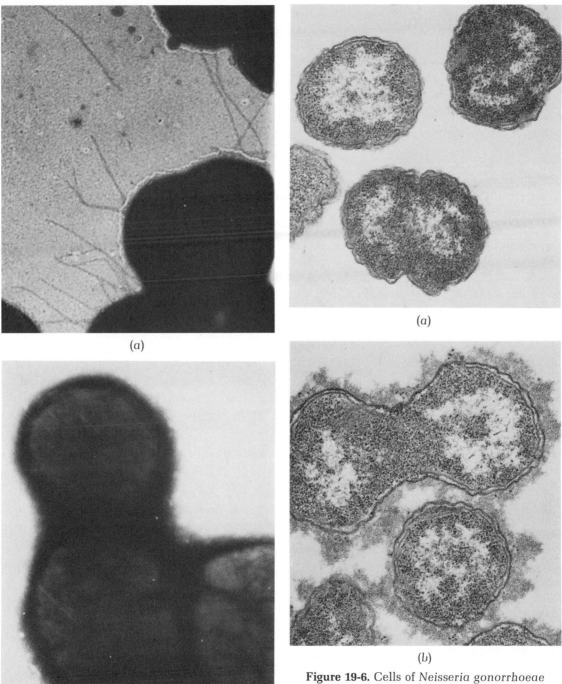

(a)

(a)

(b)

(b)

**Figure 19-5.** Negatively-stained cells of *Neisseria gonorrhoeae* (about × 34,000). *a.* Cells from a T1 colony showing numerous pili. *b.* These cells from a T4 colony lack pili.

**Figure 19-6.** Cells of *Neisseria gonorrhoeae* strain Cd (× 36,000). *a.* Cells mixed with normal preimmune serum. *b.* Cells mixed with hyperimmune serum obtained from a rabbit immunized with the Cd strain of *N. gonorrhoeae.* Note that the capsule becomes visible only after it interacts with its specific antibodies.

either the virulence of the organism or as the target for antigonococcal humoral antibodies is yet to be established. Several laboratories, however, are now investigating the biological significance of the gonococcus capsule, as well as the potential use of this capsular material for use as a vaccine.

## Epidemiology and Pathogenesis of Gonorrhea

Gonorrhea is a venereal disease which, with few exceptions, is acquired through sexual contact with an infected individual. The organisms penetrate the mucous membranes of the genital tract causing a localized infection initially. In the male, the infection may be asymptomatic, but it usually causes an acute urethritis, resulting in a purulent discharge and painful urination. The gonococci may also infect the prostate gland and epididymis. In the female, the infection is much more likely to be asymptomatic or accompanied by a minor discharge which usually goes unnoticed. The organisms, however, may infect the urethra, vagina, cervix, and fallopian tubes, causing a chronic disease resulting in sterility. Bacteremia may also occur, leading to lesions in the skin, heart, eye, meninges, or joints, resulting in a gonococcal arthritis. Pregnant women are especially susceptible to the disseminated form of gonorrhea.

Opthalmia neonatorum is a gonococcal infection of the eye acquired by a newborn during passage through the birth canal of an infected mother. Such infections often result in blindness, but have been largely eliminated by the legal requirement that silver nitrate, bactericidal for these bacteria, be dropped into a baby's eyes at birth.

## Laboratory Diagnosis of Gonorrhea

In the purulent stage, particularly in the infected male, a stain of the urethral exudate will show numerous leukocytes containing intracellular gram-negative diplococci, but a positive laboratory diagnosis of gonorrhea requires that the organism be grown and identified as an oxidase positive, gram-negative diplococcus that ferments glucose but fails to ferment maltose or sucrose.

Chronic gonorrhea, particularly in the female, can be difficult to diagnose by smear since there is little or no discharge and few organisms. Fluorescently-labeled antibody can be used to identify organisms in smears, but frequently gonococci cannot be observed or isolated from such cases. A great deal of effort is currently directed toward the discovery of serologic techniques that will demonstrate the presence of specific antibodies in infected persons. Complement fixation has not been successful; however, in some cases the use of an indirect immunofluorescence test whereby the patient's serum is reacted with known type 1 gonococci followed by fluorescently-labeled rabbit anti-human gamma globulin appears to be of value for a serologic diagnosis. Thus, the only reliable diagnosis of gonorrhea in the female requires that the organisms be grown and identified.

## Treatment and Control of Gonorrhea

Before the middle 1930's gonorrhea was treated by irrigation of the urethra with antiseptics. Then came the sulfonamides, and it was thought that this disease could be completely eradicated. However, joy was short-lived, because by the early 1940's many strains of gonococci were resistant to sulfonamide therapy. Fortunately penicillin became available at this time and it has been the treatment of choice for over 30 years. In 1976, however, penicillinase-producing gonococci were isolated from widely-separated areas in the United States and in England, and it is likely that such strains will eventually supplant the penicillin-sensitive strains. Until this becomes more of a problem, the Center for Disease Control still recommends treatment of uncomplicated gonorrhea with aqueous procaine penicillin accompanied by oral probenecid or oral ampicillin together with probenecid. The latter drug is not antibacterial; it merely retards the urinary excretion of the penicillin. It is recommended, however, that follow-up cultures be made 7–14 days after completion of therapy and that those individuals with positive cultures for the gonococcus receive two grams of spectinomycin intramuscularly. Tetracycline or erythromycin may be used for patients who are allergic to penicillin, but because of the potential toxic effects on mother and fetus, tetracycline should not be used in pregnant women. Disseminated or chronic cases may require treatment with several antibiotics for at least ten days.

The major problem in control of gonorrhea is finding infected females who have asymptomatic infections. Several very large screening tests for gonorrhea were carried out in the United States during the early 1970's. Some aspect of the magnitude of this problem can be seen in Table 19-3 which shows that of almost 9 million women examined by cultures of specimens, 4.2% were found to be infected with the gonococcus.

Great effort has been directed to produce an effective vaccine for gonorrhea, and, although success is "still around the corner," antibodies against the pili, particularly of the IgA type, seem to have the potential of providing effective immunity. In vitro studies have shown that anti-pili antibodies prevent the attachment of virulent gonococci to cells, as well as serving as opsonins for their phagocytosis and destruction.

## OTHER MEMBERS OF THE NEISSERIACEAE

A large group of very short, gram-negative rods occurring both as free-living organisms in soil and water as well as parasites of the human body—particularly the skin, saliva, eyes, ears, urine, and feces—tend to occur in pairs. Thus, a stained smear can be easily confused with Neisseria, and as a result (in 1939) they were grouped together into a tribe named "Mimeae" to indicate that they mimicked Neisseria in appearance. Within this tribe, two genera were proposed, Mima and Herellea, but subsequent decisions by an international committee abandoned this tribe and its genera and classified these organisms in the genera Acinetobacter and Moraxella.

### Acinetobacter

Organisms in the genus Acinetobacter are characterized as obligate aerobes that are oxidase negative. For the most part, they are free-living saprophytes, but, with increasing frequency, have been reported as etiologic agents of nongonococcal urethritis, meningitis, septicemia, and wound infections. Actually, there is not unanimous agreement as whether such isolates represent the true etiologic agents of these diseases or whether they are normal flora that become either contaminants or secondary invaders.

Acinetobacter varies in its sensitivity to antibiotics; organisms are usually resistant to penicillin therapy but may be sensitive to kanamycin, polymyxin B, colistin, or the tetracyclines.

### Moraxella

Moraxella comprises organisms morphologically similar to those of Acinetobacter, but all are oxidase positive and there are no serological cross-reactions between the two genera. Furthermore, Moraxella appears to be an obligate parasite of the eye, upper respiratory tract, and the genital tract. Many are not known to be associated with disease, but some species (such as M. lacunata) may cause a conjunctivitis in humans, and others may be secondary invaders of the respiratory tract (M. nonliquefaciens). There seems to be a general consensus that eye infections by these organisms occur only after predisposing conditions of poor hygienic conditions.

Unlike the Acinetobacter, Moraxella is very sensitive to penicillin therapy.

Several other species of bacteria that are

### Table 19-3. Results of Gonorrhea Culture Tests on Females United States*—July 1974–June 1975**

| Source of Test | Number Tested | Number Positive | Percent Positive |
|---|---|---|---|
| HEALTH CARE PROVIDERS (MINUS VD CLINICS) | 8,046,589 | 220,199 | 2.7 |
| HEALTH DEPT. NON-VD CLINIC | 1,743,155 | 57,214 | 3.3 |
|    Family Planning | 1,242,371 | 40,259 | 3.2 |
|    Prenatal, Ob-Gyn | 182,084 | 5,893 | 3.2 |
|    Cancer Detection | 37,174 | 355 | 1.0 |
|    Combinations or Other | 281,526 | 10,707 | 3.8 |
| PUBLIC/PRIVATE HOSPITAL —OUTPATIENT | 1,487,024 | 61,619 | 4.1 |
|    Family Planning | 154,743 | 4,603 | 3.0 |
|    Prenatal, Ob-Gyn | 355,402 | 12,387 | 3.5 |
|    Cancer Detection | 15,977 | 352 | 2.2 |
|    Combinations or Other | 960,902 | 44,277 | 4.6 |
| PUBLIC/PRIVATE HOSPITAL —INPATIENT | 63,838 | 1,720 | 2.7 |
|    Obstetric | 7,423 | 236 | 3.2 |
|    Gynecologic | 1,801 | 61 | 3.4 |
|    Combinations or Other | 54,614 | 1,423 | 2.6 |
| COMMUNITY HEALTH CENTERS | 708,448 | 20,664 | 2.9 |
|    Family Planning | 280,557 | 4,879 | 1.7 |
|    Prenatal, Ob-Gyn | 44,737 | 965 | 2.2 |
|    Cancer Detection | 5,918 | 128 | 2.2 |
|    Combinations or Other | 377,236 | 14,692 | 3.9 |
| PRIVATE PHYSICIANS | 2,492,435 | 48,683 | 2.0 |
| PRIVATE FAMILY PLANNING GROUPS | 872,811 | 15,048 | 1.7 |
| GROUP HEALTH CLINICS | 121,509 | 2,758 | 2.3 |
| STUDENT HEALTH CENTERS | 233,316 | 4,081 | 1.7 |
| MANPOWER TRAINING AGENCIES | 15,612 | 716 | 4.6 |
| INDUSTRIAL SCREENING | 5,538 | 104 | 1.9 |
| MILITARY/DEPENDENTS | 143,677 | 2,445 | 1.7 |

**Table 19-3 (continued)**

| Source of Test | Number Tested | Number Positive | Percent Positive |
|---|---|---|---|
| CORRECTION OR DETENTION CENTERS | 46,363 | 2,359 | 5.1 |
| NOT SPECIFIED | 112,863 | 2,788 | 2.5 |
| VENEREAL DISEASE CLINICS | 817,310 | 155,664 | 19.0 |
| TOTAL (ALL CLINICS) | 8,863,899 | 375,863 | 4.2 |

*Includes reports from Puerto Rico and Trust Territories

**Excludes reports from Guam (July 1974–June 1975), Iowa (April–June 1975), and Pennsylvania (January–March 1975)

part of the normal flora of the mouth and upper respiratory tract bear a morphological resemblance to the pathogenic *Neisseria*. However, the fact that these nonpathogens such as *Neisseria sicca, Neisseria subflava,* and *Branhamella catarrhalis* (formerly *Neisseria catarrhalis*) can be readily grown at room temperature on simple media allows for the easy differentiation of these organisms from the pathogens. None of these has been implicated in human disease.

# REFERENCES

Arko, R. J., W. P. Duncan, W. J. Brown, W. L. Peacock, and T. Tomizawa. 1976. Immunity in infections with *Neisseria gonorrhoeae:* Duration and serological response in the chimpanzee. *J. Infect. Dis.* **133**:441–447.

Biswas, G., S. Comer, and P. F. Sparling. 1976. Chromosomal location of antibiotic resistance genes in *Neisseria gonorrhoeae. J. Bacteriol.* **125**:1207–1210.

Buchanan, T. M., and W. A. Pearce. 1976. Pili as a mediator of the attachment of gonococci to human erythrocytes. *Infect. Immun.* **13**:1483–1489.

Center for Disease Control. 1975. Gonorrhea: Recommended treatment schedules. *Ann. Internal Med.* **82**:230–233.

Gaafar, H. A., and D. C. D'Arcangelis. 1976. Fluorescent antibody test for the serological diagnosis of gonorrhea. *J. Clin. Microbiol.* **3**:438–442.

Goldschneider, I., M. L. Lepow, and E. C. Gotschlich. 1972. Immunogenicity of the group A and group C meningococcal polysaccharides in children. *J. Infect. Dis.* **125**:509–519.

Hebeler, B. H., and F. E. Young. 1976. Mechanism of autolysis of *Neisseria gonorrhoeae. J. Bacteriol.* **126**:1186–1193.

Hendley, J. O., K. R. Powell, R. Rodewald, H. H. Holzgrefe, and R. Lyles. 1977. Demonstration of a capsule on *Neisseria gonorrhoeae. N. Engl. J. Med.* **296**:608–611.

Henriksen, S. D. 1976. *Moraxella, Neisseria, Branhamella* and *Acinetobacter. Annu. Rev. Microbiol.* **30**:63–83.

Irwin, R. S., W. K. Woelk, and W. L. Coudon III. 1975. Primary meningococcal pneumonia. *Ann. Internal Med.* **82**:493–498.

Jacobs, N. F., and S. J. Kraus. 1975. Gonococcal and nongonococcal urethritis in men. *Ann. Internal Med.* **82**:7–12.

Johnston, K. H., K. K. Holmes, and E. C. Gotschlich. 1976. The serological classification of *Neisseria gonorrhoeae. J. Exp. Med.* **143**:741–758.

Wilson, C., D. L. Rose, and E. C. Tramont. 1976. Increased antibiotic resistance of *Neisseria gonorrhoeae* in Korea. *Antimicrob. Agents Chemother.* **9**:716–718.

# 20

# Enterics and Related
# Gram-Negative Organisms

The organisms forming the tremendously large and heterogenous group of gram-negative bacteria that are either part of the normal flora of the intestine or may cause gastrointestinal diseases are collectively called the "enterics." As we shall see, this designation includes the facultatively anaerobic bacteria in the families Enterobacteriaceae and Vibrionaceae, the obligately aerobic *Pseudomonas,* and the obligately anaerobic organisms in the family Bacteroidaceae.

## Enterobacteriaceae

Some of the members of the Enterobacteriaceae are always considered to be pathogens, while others are routinely found as part of the normal flora of the intestinal tract or as saprophytes living on decaying plant matter. All, however, have the potential to produce disease under appropriate conditions and must be considered opportunists.

The Enterobacteriaceae contain gram-negative rods, which, if motile, are peritrichously flagellated. Because members of this family are morphologically and metabolically similar, much effort has been expended to develop techniques for their rapid identification. In general, biochemical properties are used to define a genus, and further subdivision is frequently based on sugar fermentations and antigenic differences. There are, however, many paradoxes which, for example, have resulted in the naming of over 1,000 species of *Salmonella,* while the equally complex genus *Escherichia* contains a single species divided into over a thousand serotypes. It is obvious that over the years many taxonomists with different ideas have been involved in the classification of these bacteria, and it is not surprising that there is still disagreement concerning family and generic names. Table 20-1 gives an outline of the taxonomic scheme proposed by Ewing and Martin for the Enterobacteriaceae, compared to that proposed in the 8th edition of *Bergey's Manual of Determinative Bacteriology.* Both schemes are used in various

**Table 20-1. Classification of the Enterobacteriaceae**

| EWING AND MARTIN | | 8TH ED. BERGEY'S MANUAL | |
| --- | --- | --- | --- |
| Tribe | Genus | Tribe | Genus |
| Escherichieae | Escherichia | Escherichieae | Escherichia |
| | Shigella | | Shigella |
| Edwardsielleae | Edwardsiella | | Edwardsiella |
| Salmonelleae | Salmonella | | Salmonella |
| | Arizona | | Citrobacter |
| | Citrobacter | Klebsielleae | Klebsiella |
| Klebsielleae | Klebsiella | | Enterobacter |
| | Enterobacter | | Hafnia |
| | Serratia | | Serratia |
| Proteeae | Proteus | Proteeae | Proteus |
| | Providencia | Yersineae | Yersinia |
| Erwineae | Erwinia | Erwineae | Erwinia |
| | Pectobacterium | | |

diagnostic laboratories, but we shall adhere more closely to the Bergey classification in this chapter.

## BIOCHEMICAL PROPERTIES USED FOR THE CLASSIFICATION OF THE ENTEROBACTERIACEAE

Early taxonomic schemes relied heavily on the ability to ferment lactose, and numerous differential and selective media have been devised to allow one to recognize either a lactose-fermenting or a nonlactose-fermenting colony on a solid medium. The effectiveness of such differential media is based on the fact that organisms fermenting the lactose form acid, while nonlactose fermenters utilize the peptones present and do not form acids. The incorporation of an acid-base indicator into the agar medium thus causes a color change around a lactose-fermenting colony (see Figure 20-1). This has been a valuable technique for selecting the major non-lactose-fermenting pathogens that cause salmonellosis or shigellosis; we shall see,

**Figure 20-1.** Lactose-positive (left) and lactose-negative (right) enteric organisms grown on Hektoen enteric agar plates. Lactose-positive colonies are larger and become salmon to orange in color, whereas lactose-negative colonies remain colorless on the green agar medium.

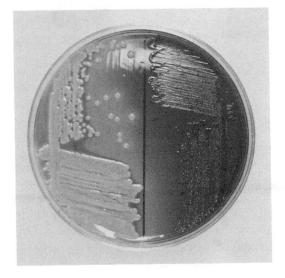

however, that under special conditions many lactose fermenters also cause a variety of infectious diseases.

In addition, many enterics ferment lactose only slowly, requiring several days before sufficient acid is formed to change the indicator. Such organisms were at one time all placed into a large category called the "paracolon" bacteria. However, it is now known that these bacteria are a heterogenous group, all of which synthesize beta-galactosidase, the enzyme which splits lactose into glucose and galactose, but lack the specific permease necessary for the transport of lactose into the cell. One can easily determine whether an organism is a slow or non-lactose fermenter by mixing a loopful of bacteria with ortho-nitrophenyl-beta-galactoside (ONPG) dissolved in a detergent. The linkage of the galactose in ONPG is the same as its linkage in lactose; inasmuch as the ONPG can enter the cell in the absence of a permease, an organism possessing beta-galactosidase will hydrolyze ONPG to yield galactose and the very bright yellow compound, ortho-nitrophenol. Thus, a slow lactose fermenter is an ONPG-positive organism that does not possess a specific lactose permease but does possess beta-galactosidase.

In addition, a number of selective media have been devised, containing bile salts, dyes such as brilliant green and methylene blue, and chemicals such as selenite and bismuth. The incorporation of such compounds into the growth medium has allowed for the selective growth of the enterics while inhibiting the growth of gram-positive organisms.

Some other biochemical properties used to classify members of the Enterobacteriaceae include the ability to: (1) form $H_2S$; (2) decarboxylate the amino acids lysine, ornithine, or phenylalanine; (3) hydrolyze urea into $CO_2$ and $NH_3$; (4) form indole from tryptophan; (5) grow with citrate as a sole source of carbon; (6) liquify gelatin; and (7) ferment a large variety of different sugars.

## SEROLOGIC PROPERTIES USED FOR THE CLASSIFICATION OF THE ENTEROBACTERIACEAE

No other group of organisms has been so extensively classified on the basis of cell surface antigens as the Enterobacteriaceae. These antigens can be divided into three types, designated O, K, and H antigens.

### O Antigens

As described in Chapter 3, all gram-negative bacteria possess a lipopolysaccharide (LPS) as a component of their outer membrane. This toxic LPS, or as it is also called, endotoxin, is composed of three regions—lipid A, core, and a repeating sequence of carbohydrates called the O antigen (see Figure 20-2). Based on different sugars, alpha- or beta-glycosidic linkages, and the presence or absence of substituted acetyl groups, *Escherichia coli* can be shown to possess over 150 different O antigens, and 64 have been described in the genus *Salmonella*.

Sometimes, after continuous laboratory growth, strains will mutate so as to lose the ability to synthesize or attach this oligosaccharide O antigen to the core region of the LPS. This loss results in a change from a smooth colony to a rough colony type, and it is referred to as an S to R transformation. Interestingly, the R mutants have lost the ability to produce disease.

### K Antigens

These antigens exist as capsule or envelope polysaccharides and cover the O antigens when present, inhibiting agglutination by specific O antiserum. Most K antigens can be removed by boiling the organisms in water, and, based on their lability to heat, they have been designated as A, B, or L type K antigens.

### H Antigens

Only those organisms that are motile will possess H antigens, since these determinants

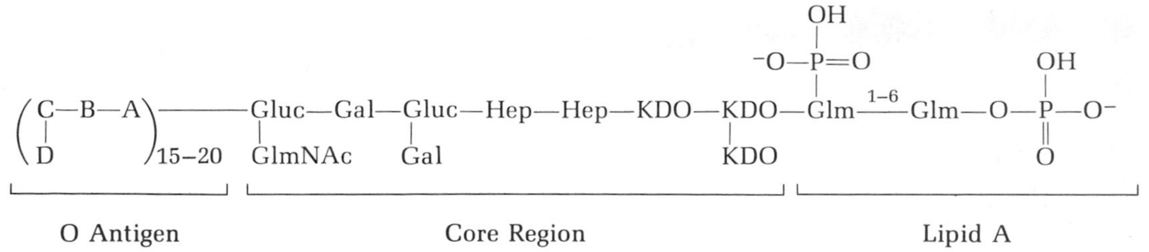

OH
|
-O—P=O    OH
|         |
$\left(\begin{array}{c} C-B-A \\ | \\ D \end{array}\right)_{15-20}$ —— Gluc—Gal—Gluc—Hep—Hep—KDO—KDO—Glm$\xrightarrow{1-6}$Glm—O—P—O⁻

GlmNAc  Gal              KDO              O

⌊_____⌋  ⌊_____⌋  ⌊_____⌋
   O Antigen              Core Region                    Lipid A

Glm      —Glucosamine
KDO      —Ketodeoxyoctonic acid
Hep      —Heptose
Gluc     —Glucose
Gal      —Galactose
GlmNAc—N-acetyl glucosamine
A,B,C,D —Monosaccharides such as mannose, galactose, rhamnose, fucose, glucose, abequose, and colitose. These sugars exist in a repeating sequence of 15 to 20 units of 3 or 4 sugars.

**Figure 20-2.** Schematic structure of one unit of *Salmonella* cell wall lipopolysaccharide (endotoxin). The structure of the cell wall LPS may vary slightly from one genus of gram-negative organism to another, but, as far as is known, all contain three general regions, as shown above. Although not shown here, all free hydroxyl groups of the glucosamines in lipid A are esterified with fatty acids. The serologic differences between different strains within a genus lie in the kinds of sugars and their linkages that exist in the O-antigen region.

are the proteins which make up the flagella. However, to complicate matters, members of the genus *Salmonella* will mutate back and forth to form different H antigens. The more specific ones are called phase 1 antigens and are designated by lower case letters (a, b, c, . . . ), while the less specific phase 2 H antigens are given letters and numbers.

After obtaining the serological data, one can write an antigenic formula such as: *Escherichia coli* O111:K58:H2, meaning this *E. coli* possesses O antigen 111, K antigen 58, and H antigen 2. *Salmonella togo* 4,12:l,w:1,6 indicates this serotype of *Salmonella* possesses O antigens 4 and 12, phase 1 H antigens l and w, and phase 2 H antigens 1 and 6.

## COLIFORMS

The meaning of the term "coliform" is somewhat arbitrary, but it usually includes those members of the Enterobacteriaceae that are normal inhabitants of the intestinal tract. With a few exceptions, these do not cause gastrointestinal-type diseases, and using this definition, the coliforms can be separated into two major groups: (1) *Escherichia* and (2) *Klebsiella, Enterobacter, Serratia,* and *Hafnia.*

*Escherichia coli* is an obligate intestinal parasite that cannot live free in nature, and its presence in water supplies is, therefore, evidence of recent fecal contamination.

### Presumptive Test for *E. coli*

To determine the presence of *E. coli* in water, test tubes of nutrient broth containing lactose are inoculated with measured quantities of water samples. These tubes also contain an inverted vial to trap gas produced and an acid-base indicator to show acid production (see

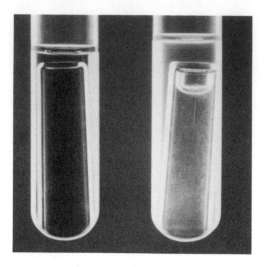

**Figure 20-3.** Fermentation tubes with inverted vials and acid indicator to test for *E. coli*. In the right-hand tube note the light color (actually yellow) due to the presence of acid and the bubble in the vial due to the evolution of gas.

Figure 20-3). Since *E. coli* ferments lactose, the presence of acid and gas in the inoculated tubes after 24 hours of incubation is presumptive evidence for its presence. If the lactose is not fermented, it is concluded that *E. coli* is not present, and the water is free from recent fecal contamination. The fermentation of lactose may, however, result from non-enteric organisms, and for a positive conclusion of fecal contamination it is necessary to show that the lactose-fermenting organisms are from fecal origin.

**Confirmed Test**

Because fecal coliforms can grow at 44.5°C whereas nonfecal coliforms cannot, differential agar media (containing lactose as a carbon source) can be streaked with known amounts of water and incubated at both temperatures. A comparison of the number of lactose-fermenting colonies growing at 37°C and 44.5°C will provide information concerning the origin of the coliforms. More

precise results, however, can be obtained by carrying out the following two tests. Eosine methylene blue (EMB) agar is streaked from the positive lactose broth fermentation grown at 37°C. *E. coli* grows as a very characteristic small flat colony that has a definitie metallic green sheen.

**Completed Test**

Colonies from the confirmed test that show a metallic green sheen are reinoculated into lactose broth, and if acid and gas are produced, the organism is identified as *E. coli*.

## DIFFERENTIATION OF *ESCHERICHIA* AND *ENTEROBACTER*

A number of biochemical tests, collectively referred to as the IMViC tests, are routinely used to differentiate between the two major groups of coliforms, and as an aid for the identification of other members of the Enterobacteriaceae.

<u>I</u>ndole is produced from tryptophan by *Escherichia,* but not *Enterobacter.* To test for the presence of indole one adds about 1 ml of diethyl ether to a broth culture of *E. coli* that has been grown in a medium containing a protein digest of high tryptophan content. The indole will be extracted from the aqueous broth and will be present in the colorless surface ether layer. The gentle addition of 0.5 ml of Kovac's reagent (5 grams of paradimethyl aminobenzaldehyde dissolved in 75 ml of amyl alcohol and 25 ml of concentrated HCl) will turn the ether layer pink if indole is present.

<u>M</u>ethyl red is an acid-base indicator that turns red below pH 4.5. *Escherichia* will ferment glucose broth to form considerable acid (see discussion of mixed acid fermentation in Chapter 3) and is methyl-red positive. *Enterobacter* carries out a butylene glycol fermentation (Chapter 3) and, hence, does not produce sufficient acid from glucose to be methyl-red positive.

<u>V</u>oges-Proskauer is the name of a test

used to detect the presence of acetoin (also called acetylmethylcarbinol), the immediate precursor of 2,3 butylene glycol. It is, thus, positive for *Enterobacter* and negative for *Escherichia*. One can assay for the presence of acetoin by taking advantage of the fact that acetoin is oxidized to diacetyl in the presence of excess alkali, and this compound reacts with creatinine (which is present in the medium) to form a red compound. Additional creatinine and α-naphthol accelerate the reaction.

Citrate utilization is negative for *Escherichia* because it lacks the permease to transport citrate into the cell. *Enterobacter* can both transport and utilize citrate as a sole carbon source.

## PATHOGENICITY OF THE COLIFORMS

### Escherichia coli

Although E. *coli* is part of the normal flora of the intestinal tract, it was suspected for years of being capable of causing a moderate to severe gastroenteritis in humans and animals. However, this was difficult to prove unequivocally, even though certain serotypes such as O111,B4 and O55,B5 appeared to be frequently associated with diarrhea. There are still some unknown factors associated with E. *coli* diarrhea, but it is now established that various E. *coli* strains may cause gastroenteritis by two seemingly different mechanisms: (1) by the production of one or two enterotoxins that indirectly result in fluid loss, or (2) by the actual invasion of the epithelial lining of the intestinal wall causing inflammation and fluid loss.

Enterotoxin-producing E. *coli*, called enteropathic E. *coli*, produce one or both of two different toxins. Some strains synthesize a heat-stable toxin called ST, while others produce in addition a heat-labile toxin referred to as LT. No strain is known that produces only LT. Both toxins cause diarrhea, but little is known concerning the chemistry or the mode of action of ST. It appears to be

a small protein which will retain its toxic activity even when heated to 100°C for 30 minutes.

LT, which is destroyed by heating at 65° C for 30 minutes, has been extensively purified, and its mode of action is identical to that described for cholera toxin. Thus, LT stimulates (in an as yet unknown manner) the activity of a membrane-bound adenyl cyclase. This results in the conversion of ATP to cyclic AMP (cAMP) as shown below:

$$ATP \xrightarrow[\text{cyclase}]{\text{adenyl}} cAMP + PP_i$$

Extremely minute amounts of cAMP will induce the active excretion of $Cl^-$ and inhibit the absorption of $Na^+$, creating an electrolyte disbalance across the intestinal mucosa that causes the loss of copious quantities of fluid from the intestine.

Interestingly, the genetic ability to produce both ST and LT resides on a single transmissible plasmid. Because of the ready conjugal transmission of this plasmid to other strains of E. *coli*, it seems that any serotype may become an enteropathic organism.

Animals are also subject to infections by their own strains of enteropathic E *coli*, and such infections in the newborn may result in death from the loss of fluids and electrolytes. Extensive studies of strains infecting newborn calves and piglets have revealed that, in addition to producing an enterotoxin, such strains possess a capsule (called a K antigen) that specifically adheres to the epithelial cells lining the small intestine. This capsule (K-88 for swine strains, and K-99 for cattle) is a pilus-like structure which provides very intimate contact between the toxin-producing organisms and the cells lining the small intestine. The requirement for this close association is supported by the fact that antibodies directed against the capsule are protective. Preliminary evidence now supports the fact that human enteropathic E. *coli* strains also possess pilus-like structures, and that antibody specific for these structures is protective (see Figure 20-4).

Those *E. coli* that produce diarrhea by the direct invasion of the epithelial cell lining of the intestinal wall have not been extensively studied. The examination of biopsy material, however, leaves no doubt that such an invasion does occur, but the specific property that provides these organisms with their invasive potential is far from understood. It certainly appears possible, though, that once an invasion of the intestinal lining has occurred, diarrheal disease may result from the toxic effects of the cell wall lipopolysaccharide (endotoxin). A more complete explanation for this disease must await a better understanding of the properties that confer the invasive abilities on these organisms.

Infection with pathogenic *E. coli* may cause a severe and sometimes fatal infection in newborns. The disease in adults, known by many names such as traveler's diarrhea or Montezuma's revenge, may vary from a mild disease with several days of loose stools, to a severe and fatal cholera-like disease. Oddly, the latter type of disease appears to occur almost exclusively in the Middle East, and it has been postulated that this unusual severity may be correlated with the nutritional condition of the infected individual.

*E. coli* is also a frequent cause of urinary tract infections of the bladder (cystitis) and, less frequently, of the kidney (pyelonephritis). In either case, infections are usually of an ascending type (enter the bladder from the urethra and enter the kidneys from the bladder). Many infections occur in young females, in persons with urinary tract obstructions, or in persons requiring urinary catheters, but they are also not infrequent in otherwise healthy women.

*E. coli* causes bacteremia and meningitis in the newborn, the debilitated patient, patients with leukemia, or those receiving immunosuppressive drugs.

### *Klebsiella pneumoniae* (Friedländers Bacillus)

This organism can be isolated from the respiratory or intestinal tract of about 5% of healthy individuals. The organism is nonmotile and can be subdivided into many types based on the antigenicity of its capsule. *K. pneumoniae* (types 1 and 2) may cause a severe and destructive bacterial pneumonia, but klebsiellae in general are more frequently involved in hospital-acquired urinary tract infections or as secondary invaders in other respiratory infections. Since *Klebsiella* can acquire the plasmids from *E. coli* that code for the heat-labile and heat-stable enterotoxins, it is not surprising that there has been a report linking it to an epidemic of diarrhea in a newborn nursery.

### *Enterobacter*

The bacteria in the genus *Enterobacter* can be differentiated from those in *Klebsiella* by the fact that they are motile. They occur as normal flora of the intestinal tract, but are also found on plant material as free-living organisms. *Enterobacter* is rarely a primary pathogen except in hospital-acquired urinary tract infections.

**Figure 20-4.** Cells of enterotoxigenic *E. coli* isolated from a patient with diarrhea and bearing a large number of pilus-like structures, or fimbriae (× 8,000).

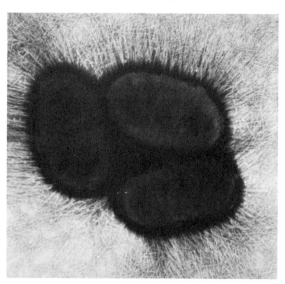

## Serratia

This genus was, in the past, considered to be totally innocuous, and because many strains synthesize a bright red pigment, the organisms were used to demonstrate bacteremia following dental extraction or the spread of organisms through a room by shaking hands. However, *Serratia* is now found to cause serious hospital-acquired infections—particularly in the newborn, the debilitated, or the patient receiving immunosuppressive drugs, and these organisms must be considered as opportunistic pathogens.

## Hafnia

The segregation of these organisms into a separate genus is disputed by some taxonomists who believe that they all should be included as a species of *Enterobacter*, particularly since the distribution and disease potential of their 197 serotypes are essentially identical to those of *Enterobacter*.

## EDWARDSIELLA AND CITROBACTER

*Edwardsiella* is a recently established genus of motile, $H_2S$-producing, non-lactose-fermenting enterics. They are occasionally isolated from the stools of humans with diarrhea, but they are also found in healthy humans. Metabolically, they are similar to the *Salmonella*.

*Citrobacter* is a genus of the Enterobacteriaceae that contains citrate-utilizing bacteria; they may be either slow or fast lactose fermenters. They appear to be antigenically similar to the *Salmonella* but are not true pathogens, even though they have occasionally been isolated from individuals with diarrhea or urinary tract infections. A group of organisms that was previously known as the Bethesda-Ballerup group is now classified within *Citrobacter*.

## PROTEUS AND PROVIDENCIA

This heterogenous group consists of very motile, non-lactose-fermenters which possess the ability to deaminate phenylalanine to phenylpyruvic acid.

*Proteus* is differentiated from *Providencia* by its ability to hydrolyze urea to $CO_2$ and $NH_3$; however, a recent classification has placed all of the non-urea-splitting *Providencia* into a single species named *Proteus inconstans*. Some taxonomists would prefer to subdivide the *Providencia* into two species, *Proteus alcalifaciens* and *Proteus stuartii*. Also, since the species *Proteus morganii* has a G + C ratio that is considerably higher than the other members of the genus *Proteus*, it has been suggested that it be placed in a new genus to be named *Morganella*. As can be seen, the taxonomy of this group is still in a rather fluid state.

In general, bacteria in the genus *Proteus* are noted for their rapid motility, which may result in their "swarming" over an agar plate rather than forming distinct colonies. Some strains of *Proteus*, designated OXK, OX2 and OX19, have antigens in common with some of the pathogenic rickettsia, and therefore the presence of antibodies to these strains of *Proteus* is used as a diagnostic aid for the diseases caused by certain rickettsiae (see Chapter 28).

*Proteus* is found in feces, sewage, and soil. Its species cause a number of opportunistic infections and probably rank close to *E. coli* in the frequency of urinary tract infections caused. *Proteus mirabilis* is the most frequent agent of *Proteus* bacteremias; *Proteus morganii* is believed to be responsible for occasional epidemics of infantile diarrhea, but the actual cause and effect relationship is not definite.

## ERWINIA

Although the members of this genus are included in the family Enterobacteriaceae, the fact that they are plant pathogens makes their inclusion in a textbook on medical microbiology somewhat unusual. However, during the early 1970's, a large series of "supposedly sterile" glucose-saline infusion bottles became contaminated with a gram-negative bacterium, and a number of patients died as a result of endotoxic shock following the intravenous use of this contaminated solution. The organism was originally identified as a member of the genus *Erwinia*, but later taxonomists decided that it should be classified as *Enterobacter agglomerans*. The 1974 edition of *Bergey's Manual of Determinative Bacteriology*, however, designates this organism as *Erwinia herbicola*.

The lessons to be learned from this tragic experience are that a solution can appear crystal clear and still contain on the order of a million bacteria per ml and, second, that no matter how innocuous the organism, the intravenous administration of large numbers of gram-negative bacteria will result in serious shock and possibly death of a patient.

## TREATMENT AND CONTROL OF THE NORMAL FLORA ENTERICS

Because of the many conjugations and transductions that occur among the members of the Enterobacteriaceae, susceptibility to any specific antibiotic will vary from strain to strain. In general, ampicillin has been effective for the treatment of many of the infections mentioned above. However, kanamycin, gentamycin, chloramphenicol, cephalothin, polymyxin, and streptomycin are also used in situations where the organisms are resistant to ampicillin.

Since many of these organisms found as "normal flora" are opportunists, control measures are directed more toward the prevention of nosocomial infections in the individual who is most susceptible to infection.

It is apparent from the brief descriptions of these "normal flora" enterics that all can cause disease under certain circumstances and that these circumstances occur most frequently in hospitalized patients whose specific and nonspecific immune systems are no longer fully functional. Most of us will probably go through a large portion (if not all) of our lives without experiencing an infection caused by these organisms. The following

two genera of the Enterobacteriaceae to be discussed in this chapter, the *Salmonella* and the *Shigella*, cannot, however, be considered as normal flora at any time.

## SALMONELLA

The term salmonellosis may be used to describe any infection caused by members of the genus *Salmonella*. This is an extremely large group of gram-negative rods that can be distinguished from the normal flora of the intestine using biochemical and antigenic criteria.

The Kauffman-White scheme is a complex antigen classification in which each *Salmonella* is assigned to a group based on the O antigens present in its cell wall lipopolysaccharide. Thus, each organism possessing O antigen 2 is placed into group A. All those possessing O antigen 4 are in group B, and so on; groups are lettered A to Z, and then the remaining groups are numbered 51 through 65. Table 20-2 lists a few examples of some of the more frequent human pathogens, showing their group placement and O antigen designation. As you can see from this table, the group designation is based on the presence of one dominant antigen, even though other O antigens are present in the organism. Also, notice the subgroups which depend on the over-all complement of O antigens possessed by a species.

The salmonellae in any one group can be further divided into serotypes on the basis of the H antigens that occur in both phase 1 and phase 2. Also, some salmonellae form a polysaccharide antigen on the outer surface of the cell that covers up the O antigen layer of the organism. Since this antigen has been found most frequently in recently isolated virulent organisms, it is called the Vi antigen, indicating virulence. Because the Vi antigen surrounds the O antigen, organisms possessing a Vi antigen will not agglutinate in specific O antiserum unless the Vi antigen is first destroyed by placing the bacteria in a boiling water bath.

## Table 20-2. Kauffman-White Classification of Selected Salmonellae

| Species or Serotype | O ANTIGENS[A] | H ANTIGENS | |
|---|---|---|---|
| | | Phase 1 | Phase 2 |
| GROUP A | | | |
| Sal. paratyphi | 1, **2**, 12 | a | — |
| GROUP B | | | |
| Sal. schottmuelleri | 1, **4**, 12 | b | 1, 2 |
| GROUP C₁ | | | |
| Sal. cholerasuis | **6**, 7 | c | 1, 5 |
| Sal. montevideo | **6**, 7 | g, m, s | — |
| GROUP C₂ | | | |
| Sal. manhattan | **6**, 8 | d | 1, 5 |
| GROUP D₁ | | | |
| Sal. typhi | **9**, 12, (Vi) | d | — |
| Sal panama | 1, **9**, 12 | l, v | 1, 5 |
| GROUP D₂ | | | |
| Sal. strasbourg | **9**, 46 | d | 1, 7 |
| GROUP E₁ | | | |
| Sal. anatum | **3**, 10 | e, h | 1, 6 |
| GROUP E₂ | | | |
| Sal. new-brunswick | **3**, 15 | l, v | 1, 7 |
| GROUP E₃ | | | |
| Sal. minneapolis | **3**, 15, 34 | e, h | 1, 6 |
| GROUP H | | | |
| Sal. florida | 1, 6, **14**, 25 | d | 1, 7 |

[A]O antigen in bold type is common to all members of the group.

Salmonellae do not ferment lactose, but most form $H_2S$, form gases from carbohydrates, and will decarboxylate lysine. *Salmonella typhi* is an exception, in that it produces very little $H_2S$ or gas from carbohydrate fermentation. *Sal. arizonae,* which consists of over 300 serotypes, is a second exception in that these organisms are slow lactose fermenters. Many taxonomists prefer to place the organisms in this group into a separate genus called *Arizona.*

Originally, the salmonellae were given species names that were descriptive of the disease they caused. Later, as more antigenic types were described, a system of nomenclature was used which named each new antigenic type according to the geographical area where it was isolated. So, we have names such as *Sal. typhi, Sal. cholerasuis, Sal. minneapolis,* and *Sal. arizonae.* Current practice, however, tends to use only three species of Salmonella: (1) *Sal. typhi,* (2) *Sal. cholerasuis,* and (3) *Sal. enteriditis.* More than 1000 additional antigenic types are listed as serotypes of *Sal. enteriditis,* such as *Sal. enteriditis* serotype alabama or *Sal. enteriditis* serotype miami.

### Epidemiology and Pathogenesis of Salmonellosis

The primary reservoir for the salmonellae are the intestinal tracts of many animals, including birds, farm animals, and reptiles. Humans become infected through the ingestion of contaminated water or food. Water, of course, becomes polluted by the introduction of feces from any animal excreting salmonellae. Infection via food usually results either from the ingestion of contaminated meat or via the hands, which act as intermediates in the transfer of salmonellae from an infected source. Thus, the handling of an infected though apparently healthy dog or cat can result in contamination with salmonellae. Another major source of *Salmonella* infections is pet turtles. In fact, it is estimated that in the early 1970's there were almost 300,000 cases of turtle-associated salmonellosis annually in the United States, and, as a result, it is now illegal to import turtles or turtle eggs or even to ship domestic turtles with shells less than four inches in diameter across state lines.

On an industrial scale, slaughterhouse workers are faced with salmonellosis as an occupational hazard, primarily from poultry and pigs. Because humans can become asymptomatic carriers of *Salmonella*, infected food handlers also are responsible for the spread of these organisms.

The general types of infections which may be caused by the salmonellae usually are grouped into three categories: enteric fevers, septicemias, and gastroenteritis.

### Enteric Fevers

Typhoid fever, caused by *Salmonella typhi*, is the classical enteric fever. Following an incubation period of one to three weeks after ingestion of the organisms, there is inflammation in the small intestine which is followed by invasion of the regional lymph nodes. From the lymphatic system, the organisms enter the blood and infect various organs and tissues, including the liver, kidneys, spleen, bone marrow, gall bladder, and sometimes the heart. Enlargement of the spleen is characteristic, and multiplication of the organisms in the skin may result in the presence of rose spots, particularly on the abdomen. Symptoms may also include headache, loss of appetite, abdominal pain, weakness, stupor, and a continued fever.

Other species of *Salmonella* also cause enteric fevers, but usually these "paratyphoid" fevers are milder than that caused by *Salmonella typhi*.

LABORATORY DIAGNOSIS OF TYPHOID FEVER. The organisms can be isolated from the blood during the first two weeks of the illness and from the urine usually between the first and fourth week. Stool specimens may remain positive for indefinite periods of time. Preincubation in selenite or tetrathionate broth is occasionally used to enrich the growth of the *Salmonella* over the coliforms prior to streaking the organisms on various selective and differential media.

A retrospective diagnosis, also, can be made by demonstrating a rise in agglutinating antibodies to *Salmonella typhi*. To be valid, this test (known as the Widal test) must show at least a four-fold increase in titer between the acute and convalescent phase serum.

TREATMENT AND CONTROL OF TYPHOID FEVER. Chloramphenicol is the major antibiotic effective against *Sal. typhi*. It causes a reduction in the febrile (fever) period, but, since many organisms grow intracellularly in monocytes, the administration of chloramphenicol must be continued for at least two weeks to avoid recurrent febrile attacks. However, because aplastic anemia (inability to make red blood cells because of a defect in the bone marrow) can result from the use of this antibiotic, many physicians are reluctant to prescribe it unless absolutely necessary. Ampicillin also may be effective, but results may not be as dramatic as those seen with chloramphenicol.

Proper sewage disposal and the periodic examination of food handlers, to ascertain that they are not carriers, remain our best method of control of typhoid fever. Convalescent patients may remain carriers for long periods of time, and ridding them of the organisms is sometimes extremely difficult. In 1971 British officials banned from their schools for life two children who were persistant carriers of *Sal. typhi.* Health officials stated that they had tried every known drug treatment on the children, and one official predicted that they would remain carriers the rest of their lives. Since the organisms tend to grow in the bile ducts, some carriers have been cured by the surgical removal of their gall bladder.

Active immunization against *Sal. typhi* has been carried out for years using a killed vaccine containing *Sal. typhi* and two additional paratyphoid organisms. However, the procedure is only moderately effective, and it is not used routinely in the United States. A newer acetone-inactivated vaccine has been used in Eastern Europe and is reported to be quite effective.

### *Salmonella* Septicemia

Septicemia caused by *Salmonella* is a fulminating blood infection that does not involve the gastrointestinal tract. Most cases are caused by *Salmonella cholerasuis* and are characterized by supporative lesions throughout the body. Pneumonia, osteomyelitis, or meningitis may result from such an infection. *Salmonella* osteomyelitis is especially prevalent in persons who have sickle cell anemia.

### Gastroenteritis

Gastroenteritis is, without doubt, the most common type of *Salmonella* infection. It may be caused by any one of the thousands of serotypes of *Salmonella,* and it is characterized by the fact that organisms remain localized in the gut. In the average case, symptoms occur 10 to 28 hours after ingesting contaminated food, and the headache, abdominal pain, nausea, vomiting, and diarrhea may continue for two to four days.

Unless it is unusually severe, most cases of *Salmonella* gastroenteritis are not treated with antibiotics.

### SHIGELLA

Members of the genus *Shigella* are pathogens that cause a serious disease known as bacillary dysentery. The genus is divided into four subgroup species, and (as shown in Table 20-3) each species may be additionally divided into serotypes. Since all *Shigella* are nonmotile, H antigens are not involved in their serological classification. *Shigella sonnei* is a slow lactose fermenter, but no other species of *Shigella* can ferment lactose. *Shigella* organisms are unable to form $H_2S$.

Shigellae are serologically related to *Escherichia coli,* probably because of intergeneric conjugation resulting in considerable genetic mixing. Both carry out a mixed acid fermentation of glucose, but the *Shigella* do not metabolize the formic acid produced and hence do not form gas.

### Epidemiology and Pathogenesis of Infections Caused by *Shigella*

Humans appear to be the only natural host for the shigellae, and they become infected following the ingestion of contaminated food or water. Unlike *Salmonella,* the organisms remain localized in the gut, and the debilitating effects of shigellosis are largely attributable to the loss of fluids and electrolytes.

*Shigella dysenteriae* type 1 (sometimes called Shiga's bacillus) excretes a potent neurotoxin and enterotoxin. The neurotoxin is characterized by the paralysis and death it causes when injected into experimental animals such as rabbits or guinea pigs. The enterotoxin can be readily demonstrated by fluid accumulation in ligated segments of

Table 20-3. Classification of *Shigella*

| Subgroup Species | Number of Serotypes |
| --- | --- |
| Shigella dysenteriae | 10 |
| Shigella flexneri | 8 |
| Shigella boydii | 15 |
| Shigella sonnei | 1 |

rabbit ileum. Attempts to separate these toxins have been unsuccessful, and it is thought that both toxic effects may reside in the same molecule.

No other serotype of *Shigella* is known to produce an exotoxin, but all possess some (as yet unknown) virulence factor which permits them to invade the epithelial cells and lamina propria of the intestine to cause ulcerative lesions. It seems possible that endotoxin is, in part, responsible for the actual lesion and that the loss of fluids and electrolytes is a result of the death of the epithelial cells.

### Laboratory Diagnosis of Shigellosis

Isolation and identification of the etiologic agent is necessary for a definitive diagnosis. The organisms are not particularly hearty, and best results are obtained when a direct swab of the ulcerative lesions is streaked out on selective media such as MacConkey or eosin methylene blue (EMB) plates.

### Treatment and Control of Shigellosis

Intravenous replacement of fluids and electrolytes plus antibiotic therapy are used for severe cases of shigellosis. Ampicillin is frequently not effective, and alternative therapies employ chloramphenicol and sulfa trimethoprim. In the Far East where shigellosis is more common than in the United States, multiple antibiotic resistance due to the acquisition of plasmids called resistance transfer factors (RTF) has become common (see Chapter 10). Shigellosis is also very common in Latin America.

Control is usually directed toward sanitary measures designed to prevent the spread of the organisms. The injection of killed vaccines is worthless, since humoral IgG does not appear to be involved in immunity to the localized intestinal infection. Live vaccines that have lost the ability to invade the epithelial cells of the gut have been shown to be effective—probably by stimulating the formation of IgA antibodies.

# Vibrionaceae

### VIBRIO CHOLERAE

*Vibrio cholerae* is a small, curved, (comma-shaped) gram-negative organism possessing a single polar flagellum (see Figure 20-5). The organisms have many similarities to the members of the Enterobacteriaceae but can be readily differentiated by their positive oxidase reaction and their ability to grow at a pH between 9.0 and 9.5.

A number of serologic types have been reported based on antigenic differences in their O antigen. Of these, three strains have been given specific names: Inaba, Ogawa, and Hikojima. The occurrence of the Hikojima strain as a valid serotype, however, has been disclaimed by some investigators who state that it is merely an intermediate between the Inaba and Ogawa serotypes. In addition,

there is a strain which produces a soluble hemolysin that has been designated the El Tor strain of *V. cholerae*. Other vibrios that are either serologically unrelated or share partial antigenicity with the above strains may also cause diarrheal disease. Because these latter strains fail to agglutinate when

**Figure 20-5.** *Vibrio cholerae,* Leifson flagellar stain (about × 1000).

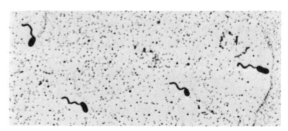

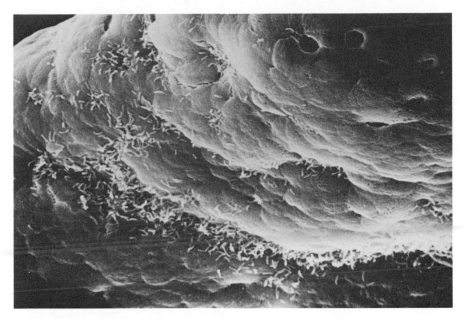

**Figure 20-6.** Numerous cells of *Vibrio cholerae* attached to rabbit intestinal villus ($\times$ 1400).

mixed with antiserum to the classical strains, they have been collectively referred to as either non-agglutinable (NAG) or non-cholera vibrios (NCV). It has been recommended that these organisms be included in the species *V. cholerae* and designated by serotypes. However, since they have not been incriminated in devastating outbreaks of cholera, some experts object to their inclusion in the species designation *V. cholerae*.

### Epidemiology and Pathogenesis of Cholera

Cholera, the disease caused by *V. cholerae*, is spread as a fecal-oral disease, and people acquire the infection by the ingestion of fecally contaminated water and food. The organisms do not spread beyond the gastrointestinal tract, where they multiply to very high concentrations in the small and large intestine. Unlike the shigellae, they do not penetrate the epithelial layer, but remain adhered to the intestinal mucosa (see Figure 20-6).

The major symptom is a severe diarrhea in which a patient may lose as much as 10 to 15 liters of liquid per day. The feces contain mucous, epithelial cells, and large numbers of vibrios and have been referred to as "rice water stools." Death, which may occur in as many as 60% of cases, results from severe dehydration and loss of electrolytes.

*Vibrio cholerae* produces diarrhea as a result of the secretion of an enterotoxin that acts to stimulate the activity of the enzyme adenyl cyclase. This, in turn, converts ATP to cyclic AMP (cAMP) which stimulates the secretion of $Cl^-$ and inhibits the absorption of $Na^+$. The copious fluid that is lost also contains large amounts of bicarbonate and $K^+$. Thus, the patient has both a severe fluid loss and an electrolyte disbalance.

The enterotoxin has been shown to bind specifically to a membrane ganglioside, designated $GM_1$ (shown in Figure 20-7). Interestingly, *V. cholerae* produces a neuraminidase that is unable to remove the N-acetylneuraminic acid (NANA) from $GM_1$, but it is able

$$\left(\text{Cer} \longrightarrow 1\,\text{gluc}\,4 \xrightarrow{\;\beta\;} 1\,\text{gal}\,4 \xrightarrow{\;\beta\;} 1\,\text{gal NAc}\,3 \xrightarrow{\;\beta\;} 1\,\text{gal}\right)$$
$$\underset{2\,\text{NANA}}{\overset{\alpha}{\uparrow}}\;\;\;\;\;\;\;3$$

**Figure 20-7.** Repeating sequence of the ganglioside $GM_1$. Although other gangliosides also bind cholera toxin in varying amounts, $GM_1$ is at least 35-fold more efficient than the next best. Cer = ceramide; gluc = glucose; gal = galactose; NANA = N-acetylneuraminic acid; gal NAc = N-acetylgalactosamine.

**Figure 20-8.** Giemsa stain of Chinese hamster ovary cells ($\times$ 500) 24 hours after exposure to the culture filtrate of nontoxigenic control *Escherichia coli* (a) and that the enterotoxigenic *E. coli* strain 334 (b).

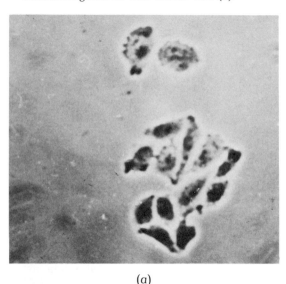

(a)

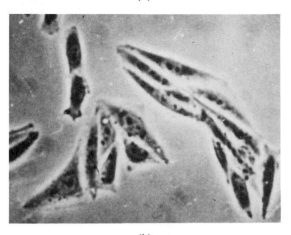

(b)

to convert other gangliosides to $GM_1$, thus synthesizing even more receptor sites to which its enterotoxin can bind.

Cholera toxin (as well as the LT toxin produced by enteropathic *E. coli*) can be quantitated by two techniques. In one method a segment of rabbit small intestine is tied so as to form a loop. Enterotoxin is serially diluted and an aliquot of each dilution is injected into the loop. The highest dilution that stimulates fluid accumulation in the loop is recorded as the titer of the enterotoxin. A second method takes advantage of the fact that cAMP causes a morphologic response in cultured Chinese hamster ovary cells and that enterotoxin will induce such cells to produce cAMP. Figure 20-8 illustrates the changes induced by a toxigenic strain of *E. coli*. To quantitate enterotoxin using this assay, one establishes a standard curve (with purified enterotoxin) which can be used subsequently to assay an unknown enterotoxin from *E. coli* or *V. cholerae* (see Figure 20-9).

### Laboratory Diagnosis of Cholera

The organisms can be viewed directly in the stools, particularly with a dark-field microscope. Additionally, because *Vibrio cholerae* is able to grow at a higher pH than other enterics, selective media at alkaline pH values are used. Fluorescently-labeled antiserum can be used to confirm the identification of the observed organisms.

### Treatment and Control of Cholera

The mortality of cholera can be dropped to less than 1% by the adequate replacement of

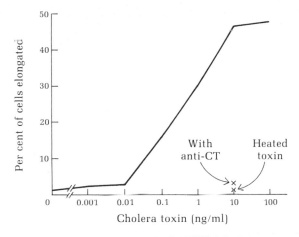

**Figure 20-9.** A standard curve to equate *E. coli* enterotoxin with purified cholera toxin. The percent of Chinese hamster ovary cells that have elongated after growing 24 hours in the presence of cholera toxin in 1% fetal calf serum is plotted against the concentration of cholera toxin present in the culture. As shown, heated toxin or toxin preincubated with antitoxin (anti-CT) have no effect on the morphology of the cells.

fluids and electrolytes. The recent observation that the inclusion of glucose in the salt solution allows oral replacement of electrolytes has made treatment of this disease (particularly in rural areas) much more effective. An epidemic in Portugal that ended in 1974 reported 2241 cases but only 38 deaths. Antibiotics, particularly tetracycline, reduce the number of intestinal vibrios and should be used along with fluid replacement.

Control of cholera requires proper sewage disposal and adequate water sanitation. Although it has become practically nonexistent in much of the Western world, cholera is still endemic in parts of Asia and India.

Immunization with cholera organisms appears to give some protection, and recovery from the disease imparts immunity of an unknown degree or duration. Chemical degradation of the enterotoxin has shown that it can be dissociated into one polypeptide of 28,000 daltons (H polypeptide) and seven polypeptides of 8,000 to 9,000 daltons (L polypeptide). Only the L polypeptide will bind to the specific receptor sites on the $GM_1$ ganglioside; thus, if one could stimulate IgA antibody production to the L polypeptide, production of an effective vaccine might be possible.

### VIBRIO PARAHEMOLYTICUS

*V. parahemolyticus* is a marine bacterium that requires a high NaCl concentration for growth. It has attained major importance as the etiologic agent of food poisoning following the ingestion of uncooked or partially cooked seafood, particularly shellfish.

The organisms appear to be distributed worldwide and to have caused a multitude of cases of acute enteritis in the United States. In countries such as Japan where seafoods comprise a high percentage of the normal diet, *V. parahemolyticus* is estimated to be the etiologic agent of about half of all cases of bacterial food poisoning. The best means of prevention is to eat only seafood that is well cooked.

## Pseudomonas

Most members of this vast genus of obligately aerobic gram-negative rods are free-living organisms, joined by some plant pathogens and only a very few species associated with human diseases. Prior to the 1940's, *Pseudomonas* infections were rare,

but these organisms have become among the more common opportunists that infect debilitated, burned, or immunosuppressed individuals.

Human diseases have been caused by *Ps. cepacia*, *Ps. multivorans*, *Ps. fluorescens*, *Ps.*

### Table 20-4. Protein Synthesis in the Liver of Normal and Toxin-Treated Mice

| Injection | Time after injection (h) | Amino acid incorporation[a] | Percent, toxin-treated saline-treated |
|---|---|---|---|
| Saline | 1–3[b] | 2,765 ± 252 | |
| Toxin | | 1,822 ± 304 | 66.0 |
| Saline | 2–4 | 2,933 ± 444 | |
| Toxin | | 1,418 ± 508 | 48.3 |
| Saline | 16–18 | 2,989 ± 354 | |
| Toxin | | 564 ± 41 | 18.8 |

[a]Mean counts per minute per milligram of protein ± the standard deviation.
[b]First number indicates the time of amino acid injection post-toxin; second number indicates the end of the pulse.

putida, Ps. pseudomallei, Ps. stutzeri, and Ps. maltophilia, but by far the most common human pathogen is Ps. aeruginosa.

## PSEUDOMONAS AERUGINOSA

Pseudomonas aeruginosa is found in stools of 5% of healthy individuals, but this figure may approach 50% during hospitalization. The organism usually produces two water-soluble pigments, a bluish pigment named pyocyanin and a greenish fluorescent pigment called fluorescein. In addition, Ps. aeruginosa may produce a number of other extracellular products and toxins, but most have not been studied sufficiently to pinpoint their role in the pathogenesis of infection. One product, however, that has been extensively studied is an exotoxin designated PA toxin. The potency of this toxin can be attested by the fact that it has an $LD_{50}$ (lethal dose for 50% of the population) of less than one microgram for the mouse and, on a weight basis, shows a similar $LD_{50}$ for monkeys, dogs, and cats. It has been shown to inhibit protein synthesis, as illustrated in Table 20-4. Note that the protein synthesis was markedly inhibited as the time the cells were in contact with the toxin increased. It is also lethal for various cell cultures, as shown in Table 20-5, apparently due to inhibition of protein synthesis. Surprisingly, the mechanism of action of PA toxin is identical to that of diphtheria

toxin (see Chapter 24) in which the toxin acts enzymatically to cleave the nicotinamide moiety from NAD, and then to catalyze the transfer of the resulting ADP-ribose to form a covalent bond with elongation factor 2 (EF-2). Because EF-2 is required for the ribosome to move to the next codon, its inactivation freezes the ribosome and protein synthesis stops.

Although the PA toxin from Pseudomonas aeruginosa is reported to act by the same intracellular mechanism as diphtheria toxin, the two toxins are not identical. Antisera to either toxin will neutralize the homologous product, but, as shown in Table 20-6, there is no cross reaction between PA and diphtheria toxin. In addition, PA toxin cannot be cleaved into two components by mild trypsin

### Table 20-5. Effect of Pseudomonas aeruginosa Toxin on Various Mammalian Cell Cultures.

| Cell Line | Percent of $^{14}C$ Amino Acid Uptake After 5-Hour Exposure | Percent Viable Cells After 24-Hour Exposure |
|---|---|---|
| L cells | 20 | 0–10 |
| Vero | 25 | 0–10 |
| PSY-15 | 60 | 40–60 |
| HeLa | 72 | 20–30 |
| KB | 85 | Not done |

treatment and disulfide bond reduction as can diphtheria toxin, nor is there any evidence that the production of PA toxin occurs as a result of lysogenic conversion as occurs in diphtheria. The fact that two different toxins from entirely unrelated organisms are both able to ADP-ribosylate mammalian EF-2 make it appear that this reaction must play some functional role in bacteria and that the site on mammalian EF-2 serves as a cross-reacting protein. It is interesting to speculate as to why *Pseudomonas aeruginosa* rarely infects a healthy person while literally millions of individuals have died from diphtheria. The answer is not known at this time, but the low invasive ability of *Pseudomonas aeruginosa* may result from differences in cell specificity between the PA toxin and diphtheria toxin.

In spite of its lack of invasiveness, *Pseudomonas aeruginosa* does cause infections and severe disease under the following circumstances: (1) it can cause infections when it is mechanically placed into the urinary tract during catheterization or into the meninges during a lumbar puncture; (2) it is able to infect respiratory ventilators and deliver large numbers of organisms directly into the lungs of an already debilitated person; (3) it may cause a fatal sepsis in persons with leukemia or persons who are receiving immunosuppressive drugs, or it may cause a septic arthritis or endocarditis in heroin addicts; and (4) because of its resistance to many antibiotics, it can cause severe infections in persons receiving antibiotic therapy for burns, wounds, cystic fibrosis, and so forth. Table 20-7 provides data for the incidence of *Pseudomonas* infections in a large number of hospitalized individuals. As can be seen, burn patients are by far the most susceptible in that approximately 25% become infected.

Current therapy uses tobramycin, carbenicillin, colistin, gentamicin, and polymyxin B. However, because of the frequency with which these organisms become resistant to antibiotics, new antimicrobials will, undoubtedly, soon become the therapy of choice.

**Table 20-6. Effect of Specific Antiserum on the NAD Transferase Activity of Fragment A of Diphtheria Toxin and on *Pseudomonas aeruginosa* Exotoxin**

| PREINCUBATION SERUM | ACID-INSOLUBLE RADIOACTIVITY (CPM) | | |
|---|---|---|---|
| | $H_2O$ | 0.02 µg of fragment A | 0.02 µg of P.A. Toxin |
| $H_2O$ | 164 | 1328 | 1651 |
| Normal rabbit serum | | 1556 | 1080 |
| Rabbit anti-fragment-A serum | | 284 | 1545 |
| Normal horse serum, 1:10 | | 1684 | 1309 |
| Pony anti-P.A.-toxin serum, 1:10 | | 1544 | 168 |

**Table 20-7. Risk of Infection Due to *Pseudomonas* in 90,000 Patients Under Surveillance in Community Hospitals**

| Hospital Service or Area | Site of Infection | Patients at Risk/ 1,000 |
|---|---|---|
| Burn unit | Burn | 246 |
| Burn unit | Urinary tract | 16 |
| Burn unit | Surgical wound | 11 |
| Urology | Urinary tract | 6 |
| Burn unit | Lower respiratory tract | 5 |
| General surgery | Surgical wound | 4 |
| Medicine | Urinary tract | 4 |
| General surgery | Urinary tract | 4 |
| General surgery | Lower respiratory tract | 3 |
| Gynecology | Urinary tract | 2 |

## Obligately Anaerobic Enterics

It may seem paradoxical that the largest part of our normal flora is so obligately anaerobic that even short periods of exposure to air will result in their death. We often think that the coliforms make up the majority of our normal intestinal flora, but in truth they are outnumbered more than 100 to one by the obligately anaerobic gram-negative rods in the family Bacteroidaceae. Two genera of this family, *Bacteroides* and *Fusobacterium*, are also found to a lesser extent in the mouth, vagina, and external genitalia.

Both of these genera can be considered opportunists with little invasive ability; however, accidental trauma or surgical proce-dures can provide the opportunity for these organisms to invade and multiply. Common infections include peritonitis and bacteremia with serious abscess formation in many organs of the body, particularly the lungs and brain. *Bacteroides fragilis* is the most common species involved, but many infections are mixed infections which include both the anaerobic streptococci and *Fusobacterium*.

Treatment almost always requires surgical drainage, together with antibiotic therapy. Clindamycin, penicillin, and chloramphenicol are all useful in treating infections caused by the obligate anaerobes.

## REFERENCES

Abe, P. M., E. S. Lennard, and J. W. Holland. 1976. *Fusobacterium necrophorum* infection in mice as a model for the study of liver abscess formation and induction of immunity. *Infect. Immun.* **13**:1473–1478.

Callahan, L. T., III. 1974. Purification and characterization of *Pseudomonas aeruginosa* exotoxin. *Infect. Immun.* **9**:113–118.

Elin, R. J., and S. W. Wolff. 1976. Biology of endotoxin. *Annu. Rev. Med.* **27**:127–141.

Evans, D. G., R. P. Silver, D. J. Evans, D. G. Chase, and S. L. Gorbach. 1975. Plasmid-controlled colonization factor associated with virulence in *Escherichia coli* enterotoxigenic for humans. *Infect. Immun.* **12**:656–667.

Finkelstein, R. A. 1975. Immunology of cholera. *Curr. Topics Microbiol. Immunol.* **69**:137–195.

Fisher, M. 1975. Polyvalent vaccine and human γ-globulin for controlling *Pseudomonas aeruginosa* infections. In David Schlessinger, ed. *Microbiology 1975.* Amer. Soc. Microbiol., Washington, D.C.

Fukumi, H., and M. Ohashi, eds. 1971. *Symposium on Cholera.* Japanese Cholera Panel: U.S.–Japan cooperative science program. Natl. Inst. of Health, Tokyo 141, Japan.

Guerrant, R. L., L. L. Brunton, T. C. Schnaitman, L. I. Rebhun, and A. G. Gilman. 1974. Cyclic adenosine monophosphate and alteration of Chinese hamster ovary cell morphology: A rapid sensitive *in vitro* assay for the enterotoxins of *Vibrio cholerae* and *Escherichia coli*. *Infect. Immun.* **10**:320–327.

Hirschhorn, N., and W. B. Greenough, III. 1971. Cholera. *Sci. American* **225**:15–21.

Holdeman, L. V., I. J. Good, and W. E. C. Moore. 1976. Human fecal flora: Variation in bacterial composition within individuals and a possible effect of emotional stress. *J. Appl. Microbiol.* **31**:359–375.

Iglewski, B. H., and D. Kabat. 1975. NAD-dependent inhibition of protein synthesis by *Pseudomonas aeruginosa* toxin. *Proc. Nat. Acad. Sci. U.S.A.* **72**:2284–2288.

Iglewski, B. H., P. V. Liu, and D. Kabat. 1977. Mechanism of action of *Pseudomonas aeruginosa* exotoxin A: Adenosine diphosphate-ribosylation of mammalian elongation factor 2 *in vitro* and *in vivo*. *Infec. Immun.* **15**:138–144.

Isaacson, R. E., and H. W. Moon. 1975. Induction of heat-labile enterotoxin synthesis in enterotoxigenic *Escherichia coli* by mitomycin C. *Infect. Immun.* **12**:1271–1275.

Levine, M. M., H. L. Dupont, R. B. Hornick, M. J. Snyder, W. Woodward, R. H. Gilman, and J. P. Libonati. 1976. Attenuated streptomycin-dependent *Salmonella typhi* oral vaccine: Potential deleterious effects of lyophilization. *J. Infect. Dis.* **133**:424–429.

Liu, P. V., S. Yoshii, and H. Hsieh. 1973. Exotoxins of *Pseudomonas aeruginosa*. II. Concentration, purification and characterization of exotoxin A. *J. Infect. Dis.* **128**:514–519.

Meyers, B. R., E. Bottone, S. Z. Hirschman, and S. S. Schneierson. 1972. Infections caused by microorganisms of the genus *Erwinia*. *Ann. Internal Med.* **76**:9–14.

Pavolovskis, O. R., L. T. Callahan, III, and M. Pollack. 1975. *Pseudomonas aeruginosa* exotoxin. In David Schlessinger, ed. *Microbiology 1975*. Amer. Soc. Microbiol., Washington, D.C.

Poupard, J. A., I. Husain, and R. F. Norris. 1973. Biology of the bifidobacteria. *Bacteriol. Rev.* **37**:136–165.

Ryder, R. W., M. H. Merson, R. A. Pollard, Jr., and E. J. Gangarso. 1976. Salmonellosis in the United States, 1968–1974. *J. Infect. Dis.* **133**:483–485.

Sack, R. B. 1975. Human diarrheal disease caused by enterotoxic *Escherichia coli*. *Annu. Rev. Microbiol.* **29**:333–353.

Sanderson, K. E. 1976. Genetic relatedness in the family Enterobacteriaceae. *Annu. Rev. Microbiol.* **30**:327–349.

Siebeling, R. J., P. M. Neal, and W. D. Granberry. 1975. Treatment of *Salmonella-Arizona* infected turtle eggs with terramycin and chloromycetin by the temperature-differential egg dip method. *J. Appl. Microbiol.* **30**:791–799.

Stirm, S., F. Ørskov, I. Ørskov, and A. Birch-Anderson. 1967. Episome-carried surface antigen K88 of *Escherichia coli*: III. Morphology. *J. Bacteriol.* **93**:740–748.

# 21

# Brucella, Yersinia, Francisella, and Pasteurella

All the organisms discussed in this chapter are animal pathogens with which humans become infected after contact with an infected animal or animal product or from the bite of an infected insect or arthropod vector. Thus, with the possible exception of epidemics of human plague by *Yersinia pestis,* these bacteria reach the end of the line when they infect humans because transmission among humans is unusual.

## BRUCELLA

At one time, there were a number of synonyms for *Brucella* infections, including Malta fever, Mediterranean fever, Gibraltar fever, Cyprus fever, and undulant fever, but now all infections by species of *Brucella* are usually referred to as "brucellosis."

The causative agent was first characterized during the late 1800's on the island of Malta, a British base where troops from England were acclimated enroute to India. At the time that Dr. David Bruce arrived from Scotland to take care of the troops, about 1000 cases of "Malta fever" (military and civilian) occurred each year, resulting in 75 to 80 deaths. In 1887, Bruce isolated the etiologic agent from the spleens of four fatal cases and fulfilled

Koch's postulates by transmitting the disease to monkeys.

Shortly afterwards, a young Maltese physician named Zammit showed that many of the more than 20,000 goats on Malta were excreting the disease organisms in their milk, and exclusion of goats' milk and cheeses essentially eliminated the disease from the military base. This organism from goats has now been named *Brucella melitensis.*

Meanwhile, a Danish veterinarian named Bang isolated a related organism which caused abortions in infected cows and was excreted in the cows' milk. This organism has been given the name *Brucella abortus.* Still later a third organism was isolated that normally infects swine, and this species has been designated *Brucella suis.*

Recently, three additional species of *Brucella* have been isolated—*B. canis* from dogs, *B. ovis* from sheep, and *B. neotamae* from the wood rat.

### Classification and Antigenic Structure of *Brucella*

All *Brucella* are aerobic organisms and can be differentiated from each other on the basis of both metabolic properties and antigenic

308

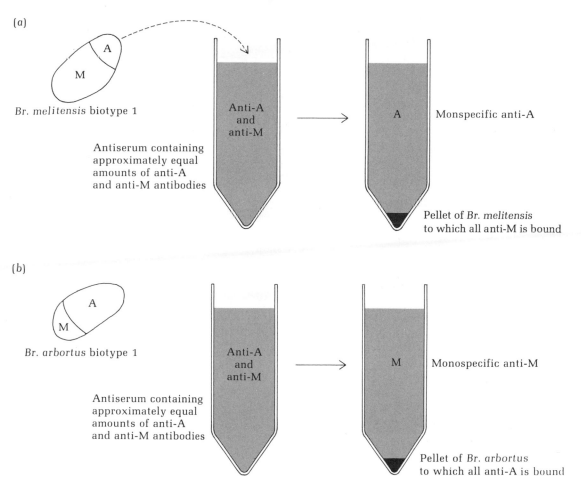

**Figure 21-1.** Preparation of *Brucella* monospecific antiserum. Antiserum containing approximately equal amounts of anti-A and anti-M antibodies is used with *Brucella* organisms that possess considerably more of one antigen than the other. The addition of limiting amounts of organisms to the antiserum results in the complete reaction of the antibody directed to the major antigen and leaves the antibody to the minor antigen unreacted in the serum. Thus, in (a) the organism contains far more M than A antigen and will, as a result, react with more anti-M antibodies, leaving pure anti-A antiserum. In (b) is the opposite situation, resulting in pure anti-M antiserum.

differences, as shown in Table 21-1. As can be seen in the table, the three major species can be subdivided into varying numbers of biotypes, based primarily on the production of H$_2$S, the ability to grow in a medium containing the dyes basic fuchsin or thionin, and their agglutination by monospecific antiserum.

The three major species of *Brucella* contain two antigens, designated as A and M, as surface determinants, but the relative proportion of each antigen varies considerably from one species or biotype to another. Thus, monospecific A or M antiserum can be prepared by adsorbing out cross-reacting antibodies (Figure 21-1), and differences in the agglutination reactions among the various brucellae can be shown (see Table 21-1).

**Table 21-1. Differential Characters of the Species and Biotypes of the Genus Brucella**

| Biotype | $CO_2$ Required | $H_2S$ Produced | Growth on Dye Media[a]: Basic Fuchsin b. | Thionin a. | Thionin b. | Agglutination in Mono-specific Sera A | Agglutination in Mono-specific Sera M | Anti-rough Serum | Lysis by phage Tb, RTD[b] | L-Alanine | L-Aspara-gine | L-Glutamic acid | L-Arabinose | D-Galactose | D-Ribose | D-Glucose | L-Erythritol | | L-Arginine[c] | L-Lysine |
|---|---|---|---|---|---|---|---|---|---|---|---|---|---|---|---|---|---|---|---|---|
| *B. melitensis* 1 | − | − | + | − | + | − | + | − | − | + | + | + | − | − | − | + | + | − | − | − |
| 2 | − | − | + | − | + | + | − | − | − | + | + | + | − | − | − | + | + | − | − | − |
| 3 | − | − | + | − | + | + | + | − | − | + | + | + | − | − | − | + | + | − | − | − |
| *B. abortus* 1 | d[d] | + | + | − | + | + | − | − | + | + | + | + | + | + | + | + | + | − | − | − |
| 2 | d | + | − | − | + | + | − | − | + | + | + | + | + | + | + | + | + | − | − | − |
| 3 | d | + | + | + | + | + | − | − | + | + | + | + | + | + | + | + | + | − | − | − |
| 4 | d | + | + | − | + | − | + | − | + | + | + | + | + | + | + | + | + | − | − | − |
| 5 | − | − | + | − | + | − | + | − | + | + | + | + | + | + | + | + | + | − | − | − |
| 6 | − | − | + | − | + | + | − | − | + | + | + | + | + | + | + | + | + | − | − | − |
| 7 | − | d | + | − | + | + | + | − | + | + | + | + | + | + | + | + | + | − | − | − |
| 8 | + | − | + | − | + | − | + | − | + | + | + | + | + | + | + | + | + | − | − | − |
| 9 | − | + | + | − | + | − | + | − | + | + | + | + | + | + | + | + | + | − | − | − |
| *B. suis* 1 | − | + | − | + | + | + | − | − | − | − | − | − | + | + | + | + | + | + | + | + |
| 2 | − | − | − | − | + | + | − | − | − | − | + | + | + | + | + | + | + | + | + | − |
| 3 | − | − | + | + | + | + | − | − | − | − | − | + | − | − | + | + | + | + | + | + |
| 4 | − | − | + | + | + | + | + | − | − | − | − | + | + | + | + | + | + | + | + | + |
| *B. neotomae* | − | + | − | − | + | + | − | − | − | − | + | + | + | + | d | + | + | + | − | − |
| *B. ovis* | + | − | + | + | + | − | − | + | − | + | + | + | − | − | − | − | − | − | − | − |
| *B. canis* | − | − | − | + | + | − | − | + | − | − | − | − | + | − | + | + | d | − | + | + |

(Substrate columns grouped under "SUBSTRATES METABOLIZED OXIDATIVELY.")

[a] Certified dyes (National Aniline Division, Allied Chemical and Dye Co., New York) at concentrations a. = 1:25,000; b. = 1:50,000
[b] RTD, routine test dilution
[c] Same reactions with DL-citrulline and DL-ornithine
[d] 11–89% strains positive

## Epidemiology and Pathogenesis of *Brucella*

The portal of entry for most human infections is the skin or conjunctiva, following direct contact with infected animals or aborted fetuses. Some persons contract the disease by the ingestion of contaminated dairy products; but since the organisms are very sensitive to the acidity of the stomach, infection probably occurs by way of the mucous membranes of the throat.

Primary invasion spreads via the lymphatics, with localization in the regional lymph nodes. The organisms are phagocytosed by macrophages but are able to survive and multiply within this protected environment (see Figure 21-2).

Blood stream invasion follows, and as some macrophages die, the brucellae are released to form lesions in the liver, spleen, bone marrow, and kidney. In some mammals (but not humans) the organisms may infect the mammary glands and be shed in the milk. The brucellae will also infect the placenta in cows, sheep, pigs, or goats (but again not humans) and cause abortions. Animals that are susceptible to this type of abortion contain large amounts of the four-carbon sugar alcohol erythritol in their placenta, and erythritol markedly stimulates the growth of the brucellae.

In humans the incubation period may vary from one to six weeks, followed by malaise, weakness, and an undulating diurnal fever (undulant fever). Relapses, during a 2–4 month convalescence, are frequent, and in rare cases the disease is thought to become chronic, extending over periods of many years, resulting in variable symptoms of weakness and malaise, and characterized by emotional disturbances. However, some clinicians doubt that this chronic state even exists because it is not possible to isolate the brucellae during this stage.

## Laboratory Diagnosis of Brucellosis

A definitive diagnosis of brucellosis requires the isolation and identification of the etiologic agent. Most human cases are caused by *B. abortus*, *B. melitensis*, and *B. suis*, although human infections with *B. canis* have been reported.

**Figure 21-2.** *a.* Phagocyte infected with *Brucella abortus* for 48 hours. The brucellae are in a large vacuole. ($\times$ 21,170.) *b.* Phagocytosis of *Brucella abortus* by a phagocyte in a 48-hour infection mix. Pseudopodia engulf the brucella. ($\times$ 75,300.)

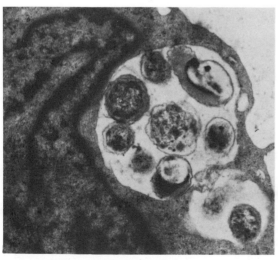

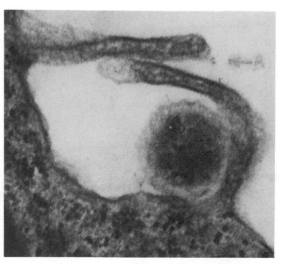

(a)                                             (b)

**Table 21-2. 309 Cases of Brucellosis by Occupation and Most Probable Source of Infection, U.S., 1975**

| Classification | Occupation | Domestic Animals | | | | Wild Animals | | | Unpasteurized Dairy Products | | Accidents | | Unknown | Total | % of Total |
|---|---|---|---|---|---|---|---|---|---|---|---|---|---|---|---|
| | | Swine | Cattle | Swine or Cattle | Unspecified Farm Animals | Deer | Caribou | Feral Swine | Domestic | Foreign | Strain 19 Vaccine | Laboratory | | | |
| Meat processing industry | Packing house employee | 77 | 47 | 44 | 2 | — | — | — | — | — | — | — | — | 170 | 55.2 |
| | Government inspector | 2 | 6 | 4 | 1 | — | — | — | — | — | — | — | — | 13 | 4.2 |
| | Rendering plant employee | — | — | 1 | 1 | — | — | — | — | — | — | — | — | 2 | 0.6 |
| Livestock industry | Livestock market employee | — | 1 | — | — | — | — | — | — | — | — | — | — | 1 | 0.3 |
| | Livestock producer | 11 | 39 | 1 | — | — | — | — | 2 | — | 1 | — | — | 54 | 17.5 |
| | Veterinarian | — | 2 | 1 | — | — | — | — | — | — | 1 | — | — | 4 | 1.3 |
| Other categories | Laboratory worker | — | — | — | — | — | — | — | — | — | — | 1 | — | 1 | 0.3 |
| | Homemaker | — | 1 | — | — | — | — | — | 2 | 1 | — | — | 1 | 5 | 1.6 |
| | Student or child | — | 2 | — | 2 | — | — | — | 2 | 5 | — | — | 3 | 14 | 4.5 |
| | Other | 3 | 6 | 2 | — | — | 1 | 4 | 2 | 9 | — | — | 9 | 36 | 11.6 |
| | Unknown | 1 | — | — | — | 1 | — | — | — | 1 | — | — | 6 | 9 | 2.9 |
| Total | | 94 | 104 | 53 | 6 | 1 | 1 | 4 | 8 | 16 | 2 | 1 | 19 | 309 | 100.0 |
| % of Total | | 30.5 | 33.7 | 17.2 | 1.9 | 0.3 | 0.3 | 1.3 | 2.6 | 5.2 | 0.6 | 0.3 | 6.1 | 100.0 | |

Blood or biopsy material from bone marrow, liver, or lymph nodes should be inoculated into trypticase soy broth and incubated at 37°C in a candle jar or a $CO_2$ incubator with an aerobic atmosphere containing 10% $CO_2$. The initial isolates may grow very slowly and it may require as long as six weeks before organisms can be subcultured on solid media.

The presence of agglutinating antibodies may be of aid in the diagnosis of brucellosis, but because other organisms contain antigens that induce cross-reacting antibodies, one should obtain an agglutinating titer of at least 1:80, or ideally see at least a four-fold increase in the agglutination titer arising during the convalescent phase of the disease.

Occasional individuals will form high levels of nonagglutinating serum IgA, which inhibits the agglutination of the test suspension. The interference of these blocking antibodies may be eliminated by diluting the patient's serum with saline or albumin to the point where the blocking antibodies are ineffective and the IgG antibodies will agglutinate the organisms.

Since the brucellae induce a cellular-type immunity, a protein extract of the organisms, called brucellergin, will give a delayed-type skin reaction in individuals who are hypersensitive to the antigens of the brucellae. However, a positive reaction does not mean active disease but only a past history of exposure to brucellosis. Further, since brucellergin is itself antigenic, repeated skin tests may induce a positive skin reaction.

**Treatment and Prevention of Brucellosis**

The incidence of brucellosis in the United States has decreased during the past several decades from a quite common infection to only 266 reported cases during 1975. This drop has been due primarily to an extensive program of testing and immunization of cattle by the U.S. Department of Agriculture. It is required that all cattle be immunized with a living, attenuated strain of *Brucella abortus* (strain 19), and brucellergin-positive animals that have not been immunized are destroyed. Pasteurization of milk is also designed to kill brucellae, and this procedure alone has undoubtedly prevented many human infections.

Most human cases in the United States occur in workers—such as slaughterhouse employees, veterinarians, and farmers—who have direct contact with infected animals or result from eating unpasteurized dairy products or imported cheeses (see Table 21-2). Active immunization of humans has not been done in the United States, although some Eastern European countries have used attenuated avirulent strains to immunize high-risk groups of individuals.

Treatment of brucellosis is difficult—probably because the organisms exist intracellularly in the monocytes (see Figure 21-2) and are protected from the effect of antibiotics. However, prolonged use of a combination of streptomycin and tetracycline is the treatment of choice.

## YERSINIA

The designation of the genus *Yersinia* was set forth in 1970 by a subcommittee studying the taxonomic position of members of the genus *Pasteurella*. It was noted that some organisms then in the genus *Pasteurella* possessed properties which related them more closely to the enteric bacteria than to the *Pasteurella*. As a result, the new genus *Yersinia* was created in commemoration of Yersin, the discoverer of the plague bacillus. It has been shown that yersiniae can conjugate with *E. coli* and accept various episomes, such as resistance transfer factors. In addition, *Yersinia* has several antigens in common with some of the enterics and thus appears to be better positioned taxonomically as a member of the Enterobacteriaceae.

### Bubonic Plague

Bubonic plague, caused by *Yersinia pestis*, is an ancient disease that has killed untold millions of people over the centuries. For example, it is believed to have killed more than 100 million persons in an epidemic in the sixth century. Another epidemic in the fourteenth century killed one-fourth of the European population, and the London plague in 1665 killed over 70,000 persons. In 1893, an epidemic began in Hong Kong and spread to India where more than 10 million individuals died over a 20-year period. This epidemic eventually reached San Francisco about 1900, and the disease is now firmly established in the rodent population in the southwestern United States (in, for example, prairie dogs, ground squirrels, wood rats, and mice—see Figure 21-3) as well as in many other areas of the world.

MORPHOLOGY AND ANTIGENIC STRUCTURE OF *Yersinia pestis.* Y. *pestis* is a small, gram-negative, nonmotile coccobacillus which becomes rather pleomorphic if grown under suboptimal conditions, such as a high salt concentration. The organisms have a tendency for bipolar staining (in which the ends of the bacilli stain darker than the central part—see Figure 21-4), but are not particularly fastidious since they can easily be grown in a routine peptone medium.

Y. *pestis* produces a variety of different antigens, but only a few have been characterized sufficiently well to postulate their role in production of disease: (1) a capsular antigen, designated Fraction 1 (F1) is antiphagocytic; (2) V/W antigens, consisting of a protein (V) and a lipoprotein (W) are produced together and act to prevent phagocytosis; and (3) an intracellular murine toxin which is lethal for the mouse ($LD_{50} < 1 \mu g$) and rat, apparently by acting on the vascular system causing irreversible shock and death. Also described have been two bacteriocins, Pesticin I and II, which have a lethal effect on *Yersinia pseudotuberculosis* and some *E. coli* strains. No role in virulence, however,

**Figure 21-3.** Counties of the United States reporting one or more cases of human bubonic plague, 1900–1972.

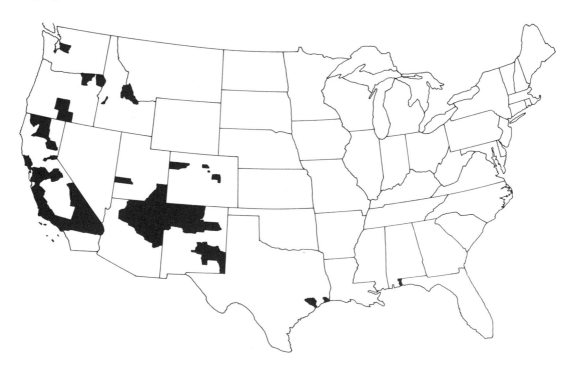

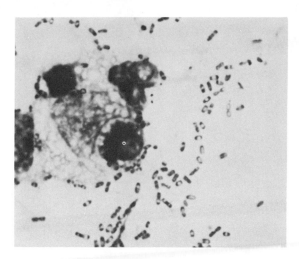

**Figure 21-4.** Wayson-stained smear of spleen from an experimentally infected mouse showing bipolar staining of cells of Yersinia pestis ($\times$ 1000).

can be assigned to either of these substances. In addition, Y. pestis possesses an outer membrane endotoxin, but since it is similar to that of the enterics, any role that it would play in the pathogenesis of plague would be of secondary importance.

EPIDEMIOLOGY AND PATHOGENESIS OF BUBONIC PLAGUE. Plague is normally a disease of rodents which exists in two kinds of epidemic centers, namely the permanent but relatively resistant rat population where the organisms reside in inter-epidemic periods and the temporary but susceptible rodents, particularly the domestic rat population.

The spread of plague to humans is a function of the relative balance between resistant and susceptible species of rats. Thus, when the domestic rat population overlaps into the wild rat population, the domestic rats become infected by the bite of an infected rat flea. The domestic rat fleas then become infected, and when biting other rats, regurgitate the plague bacilli into the new host, instituting a new epidemic. As the domestic rats continue to die, the rat fleas will bite humans —intruders in the normal rat-rat flea cycle.

Since epidemics of plague usually occur in crowded areas with poor sanitation, it has been proposed that once started, human-to-human spread occurs also by human fleas.

Following the flea bite, Y. pestis is transported in the human body to the regional lymph nodes (usually in the groin) causing them to become enlarged tender nodes called "buboes." Oddly, the organisms entering from the flea bite possess neither the F1 capsule, nor the antiphagocytic V/W antigens because these antigens are not formed at 28° C, the normal flea temperature. As a result, the bacilli that are phagocytosed by polymorphonuclear neutrophils (PMN) are destroyed. But those that are phagocytosed by macrophages are able to grow; and since they are now at 37° C, both F1 and V/W antigens are synthesized, and the bacilli can leave the macrophage as fully virulent organisms resistant to phagocytosis.

After leaving the regional lymph nodes, Y. pestis disseminates via the blood stream to the spleen, liver, lungs, and other organs and may cause subcutaneous hemorrhages, which gave bubonic plague the name "Black Death." If lung involvement occurs, the resulting pneumonia can also be spread via respiratory discharges.

The mechanism by which the plague bacillus produces death is not entirely clear. All virulent organisms produce the antiphagocytic V/W antigens and the intracellular toxin. However, in untreated cases, even with a case fatality approaching 75% for bubonic plague and 100% for pneumonic plague, the precise property of the plague bacillus which confers this high virulence is not known.

LABORATORY DIAGNOSIS OF BUBONIC PLAGUE. Ideally, the organisms can be grown from aspirates of enlarged buboes, or from sputum in the case of pneumonic plague. Stained smears should show bipolar staining (Figure 21-4) and specifically labeled fluorescent antibody is available for a definitive identification.

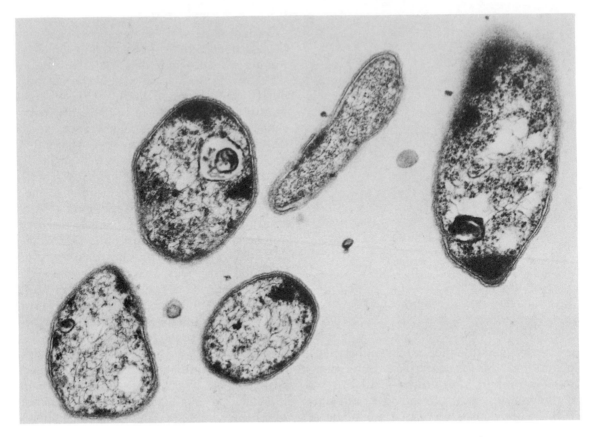

**Figure 21-5.** Pleomorphic cells of *Francisella tularensis* (× 42,000).

The aspirates or sputum can be injected into guinea pigs or mice, but such procedures can be dangerous to the investigator unless very specialized isolation equipment is available.

The appearance of agglutinating antibodies to Y. *pestis* during convalescence of the patient is of value as a confirming retrospective diagnosis of plague.

TREATMENT AND CONTROL OF BUBONIC PLAGUE. Rapid treatment of plague with streptomycin, chloramphenicol, or the tetracyclines is quite effective.

Prevention is directed at minimizing the domestic rat population, but once an epidemic has begun, efforts are switched to eliminate the human fleas as well as the rat fleas. Thus, the liberal use of DDT after World War II is credited with preventing major epidemics of plague (and also typhus) in parts of Europe and Africa.

Vaccines containing killed organisms have been used to provide short-term protection, and an avirulent living vaccine has been used with apparent success in humans.

### Other *Yersinia*

*Yersinia pseudotuberculosis* is primarily a pathogen of animals and birds in which it may cause gastroenteritis, an infection of the lymph nodes, or an acute septicemia. Infections in humans frequently involve the mesenteric lymph nodes, resulting in symptoms that are easily confused with acute appendicitis. These organisms may also invade the blood stream, causing a severe septicemia.

Yersinia enterocolitica has been isolated from humans with acute abdominal disease, and the resulting mesenteric lymphadenitis (swollen lymph nodes) may also mimic the symptoms of acute appendicitis. It is highly pathogenic for guinea pigs and hares but not for other laboratory animals.

## FRANCISELLA TULARENSIS

Although tularemia occurs throughout the world, the organisms causing it, Francisella tularensis, were first described and grown in the United States in the early 1900's. Members of this species are extremely pleomorphic, small, gram-negative rods which may vary from coccoid to filamentous forms (see Figure 21-5). Nutritionally, F. tularensis requires a rich medium to which the amino acid cystine has been added; and although it is a facultative anaerobe, better growth is obtained when it is grown aerobically.

### Epidemiology and Pathogenesis of Tularemia

The chronology of events which explain the epidemiology of tularemia began in 1912 when the organisms were isolated from rodents in Tulare County, California. In 1919, Dr. Edward Francis isolated the same organism in Utah from a fatal case of deer fly fever, and during this same period, F. tularensis was shown to be the etiologic agent of "market fever," a severe illness occasionally contracted by butchers after cleaning wild rabbits. Also, the organism was shown to exist in the wood tick where it is passed transovarily from generation to generation, providing both a reservoir and a vector for the transmission of the disease. Thus, there is a varied epidemiology in which the disease may be transmitted by the deer fly in the southwestern United States, by the wood tick in the Northwest and Midwest, and all over

the world by direct contact with infected animals—especially rabbits, which account for about 90% of all infections in the United States.

There are, in general, three major manifestations of tularemia, depending in part on the route of entry of the organisms:

Ulceroglandular tularemia, which follows direct contact with infected animals, is by far the most common type of this disease. It is characterized by the appearance of a primary lesion at the point of entry (usually the fingers) which may become an open ulcer after seven or eight days. In those cases where the eye has been the portal of entry, a severe conjunctival ulcer may develop and the disease may be referred to as ulcero-ocular tularemia. The organisms reach the regional lymph nodes, which become swollen and tender and may on occasion break open and drain. They can then spread via the blood stream to cause lesions in other organs, particularly the liver, spleen, and, occasionally, the lungs.

When the organisms reach the lungs, whether by hematogenous spread or by the respiratory route, the infection is called pneumonic tularemia. This manifestation of tularemia can result in the direct spread from person to person and is associated with a high mortality rate.

One may also acquire tularemia by the ingestion of contaminated food or by drinking water which has been contaminated by animals that have died from tularemia. In these instances, there is no primary lesion, and the disease, known as typhoidal tularemia, has many of the gastrointestinal and high-fever symptoms associated with typhoid fever.

Francisella tularensis is considered to be among the more virulent organisms that infect humans, and yet it is still not possible to pinpoint the factors which contribute to this virulence. Certainly, its ability to grow and survive in monocytes protects the organisms from destruction by polys or lysis by humoral antibody and complement. However, no toxic factors have been described that can explain the extreme virulence of these organisms.

### Laboratory Diagnosis of Tularemia

Smears from skin lesions can be stained with fluorescently-labeled specific antibody to provide a diagnosis, or one can determine the agglutination titer of the patient's serum to the specific organisms for a retrospective diagnosis.

Ideally, one should grow and identify the causative organism, using fluorescent antibody or agglutination with specific antiserum, but to do so a special cystine-glucose-blood medium is required. In actual practice, many diagnostic laboratories are reluctant to grow this organism because of the danger to laboratory personnel. As a consequence, most diagnoses of tularemia are based on the history, the clinical picture, and either examining the exudate with labeled antibody or noting the appearance of agglutinins eight to ten days after the initial symptoms.

### Treatment and Control of Tularemia

Treatment with any antibiotic is difficult, probably because of the intracellular existence of the organisms. However, streptomycin seems to be the antibiotic of choice, although the tetracyclines or chloramphenicol are efficacious, also. Relapses are not uncommon, and prolonged treatment may be necessary.

Control is virtually impossible in the wild animal population, but since the majority of human cases result from direct contact with infected rabbits, one should either use rubber gloves when cleaning wild rabbits or, for absolute protection, follow the advice given in Leviticus XI, verses 6–8, which, in part, states, ". . . and of the hare . . of their flesh shall ye not eat, and their carcass shall ye not touch; they are unclean to you."

### PASTEURELLA MULTOCIDA

*Pasteurella multocida* exists as part of the normal flora of the respiratory tract of many animals and birds. They are small, gram-negative coccobacilli which appear to cause disease in animals, primarily when the animals are under stress, such as while being shipped to market. The manifestations of disease are usually a pneumonia or a hemorrhagic septicemia, and this is referred to as "shipping fever" or "fowl cholera."

Humans can become infected—particularly following the bite by an animal such as a dog or cat—resulting in a localized tissue infection, a systemic septicemia or meningitis, or a respiratory infection.

Killed vaccines are used for animal protection, and most strains are sensitive to penicillin and tetracycline.

### REFERENCES

Bibel, D. J., and T. H. Chen. 1976. Diagnosis of plague: An analysis of the Yersin-Kitasato controversy. *Bacteriol. Rev.* **40**:633–651.

Center for Disease Control. 1976. Human plague—Arizona, California, New Mexico. *Morbid. Mortal. Weekly Rep.* **25**:155.

Center for Disease Control. 1976. Plague—Arizona, Colorado, New Mexico. *Morbid. Mortal. Weekly Rep.* **25**:189.

Chester, B., and G. Slotzky. 1976. Temperature-dependent cultural and biochemical characteristics of rhamnose-positive *Yersinia enterocolitica*. *J. Clin. Microbiol.* **3**:119–127.

Francis, E. 1919. Deer fly fever: A disease of man of hitherto unknown etiology. *Pub. Health Rep.* **34**:2061–2062.

Francis, E. 1922. Tularemia: A new disease of man. *J. Amer. Med. Assoc.* **78**:1015–1018.

Gutman, L. T., E. A. Ottesen, T. J. Quan, P. S. Noce, and S. L. Katz. 1973. An interfamilial outbreak of *Yersinia enterocolitica* enteritis. *New Engl. J. Med.* **288**:1372–1377.

Holland, J. J., and M. J. Pickett. 1958. A cellular basis of immunity in experimental *Brucella* infections. *J. Exp. Med.* **108:**343–359.

Iannelli, D., R. Diaz, and T. M. Bettini. 1976. Identification of *Brucella abortus* antibodies in cattle serum by single radial diffusion. *J. Clin. Microbiol.* **3:**119–127.

Keppie, J., A. E. Williams, K. Witt, and H. Smith. 1965. The role of erythritol in the tissue localization of the brucellae. *Br. J. Exp. Pathol.* **46:**104–108.

Klock, L. E., P. F. Olsen, and T. Fukushima. 1973. Tularemia epidemic associated with the deerfly. *JAMA* **226:**149–152.

Palmer, D. L., A. L. Kisch, R. C. Williams, Jr., and W. P. Reed. 1971. Clinical features of plague in the United States: The 1969–1970 epidemic. *J. Infect. Dis.* **124:**367–371.

Rabson, A. R., A. F. Hallett, and H. J. Koornhof. 1975. Generalized *Yersinia enterocolitica* infection. *J. Infect. Dis.* **131:**447–451.

Reddin, J. L., R. K. Anderson, R. Jenness, and W. Spink. 1965. Significance of 7S and macroglobulin *Brucella* agglutinins in human brucellosis. *New Engl. J. Med.* **272:**1263–1268.

Spink, W. W. 1956. *The Nature of Brucellosis.* University of Minnesota Press, Minneapolis.

Street, L., W. W. Grant, and J. D. Alva. 1975. Brucellosis in childhood. *Pediatrics* **55:**416–420.

# 22

# Haemophilus and Bordetella

Organisms included in the genera *Haemophilus* and *Bordetella* are frequently referred to as the hemophilic bacteria because they either require fresh blood or are stimulated if blood is added to their growth medium. The major pathogen in each genus is characterized by causing respiratory or meningeal infections in young children but only rarely in adults. *Haemophilus influenzae* is the principal etiologic agent of meningitis in children under the age of 3 years, and *Bordetella pertussis* is the cause of whooping cough.

## HAEMOPHILUS

The generic name of *Haemophilus* evolved from the fact that for growth these organisms have an absolute requirement for a blood-containing medium. This need for red blood cells is based on two essential substances: (1) a heat-stable material originally designated as X factor, and (2) a heat-labile component that was given the name V factor. Subsequent research has shown that X factor is hematin, which is required for the synthesis of *Haemophilus'* heme-containing cytochrome system and the enzyme catalase. The V factor can be replaced by either NAD or NADP, although if nicotinamide riboside is supplied, the organisms can synthesize their own NAD and NADP. Not all species of *Haemophilus* need both factors, but (as suggested by Table 22-1) all species require the addition of at least one of these components for growth.

It should be noted that, although red blood cells contain the required X and V factors, only *H. hemolyticus,* a nonpathogen of the respiratory tract, is β-hemolytic and able to hemolyze the erythrocytes. The other *Haemophilus* species do not grow well on blood agar media unless it has been heated to 80°C for 15 minutes to lyse the red blood cells and inactivate enzymes that may destroy V factor. As noted previously, the resulting brown agar medium is commonly called chocolate blood agar.

### Haemophilus influenzae

*Haemophilus influenzae* (sometimes called Pfeiffer's bacillus) is a small gram-negative, rather pleomorphic coccobacillus (see Figure 22-1) and a facultative anaerobe that prefers aerobic conditions. These organisms utilize

**Table 22-1. Growth Characteristics of Some Species of *Haemophilus* and *Bordetella***

| Organism | Requires X (hematin) | Requires V (NAD) | Beta-hemolytic |
|---|---|---|---|
| *Haemophilus influenzae* | + | + | − |
| *Haemophilus parainfluenzae* | − | + | − |
| *Haemophilus hemolyticus* | + | + | + |
| *Haemophilus suis* | + | + | − |
| *Bordetella pertussis* | − | − | + |

carbohydrates very poorly, and differential sugar fermentation reactions are of no value for their identification.

ANTIGENIC STRUCTURE OF *Haemophilus influenzae*. The organisms in *H. influenzae* are divided into six types designated a, b, c, d, e, and f, on the basis of antigenic differences in their capsular material. Antibodies to the capsular material are protective since they enhance phagocytosis as well as stimulate a complement-requiring bactericidal effect.

Type b, the one most often associated with serious disease in children, possesses a capsule that is a polymer of ribose phosphate. Nonencapsulated strains of *H. influenzae* are antigenically heterogeneous, although all types appear to contain a similar protein M antigen. Like the pneumococcus, transformation of capsular types, as well as transfer of streptomycin resistance, has been accomplished with free DNA. Moreover, strains resistant to ampicillin are found with increasing frequency, and this resistance

**Figure 22-1.** Electron micrographs of thin sections of nonencapsulated and encapsulated *Haemophilus influenzae* type b. *a*. Nonencapsulated cells (× 38,000). *b*. Encapsulated cells with dense matted capsular antigen visible on their surfaces (× 27,000). *c*. Encapsulated cells exposed to type b specific antiserum before fixation (× 30,000). Note the complete enveloping of the cells and the fibrillar nature of the antigen-antibody complex, which seems to emanate from discrete points in the cell wall.

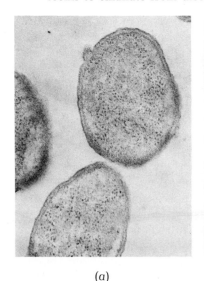
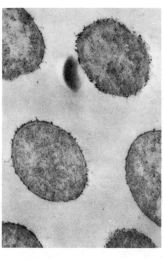
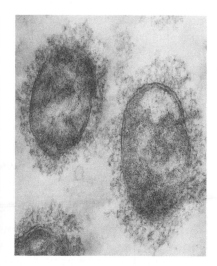

(a)                                   (b)                                   (c)

appears to be encoded in a transmissible plasmid.

EPIDEMIOLOGY AND PATHOGENICITY OF *Haemophilus influenzae*.  The somewhat misleading name of *Haemophilus influenzae* stems from uncertainty about the role of this organism as the etiologic agent of the influenza pandemics of 1890 and 1918. It is now recognized that influenza is a viral disease (see Chapter 39), but the fact that this organism is a common secondary invader of viral influenza victims led to the erroneous conclusion that *H. influenzae* was the etiologic agent. There is a possibility that this organism can act synergistically with the human influenza virus, but this hypothesis is supported primarily by the observation that a combination of *Haemophilus suis* and swine influenza virus produce a swine disease more severe than that which either agent could cause alone.

*Haemophilus influenzae* is an obligate human parasite which is passed from person to person via the respiratory route. It is reported that 30–50% of all children carry the bacillus asymptomatically in the nasopharynx, generally as avirulent, nonencapsulated organisms.

Meningitis is the most severe type of infection caused by *H. influenzae*, and it is interesting that the majority of such infections occur between the ages of six months and three years of age. In fact, barring an epidemic of meningococcal meningitis, *H. influenzae* is the chief cause of meningitis in young children, with an annual attack rate of about 1 in 2000 in persons from three months to six years of age.

The pathogenesis of the disease is not unlike that of meningococcal meningitis, in which the organisms travel from the nasopharynx to infect the regional lymph nodes, enter the blood stream, and invade the meninges. The precipitating event that determines whether an individual will be an asymptomatic carrier or succumb to an overt infection is not understood, but this may well be initiated by other respiratory infections. As we shall see, the severity of the infection is inversely proportional to the presence of circulating antibodies to the specific capsular carbohydrate.

Acute epiglottitis is another serious disorder produced by type b *H. influenzae*. Here, an apparently healthy child suddenly has acute respiratory distress and may need immediate hospitalization for relief from the obstruction of the air passages. Usually, the epiglottis is markedly swollen, red, and edematous (filled with fluid). If acute epiglottitis is not treated promptly, commonly by tracheotomy, the child may suffocate.

LABORATORY DIAGNOSIS OF *Haemophilus influenzae* INFECTIONS.  Suspected cases of *H. influenzae* meningitis must have immediate treatment; untreated cases have a high mortality rate. Survivors suffer a high incidence of neurological disorders, including mental retardation, blindness, hydrocephalus, and convulsions. Gram stains of sedimented spinal fluid that show pleomorphic gram-negative rods are assumed to be *H. influenzae*, but they should be mixed with specific type b antiserum and observed for a positive quellung reaction.

Both blood and spinal fluid should be cultured on chocolate blood agar and incubated at 37°C in a candle jar or in a $CO_2$ incubator. Isolated organisms can be assayed for X and V factor requirements: a trypticase soy agar plate is streaked and sterile discs (available commercially) containing X factor, V factor, and a combination of X and V factors are placed onto the surface of the agar. Growth that is limited to the vicinity of the paper discs will make obvious any X or V factor requirement (see Figure 22-2). One can also demonstrate a satellite phenomenon if a blood agar plate is streaked with the unknown organisms, and a small loopful of *Staphylococcus aureus* is pinpointed on the plate. The hemolytic staphylococci will release both X and V factors from the red blood cells, and satellite growth of the *Hae-*

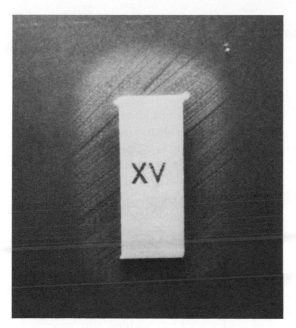

**Figure 22-2.** In this preparation colonies of *Haemophilus influenzae* on tryptic soy agar grow only around a paper strip impregnated with X and V factors.

mophilus occurring only in the vicinity of the *Staphylococcus* colony will be seen.

PREVENTION AND CONTROL OF INFECTIONS BY *Haemophilus influenzae.* Because of the ubiquity of *H. influenzae,* most persons acquire protective antibodies between the ages of three to eight years. The newborn is protected for three to six months by passively acquired maternal antibody, and the danger period begins at about six months and lasts until the acquisition of bactericidal antibody. Obviously, most individuals acquire such antibody either by becoming asymptomatic carriers or from an undiagnosed respiratory disease. There is no commercially available vaccine to stimulate active immunity to type b *H. influenzae,* but the mortality rate and the permanent neurological damage incidence have provoked much investigation for such a vaccine.

Until recently, ampicillin was the therapy of choice for *H. influenzae* infections; with the increase in reported ampicillin-resistant organisms, one can no longer rely on ampicillin sensitivity. Chloramphenicol is also usually effective and is used when ampicillin resistance is suspected. Chloramphenicol-resistant strains have, however, been reported.

### Haemophilus aegyptius

*H. aegyptius* (also called the Koch-Weeks bacillus) is the etiologic agent of a common conjunctivitis informally referred to as "pink-eye." The illness may be mild or severe, varying from vascular infection of the conjunctiva with a slight discharge to severe irritation with lacrimation, swelling of the lids, photophobia, and a mucopurulent discharge.

The infection can be diagnosed by microscopic examination of smears and growth of the organism on chocolate blood agar. Topical application of tetracycline ointment usually provides effective treatment.

### Haemophilus ducreyi

*Haemophilus ducreyi* is the cause of the venereal disease chancroid (soft chancre), which is characterized by a ragged ulcer on the genitals, with marked swelling and pain. Regional lymph nodes swell and may suppurate. Autoinoculation may occur, resulting in multiple lesions.

The infection is transmitted sexually, and the diagnosis is confirmed by smears and cultures. Both sulfonamides and streptomycin have been used to treat the infections.

### BORDETELLA

### Bordetella pertussis

*Bordetella pertussis,* the causative agent of whooping cough, was isolated and described in 1906 by Bordet and Gengou. It is a very fragile, gram-negative coccobacillus which is nonmotile, but may be encapsulated.

*Bordetella pertussis* does not require either the X or V factors but does need an enriched medium to which have been added such substances as blood or starch. The organisms are most commonly grown on a potato-blood-glycerol agar called Bordet-Gengou's medium.

ANTIGENIC STRUCTURE OF *Bordetella pertussis.* Freshly isolated organisms are of a single antigenic type that is encapsulated and possesses what appear to be pili. These virulent organisms have been designated as phase 1(see Figure 22-3), but after cultivation in the laboratory on artificial media, the organisms lose their capsule and pili and the O-specific antigen undergoes an S → R mutation. The exact molecular events that occur during these stepwise changes are unknown,

**Figure 22-3.** Negatively-stained portion of a spheroplast of phase 1 *Bordetella pertussis* in which the protoplast is retracted from the cell wall (× 140,000). The surface projections and barely visible pili appear to originate in the wall.

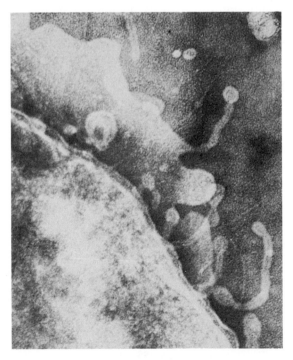

but they have been designated as phases 2, 3, and 4; phase 4 is entirely avirulent.

Other antigens of phase 1 have been reported, but none have been completely characterized. The chemical nature of the specific phase 1 antigen (which may be either in the capsule or pili) is not known. The organisms excrete a hemagglutinin, and disrupted cells release both a heat-stable toxin (probably endotoxin) and a heat-labile toxin that is destroyed by heating at 56°C for 30 minutes.

EPIDEMIOLOGY AND PATHOGENESIS OF WHOOPING COUGH. Whooping cough is an acute infection of the respiratory tract involving primarily the ciliated epithelial cells of the bronchi and trachea. It begins with a catarrhal stage characterized by sneezing and a mild, but irritating, cough. After one to two weeks, the disease enters the spasmodic stage in which the cough may become very violent. These episodes of violent coughing frequently are followed by a "whoop" on inspiration, and it is this characteristic whoop that gives the disease its name. The paroxysms of coughing may be so severe that cyanosis, vomiting, and convulsions follow, completely exhausting the patient. The spasmodic state persists for about two weeks and is followed by a convalescent state which lasts an additional two weeks.

Endotoxins, as well as the heat-labile toxin, are undoubtedly released from disintegrating organisms, causing local necrosis, inflammation, and fever. As the organisms grow on the membranes of the trachea and bronchi, a thick, ropy exudate is formed which is expelled with great difficulty. No doubt, this accounts for the severity of the cough. The organisms do not invade the bloodstream but remain localized in the respiratory tract.

The incubation period is usually seven to ten days after contact with the respiratory discharges of an infected individual. The organisms may be transmitted either by direct contact, by droplets, or from freshly contaminated articles. Major spread probably occurs in the catarrhal stage before the disease is diagnosed. In this stage the organisms are present in the nasopharynx, and when the individual coughs (even though the cough is not severe) the organisms are expelled and sprayed through the air. Unfortunately, as a rule, a person is isolated only after whooping begins, past the stage at which an individual is an important source of spread of the disease. Healthy carriers have not been recognized.

LABORATORY DIAGNOSIS OF WHOOPING COUGH. To establish a diagnosis, a cough plate containing Bordet-Gengou medium can be held in front of a patient's mouth during a coughing episode. The plate is then incubated and examined for colonies of B. pertussis. A better technique is the use of a sterile cotton swab to obtain a specimen from the nasopharyngeal area while the patient coughs. Since B. pertussis is resistant to penicillin, the swab is usually mixed with a drop of penicillin to limit the growth of throat contaminants.

Organisms growing on the culture plates may be identified by employing specific antiserum for an agglutination test or by staining with fluorescently-labeled specific antibody. This latter staining technique can also be used to stain smears taken from the nasopharynx.

TREATMENT AND CONTROL OF WHOOPING COUGH. Several antibiotics are of value, although treatment is not entirely satisfactory. For severe whooping cough tetracyclines, erythromycin, or chloramphenicol can be used. Antibiotic therapy also lessens the number of secondary infections, such as bronchitis or pneumonia.

The introduction of an effective vaccine has markedly reduced the incidence of whooping cough. Formerly, almost every child had this disease during the early years of life, while in 1975 only 1563 cases of pertussis were reported in the United States. The vaccine consists of killed, encapsulated phase-1 organisms that are usually incorporated with diphtheria and tetanus toxoids.

Because of the high mortality of the disease in infants under one year of age, the vaccine should be administered at two months of age with two additional booster injections given at three and four months of age. Another booster is given at the time the child begins school.

**Other Bordetella**

Both *Bordetella parapertussis* and *Bordetella bronchiseptica* have been isolated from children with the whooping cough syndrome; however, neither organism causes the severe infections characterized by *B. pertussis*.

## REFERENCES

Aftandelians, R. V., and J. D. Connor. 1974. *Bordetella pertussis* serotypes in a whooping cough outbreak. *Amer. J. Epidemiol.* **99**:343–346.

Bass, J. W., E. L. Klenk, J. B. Kotheimer, C. C. Linnemann, and M. H. D. Smith. 1969. Antimicrobial treatment of pertussis. *J. Pediat.* **75**: 768–781.

Elwell, L. P., J. DeGraaff, D. Seibert, and S. Falkow. 1975. Plasmid-linked ampicillin resistance in *Haemophilus influenzae* type b. *Infect. Immun.* **12**:404–410.

Honig, P. J., P. S. Pasquariello, and S. E. Stool. 1973. *H. influenzae* pneumonia in infants and children. *J. Pediat.* **83**:215–219.

Kendrick, P. L. 1975. Can whooping cough be eradicated? *J. Infect. Dis.* **132**:707–712.

Robbins, J. B. 1975. Acquisition of "natural" and immunization-induced immunity to *Haemophilus influenzae* type b diseases. In David Schlessinger, ed. *Microbiology 1975.* Amer. Soc. Microbiol., Washington, D.C.

Schneerson, R., and J. B. Robbins. 1975. Induction of serum *H. influenzae* type b capsular antibodies in adult volunteers fed cross-reacting *Escherichia coli* O75:K100:H5. *New Engl. J. Med.* **292**:1093–1096.

Thorne, G. M., and W. E. Farrar Jr. 1975. Transfer of ampicillin resistance between strains of *Haemophilus influenzae* type b. *J. Infect. Dis.* **132:** 276–281.

Vega, R., H. L. Sadoff, and M. J. Patterson. 1976. Mechanisms of ampicillin resistance in *Haemophilus influenzae* type b. *Antimicrob. Agents Chemother.* **9:**164–168.

Whisnant, J. K., G. N. Rogentine, M. A. Gralnick, J. K. Schlesselman, and J. B. Robbins. 1976. Host factors and antibody response in *Haemophilus influenzae* type b meningitis and epiglottitis. *J. Infect. Dis.* **133:**448–455.

# 23

## Gram-Positive Spore-Forming Bacilli

Five different genera of bacteria produce endospores (see Chapter 3) but only two are of medical importance, *Bacillus* and *Clostridium*.

### BACILLUS

The genus *Bacillus* contains a heterogeneous group of organisms which are gram-positive, endospore-forming rods whose metabolism is either aerobic or facultatively anaerobic. Metabolically, some species carry out a homolactic fermentation, some a butanediol fermentation, and others a modified mixed-acid fermentation. In all likelihood, future taxonomists will subdivide this genus into several genera, but since *Bacillus anthracis* is the only species that is pathogenic for humans, an additional subdivision should not provide undue hardship for the medical microbiologist.

### Bacillus anthracis

*Bacillus anthracis* is a large, facultatively anaerobic rod (see Figure 23-1). Its isolation by Robert Koch in 1877 marked the beginning of modern medical microbiology, since it was, in part, Koch's work with this organism that was responsible for the well-known Koch's postulates.

ANTIGENIC CLASSIFICATION. There is only one antigenic type of *B. anthracis,* and it contains two major cell antigens: (1) a cell wall polysaccharide made up of N-acetyl glucosamine and D-galactose, and (2) a capsular polypeptide which is a polymer of γ-D-glutamic acid. The capsule is rather unusual in that it contains only the D (or "unnatural") isomer of the amino acid; furthermore, the virulence of the organism depends in part upon the antiphagocytic activity of this capsular material.

EPIDEMIOLOGY AND PATHOGENESIS OF ANTHRAX. Anthrax is primarily a disease of sheep, goats, cattle, and, to a lesser extent, other herbivorous animals. Although it is found in only a few parts of the United States (Louisiana, Texas, California, Nebraska, and South Dakota), it is a worldwide problem, especially in parts of Europe, Asia, and Africa. Once the disease is established in an area, bacterial endospores from a dead infected animal are able to contaminate the

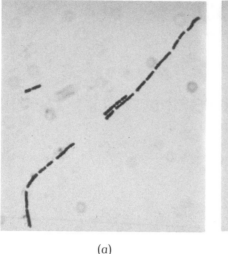
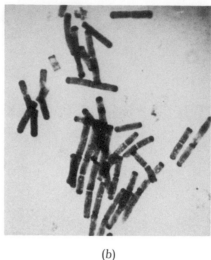

(a)                    (b)

**Figure 23-1.** Giemsa-stained cells of *Bacillus anthracis* (about × 2000). *a.* Chains of cells after 18 hours in nutrient broth. *b.* *B. anthracis* as it appears when growing in animals (media was supplied with all constituents necessary for antigen production). Note broader cells, square corners, and irregularly-stained cytoplasm.

soil, and the resistant endospores keep the pasture area infectious for other animals for many years. In most animal infections, the spores enter the body via abrasions in the oral or intestinal mucosa, and after entering the blood stream, they germinate and multiply to tremendous numbers, causing death in two to three days.

Humans become infected through the skin by contact with hides of infected animals or by inhaling the spores from infected hides. Since the pulmonary form of the disease occurs frequently in those persons engaged in sorting sheep's wool or goats' hair, it has been referred to as "woolsorter's" disease. The lesion from the skin inoculation (cutaneous infection route) is sometimes called a malignant pustule.

Cutaneous infection is an occupational hazard for persons who handle livestock or work with items derived from contaminated wool or hides. The organisms gain entrance into the body through small cuts or abrasions —usually on the hands. An initial lesion occurring at the site of entry soon develops into a black necrotic area (see Figure 23-2). If the lesion is not treated, the organisms will invade the regional lymph nodes and blood stream, causing death within five to six days. The pulmonary form of the disease occurs less frequently than the cutaneous form, but it is more serious and carries a higher mortality rate.

**Figure 23-2.** Lesion of cutaneous anthrax (8th day of illness) on the arm of a woman who had been a carder in a wool factory.

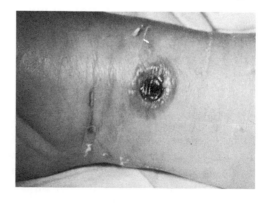

Until 1955, it was believed that anthrax caused death by its ability to resist phagocytosis, allowing it to grow to tremendous numbers of bacilli that clogged capillaries. This explanation had been termed the "log jam" theory. Now, it is known that this concept is incorrect and that *B. anthracis* secretes a very toxic exotoxin.

There are a number of reasons why the production of this toxin was missed for so many years, but perhaps most important was that *in vitro* the toxin is not liberated, or even produced, in the absence of added bicarbonate. Furthermore, the toxin is quite labile and rapidly destroyed.

The toxin is a complex which has been separated into three components named edema factor (EF), lethal factor (LF), and protective antigen (PA). Some biological activity can be demonstrated with PA or LF alone, but PA and EF must be combined to show a dermonecrotic effect.

There are important gaps in our knowledge concerning the mode of action of this toxin, but it seems most likely that the toxin interacts with the central nervous system, resulting in acute respiratory failure, and that other physiologic changes are nonspecific and secondary to the involvement of the central nervous system.

LABORATORY DIAGNOSIS OF ANTHRAX. Direct smears and cultures from cutaneous lesions may aid in making a diagnosis; sputum is not usually a good source of organisms. Blood should be cultured from a suspected case of either cutaneous or pulmonary anthrax. Blood can be injected into a guinea pig or a mouse, and the chains of gram-positive rods isolated from the animal's blood in 24 to 36 hours.

PREVENTION AND CONTROL OF ANTHRAX. Ever since Pasteur's celebrated field trial in which animals were successfully immunized with a living attenuated suspension of *B. anthracis,* efforts have been directed toward the production of effective vaccines which possess little or no toxicity. Since killed vaccines are worthless, this has resulted in two different approaches to the stimulation of artificial immunity: (1) the isolation and use of the protective antigenic component of the anthrax toxin, and (2) the use of attenuated living bacteria to induce both anticapsular and antitoxic immunity.

Recovery from anthrax provides an animal with a good immunity against subsequent infections, and therefore the use of attenuated vaccines stimulates a more effective and longer-lasting immunity than do the toxin preparations. However, all effective living vaccines possess some toxicity, and they have not been used in the United States for humans. The vaccine used for humans is a preparation of alum-precipitated protective antigen that induces a short-lived immunity and requires annual boosters.

Control of anthrax in humans is, therefore, not a simple matter, particularly for those who are occupationally exposed, but sterilization of wool, hair, and other animal materials capable of transmitting the disease does prevent the spread of the bacilli to persons not normally exposed to infected hides. However, not all such products are currently sterilized, as recently exemplified by the individual who contracted anthrax from contaminated goat hair fringe on a souvenir drum purchased in Haiti. Other Haitian products using goat hair have been found contaminated with anthrax spores (see Table 23-1) and the Center for Disease Control in Atlanta has recommended that all such items be considered potentially contaminated and that they be given to local health authorities for disposal.

## CLOSTRIDIUM

The clostridia are large gram-positive, endospore-forming rods that are unable to utilize molecular oxygen as a final electron acceptor. They are also unable to synthesize the prosthetic heme component necessary for a cytochrome system and the enzyme catalase

**Table 23-1.** *Bacillus anthracis* **Culture Results for Haitian Goatskin Products Imported into the U.S., 1974**

| Item | No. Cultured | No. Positive | % Positive |
|---|---|---|---|
| Drums | 219 | 22 | 10 |
| Rugs | 58 | 45 | 78 |
| Mosaic pictures | 55 | 20 | 36 |
| Voodoo dolls | 13 | 3 | 23 |
| Goatskins | 10 | 4 | 40 |
| Purses | 10 | 1 | 10 |
| Stool | 1 | 1 | 100 |
| Hat | 1 | 0 | 0 |
| Bottle holder | 1 | 0 | 0 |
| Total | 368 | 96 | 26 |

or superoxide dismutase, and must, therefore, be grown under anaerobic conditions. This can be done by placing cultures in a container and replacing the air with $N_2$ or $H_2$ or by using a liquid medium containing 0.1% agar and a reducing agent such as sodium thioglycollate or dithiothreotol.

The natural habitat of the clostridia is soil and the intestinal tract of humans and animals. Some are saccharolytic and will ferment carbohydrates to form products such as butyric acid, butanol, isopropanol and acetone, while others are proteolytic and will metabolize proteins, often yielding rather foul-smelling amines as end products.

In general, the clostridia are not invasive organisms, and those that produce disease do so as a result of the formation and liberation of destructive enzymes and toxic exotoxins.

### Tetanus

*Clostridium tetani,* the causative agent of tetanus, is widely distributed in the soil and feces of many animals. The organisms are morphologically characterized by swollen, terminally located endospores which give the sporulating organism a drumstick appearance (see Figure 23-3).

ANTIGENIC CLASSIFICATION OF *Clostridium tetani. Cl. tetani* can be divided into a number of serological types, but the exotoxin released by all of them is serologically identical. Since immunity is directed only against the exotoxin, the antigenic characterization of the species is of little value.

EPIDEMIOLOGY AND PATHOGENESIS OF TETANUS. Although widely distributed in soil, *Clostridium tetani* has essentially no invasive abilities. To produce tetanus, the spores must be introduced into the body via a wound, such as a puncture, gunshot, burn, or even an animal bite.

Once inside the body, the presence of necrotic cells (that are no longer receiving oxygenated blood) provides a sufficiently anaerobic environment to allow the germination of the tetanus spores and the subsequent formation of the toxin. The incubation period may vary considerably, and it is possible for the endospores to remain dormant for long periods of time before germinating and producing toxin.

The toxin is a potent neurotoxin which is apparently released by lysis of the cells.

**Figure 23-3.** Cells of *Clostridium tetani* after 24 hours on a cooked-meat glucose medium ($\times$ 4500). Note spherical terminal endospores.

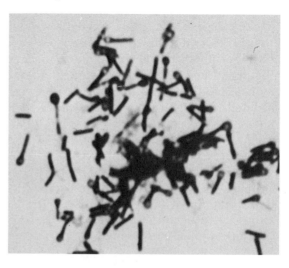

It is believed to travel from the wound along the nerve fibers to the anterior horn cells of the spinal cord, where it causes convulsive contractions of voluntary muscles. Since the spasms frequently involve the neck and jaws, the disease has been referred to as "lockjaw." Death ordinarily results from muscular spasms affecting the mechanics of respiration.

LABORATORY DIAGNOSIS OF TETANUS. A clinical picture of tetanus with a history of injury is usually sufficient to provide a working diagnosis. A more specific diagnosis requires the isolation and identification of the organisms, as well as the demonstration of tetanus toxin production by the bacterium. However, since the clinical picture is usually conclusive, a complete laboratory diagnosis is not ordinarily done.

PREVENTION AND CONTROL OF TETANUS. Characteristically, tetanus can occur following wounds that are so minor they are soon forgotten. Untreated tetanus may have a fatality rate as high as 60%, and even with therapy, the mortality may be 20–30%.

Prevention relies almost entirely on the presence of neutralizing antibodies to the toxin. Good active immunity can be acquired by the injection of a formalin-inactivated toxin (toxoid) which may or may not be precipitated with alum. The initial immunization requires three injections (usually begun at about three months of age along with diphtheria toxoid and pertussis vaccine). Booster doses are probably not necessary for five to ten years, although in the event of a traumatic injury in which the introduction of tetanus organisms is a possibility most physicians give a booster shot if the patient has not been immunized within the past two or three years. Rare individuals do form an IgE response, and excessively frequent boosters are, therefore, not recommended.

Following an injury, tetanus antitoxin is usually administered to those individuals who have never been previously immunized with tetanus toxoid. The organisms are sensitive to penicillin, but the antibiotic has no effect on the neutralization of the toxin. However, after surgical cleansing of the wound, antibiotic therapy can be helpful in preventing any additional growth of the organisms.

**Gas Gangrene**

There are a number of different species of the genus Clostridium that can infect wounds to produce the clinical syndrome known as gas gangrene. All of these species are morphologically similar—they are gram-positive, spore-forming rods, and all are obligate anaerobes. Furthermore, they are pervasive in the soil, so that contamination of a wound with dirt may very likely mean contamination with one or more of the gas-gangrene clostridia.

CLASSIFICATION OF THE GAS-GANGRENE CLOSTRIDIA. The organisms causing this syndrome can be thought of as the "gas-gangrene group," since, under most circumstances, any specific infection will contain several species of clostridia. Clostridium perfringens is the most frequent agent of gas gangrene, but other active species include C. novyi, C. septicum, and C. histolyticum, as well as a number of less common species such as C. bifermentans.

EPIDEMIOLOGY AND PATHOGENESIS OF GAS GANGRENE. Gas gangrene results from the contamination of wounds with Clostridium spores which are universally present in the soil. Since all of these organisms are anaerobic, they are able to germinate and grow in deep wounds that become necrotic as a result of a diminished blood supply. After germination, the organisms secrete their exotoxins and enzymes into the surrounding environment, causing more tissue destruction and resulting in a rapid and fulminating spread of the organism in the necrotic environment. In addition, carbohydrates are fermented, resulting in the production of large quantities of gas in the tissues. The pressures resulting from the gas formation may cause still more restriction of the blood supply to adjoining tissue, and, hence, still more necrosis. In the absence of surgical and antitoxic treatment, severe toxemia and death frequently ensue.

The toxins and enzymes produced by the various species of the gas gangrene group are similar but not identical from one species to another. Actually, most of them have not been purified or characterized and are lumped under the general name "lethal toxins." The products produced by *Clostridium perfringens* have received the most study; at least 12 different toxins and enzymes have been described and named by Greek letters (see Table 23-2). Not all serological strains of *C. perfringens* produce all 12 products or even similar quantities of certain toxins and enzymes.

The most extensively studied toxin is the $\alpha$ toxin, a lecithinase that hydrolyzes the phospholipid lecithin to a diglyceride and phosphorylcholine (see Figure 23-4). Since lecithin is a component of cell membranes, its hydrolysis can result in cell destruction throughout the body. Another toxin produced by this group is the $\theta$ toxin, a lethal hemolytic product characterized by its effect on the heart, more precisely its cardiotoxic properties. Other toxic enzymes produced by the gas gangrene group include a collagenase that hydrolyzes the body's collagen, a hyaluronidase, a fibrinolysin that breaks down blood clots, a DNase, and a neuraminidase that can remove the neuraminic acid from a large number of glycoproteins. With such a vast array of toxic substances, it is no wonder that gas gangrene was one of the major causes of death in the American Civil War—and, undoubtedly, in many other wars.

In addition to battlefield casualties, automobile and farm equipment accidents may also cause traumatic wounds resulting in gas gangrene. Because *C. perfringens* can be part of the normal flora of the female genital tract, induced abortions may also result in severe infections.

**Table 23-2. Toxins and Toxigenic Types of *Clostridium perfringens***

| TOXINS | | A | B | C | D | E |
|---|---|---|---|---|---|---|
| | | BACTERIAL TYPES | | | | |
| $\alpha$ | (lecithinase) | + + + | + + + | + + + | + + + | + + + |
| $\beta$ | (lethal, necrotizing) | — | + + + | + + + | — | — |
| $\gamma$ | (lethal) | — | + + | + + | — | — |
| $\delta$ | (lethal, hemolytic) | — | + | + + | — | — |
| $\varepsilon$ | (lethal, necrotizing) | — | + + + | — | + + + | — |
| $\eta$ | (lethal) | + | ? | ? | ? | ? |
| $\theta$ | (lethal, hemolytic) | + | + + | + + + | + + + | + + + |
| $\iota$ | (lethal, necrotizing) | — | — | — | — | + + + |
| $\kappa$ | (collagenase) | + | + | + + + | + + | + + + |
| $\lambda$ | (proteinase) | — | + | — | + + | + + + |
| $\mu$ | (hyaluronidase) | + + | + | + | + + | + |
| $\nu$ | (deoxyribonuclease) | + + | + | + + | + + | + + |

+ + + = most strains; + + = some strains; + = a few strains; — = not produced

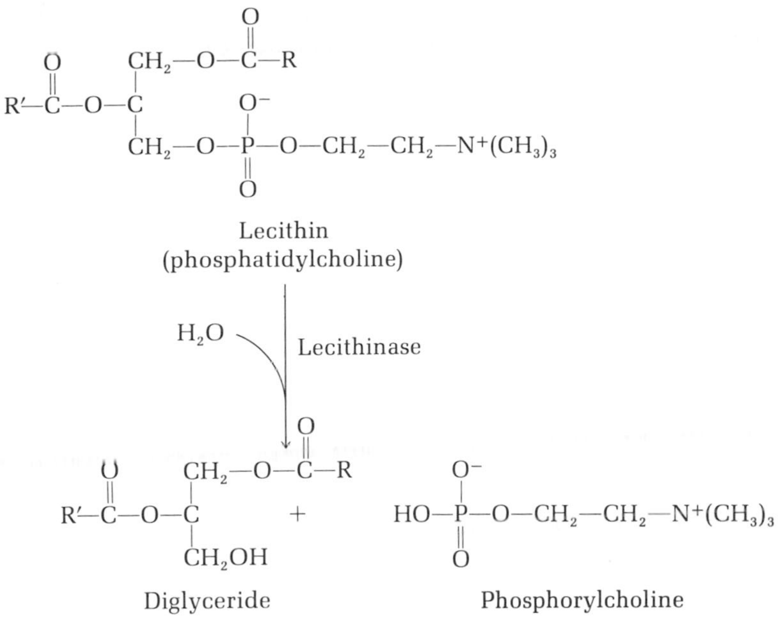

$$R'-\overset{\overset{O}{\|}}{C}-O-\underset{\underset{CH_2-O-\overset{O^-}{\underset{\|}{P}}-O-CH_2-CH_2-N^+(CH_3)_3}{|}}{\overset{\overset{\overset{O}{\|}}{CH_2-O-C-R}}{C}}$$

Lecithin
(phosphatidylcholine)

$H_2O$ ⟶ Lecithinase

$$R'-\overset{\overset{O}{\|}}{C}-O-\underset{CH_2OH}{\overset{\overset{\overset{O}{\|}}{CH_2-O-C-R}}{C}} \quad + \quad HO-\overset{\overset{O^-}{|}}{\underset{\underset{O}{\|}}{P}}-O-CH_2-CH_2-N^+(CH_3)_3$$

Diglyceride                    Phosphorylcholine

**Figure 23-4.** Hydrolysis of lecithin by $\alpha$ toxin (lecithinase) to a diglyceride and phosphorylcholine.

LABORATORY DIAGNOSIS OF GAS GANGRENE. The usual diagnosis is based on the clinical picture, but since other organisms (primarily among the *Bacteroides*) may cause similar infections, final proof of the etiology of the infection requires the isolation and identification of clostridia.

*Clostridium perfringens* is found in 70–80% of all cases of gas gangrene, and of the six serologic types of this organism, type A is the most prevalent. Any exudate is cultivated on thioglycollate broth and on blood agar plates which are incubated both aerobically and anaerobically. The presence of large gram-positive rods that grow only anaerobically is strong evidence for clostridia. *C. perfringens* is characterized by a stormy fermentation in milk (see Figure 23-5) in which the coagulated milk is blown apart by gas formed during the fermentation of the lactose in milk. Organisms producing an $\alpha$ toxin will hydrolyze the lecithin in an egg yolk medium, breaking down the lipid emulsion and, in turn, causing an opaque area to appear around the colony. Individual clostridial species are identified by a series of biochemical tests.

PREVENTION AND CONTROL. Surgical cleansing of wounds to eliminate extraneous material or necrotic tissue is undoubtedly the

**Figure 23-5.** Stormy fermentation in coagulated milk caused by *Clostridium perfringens*.

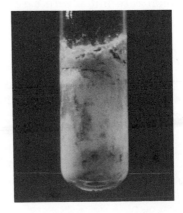

most important control mechanism for gas gangrene. Additionally, antitoxin against the bacterial filtrates can be used when complete surgical debridement is not possible. Antibiotics, such as penicillin or the tetracyclines, would be effective only in tissues still receiving a blood supply but are of little value in necrotic areas. Hyperbaric oxygen chambers, in which an infected area is placed in a chamber containing pure oxygen under pressure, have been used with some success to stop the growth of these obligate anaerobes.

### Food Poisoning Due to *Clostridium perfringens*

In addition to being the major etiologic agent in wound infections, C. perfringens is also an important cause of food poisoning. Most outbreaks are caused by C. perfringens type A strains that produce a heat-labile enterotoxin only when the vegetative cells sporulate. The most common food involved is meat (or meat products) containing large numbers of vegetative cells of C. perfringens. Following ingestion, the vegetative cells sporulate in the small intestine, releasing the newly synthesized enterotoxin. Symptoms of acute abdominal pain and diarrhea begin 8–24 hours after ingestion of the contaminated food and usually subside within 24 hours. The mechanism of action of the enterotoxin is unknown, but the effect is similar to that produced by the enteropathic E. coli.

Occasional rare but severe cases of food poisoning characterized by hemorrhagic enteritis and a high mortality are caused by C. perfringens type C. Such cases have been reported primarily from Germany and New Guinea. Those in New Guinea have been associated with the eating of pork which had been insufficiently cooked and improperly handled and cooled. Type C organisms produce a sporulation enterotoxin indistinguishable from that produced by type A C. perfringens, but they also produce large amounts of α toxin and the lethal, necrotiz-

ing β toxin. It is probable that the severe hemorrhagic enteritis may be a result of both the β toxin produced prior to sporulation and the enterotoxin produced during sporulation.

### Botulism

*Clostridium botulinum* is the causative agent of a highly fatal food poisoning that follows the ingestion of a preformed toxin produced by the organisms while growing in the food.

ANTIGENIC CLASSIFICATION. Seven immunologically distinct toxins are produced by different types of C. botulinum and are indicated by capital letters. Types A, B, E, and, to a lesser extent, F are responsible for most cases of human botulism, while type C is found most often in ducks and fowl and type D in cattle, horses, and sheep. Type G has been isolated from soil, and although it does produce toxin, it has not been reported to cause human or animal botulism.

Curiously, the toxins appear to be secreted as progenitor toxins that, even though some have been crystallized, are composed of two or more easily dissociated polypeptides. Also, although not understood at the molecular level, the toxicity of those toxins that have been extensively studied can be increased from 4- to 250-fold by treatment with trypsin.

Additionally, it has been shown that the toxins produced by types D, C, and E are a result of a lysogenic conversion. Moreover, type C organisms can be cured by heating their spores at 70°C for 15 minutes, after which they are no longer toxin producers. Reinfection of these cured bacteria with phage 3C restores type C toxigenicity, but reinfection with phage 1D converts the cured type C organism into a toxigenic C. botulinum of type D. Moreover, reinfection of the cured type C organisms with phage NA1 (isolated from C. novyi) converts the C. botulinum into a toxigenic C. novyi type A, which then produces the lethal α toxin characteristic of the gas gangrene group.

EPIDEMIOLOGY AND PATHOGENICITY. *Clostridium botulinum* is distributed in soil, lake bottoms, and decaying vegetation; thus, many foods, both vegetables and meats, become contaminated with these organisms. Numerous animals die each year after ingestion of fermenting grains. This is especially true of ducks (the disease is called "limber neck") and cattle (particularly in South Africa).

The endospores of *C. botulinum* are very resistant to heat and may withstand boiling water temperatures for several hours. Thus, botulism in humans usually occurs in food which has been inadequately sterilized and placed in an anaerobic environment where the surviving spores can germinate and produce toxin.

Most cases in Europe have resulted from eating smoked, salted, or spiced meats and fish; botulism in the United States frequently follows the ingestion of home-canned vegetables. Botulism in commercially prepared foods is rare, and when it occurs it is a result of human error. During the past several decades, botulism has occurred in commercial cheese, tuna fish, vichyssoise, mushrooms, and smoked white fish.

The toxins are among the most toxic compounds known. It is estimated that 1 ml of culture fluid is sufficient to kill two million mice and that the lethal dose for humans may be in the range of 1 microgram of toxin.

Human symptoms usually begin after an incubation period of 18 to 36 hours and may include nausea and vomiting in addition to double vision, difficulty in swallowing, and some muscle paralysis. This may be followed by muscle weakness, blurred vision, and death as a result of respiratory failure. The toxin acts primarily as a neurotoxin by interfering with the release of acetylcholine from nerve endings. Untreated botulism has a mortality of 30–65%.

Although *C. botulinum* is described as an organism with essentially no invasive abilities, about a dozen cases of wound botulism have been reported in the United States between 1972 and 1975. Usually the wounds themselves were not serious, and wound botulism should be suspected for any individuals with even minor wounds who present the typical symptoms of botulism—blurred vision, weakness, difficulty in swallowing, and so forth.

A new variety of this disease was recognized during 1976 with the report of five cases of infant botulism. These cases occurred in babies as young as five weeks, some of whom were breast-fed, although all had some exposure to other foods. The surprising aspect of infant botulism is that both organisms and toxin were present in stools but could not be demonstrated in serum. Even more surprisingly, all infants recovered without treatment with antitoxin in spite of the fact that in one case botulism toxin and organisms continued to be present in stool specimens for eight weeks after clinical recovery. There is at present no data concerning the epidemiology of infant botulism, but it has been proposed that the infants ingested viable *Clostridium botulinum* spores (which are normally present on many raw foods and are extremely heat-resistant) and that the disease resulted from the germination of the spores in the intestinal tract. The fact that four of these cases occurred in California within a six-month period suggests that infant botulism may be more common than previously recognized and that this disease should be considered in infants with unexplained weakness, difficulty in swallowing, opthalmoplegia (paralysis of the ocular muscles), or respiratory arrest.

LABORATORY DIAGNOSIS OF BOTULISM. Even after an individual develops symptoms of botulism, there may be free toxin in the blood stream. Mice are incredibly sensitive to the toxin, and the intraperitoneal injections of a patient's serum may result in death of the mouse. Usually, the implicated food is no longer available, but if it is, extracts should also be injected into mice and aliquots cultured anaerobically in an attempt to grow the organisms.

PREVENTION AND CONTROL OF BOTULISM. Any individual suspected of having botulism should be given antitoxin to types A, B, and E. The antiserum cannot neutralize any fixed toxin but can react with free residual toxin. All other individuals who possibly could have eaten the same food should also be administered antitoxin.

In contrast to the endospores of the organism, botulism toxin is very heat labile. Thus, home-canned vegetables (particularly nonacid ones such as corn, peas, and beans) should be boiled for about 10 minutes before eating. Such treatment would inactivate toxin that might be present. Home-canned foods that are prepared in a pressure cooker, where temperatures of 120°C are reached, should be completely sterile; however to be effective the cooking temperature must be maintained for sufficient time to bring all of the food to that temperature for at least 15 minutes.

Toxoids stimulate solid immunity, but because of the rarity of the disease in humans (15 cases during 1975 in the United States) their use would be unwarranted. Toxoids have, however, been used successfully for the prevention of botulism in cattle, particularly in South Africa.

## REFERENCES

Brachman, P. S. 1970. Anthrax. *Ann. New York Acad. Sci.* **174:**577–582.

Davis, J. C., J. M. Dunn, C. O. Hagood, and B. E. Bassett. 1973. Hyperbaric medicine in the U.S. Air Force. *JAMA* **224:**205–209.

Donadio, J. A., E. J. Gangarosa, and G. A. Faich. 1971. Diagnosis and treatment of botulism. *J. Infect. Dis.* **124:**108–112.

Duncan, C. L., D. H. Strong, and M. Sebald. 1972. Sporulation and enterotoxin production by mutants of *Clostridium perfringens. J. Bacteriol.* **110:**378–391.

Ecklund, W. W., F. T. Poysky, S. M. Reed, and C. A. Smith. 1971. Bacteriophage and the toxigenicity of *Clostridium botulinum* type C. *Science* **172:**480–482.

Gould, G. W., and A. Hurst, eds. 1969. *The Bacterial Spore.* Academic Press, New York.

Hatheway, C. L. 1976. Toxoid of *Clostridium botulinum* type F: Purification and immunogenicity studies. *J. Appl. Microbiol.* **31:**234–242.

Labbe, R., E. Somers, and C. Duncan. 1976. Influence of starch source on sporulation and enterotoxin production by *Clostridium perfringens* type A. *J. Appl. Microbiol.* **3:**455–457.

Lamb, R. 1973. A new look at infectious diseases: Anthrax. *Br. Med. J.* **1:**157–160.

Lincoln, R. E., and D. C. Fish. 1970. Anthrax Toxin. Chapter 9 in T. C. Montie, S. Kadis, and S. J. Ajl, eds. *Microbial Toxins*, Vol. III. Academic Press, New York.

Lowenstein, M. S. 1972. Epidemiology of *Clostridium perfringens* food poisoning. *New Engl. J. Med.* **286:**1026–1028.

Merson, M. H., J. M. Hughes, V. R. Dowell, A. Taylor, W. H. Barker, and E. J. Gangarosa. 1974. Current trends in botulism in the United States. *JAMA* **229:**1305–1308.

Nakamura, M., and J. A. Schulze. 1970. *Clostridium perfringens* food poisoning. *Annu. Rev. Microbiol.* **24:**359–372.

Sugiyama, H., and K. H. Yang. 1975. Growth potential of *Clostridium botulinum* in fresh mushrooms packaged in semipermeable plastic film. *J. Appl. Microbiol.* **30:**964–969.

Sugiyama, H., S. L. Brenner, and B. R. Dasgupta. 1975. Detection of *Clostridium botulinum* toxin by local paralysis elicited with intramuscular challenge. *J. Appl. Microbiol.* **30:**420–423.

Weinstein, L. 1973. Tetanus. *New Engl. J. Med.* **289:**1293–1296.

# 24

## Corynebacterium and Listeria

### Corynebacterium

Although diphtheria no longer is common in the United States, it still occurs as sporadic individual cases or small outbreaks (128 reported cases in 1976). Table 24-1 provides the annual case rate for the period 1967–1976. Although the morbidity rate is small, few areas of the country are completely free of the disease.

**Table 24-1. Diphtheria in the United States, 1967–1976**

| Year | No. of cases | Cases per 100,000 population |
|------|--------------|------------------------------|
| 1967 | 219 | 0.11 |
| 1968 | 260 | 0.13 |
| 1969 | 241 | 0.12 |
| 1970 | 435 | 0.21 |
| 1971 | 215 | 0.10 |
| 1972 | 152 | 0.07 |
| 1973 | 228 | 0.11 |
| 1974 | 272 | 0.13 |
| 1975 | 307 | 0.14 |
| 1976 | 128 | 0.06 |

### CHARACTERIZATION OF CORYNEBACTERIUM DIPHTHERIAE

Corynebacterium diphtheriae was isolated in 1883 by Klebs, and was shown to be the etiologic agent of diphtheria by Loeffler in 1884. Consequently, it is sometimes referred to as the Klebs-Loeffler bacillus. The generic name Corynebacterium is derived from the Greek stem kory meaning club-shaped. They are gram-positive, non-spore-forming, non-motile rods that can certainly be described as pleomorphic. Some may be straight, whereas others are curved or club-shaped. When they divide by binary fission, the newly formed bacteria have a tendency. to snap apart. Stained smears show many cells forming sharp angles with each other (see Figure 24-1).

Another outstanding characteristic of the diphtheria bacillus is its granular and uneven staining. When stained with methylene blue or toluidine blue, the granules in the cell take on a reddish appearance. These refractive granules have a variety of names, such as Babes-Ernst bodies, metachromatic granules, and volutin; they are composed of a polymer of inorganic polyphosphate. The granules are not seen during active growth, but start to

337

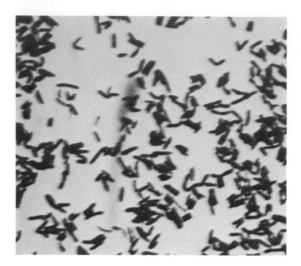

**Figure 24-1.** Gram-stained culture smear of *Corynebacterium diphtheriae* ($\times$ 4200).

appear toward the end of the logarithmic growth period. It appears that they represent storage depots for materials needed to form high-energy phosphate bonds; the bacteria possess enzymes that phosphorylate glucose to form glucose-6-phosphate and ADP to form ATP, using the phosphate present in the storage granules.

*Corynebacterium diphtheriae* grows well on blood agar medium. However, because most other bacteria in the throat also grow under these conditions, media have been devised that favor the growth of the diphtheria bacillus and restrict the growth of some of the normal flora of the throat. Two media are useful for this purpose: (1) Loeffler's coagulated blood serum, and (2) blood agar or chocolate blood agar to which potassium tellurite ($K_2TeO_3$) has been added. On the latter medium, colonies of *C. diphtheriae* become dark gray to black (see Figure 24-2). This occurs because the tellurite or tellurous ions are able to diffuse through the cell wall and membrane and are reduced to tellurium metal which is precipitated inside the cell.

The organisms in this species have been divided into three types, based primarily on the appearance of their colonies on tellurite media. Originally, it was thought that there was a correlation between the severity of the disease and the colony type. This is now known to be untrue, but the names *gravis, intermedius,* and *mitis* are still used to refer to the three types of *C. diphtheriae.*

## EPIDEMIOLOGY AND PATHOGENICITY OF DIPHTHERIA BACILLI

Basic comprehension of diphtheria came in 1888 when Roux and Yersin discovered that culture filtrates (free from diphtheria bacilli) are lethal for animals. Furthermore, the symptoms and the pathologic changes that occur as a result of the injection of the toxic filtrates are the same as those from the disease itself. In brief, diphtheria is an acute infection in which the causative organisms remain in the respiratory tract, even though on some occasions, especially in the tropics, the organisms produce wound infections. The site of the infection, usually the throat, becomes inflamed as the bacteria grow and excrete a powerful exotoxin. Dead tissue cells, along with the host's leukocytes, red blood cells, and the bacteria, form a dull, gray exudate called a diphtheritic pseudomembrane. If this pseudomembrane extends into the trachea, the air passages may become

**Figure 24-2.** Gray-black colonies of *Corynebacterium diphtheriae* from a throat swab streaked on cystine tellurite medium.

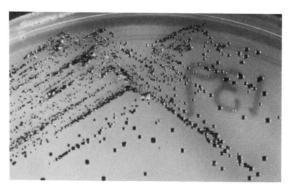

blocked, and in these cases a tracheotomy may be necessary to prevent suffocation.

Although there is no doubt as to the role of the toxin in the production of diphtheria, there are unknown virulence factors that also contribute to the ability of the diphtheria bacillus to cause infections. Thus, it is possible for non-toxin-producing strains of C. diphtheriae to be involved in a local infection with pseudomembrane formation, but these cases are mild. The severe symptoms and frequent death from diphtheria are the result of the action of the diphtheria toxin, which is transported via the blood stream to all parts of the body. Lesions may occur in the kidney, heart, and nerves, resulting in acute nephritis and serious cardiac weakness. The incubation period is two to five days.

## TOXICOGENICITY OF
## CORYNEBACTERIUM DIPHTHERIAE

The ability to produce toxin is the major difference between avirulent and virulent organisms. In 1951, Freeman discovered that this ability to synthesize toxin was possessed only by organisms that are lysogenic for phage $\beta$ or a closely related bacteriophage. Thus, all strains of diphtheria organisms that produce toxin are lysogenic, and avirulent strains of diphtheria bacilli can be made into virulent, toxin-producing strains by infecting them with the temperate bacteriophage. As noted in previous instances, this change in the properties of a bacterial cell as a result of becoming lysogenic is called lysogenic conversion (see Chapter 8).

In the commercial production of diphtheria toxin for vaccine, the amount of iron present in the growth medium is critical. Good toxin production is obtained only at very low concentrations of iron (2.0 micromolar). At concentrations as low as 10 micromolar, toxin production becomes negligible. As yet there are no absolute data to explain this phenomenon, but circumstantial evidence suggests that, normally, the bacterium forms a repressor that prevents the expression of the phage tox+ gene and that this repressor may be an iron-containing protein. Thus, when the concentration of iron is abnormally low, the repressor will not be synthesized, and the tox+ gene will be transcribed, ultimately yielding toxin.

### Mode of Action of Diphtheria Toxin

Since the toxin is effective against many cells, the use of tissue cultures provides a model for studying its mode of action. Early studies reported that, although toxin had no effect on the respiration of HeLa cells (human cervical carcinoma tissue culture cells), all protein synthesis stopped about 1 to 1.5 hours after the additon of the toxin. Surprisingly, dialyzed, cell-free, protein-synthesizing systems were entirely insensitive to the action of the toxin unless oxidized nicotinamide adenine dinucleotide (NAD) was added to the reaction.

Subsequent research has shown that the toxin possesses enzymatic activity which cleaves nicotinamide from NAD and then catalyzes the covalent attachment of the resulting ADP-ribose to elongation factor 2 (EF-2, see Figure 24-3). EF-2 is required for the translocase reaction of polypeptide synthesis in which the ribosome is moved to the next codon on the mRNA after the peptide bond is formed to the most recent amino acid to be added to the chain. When EF-2 is inactivated by the additon of ADP-ribose, the ribosome is frozen, and protein synthesis stops. Insofar as is known, EF-2 from all eucaryotic cells (those studied include vertebrate, invertebrate, wheat, and yeast) is inactivated in the presence of diphtheria toxin and NAD, whereas the corresponding factor, EF-G (which occurs in bacteria) or the analogous factor from mitochondria are not affected.

### Structure of Diphtheria Toxin

The toxin is excreted from the bacterium as a single polypeptide chain of about 63,000

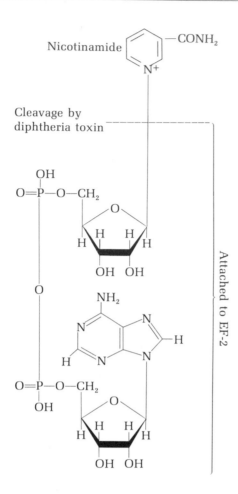

Figure 24-3. Structure of NAD, showing bond cleaved by diphtheria toxin.

daltons with two disulfide bridges. Although highly toxic for cells or animals, the pure, intact toxin is inert in cell-free protein systems, even when NAD is present. Thus, the secreted toxin is actually a "proenzyme" that in cell-free systems must be activated before it can function as an enzyme. This activation, as shown in Figure 24-4, is accomplished in two steps: (1) treatment with trypsin hydrolyzes a peptide bond between the disulfide-linked amino acids, and (2) reduction of the disulfides to sulfhydryl groups using a reducing agent such as mercaptoethanol yields two smaller peptides which have been designated fragment A (24,000 daltons) and fragment B (39,000 daltons).

Fragment A is very active in cleaving the nicotinamide moiety from NAD and in catalyzing the transfer of ADP-ribose from NAD to EF-2 when added to cell-free protein synthesizing systems, but it has no effect when given to animals or to intact HeLa cells. Thus, it appears that although fragment A is the activated enzyme (and hence contains all the toxic properties), it cannot get into intact cells.

Fragment B, on the other hand, has no enzymatic activity, but current information indicates that fragment B is needed for attachment of the toxin to specific receptor sites on cells. Cells probably possess specific receptor sites for the diphtheria toxin, as suggested by several observations: rats and mice are over 1000 times more resistant to the intact toxin than are other susceptible animals, but their cell-free protein synthesiz-

Figure 24-4. Sequence of events in the expression of enzymatic activity (ADP-ribosylation of EF-2) in diphtheria toxin. Fragment A is nontoxic because it cannot cross the cell membrane except when it is linked to the fragment B portion of the molecule.

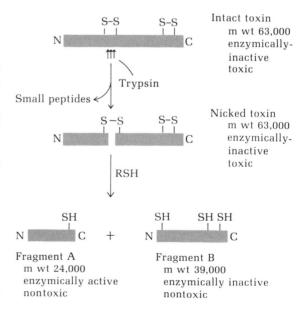

ing system is equally sensitive to the enzymatic action of fragment A; and mutant phages which code for a protein that is defective in its A fragment (and is, therefore, nontoxic) will competitively inhibit the action of normal toxin on HeLa cells.

The question of whether or not the phage genome itself codes for the toxin or merely derepresses a bacterial gene which could then synthesize the toxin was solved using a series of mutant phages. After treatment of the phages with the mutagen nitrosoguanidine, phage-infected bacteria that produced defective nontoxic proteins immunologically similar to normal diphtheria toxin were isolated. Some of these nontoxic proteins were defective in fragment B and could not attach to susceptible cells, while others were defective in fragment A and were inactive in cell-free systems even after trypsin and mercaptoethanol treatment. Furthermore, toxin can be synthesized in a cell-free system from E. coli using DNA from phage $\beta$. Thus, the data seem unequivocable that the toxin is coded directly by the phage genome.

In summary, the usual series of events leading to toxin action is as follows: (1) the toxin binds to specific receptor sites on susceptible cells; (2) the toxin enters the cell (perhaps through a phagocytic vesicle which can then fuse with a lysosome), and lysosomal proteases hydrolyze the toxin into fragments A and B; and (3) reduction of the disulfide bridges (perhaps by glutathione) releases fragment A from fragment B, and fragment A can then enzymatically inactivate EF-2.

## LABORATORY DIAGNOSIS OF DIPHTHERIA

Diagnosis of diphtheria is based on isolating Corynebacterium diphtheriae from the infected area and demonstrating its toxin-producing ability. Specimens are inoculated on Loeffler's coagulated serum slants, tellurite plates, and blood agar plates. Direct smears are stained with methylene blue and observed for volutin granules.

A definitive laboratory diagnosis requires the differentiation between the avirulent, nontoxin-producing strains and the virulent toxin-producing organisms. This can be done by the intracutaneous injection of a suspension of organisms into two guinea pigs, one of which is protected by prior receipt of specific diphtheria antitoxin. A toxin-producing organism will produce a severe inflammation in the unprotected animal but little or no inflammation in the protected animal. Also, there is an in vitro virulence test in which the unknown organism is compared with a known toxin-producing diphtheria bacillus. In this case, antiserum is placed on a piece of filter paper which is placed vertically across the streaks of the organisms on a petri dish. If toxin is produced by the unknown organisms, a line of precipitate will occur at the optimal concentration of the toxin and antitoxin, forming a line of identity with the adjacent known toxin-producing organisms (see Figure 24-5).

## TREATMENT AND CONTROL OF DIPHTHERIA

It is essential that antitoxin be administered promptly to neutralize the toxin being produced. This is because antitoxin is ineffective if given after the toxin is bound to cell receptor sites. Thus, the initial diagnosis must be made from the clinical picture, since it would be unsafe to wait for a bacteriologic confirmation before starting treatment. Most physicians agree that it is safer to err by occasionally administering antitoxin to someone who was clinically misdiagnosed than to wait for a more positive confirmation.

The organism is sensitive to penicillin and other antibiotics, but the antibiotics do not neutralize circulating toxin and therefore are of value only when used concurrently with antitoxin.

Control is based entirely on the mass immunization of children with a nontoxic

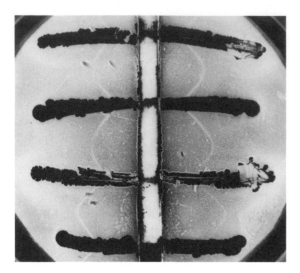

**Figure 24-5.** Curved lines of identity (precipitate) are visible between the dark streaks of organisms that cross a paper strip saturated with antitoxin. In this case, then, all four streaks are *Corynebacterium diphtheriae.*

toxoid prepared by treating toxin with formalin. This is usually administered along with tetanus toxoid and pertussis vaccine in three monthly injections beginning at three or four months of age. Immunization does not provide life-long immunity, and booster shots are necessary every three to five years—particularly for children, who appear more susceptible to overt disease.

Recent reports show that only antibodies to the fragment B portion of the toxin molecule are capable of neutralizing the toxin—supposedly by preventing the attachment of toxin to the specific receptor sites on the cell surface. Treatment of the toxin

with formalin, however, both detoxifies the toxin (by an unknown mechanism) and protects fragment B from the action of proteolytic enzymes, resulting in better protective antibody production than obtained by using untreated fragment B or defective toxins possessing a normal fragment B.

A Schick test may be used to determine whether or not an individual is susceptible to diphtheria. This test is carried out by the intradermal injection of a small amount of diphtheria toxin. A person without antibodies to the toxin (and hence, susceptible to diphtheria) will develop an inflamed area at the site of the injection that will reach a maximum level in about 48 hours. In contrast, those persons who have antibodies will neutralize the toxin and will not develop an inflammation at the site of the toxin injection. In actual practice, a control substance in which the toxin has been inactivated by heating is injected intradermally into the other arm to make certain that any inflammatory response is due to the toxin and is not a result of a hypersensitivity reaction to some extraneous component in the toxin preparation.

## OTHER CORYNEBACTERIA

Many species of *Corynebacterium* exist in the soil: a few cause animal diseases, and a large number are plant pathogens. However, *C. hofmannii,* a normal inhabitant of the throat, *C. xerosis,* found in the normal conjunctiva, and *C. acnes,* a normal skin inhabitant, are routinely isolated from humans. These are not toxigenic nor associated with disease in humans.

# Listeria

Until recently, listeriosis was considered to be a rare disease in humans, but reports of the increasing frequency of human listeriosis suggest that *Listeria* infections are not rare but have been frequently unrecognized.

## CHARACTERIZATION OF *LISTERIA MONOCYTOGENES*

*Listeria monocytogenes* is a small, gram-positive, motile diphtheroid. The organisms are facultative and produce a narrow band of beta-hemolysis when growing on blood agar plates. Colonies growing on a clear, tryptose agar appear blue-green when viewed with an oblique light held at an angle of about 45°.

Once isolated, *Listeria monocytogenes* is easily subcultured, but initial isolation may be difficult. One unusual enrichment technique is to store specimens at 4°C for extended periods of time. This may be done by inoculating blood or spinal fluid into a tenfold excess of blood culture medium. This is then stored at 4°C and subcultured weekly for three to six months by streaking onto a blood agar plate. Tissue or fecal suspensions may also be stored in screw-cap tubes at 4°C and subcultured at weekly intervals. The organisms demonstrate a tumbling type of motility if grown at 18 to 20°C.

## EPIDEMIOLOGY AND PATHOGENICITY OF LISTERIOSIS

It appears that *L. monocytogenes* is primarily an animal pathogen, and it is likely that many human infections are acquired through contact with domestic animals and birds. *L.*

*monocytogenes*, however, has also been isolated from soil, water, and sewage and from the feces of a number of asymptomatic humans, rodents, swine, and poultry. It is obvious, therefore, that it is a very ubiquitous organism, and although many human infections reportedly result from animal contact, some occur in urban residents who have little or no contact with animals.

Listeriosis can mimic a number of infectious diseases and in humans can cause meningitis, septicemia, endocarditis, urethritis, conjunctivitis, and abortions. The fatality rate for all reported *Listeria* infections in the United States between 1933 and 1966 was 42%. All age groups are susceptible to infection, but, as shown in Table 24-2, the fatality rate is much higher for the newborn under four weeks of age and for the older population than for other persons under the age of 50. Susceptibility and the corresponding high fatality rate in the older age group are frequently associated with heart disease, various types of malignancies, diabetes mellitus, and the use of immunosuppressive drugs.

Infection during pregnancy may result in abortion, stillbirth, or meningitis in the newborn. Infections occurring in the first few

**Table 24-2. Age and Sex Distribution for Human Listeriosis in the U.S., 1968–1969**

| Age Group | Male | Female | Total | Percentage of total | Fatalities | Group fatality rate |
|---|---|---|---|---|---|---|
| 0–4 weeks | 11 | 21 | 32 | 27.3 | 5[a] | 15.2 |
| 4 weeks–9 years | 3 | 4 | 7 | 6.0 | 1 | 3.0 |
| 10–19 years | 1 | 1 | 2 | 1.7 | 1 | 3.0 |
| 20–29 years | 2 | 5 | 7 | 6.0 | 0 | 0 |
| 30–39 years | 2 | 2 | 4 | 3.4 | 0 | 0 |
| 40–49 years | 8 | 7 | 15 | 12.8 | 5 | 15.2 |
| 50–59 years | 12 | 11 | 23 | 19.7 | 8 | 24.2 |
| 60–69 years | 9 | 5 | 14 | 12.0 | 6 | 18.2 |
| 70+ years | 12 | 1 | 13 | 11.1 | 7 | 21.2 |
| Total | 60 | 57 | 117 | 100.0 | 33[a] | 28.2 |
| Percentage of total | 51.3 | 48.7 | 100.0 | . . . | 28.2 | . . . |

[a]Does not include one aborted 5-month fetus or one death in which age and sex were unknown.

weeks of life are believed to be spread from the mother who acquires the organism during the third trimester of pregnancy.

## TREATMENT AND CONTROL OF LISTERIOSIS

*Listeria monocytogenes* is sensitive to penicillin, ampicillin, and the tetracyclines, and many investigators report that the tetracyclines are the drugs of choice.

Because of the ubiquity of the organisms, prevention of infections is difficult. Control appears limited to the early recognition and treatment of listeriosis.

## REFERENCES

Barksdale, L. 1970. *Corynebacterium diphtheriae* and its relatives. *Bacteriol. Rev.* **34:**378–422.

Brooks, G. F., J. V. Bennett, and R. A. Feldman. 1974. Diphtheria in the United States, 1959–1970. *J. Infect. Dis* **129:**172–178.

Busch, L. A. 1971. Human listeriosis in the United States. *J. Infect. Dis.* **123:**328–331.

Collier, R. J. 1975. Diphtheria toxin: Mode of action and structure. *Bacteriol. Rev.* **39:**54–85.

Freeman, V. J. 1951. Studies on the virulence of bacteriophage-infected strains of *Corynebacterium diphtheriae*. *J. Bacteriol.* **61:**675–678.

Gantz, N. M., R. L. Myerowitz, A. A. Medeiros, G. F. Carrera, R. E. Wilson, and T. F. O'Brien. 1975. Listeriosis in immunosuppressed patients. *Amer. J. Med.* **58:**637–643.

Gill, D. M., A. M. Pappenheimer, Jr., R. Brown, and J. T. Kurnick. 1969. Toxin-stimulated hydrolysis of nicotinamide adenine dinucleotide in mammalian cell extracts. *J. Exp. Med.* **129:**1–21.

Medoff, G., L. J. Kunz, and A. N. Weinberg. 1971. Listeriosis in humans: An evaluation. *J. Infect. Dis.* **123:**247–250.

Moehring, T. J., and J. M. Moehring. 1976. Interaction of diphtheria toxin and its active subunit, fragment A, with toxin-sensitive and toxin-resistant cells. *Infec. Immun.* **13:**1426–1432.

Pappenheimer, A. M., Jr., and D. M. Gill. 1973. Diphtheria. *Science* **182:**353–358.

Uchida, T., A. M. Pappenheimer, Jr., and A. A. Harper. 1972. Reconstitution of diphtheria toxin from two nontoxic cross-reacting mutant proteins. *Science* **175:**901–903.

Weis, J., and H. P. R. Seeliger. 1975. Incidence of *Listeria monocytogenes* in nature. *J. Appl. Microbiol.* **30:**29–32.

# 25

# Mycobacterium

The most obvious characteristic of the mycobacteria is the large amount of lipid present in their cell walls—approximately 40% of the total cell dry weight—causing them to grow as extremely rough, hydrophobic colonies. Mycobacteria are also difficult to stain, but once stained, they resist decolorization—even when washed with 95% ethanol containing 3% hydrochloric acid. Organisms with the ability to retain a stain in spite of washing with acid alcohol are referred to as acid-fast. Only the members of the genus *Mycobacterium* and a few species of *Nocardia* possess this property, and this characteristic helps in detecting mycobacteria in body fluids, such as sputum or gastric washings.

There are many nonpathogenic mycobacteria as well as many pathogens whose range of host animals is narrowly restricted. Human mycobacterial infections are primarily of two types: (1) tuberculosis, usually a respiratory infection but occasionally acquired by ingestion of the organisms, and (2) leprosy, primarily a disease of the skin. Both diseases are chronic infections and may last for many years, causing destructive lesions as a result of a cellular immune response to the organisms and their products.

## MYCOBACTERIUM TUBERCULOSIS

In 1882 *Mycobacterium tuberculosis* (commonly called the tubercle bacillus) was shown by Robert Koch to be the causative agent of tuberculosis. This human disease may occur as a brief, completely asymptomatic incident in the life of one individual, while in another it may produce a chronic, progressive pulmonary disease that results in the loss of almost all functional lung tissue.

### Properties of Tubercle Bacilli

In an effort to define the factors responsible for their virulence, few microorganisms have been as intensively studied from a chemical standpoint as the tubercle bacilli. Although a number of factors have been characterized, no one component that accounts for their disease-producing potential has been discovered.

STRUCTURE AND GROWTH OF *Mycobacterium tuberculosis*. The tubercle bacilli are thin rods, usually straight but sometimes bent or club-shaped. They are nonmotile, do not form spores, do not form capsules, and, when stained, often appear beaded or granular (see Figure 25-1).

345

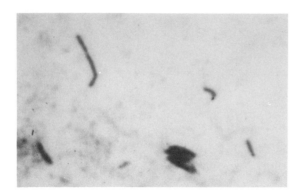

**Figure 25-1.** Short and long cells, chains, and a clump of acid-fast mycobacteria in a sputum smear (about × 5000). (The "dark" cells are actually red against a blue background.) Chemical and cultural tests would be needed to confirm these as *Mycobacterium tuberculosis*.

Routinely, tubercle bacilli are stained using the Ziehl-Neelsen technique in which a smear is covered with the red stain carbolfuchsin and the dye-covered smear is heated to steaming for a few minutes to aid the penetration of the dye into the bacterium. A cold-stain modification of this procedure, in which the carbol-fuchsin is first dissolved in a detergent, is also used to stain these organisms. In either case the stained smear is washed with acid alcohol and counterstained with methylene blue. The acid-fast mycobacteria retain the original red stain, whereas all non-acid-fast organisms will appear blue.

*Mycobacterium tuberculosis* is an obligate aerobe that can be grown in a simple medium composed of only inorganic salts, asparagine, and glycerol. Because of their high lipid content, the bacteria grow in tightly-matted colonies, or as surface pellicles in a liquid medium (see Figure 25-2). Mycobacteria will grow evenly dispersed in a medium (described by Dubos) which contains a nonionic detergent called Tween 80.

The growth of *M. tuberculosis* is considerably slower than that of most other bacteria, and even under optimal conditions cell division requires 12 to 20 hours. It may therefore take as long as six weeks before growth is visible following a small inoculum.

The organisms are readily killed by heat, and the conditions of pasteurization practiced in the United States are sufficient to kill tubercle bacilli that might be present in milk. On the other hand, they are quite resistant to chemical agents and are particularly resistant to drying, making it possible for *M. tuberculosis* to remain alive for long periods in rooms, bedding, sputum, and similar environments.

CHEMICAL COMPOSITION OF TUBERCLE BACILLI. The fact that as much as 40% of the dry weight of a mycobacterium may consist of lipid undoubtedly accounts for many of their unusual growth and staining characteristics. A comprehensive discussion of mycobacterial lipids is beyond the scope of this text, but one class of lipids, the mycosides, is unique to acid-fast organisms and involved in some manner with the pathogenicity of the mycobacteria.

Mycolic acid (Figure 25-3) is a large α-branched, β-hydroxy fatty acid that varies

**Figure 25-2.** *a.* A single, tightly-matted colony of *Mycobacterium tuberculosis* on a solid medium. *b.* A surface pellicle of *M. tuberculosis* grown on a liquid medium.

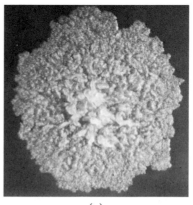

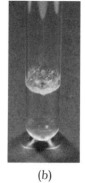

(b)

(a)

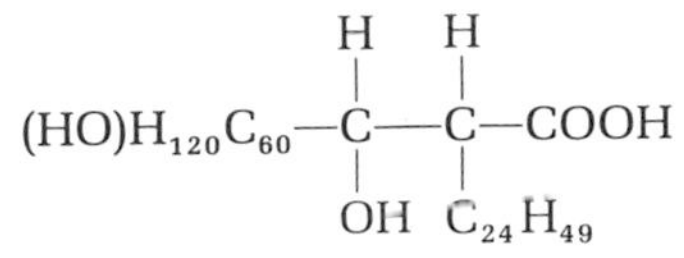

$$\text{(HO)H}_{120}\text{C}_{60}\underset{\overset{|}{\text{OH}}}{\overset{\overset{|}{\text{H}}}{-}\text{C}-}\underset{\overset{|}{\text{C}_{24}\text{H}_{49}}}{\overset{\overset{|}{\text{H}}}{-}\text{C}-}\text{COOH}$$

**Figure 25-3.** Structure of mycolic acid from *M. tuberculosis*. The length of the two side chains varies among the different species of mycobacteria.

slightly in size from one species of mycobacterium to another. These acids occur free or bound to carbohydrates as glycolipids that are referred to as mycosides. Free mycolic acid is, by itself, acid-fast, but the observation that acid-fastness is lost following the destruction of the cell integrity by sonication makes it unlikely that mycolic acid alone accounts for this property.

Cord factor is a mycoside that contains two molecules of mycolic acid esterified to the disaccharide, trehalose (see Figure 25-4a). It is found in virulent mycobacteria, and its presence is responsible for a phenomenon in which the individual bacteria grow parallel to each other forming large serpentine cords (see Figure 25-4b). Avirulent mycobacteria do not grow in such cords. Purified cord factor is lethal for mice, and although it

seems obvious that it is involved in virulence, its precise role in the pathogenesis of tuberculosis is unknown.

Wax D is a very complicated mycoside in which 15 to 20 molecules of mycolic acid are esterified to a large polysaccharide composed of arabinose, galactose, mannose, glucosamine, and galactosamine—all of which appear to be linked to the peptidoglycan of the cell wall. When emulsified with water and oil, Wax D acts as an adjuvant to increase the antibody response to an antigen, and it is probably the active component in Freund's complete adjuvant, which employs intact tubercle bacilli emulsified with water, oil, and antigen. Wax D also seems to be the component responsible for the induction of a cellular type of immune response to the tubercle bacilli. If Wax D is mixed with mycobacterial proteins, one obtains a cellular immune response to the proteins, while this does not occur using the proteins alone.

*Mycobacterium tuberculosis* also possesses a number of protein antigens which by themselves do not appear to be toxic or involved in virulence. However, the host's cellular immune response to certain of these mycobacterial proteins apparently accounts

**Figure 25-4.** *a.* Structure of cord factor (6,6′-Dimycolyltrehalose). *b.* Young colony of virulent *Mycobacterium tuberculosis* on brain-heart infusion showing typical parallel growth.

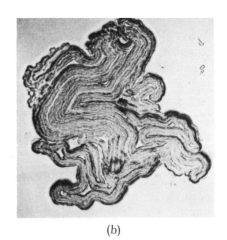

(a)

(b)

for the acquired immunity and allergic response to the tubercle bacilli.

## Pathogenesis of
### *Mycobacterium tuberculosis*

Humans tend to vary considerably in their response to infection by tubercle bacilli, and active disease can, in general, be thought of as resulting either from a primary infection or from a subsequent reactivation of a quiescent infection.

PRIMARY INFECTION. Following inhalation, tubercle bacilli initiate small lesions in the lower respiratory tract and drain from these lesions to the regional lymph nodes. This primary complex, as these lesions are called, frequently heals to form tiny "tubercles" which are too small to be seen by X-rays but may continue to harbor the viable tubercle bacilli indefinitely. In other cases, multiplication of the bacilli continues and the lesion expands, destroying the normal tissue and leaving the necrotic tissue in a semisolid, cheesy state. This process, called caseation necrosis, may eventually heal and become infiltrated with fibrous tissue and calcium deposits; or the lesion may continue to expand, leaving cavities in the lung after the clearance of necrotic tissue. The lesion might also involve a pulmonary vein, allowing the organisms to spread via the blood stream. This development causes miliary tuberculosis, with lesions in every organ of the body. When a lesion ruptures into the meninges, a tuberculous meningitis will occur.

During the early part of the infection, the organisms encounter little, if any, host resistance, and the lesions, called exudative lesions, are characterized by the presence of polymorphonuclear leukocytes, fluid, and inflammation. At this time most tubercle bacilli are found growing intracellularly in macrophages. Later, as the host develops a cellular immunity or allergy to the tubercle bacilli, the lesions are called productive lesions, or tubercles, and the organisms, which are few in number, are now mostly extracellular, surrounded by necrotic tissue and large mononuclear macrophages known as epithelioid cells. Some of the epithelioid cells have fused to form large, multinucleate giant cells. The necrotic tissue and epithelioid cells are, in turn, surrounded by lymphocytes and fibrous tissue, which wall off the tubercle from the normal tissues of the lung.

REACTIVATION INFECTION. Whether or not the primary infection heals early or late, the walled-off tubercle is believed to contain viable organisms, which probably persist for the remaining life of the host. It is estimated that two-thirds of all new active cases of tuberculosis represent a reactivation of a healed primary infection. This postulation is difficult to prove, but it is strongly supported by the observation that over 80% of all new cases reported occur in persons over 25 years of age. Also, it has been shown that the majority of new cases of active tuberculosis among Navy recruits occur in persons who exhibited positive skin reactions to tuberculin at the time of their enlistment.

## Immunity and Host Response to
### *Mycobacterium tuberculosis*

Immunity to tuberculosis is an elusive concept, and although no one doubts its existence, there is no easy way that it can be quantitated. The earliest demonstration of immunity occurred when Koch showed that a second injection of tubercle bacilli into a guinea pig produced a different host response from that of the initial injection. In essence, Koch's initial injection resulted in an ulcer that failed to heal at the injection site, followed by spread to regional lymph nodes. A subsequent injection several weeks later was characterized by a more localized ulcer that eventually healed and by the guinea pig's ability to kill the tubercle bacilli before they reached the regional lymph nodes. This observation, called the Koch phenomenon, certainly demonstrates some immunity, since the lymph nodes draining the site of the second injection do not routinely become infected. However, the guinea pigs in such experiments die from the initial infection.

Subsequently, Koch found that the injection of a culture filtrate into an animal that had been previously infected with tubercle bacilli evoked an allergic response which was characterized by induration (a hardened area that becomes maximal in 48 hours), erythema, and (in severe reactions) by an ulcerative necrosis at the site of injection. Koch named this culture filtrate tuberculin, and since the reaction was slower than the antibody-mediated arthus reaction (see Chapter 16), similar reactions have been referred to as delayed-type hypersensitivity or tuberculin-type hypersensitivity. The proteins in the culture filtrate that evoke this allergic response have been partially purified and are available commercially as a purified protein derivative (PPD), while Koch's original type preparation is called old tuberculin or O.T.

The question of whether or not this allergic response to tuberculin is synonymous with the immune response characterized by the Koch phenomenon has activated considerable controversy among immunologists. However, the fact that allergy to tuberculin and immunity to tuberculosis can be passively transferred only with cells makes it probable that both are manifestations of a typical cellular-type immunity to the tubercle bacillus.

## Laboratory Diagnosis of Tuberculosis

A tentative diagnosis of tuberculosis can be made by observing acid-fast rods in smears of sputum, gastric washings, or urine, but a definite diagnosis is established only after the isolation and the identification of tubercle bacilli from the patient.

Direct smears are stained by either the Ziehl-Neelson technique and observed for acid-fast rods or by a fluorescent rhodamine-auramine dye and observed with a special microscope employing ultraviolet light. Since tubercle bacilli are strongly resistant to alkali, sputum is usually first thinned by

shaking in 0.1 N NaOH, following which the mixture is centrifuged to concentrate the organisms.

Cultural methods are considerably more reliable than staining direct smears because only a few organisms are necessary for growth. Most cultures are grown on a medium containing egg yolk or oleic acid and albumin, and dyes such as malachite green or antibiotics such as penicillin may be added to inhibit the growth of contaminating organisms.

Guinea pig inoculation is also a sensitive (but expensive) procedure for the demonstration of small numbers of tubercle bacilli. Samples of concentrated sputum or other body fluids are injected subcutaneously into a guinea pig and after several weeks the animal is tested for tuberculin hypersensitivity. At that time the resulting lesion can also be cultured and examined for acid-fast organisms.

## Clinical Management of Tuberculosis

TREATMENT. Before the antibiotic era complete bed rest was the primary treatment for tuberculosis, and every state had a number of sanatoriums that were used exclusively for tuberculosis patients. The discovery of streptomycin in the mid-1940's marked the beginning of the chemotherapeutic treatment of tuberculosis. But, a cure was neither quick nor easy, and it was soon found that long-term therapy with streptomycin resulted in damage to the eighth cranial nerve (involved in hearing) and in the occurrence of mutants of M. tuberculosis which were resistant to streptomycin. Currently, isoniazid (INH) is the treatment of choice, since it is inexpensive, effective, relatively nontoxic to the patient, and can be administered orally. However, INH-resistant mutants also occur, and it is routine to treat active tuberculosis simultaneously with INH plus a companion agent to kill any INH-resistant mutants. Companion drugs include para-aminosalicylic acid (PAS), ethambutol, and rifampin. In all cases treatment must be continued for up to a year. Reasons for such long treatments probably include the fact that many organisms are intracellular, their rate of metabolism is very slow, and the chemotherapeutic drug does not easily penetrate the fibrotic or caseous lesions.

CONTROL OF TUBERCULOSIS. The control of tuberculosis in a population requires the location and treatment of infected individuals who spread tubercle bacilli via pulmonary secretions. However, even though there are annually over 30,000 new cases and 3600 deaths reported in the United States, tuberculosis is usually a slow, chronic disease, and it is exceedingly difficult to find infected persons until after months or years of active infection. For early detection, therefore, one must rely on the tuberculin skin test, and a positive reaction is interpreted as denoting an infected person, whether or not the disease is quiescent or active. For this reason control now relies heavily on the preventive therapy of tuberculosis, and the Tuberculosis Advisory Committee to the Center for Disease Control has recommended that the following types of persons be considered as potential candidates for active disease (in the order listed) and that they be treated with daily oral INH for one year: (1) household members and other close associates of persons with recently diagnosed tuberculosis; (2) positive tuberculin reactors with findings on a chest roentgenogram consistent with nonprogressive tuberculosis even in the absence of bacteriologic findings; (3) all persons who have converted from tuberculin negative to tuberculin positive within the past two years; (4) positive tuberculin reactors undergoing prolonged therapy with adrenocorticoids, receiving immunosuppressive therapy, having leukemia or Hodgkin's disease, having diabetes mellitus, having silicosis, or following a gastrectomy, and (5) all persons under 35 years of age who are positive tuberculin skin reactors. INH therapy is not recommended for positive tuberculin reactors 35 years of age

or older because prolonged treatment with INH causes occasional progressive liver disease; although the risk is very low below 35 years, the incidence increases to 1.2% of persons between 35 and 49, and to 2.3% for individuals over the age of 50.

IMMUNIZATION FOR TUBERCULOSIS. A living, avirulent bovine strain named BCG (bacillus of Calmette and Guerin) has been widely used throughout the world to immunize negative tuberculin reactors; in England, a murine mycobacterium called the Vole bacillus has been used. As one might surmise, the resulting immunity is not solid, but statistics on immunized and nonimmunized persons indicate a four- to five-fold reduction of active tuberculosis in the immunized group.

In spite of the apparent benefit in eliminating tuberculosis, vaccines are rarely used in the United States. Many have worried that avirulent organisms could revert to a virulent strain (even though there have been no such reports in over 50 years of vaccine use), and, more important, a successful immunization converts an individual to a positive tuberculin reactor, eliminating the only good method for finding early infections. Thus, the general procedure in the United States is to wait until a person becomes tuberculin positive and then carry out preventive therapy with INH.

The U.S. Public Health Service Advisory Committee on Immunization Practices has recommended that BCG immunization should, however, be seriously considered for persons who are negative for the tuberculin skin test and who have repeated exposure to persistently untreated or ineffectively treated sputum-positive tuberculosis patients.

## MYCOBACTERIUM BOVIS

Mycobacterium bovis is closely related to M. tuberculosis in growth characteristics, chemical composition, and potential for virulence. Since it is normally a pathogen of cattle, human infections ordinarily result from the ingestion of contaminated milk. The organisms do not usually infect the lungs, but rather produce lesions primarily in the bone marrow of the hip, knee, and vertebrae, and in the cervical lymph nodes. However, if inhaled, M. bovis produces a pulmonary disease indistinguishable from that of M. tuberculosis.

Bovine tuberculosis has been essentially eradicated in many countries—including the United States—by a strict program for destruction of tuberculin-positive cattle and by the widespread use of pasteurized milk.

## MYCOBACTERIUM ULCERANS

This unusual organism appears to be very closely related to M. tuberculosis, but it is unable to grow above 33°C. As a result, it cannot cause a systemic infection but is the etiologic agent for a rare skin infection seen primarily in Australia and Africa.

## ATYPICAL MYCOBACTERIA

During the past several decades, it has become obvious that there is an extremely large group of mycobacteria that are apparently normal inhabitants of soil and water. In the United States, such organisms are found predominantly in the South where, as judged by specific tuberculin reactions (using tuberculin prepared from these organisms), between one-third and one-half of the population has been infected with them. The pulmonary disease in diagnosed cases is milder than that caused by M. tuberculosis and, strangely, does not appear to be communicable from person to person.

This over-all group of organisms has had several names, such as the anonymous mycobacteria (because no one knew enough about them to name them) or the atypical mycobacteria (because, unlike M. tuberculosis or M. bovis, they are completely avirulent for guinea pigs). Currently, the popular classification divides them into the following three groups: (1) photochromogens, which produce a yellow pigment only if grown in the light; (2) scotochromogens, which produce an orange pigment whether grown in the light or dark; and (3) nonchromogens, which do not produce pigment under any circumstances.

All are acid-fast bacilli, but infection does not induce a strong skin reaction to the usual tuberculin prepared from M. tuberculosis. However, tuberculin prepared from the atypical mycobacteria reacts intensely when injected into individuals with the homologous infection. Some, such as M. kansasii and M. intracellulare, are most often associated with a mild pulmonary infection, although they may cause severe pulmonary disease that is similar to classical tuberculosis, while others may cause skin infections (M. marinum), lymphadenitis (M. scrofulaceum), or small abscesses (M. fortuitum).

## MYCOBACTERIUM LEPRAE

Leprosy is probably the most feared chronic infectious disease known. Even though it is an ancient disease of humans, the etiologic agent has never been grown in an artificial medium. Moreover, the epidemiology of the disease is still unclear, and only during the past few years has there been a good comprehension of the events involved in the pathogenesis of leprosy.

### Properties of Leprosy Bacilli

The etiologic agent of leprosy is morphologically similar to M. tuberculosis. The organisms appear in lesions as acid-fast rods 3 to 5 $\mu$m long and 0.2 to 0.4 $\mu$m in diameter.

Scores of attempts to infect human volunteers with Mycobacterium leprae have been unsuccessful. It will, however, grow in the foot pad of the mouse, and recently it has been shown by Kirchheimer to produce a generalized, progressive, systemic infection in the armadillo.

### Epidemiology and Pathogenesis of Leprosy

Very little is known concerning the epidemiology of leprosy, but it is an infectious disease whose transfer may depend in large part on the susceptibility of a specific individual. Children appear to be more susceptible than adults, and, on a worldwide basis, leprosy is twice as common in males as in females. In general, it seems that infection requires only relatively brief contact for "susceptible" persons but that most persons probably cannot be infected by any means. Clinically, the disease may occur in either of two major forms, lepromatous leprosy or tuberculoid leprosy.

LEPROMATOUS LEPROSY. This is a progressive, malignant form of the disease, which, if

### Table 25-1. Comparison of Prominent Features Distinguishing Lepromatous Leprosy from Tuberculoid Leprosy

| Characteristics | Lepromatous | Tuberculoid |
|---|---|---|
| CLINICAL FEATURES | | |
| Sites of election | Skin (and nerves) | Nerves (and skin) |
| Visceral lesions | Many subclinical | (lymph nodes?) |
| Mucosal lesions | Often and early | Nose only |
| Eye lesions | Often, late | Rarely |
| Pale macules | Sometimes | Frequently |
| Annular plaques | Sometimes | Frequently |
| Fever | In reactions | Not seen |
| Eyebrow loss | Common | Not seen |
| Symmetry of lesions | Common | Often lacking |
| Nerve enlargement | Slow, symmetric | Rapid, asymmetric |
| Nerve damage | Slow | Rapid |
| Anesthesia | Glove and stocking | In macules or plaques; circumscribed |
| BACTERIOSCOPY | | |
| Acid-fast bacilli | Always abundant | Rare except in reactions |
| IMMUNOLOGY | | |
| Cellular immunity | Very low | High |
| Humoral immunity | High | Low |
| Lepromin reaction | Negative | Positive |
| False positive serology for syphilis | 40–60% | None |
| COURSE | | |
| Untreated | Progression | Spontaneous recovery often |

untreated, routinely ends in death. The organisms are found in essentially every organ of the body, although the major pathological changes occur in the skin, nerves, and testes. Skin lesions may be hypopigmented or nodular, and lesions of mucous membrane may involve the nose, causing severe nasal deformities due to the destruction of the cartilaginous septum. Nerve involvement invariably occurs and tends to be bilateral and symmetric. In advanced cases, the eye is usually infected and eventual blindness is common.

Lepromatous leprosy occurs only in individuals who have a defective cellular immune system. Thus, lepromatous patients reject skin allografts very slowly, and their lymphocytes are unable to release macrophage migration inhibition factor when exposed to lepromin. It may, however, be that the defective cellular immune system is a result of the infection.

TUBERCULOID LEPROSY. Tuberculoid leprosy is frequently a self-limiting disease which may even regress spontaneously. Skin lesions occur, and nerve involvement producing areas of anesthesia is the most conspicuous feature of this form of leprosy. Unlike the lepromatous form of leprosy, organisms are extremely rare and may not be seen in skin scrapings or biopsies. The major characteristic accounting for this form of the disease is a normal cellular immune response mounted against the leprosy bacillus. Thus, nerve damage (which occurs much more rapidly than in the lepromatous form) actually results from inflammation that occurs during a cellular immune response to the bacilli in the nerves. Table 25-1 summarizes the characteristics of both forms of leprosy.

## Laboratory Diagnosis of Leprosy

Although there are an estimated 3 million cases of leprosy in the world, including about 1000 in the United States, the rarity of the disease plus its ability to mimic other diseases makes diagnosis very difficult. The occurrence of anesthesia and the presence of acid-fast rods that cannot be cultured are actually the only criteria available for diagnosis. Lepromin, purified from infected tissues, is analogous to tuberculin, but it is of no aid in the diagnosis of leprosy for two reasons: (1) lepromatous patients have an impaired cellular immune response and hence will not react; and (2) most persons will give a positive reaction to lepromin.

## Treatment and Control of Leprosy

Patients with leprosy can be successfully treated with diamino diphenyl sulfone (dapsone), and within 50 days infectivity of their organisms for the mouse footpad disappears. However, the drug is toxic, relapses occasionally occur, and maintenance therapy must be continued for life in lepromatous cases. A repository sulfone, diacetyl diamino diphenyl sulfone (diacetyl dapsone) may also be used, and it need be given only every 75 days. Its low toxicity and impressive results from field trials are encouraging. Recent work with the antibiotic rifampin has shown that the infectivity of the organisms disappears by the seventh day of treatment, and this treatment may soon supplant the use of dapsone.

Isolation or hospitalization is no longer regarded as necessary for persons with leprosy, inasmuch as contagiousness appears to decline rapidly after the initiation of therapy.

## REFERENCES

Arnold, H. L., Jr., and P. Fasal. 1973. *Leprosy. Diagnosis and Management.* Charles C. Thomas, Springfield, Illinois.

Baker, D. C., and E. J. Hsu. 1976. Effect of a sputum digest on the viability of *Mycobacterium fortuitum. J. Appl. Microbiol.* **31:**773–777.

Browne, S. G., and T. F. Davey. 1975. What kind of strategy for leprosy. *Nature* **255:**182.

Comstock, G. W., V. T. Livesay, and S. F. Woolpert. 1974. The prognosis of a positive tuberculin reaction in childhood and adolescence. *Amer. J. Epidemiol.* **99**:131–138.

Goren, M. B. 1972. Mycobacterial lipids: Selected topics. *Bacteriol. Rev.* **36**:33–64.

Kirchheimer, W. F., and E. E. Storrs. 1971. Attempts to establish the armadillo (*Dasypus novemcictus* Linn) as a model for the study of leprosy. I. Report of lepromatoid leprosy in an experimentally infected armadillo. *Int. J. Leprosy* **39**:693–702.

Levy, L. 1976. Bactericidal action of dapsone against *Mycobacterium leprae* in mice. *Antimicrob. Agents Chemother.* **9**:614–617.

Levy, L., and J. H. Peters. 1976. Susceptibility of *Mycobacterium leprae* to dapsone as a determinant of patient response to acedapsone. *Antimicrob. Agents Chemother.* **9**:102–112.

Ramakrishnan, T., P. S. Murthy, and K. P. Gopinathan. 1972. Intermediary metabolism of mycobacteria. *Bacteriol. Rev.* **36**:65–108.

Ratledge, C. 1976. The physiology of the mycobacteria. *Adv. Microbial Phys.* **13**:116–244.

Recommendation of the Public Health Service Advisory Committee on Immunization Practices: BCG Vaccines. 1975. *Morbid. Mortal. Wkly. Rep.* **24**:69.

Rouillon, A., and H. Waaler. 1976. BCG vaccination and epidemiological situation. A decision-making approach to the use of BCG. *Adv. Tuberc. Res.* **19**:65–126.

Shepard, C. C. 1969. Chemotherapy of leprosy. *Annu. Rev. Pharmacol.* **9**:37–50.

Stodola, F. H., A. Lesuk, and R. J. Anderson. 1938. The chemistry of the lipids of tubercle bacilli. LIV. The isolation and properties of mycolic acid. *J. Biol. Chem.* **126**:505–513.

Storrs, E. E., G. P. Walsh, and H. P. Burchfield. 1974. Leprosy in the armadillo: A new model for biomedical research. *Science* **183**:851–852.

Sutherland, I. 1976. Recent studies in the epidemiology of tuberculosis based on the risk of being infected with tubercle bacilli. *Adv. Tuberc. Res.* **19**:2–63.

Walsh, G. P., E. E. Storrs, H. P. Burchfield, E. H. Cottrell, M. F. Vidrine, and C. H. Binford. 1975. Leprosy-like disease occurring naturally in armadillos. *J. Reticuloendothel. Soc.* **18**:347–351.

Wolinsky, E. 1974. Nontuberculous mycobacterial infections of man. *Med. Clin. North Am.* **58**:639–648.

# 26

# Spirochetes

The term spirochete refers to a class of bacteria that characteristically possess flexible coiled cell walls. The organisms are extremely motile, and their motion appears to result from the contraction of flagella (axial fibers) wrapped from end to end of the protoplasmic cylinder (see Figure 26-1). The flagella and the protoplasmic cylinder are both covered by a fragile membrane.

Pathogenic spirochetes are found in three genera: *Treponema, Borrelia,* and *Leptospira.*

## TREPONEMA

No pathogenic species of *Treponema* has been cultivated on artificial media, although they can be grown in laboratory animals. The tightly-coiled organisms vary from 5 to

**Figure 26-1.** One end of a free-living spirochete, showing protoplasmic cylinder, axial fiber, and surrounding sheath ($\times$ 84,000).

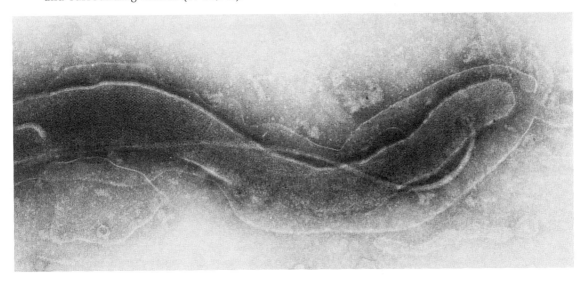

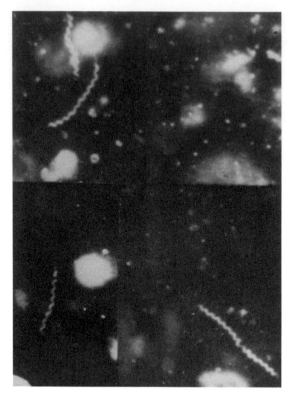

**Figure 26-2.** Dark-field micrographs of *Treponema pallidum* in fluid from a chancre (about × 2000).

15 μm in length and about 0.09 to 0.5 μm in diameter. Since this is about the limit of resolution of the light microscope, the treponemes are observed using dark-field microscopy (see Figure 26-2). There are three major human treponemal pathogens: (1) *Treponema pallidum,* the etiologic agent of syphilis, (2) *Treponema pertenue,* the cause of yaws, and (3) *Treponema carateum,* the cause of pinta.

## Syphilis

Syphilis, the disease caused by *Treponema pallidum,* does not appear to be as ancient as some other diseases discussed in this text. Early references describe its initial spread throughout Europe about the time Columbus' sailors returned from the New World. This later led to a theory that the disease was brought to Europe from the Americas. Others, however, believe the timing was mere coincidence and that syphilis evolved as a nonvenereal disease in Africa and became a venereal disease in Europe about the time Columbus returned. In any event, the disease spread through Europe in epidemic proportions during the sixteenth century. Based on accounts of the time, it is believed that syphilis was much more severe in the sixteenth century than it is at present.

EPIDEMIOLOGY AND PATHOGENESIS OF SYPHILIS. With the exception of congenitally acquired syphilis, the disease is usually acquired during sexual contact with an infected individual. Following initial contact, the organisms penetrate the mucous membranes and produce a localized ulcer, called a chancre. This primary lesion normally occurs one to four weeks after contact, although its appearance may be delayed as long as eight weeks. The lesion is teeming with treponemes, and a dark-field examination of the fluid from the chancre is the most fundamental laboratory method for an immediate clinical diagnosis (see Figure 26-2). By the time the chancre becomes recognizable, the organisms have migrated to the regional lymph nodes, causing these structures to become enlarged and firm.

After several weeks, the chancre spontaneously heals, and the disease outwardly appears quiescent. But during this period the organisms are transported throughout the body via the bloodstream, eventually resulting in widespread lesions. This condition, known as secondary syphilis, becomes manifest by the appearance of a skin rash —originally given the name of the great pox to differentiate it from smallpox. The lesions of secondary syphilis may also occur on the mucous membranes, eyes, bones, and central nervous system and, like the primary chancre, are swarming with treponemes that can be visualized using dark-field microscopy.

During secondary syphilis humoral antibodies appear, and after a period of from months to a few years, the lesions spontaneously disappear. Approximately one-fourth of these cases appear to be true cures, based on the observation that such individuals will lose their antibodies to the treponema. Another one-fourth apparently retain a latent infection for life, since they maintain antibody to the organisms but remain asymptomatic. However, about one-half of the spontaneous remissions of secondary syphilis become reactivated as tertiary syphilis. Recent data support the concept that the long duration of the secondary disease before it culminates in latency occurs because the treponemes are able to suppress a cellular immune response and that it is only after the host is able to overcome this suppression that the disease is cured or enters a latent state.

Tertiary syphilis may occur 5 to 40 years after the initial infection. Lesions may occur in the central nervous system, causing paresis, or in the cardiovascular system, resulting in aortic aneurysms. They may also arise in the eyes, skin, bones, or viscera. Tertiary lesions, called gummata, develop as painless swellings which enlarge and later rupture, resulting in ulcers. These lesions contain very few organisms, and the remarkable severity of the lesion is attributed to an intense cellular immune response to the organisms and their products.

*Treponema pallidum* can pass across the placenta to infect the fetus, and if the infection does not kill the fetus, the newborn will have congenital syphilis. Congenital syphilis often can be avoided if the infected mother is treated early in pregnancy.

LABORATORY DIAGNOSIS OF SYPHILIS. Since direct observation of the spirochetes is possible only during the active primary or secondary stages of the disease, serologic techniques are the major diagnostic tool. The magnitude of serologic tests for the diagnosis of syphilis can be appreciated by the fact that the Venereal Disease Control Division estimated that over 38,000,000 such tests were run in the United States during 1973. Undoubtedly the current figure is higher. These tests may be specific or nonspecific, depending upon the antigen employed.

The original antigen used by A. P. von Wassermann was an extract from fetal liver obtained from fetuses that had died from congenital syphilis. He mixed this material with dilutions of the patient's serum and fresh guinea pig serum, and observed for complement fixation (see Chapter 14). Subsequently, it was found that it is not necessary to use liver or other organs which have been infected with *T. pallidum* and that extracts of normal beef heart serve equally well. It is now known that the actual antigenic substance involved in the Wassermann test is a normal constituent of tissues called cardiolipin, which is diphosphatidylglycerol (see Figure 26-3). Over the years, a number of modifications of this test using the same

**Figure 26-3.** Structure of cardiolipin. This molecule consists of three molecules of glycerol joined by phosphodiester bonds; the terminal two glycerol molecules are each esterified with two long-chain fatty acids.

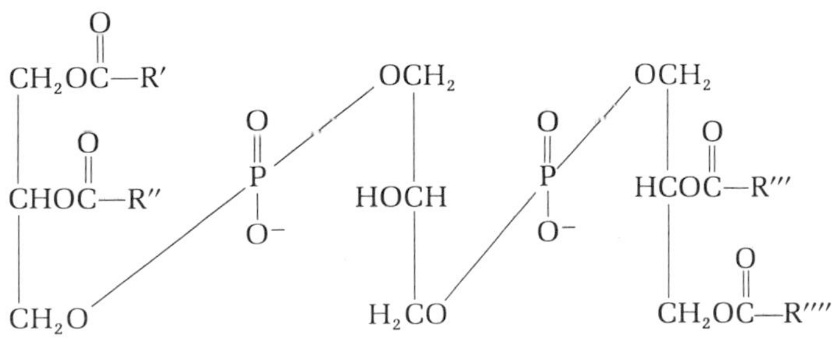

antigen have been devised. These modifications employ flocculation rather than a complement-fixation test and go by the names of their originators. Some of the more common ones are the Kolmer, Kline, Hinton, and Kahn tests. One test which is frequently used is the VDRL (Venereal Disease Research Laboratory); this test mixes a buffered saline suspension of cardiolipin, plus lecithin and cholesterol, on a slide with the patient's serum. The slide is agitated on a mechanical rotor for several minutes, and a positive test is noted by a clumping of the cardiolipin. Another widely used nonspecific test is the Rapid Plasma Reagin (RPR) card test. The RPR is performed by adsorbing the VDRL antigen on carbon particles and mixing this modified antigen with the patient's serum on a card. In a positive test, the flocculation of the carbon particles is visible to the naked eye. None of the tests employing cardiolipin as a antigen are completely specific, and other disorders occasionally give rise to antibodies resulting in false positive reactions. A more specific test to check positive results is essential.

A number of specific tests are now available for the definite diagnosis of syphilis. All require either live *T. pallidum* grown in the testes of a rabbit or the Reiter strain of *Treponema,* which is thought to be an avirulent form of *T. pallidum* and can be grown on artificial media. The TPI (*Treponema pallidum* immobilization) test uses live, testes-grown treponemes. If suspended anaerobically in the presence of specific antibody and complement, the organisms will lose their motility. The test is positive for any of the treponemal diseases (including yaws and pinta), but it requires specialized equipment and 18 hours to complete. By far the most widely used serologic test for specific treponemal antibodies is an indirect fluorescent antibody test, abbreviated FTA-ABS for "fluorescent treponemal antibody —absorption." The absorption step in this test is necessary to eliminate nonspecific reactions which occur as a result of antibodies to common antigens shared by both

pathogenic and saprophytic treponemes. The absorption is accomplished by mixing the patient's serum with a standardized extract from nonpathogenic Reiter treponemes. (This sorbant can be purchased commercially.) The absorbed serum is then used to cover a smear of pathogenic, testes-grown treponemes (Nichols strain, which can be purchased commercially as lyophilized organisms). After 30 minutes at 37° C the slide is thoroughly rinsed to remove unreacted serum proteins, and the slide is then covered with a fluorescently-labeled anti-human gamma globulin. This again is allowed to react for 30 minutes before rinsing, and the slide is examined microscopically (with an ultraviolet light source) for the presence of fluorescently stained treponemes. Because the fluorescently-labeled anti-human gamma globulin could react with the treponemes only if the organisms were coated with human antibody, the presence of fluorescently-labeled treponemes signifies the presence of specific antibodies to *Treponema pallidum*. On occasions when lesions are present, expressed material can be stained directly with specific antibodies to *T. pallidum* that have been conjugated to a fluorescent dye (DFATP —Direct Fluorescent Antibody test for *T. pallidum*).

The microhemagglutination test for *Treponema pallidum* (MHA-TP) also assays for specific treponemal antibodies. This method employs specially treated sheep's erythrocytes that have been coated with antigen from *T. pallidum*. The test has been automated and adapted to a microvolume procedure. A positive result is signified by the agglutination of the red cells.

There are a number of other procedures for determining specific treponemal antibodies, such as the TPA (*Treponema pallidum* agglutination), TPIA (*Treponema pallidum* immune adherence), and whole body *Treponema pallidum* complement fixation tests. None of these, however, is used in diagnostic laboratories; they serve primarily as research tools.

The choice of which test to use may, in

part, be dictated by personal preference. The VDRL or RPR are less expensive than procedures for determining specific antibodies and should, therefore, be used in screening low-risk populations such as individuals having premarital serologic testing. Positive results can be confirmed with one of the specific tests. When it becomes possible to grow the pathogenic treponemes in an artificial medium, the availability of an inexpensive antigen will undoubtedly influence the choice of tests used to diagnose syphilis serologically.

TREATMENT AND CONTROL OF SYPHILIS. Before the turn of the century there was no treatment for syphilis, but at that time Paul Ehrlich was carrying out his systematic search for a "magic bullet" which would selectively attack microorganisms without undue toxicity to the host. Although Ehrlich never found his universal weapon, he did develop an arsenical compound, arsphenamine, that together with bismuth was relatively effective in treating syphilis. Such treatment was long and painful and has not been used since the advent of penicillin.

Syphilis could, theoretically, be eradicated, as the organism is sensitive to low levels of penicillin. Even the tertiary stage may be arrested with adequate penicillin therapy, but in these cases therapy must be prolonged for several weeks, probably because the organisms are growing so slowly. However, in spite of the ease with which the disease may be cured, public health authorities have reported a rising incidence since 1960.

Humoral antibodies to syphilis appear several weeks after the occurrence of the primary lesion, but it is believed that a cellular immune response is responsible for the eventual regression of the lesions of secondary syphilis. Individuals with a latent infection cannot be reinfected, and even if treated, persons with long-standing infections appear to retain their immunity. It would, therefore, seem theoretically possible to produce an effective vaccine, and considerable effort is being expended toward this objective.

Initial attempts with rabbit-grown treponemes indicate that vaccines may be effective but that the antigen inducing immunity is probably quite labile. Undoubtedly, the ability to grow the pathogenic organisms in culture would provide a boost toward a potential vaccine.

### Yaws

*Treponema pertenue,* the etiologic agent of yaws, is morphologically indistinguishable from *T. pallidum,* and it is likely that they are closely related organisms.

EPIDEMOLOGY AND PATHOGENESIS OF YAWS. Yaws is restricted to the tropics, where it seems to be spread from person to person either by direct contact with open ulcers or by vectors such as flies. An initial lesion occurs three to four weeks after exposure, and, after ulcerating, spontaneously heals. Several months later, secondary lesions appear, which ulcerate, heal, and reappear in crops over a period of several years. The disease may become quiescent, only to reappear as tertiary lesions of the skin and bones—frequently resulting in considerable disfigurement of the face.

LABORATORY DIAGNOSIS, TREATMENT AND CONTROL OF YAWS. In all likelihood, the average diagnosis is based on the clinical picture occurring in an area where yaws is endemic. However, all of the serological tests for syphilis described above will yield positive results. *T. pertenue* is very sensitive to penicillin, and like syphilis, this disfiguring disease could be easily controlled if it were possible to give adequate penicillin therapy to infected persons. However, the lack of sanitation and medical personnel in areas where yaws is endemic make such eradication virtually impossible at this time.

### Pinta

Pinta is a disease which occurs mainly in Central and South America. *Treponema carateum,* the etiologic agent, also is indistinguishable from *T. pallidum,* but the skin lesions produced are flat red or blue areas which do not ulcerate and ultimately become depigmented. Lesions are usually confined to the skin.

Transmission appears to require direct person-to-person contact, and like the other species of *Treponema, T. carateum* is very sensitive to penicillin.

### Vincent's Angina

*Treponema vincentii* (older name was *Borrelia vincentii*) and *Bacteroides melaninogenicus* have been thought to be involved in a fusospirochetal (caused by both fusiform bacteria and spirochetes) disease. It is commonly referred to as Vincent's angina, or trench mouth (it was prevalent among the infantry during World War I). *T. vincentii* is an active, motile spirochete, and *Bacteroides melaninogenicus* is a nonmotile, gram-negative, straight or slightly curved rod that frequently occurs in pairs with the outer ends pointed and the blunt ends together. Both organisms are obligate anaerobes.

Vincent's angina is characterized by ulcerative lesions of the mouth or tonsilar area. There is a possibility that the real etiologic agent is a herpes virus, and for reasons not understood the two bacteria, which are normal flora of the mouth, multiply during the active disease.

Diagnosis is based on the clinical picture and smears of the lesions. Penicillin will help to control the bacterial population, but it is not particularly effective in eliminating the ulcerative lesions, perhaps because the bacteria are not the true etiologic agents.

### *BORRELIA*

Members of the genus *Borrelia* can be differentiated from those of *Treponema* by their coarse, irregular coils. Organisms may be up to 0.5 $\mu$m wide and 20 $\mu$m in length, and are, therefore, much easier to see than other spirochetes when stained with analine dyes and viewed with a light microscope (see Figure 26-4).

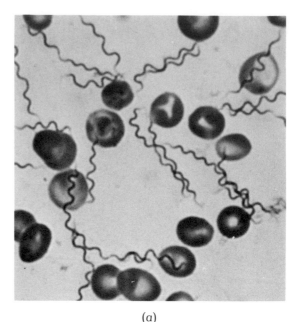

(a)

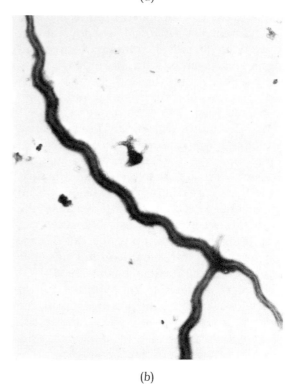

(b)

**Figure 26-4.** *a.* Giemsa stain of *Borrelia hermsii* in the blood of an experimentally infected pine squirrel ($\times$ 2,700). *B. hermsii* is one of the causes of relapsing fever in the U.S. *b.* Electron micrograph of negatively-stained *B. hermsii* ($\times$ 5,500).

## Relapsing Fever

EPIDEMIOLOGY AND PATHOGENESIS OF RELAPS-
ING FEVER. In humans any one of 11 different species of *Borrelia* may cause relapsing
fever. *B. recurrentis* is the only species that
is transmitted from human to human by
the body louse; all other species are transmitted by various species of the tick *Orni-
thodoros*. The body louse and several of the
tick species feed only on humans, and humans are therefore the sole vertebrate reservoir for the species of *Borrelia* associated
with the louse and those particular species
of tick. However, since the organisms are
passed transovarily in the tick, this vector
can also serve as a reservoir for all species
of *Borrelia* except *B. recurrentis*. Other
primary reservoirs maintained by tick species
that do not feed exclusively on humans
include rodents, ground squirrels, armadillos,
and monkeys. A few strains of *Borrelia* have
been grown on artificial media, and these
strains require a microaerophilic atmosphere
and an enriched medium.

Humans acquire the infection from the
bite of an infected vector. The microorganisms enter the blood and cause multiple
lesions in the spleen, liver, kidneys, and
gastrointestinal tract. After a fever of four
or five days, the microorganisms seem to
disappear, and the patient becomes afebrile
for a week or ten days. Then a relapse occurs,
and the organisms can again be found in
blood and internal lesions. After four or
five days, they again disappear, only to
relapse three to ten more times before complete recovery.

The mechanism of the relapse appears to
result from the spontaneous appearance of
new antigenic types. Thus, when each succeeding humoral immune response clears
the organisms, a new antigenic type is
selected and becomes responsible for the
ensuing relapse.

LABORATORY DIAFNOSIS, TREATMENT, AND
CONTROL OF RELAPSING FEVER. The diagnosis
of relapsing fever is based on clinical symptoms plus the observation of *Borrelia* organisms in stained blood smears or dark-field
microscopy. Also, blood can be injected into
mice, and the mouse blood examined for
*Borrelia* after two or three days.

Penicillin is the drug of choice, although
other antibiotics such as tetracycline and
chloramphenicol are effective. Since the
organisms are transmitted only by vectors,
tick and louse control are effective measures
for the control of relapsing fever.

## *LEPTOSPIRA*

Leptospirosis is the name given to a variety
of clinical syndromes caused by members
of the genus *Leptospira*. The *Leptospira* are
morphologically characterized as spirochetes
exhibiting a fine and tightly-coiled spiral and
usually possessing a hook on one or both
ends. They are very thin (0.1 $\mu$m), usually
quite long (10 to 20 $\mu$m), and are readily
visible with dark-field microscopy (see Figure
26-5). Their extremely active motility appears
to be due to the rhythmic contractions of
their flagella (axial fibrils), particularly at the
hooked ends.

*Leptospira* can be grown in a number of
artificial media supplemented with bovine
albumin or sterile rabbit serum, and some
strains have been cultivated in chemically
defined media. All *Leptospira* are obligately
aerobic and appear to grow best in a neutral
medium at 30° C.

### Antigenic Classification of the *Leptospira*

The taxonomy of the *Leptospira* is in a
fluid state and is currently being studied by
a Subcommittee on *Leptospira* of the International Committee on Systematic Bacteriology. Some proposals have presented
more than 18 serogroups that are further
divided into over 130 serotypes; others have
divided the entire genus into two species
—the pathogenic *L. icterohemorrhagiae*
(which is subdivided into many serotypes)
and the saprophytic *L. biflexa*. The 1974 edition of *Bergey's Manual of Determinative
Bacteriology* lists only a single species, *L.*

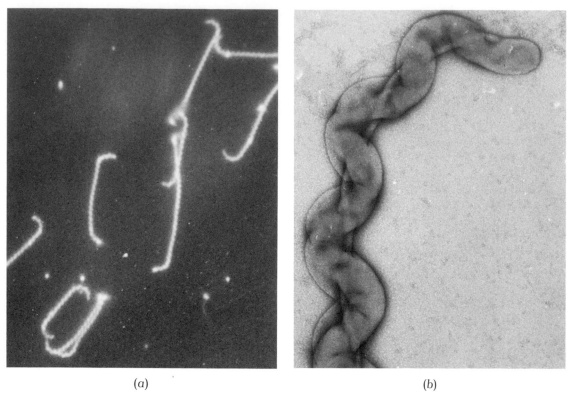

(a)                                                        (b)

**Figure 26-5.** *a.* Dark-field micrograph of *Leptospira interrogans* serotype *illini* (× 1000). *b.* Electron micrograph of one end of a negatively-stained leptospire, showing clearly the axial fibril (× 51,000).

*interrogans,* followed by a serotype designation such as "*L. interrogans* serotype *icterohemorrhagiae.*" Medical microbiologists have tended to use these serotype designations as specific names, and these names have become entrenched in medical literature during the past several decades. Suffice it to say that the differentiation of the serotypes is based primarily on agglutination and cross-agglutination studies carried out with antisera prepared in rabbits.

## Epidemiology and Pathogenesis of Leptospirosis

*Leptospira* are primarily parasites of vertebrates other than humans, such as rodents, dogs, pigs, cattle, and raccoons, in which the bacteria appear to persist in a life-long asymptomatic infection of the kidney. They are continuously shed in the urine of some infected animals. Certain serotypes are routinely associated with specific hosts, for example *icterohemorrhagiae* with rodents, *canicola* with dogs, *pomona* with pigs, and *autumnalis* and *grippotyphosa* with mice, but cross infections do occur.

Disease in humans may be caused by any one of the serotypes of *Leptospira.* The usual sequence of events begins when a person becomes infected through skin contact with urine from an infected animal or by exposure to urine-contaminated water or soil. The organisms enter the blood and then invade various tissues and organs, particularly the kidney, liver, meninges, and conjunctiva. Physical symptoms frequently include muscular pain, headache, photophobia, fever, and chills. The infections caused by the various *Leptospira* may or may not result in jaundice or meningitis. One serotype, *icterohemorrhagiae,* causes a more severe illness referred to as Weil's disease or infectious jaundice, and the fatality rate from Weil's disease may run as high as 25%. Another unusual leptospiral infection, pretibial (or Fort Bragg) fever, characterized by a rash on the shins, is caused by serotype *fort-bragg.*

### Laboratory Diagnosis of Leptospirosis

Although the observation of *Leptospira* in a dark-field examination of blood would provide strong support, an unequivocable diagnosis requires that the organisms be grown and identified as *Leptospira* by serological methods. Organisms from the patient's blood can be cultured in artificial media or the blood can be inoculated into young hamsters or guinea pigs to enrich the number of organisms present.

Convalescent serum from a patient can be used to measure agglutination of *Leptospira,* lysis of *Leptospira* in the presence of complement, or complement fixation. Identification of specific serotypes requires specialized sera that are not normally available in the diagnostic laboratory.

### Treatment and Control of Leptospirosis

Penicillin appears to provide the best therapy for leptospiral infections, but erythromycin and tetracyclines have some value. Results are not striking, particularly if treatment is instigated late in the infection.

Control is extremely difficult because the organisms are so wide-spread, especially in the rodent population. Leptospirosis is an occupational hazard for sewage workers, slaughterhouse employees, or individuals who come in contact with rat-infested areas. Because a vaccine for humans is not available, rodent control and vaccination of domestic animals provide the best means for preventing human infections. Interestingly, the most common source of human leptospirosis in the United States is the dog.

## REFERENCES

Deacon, W. E., J. B. Lucas, and E. V. Price. 1966. Fluorescent treponemal antibody absorption (FTA-ABS) test for syphilis. *JAMA* **198**:624–628.

Finn, M. A., and R. H. Jones. 1976. Growth of saprophytic and pathogenic leptospira: Evaluation of medium, temperature, inoculum and cost. *J. Appl. Microbiol.* **31**:134–137.

Hunter, E. F., W. E. Deacon, and P. E. Meyer. 1964. An improved test for syphilis—the absorption procedure (FTA-ABS). *Pub. Health Rep.* **79**:410–412.

Jaffe, H. W. 1975. The laboratory diagnosis of syphilis. *Ann. Internal. Med.* **83**:846–850.

Johnson, R. C. 1976. *The Biology of Parasitic Spirochetes.* Academic Press, New York.

Logan, L. C., and P. M. Cox. 1970. Evaluation of a quantitative automated microhemagglutination assay for antibodies to *Treponema pallidum. Amer. J. Clin. Path.* **53**:163–166.

Miller, J. N. 1973. Immunity in experimental syphilis. VI. Successful vaccination of rabbits with *Treponema pallidum,* Nichol's strain, attenuated by γ-radiation. *J. Immunol.* **110**:1206–1215.

Nelson, R. A., Jr., and M. M. Mayer, 1949. Immobilization of *Treponema pallidum in vitro* by antibody produced in syphilitic infection. *J. Exp. Med.* **89**:369–396.

Southern, P. M., and J. P. Sanford. 1969. Relapsing fever. *Medicine* **48**:129–149.

Sparling, P. F. 1971. Medical progress. Diagnosis and treatment of syphilis. *New Engl. J. Med.* **284**:642–653.

Turner, L. H. 1973. Leptospirosis. *Br. Med. J.* **1**:537–540.

United States Public Health Service. 1968. Syphilis: A Synopsis. U.S. Public Health Service Publication No. 1660, 109–116.

Wood, R. M. 1974. Tests for syphilis. In E. H. Lennette, E. H. Spaulding, and J. P. Traunt, eds. *Manual of Clinical Microbiology,* 2nd ed. American Society for Microbiology, Washington, D.C.

# 27

## Mycoplasma and L-Forms

### MYCOPLASMAS

Mycoplasmas are the smallest known organisms capable of growth and reproduction outside living host cells. Because mycoplasmas are pleomorphic, the size of individual cells is variable, ranging from 0.12–0.25 $\mu$m in diameter.

The first isolated mycoplasma was an organism that causes pleuropneumonia in cattle. Prior to its growth in 1898 the organism was thought to be a virus because of its ability to pass through filters that retained bacteria. We now know that a number of similar organisms cause disease in various animals (see Table 27-1). Since the original organism isolated from cattle was called a pleuropneumonia organism, all similar organisms subsequently isolated were referred to as pleuropneumonia-like organisms, or more commonly by the abbreviation PPLO. This abbreviation was used widely until 1967 when mycoplasmas were placed into a new class, Mollicutes ("soft skin"). This class is now subdivided into a number of genera (as shown in Table 27-2), but we shall restrict our discussion to the Mycoplasmataceae, since the members of this family are the only mycoplasmas known to cause disease in humans and other animals.

### Morphology and Reproduction of Mycoplasmas

The major morphological difference between mycoplasmas and other procaryotic cells is that mycoplasmas completely lack a cell wall. Because there is no cell wall, the major components of a mycoplasma cell are simply the plasma membrane, the cytoplasm, and chromosomal DNA. No cell wall components, such as muramic acid or diaminopimelic acid, are synthesized. As might be expected for cells so poorly protected from the osmotic vagaries of their environment, the shapes of mycoplasmas vary over a wide range—from ultramicroscopic coccoid cells to long filaments that may or may not be branched.

There is still some confusion concerning the details of mycoplasma reproduction. It appears that a coccoid cell routinely elongates into a long filament, then coccoid structures form within the filament and are

### Table 27-1. Partial List of Mycoplasmas That Infect Animals

| Organism | Host | Disease |
|---|---|---|
| M. bovigenitalium | Cattle | Mastitis & vulvovaginitis |
| M. bovirhinis | Cattle | (?) Respiratory disease |
| M. mycoides | Cattle | Pleuropneumonia |
| M. ovipneumoniae | Lambs | Pneumonia |
| M. conjunctivae | Goats and sheep | Conjunctivitis |
| M. gallisepticum | Poultry | Respiratory disease and encephalitis |
| M. pulmonis | Mice and rats | Respiratory disease |
| M. arthritidis | Rats | Polyarthritis |
| M. hyorhinis | Swine | Arthritis |
| M. hyosynoviae | Swine | Arthritis and synovitis |
| M orale | Humans | Parasite of oropharynx |
| M. pneumoniae | Humans | Atypical primary pneumonia |
| M. salivarium | Humans | Parasite of oropharynx |
| T-strains (Ureaplasma) | Humans and other animals | (?) Urethritis |

### Table 27-2. Generic Classification of Mollicutes

| Families and Genera | Major Characteristics |
|---|---|
| MYCOPLASMATACEAE | All require cholesterol |
| Genus 1 Mycoplasma | Pathogenic for animals and humans; colonies may be 600 $\mu$m diameter |
| Genus 2 Ureaplasma | Proposed name for urea-utilizing T-strains; pathogens or parasites; tiny colonies 10 to 30 $\mu$m diameter |
| ACHOLEPLASMATACEAE | None require cholesterol |
| Genus 1 Acholeplasma | Saprophyte and/or parasite for mammals and birds. |
| Genus 2 Spiroplasma | Plant/animal pathogen possessing helical and branched filaments |
| Genus 3 Thermoplasma | Saprophyte having an optimum growth temperature of 59°C at pH 1 to 3 |
| Genus 4 Anaeroplasma | Saprophyte obligately anaerobic isolated from rumen of cattle and sheep |

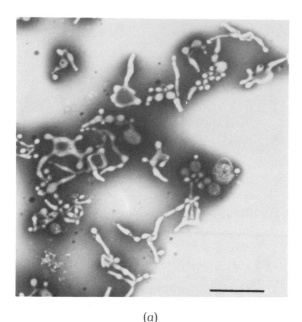

(a)

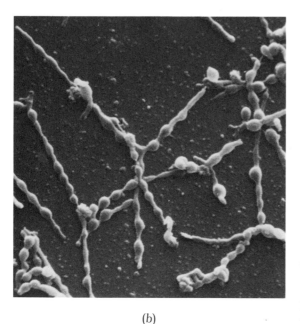

(b)

**Figure 27-1.** *a.* Electron micrograph of a negatively-stained preparation of *Mycoplasma pneumoniae* (scale = 1μm). The variable morphology, ranging from rings with lobes to beaded filaments, is evident. *b.* Scanning electron micrograph of *Mycoplasma pneumoniae* (× 10,000); note the coccoid structures within the filaments.

subsequently released by fragmentation (see Figure 27-1). Reproduction by budding may also occur.

Mycoplasmas also vary considerably in their growth requirements, but all can be grown on artificial media. Members of the family Mycoplasmataceae require cholesterol for growth. The exact function of the cholesterol is not known, but it is adsorbed to a preformed constituent in the cell membrane and is thought to be necessary for the pliability and tensile strength of the cell membrane. Members of the genus *Acholeplasma* (in the family Acholeplasmataceae) do not require added sterols for growth and synthesize carotenoids which they deposit in their cell membrane. There have been reports that *Mycoplasma* can be grown in a medium employing carotenoids as substitutes for cholesterol.

Growth of *Mycoplasma* on a solid medium routinely results in the formation of colonies so small that they cannot normally be seen with the naked eye. When cultures are viewed under the low power (10×) of the light microscope, diphasic colonies with a "fried-egg look" frequently appear. Such colonies are formed when cells in the center of the colony grow down into the medium (see Figure 27-2).

A number of strains of *Mycoplasma* will also grow in the amniotic sac or yolk of chick embryos, or as contaminants of cell cultures, causing various cytopathic effects.

### Classification of Mycoplasmas

Immunologic techniques provide the primary basis for the classification of mycoplasmas, and growth inhibition by specific antisera seems to be the easiest and most specific method for their identification. The test can be carried out using one of a variety of techniques, such as incorporating dilutions of antiserum directly into the agar medium, placing a filter-paper disc that has been soaked in antiserum onto an inoculated area of a culture plate and subsequently observing for inhibition of mycoplasma

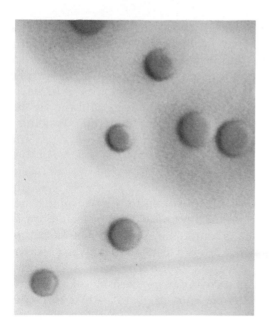

**Figure 27-2.** Colonies of *Mycoplasma fermentans* show "fried-egg" appearance; growth was on agar for 14 days (about × 185).

growth around the disc, or adding dilutions of antiserum to plastic cylinders embedded in the agar of the culture plate.

Complement fixation or agglutination tests can also be conducted, but studies have shown that growth-inhibition tests provide better correlations with accepted mycoplasma species.

### Mycoplasma pneumoniae

During the 1940's, clinical and laboratory observations provided a description of a type of pneumonia distinct from typical bacterial pneumonia. Using human volunteers, it was shown to be caused by an infectious agent, and since no bacterium could be isolated, it was assumed to be caused by a virus. The organism was named Eaton's agent for the scientist who first reported that the disease was caused by a filterable agent that could be grown in chick embryos. Not until 20 years later was Eaton's agent found to be a mycoplasma, subsequently named *Mycoplasma pneumoniae*.

*Mycoplasma pneumoniae* will adsorb to a number of different kinds of erythrocytes and mammalian cells, especially tracheal epithelial cells. The cell receptor appears to be a glycoprotein that contains a terminal neuraminic acid residue. Treatment of cells with neuraminidase removes the neuraminic acid and destroys the receptor, rendering the cells incapable of adsorption (influenza virus, which also causes a respiratory infection, adsorbs to a similar type of cell receptor).

*Mycoplasma pneumoniae* causes beta-hemolysis on a number of different types of erythrocytes, and the factor responsible for the hemolysis has been shown to be hydrogen peroxide—produced by the metabolism of *Mycoplasma*. Since erythrocytes possess an active catalase, their lysis by $H_2O_2$ is unusual, and it has been suggested that it occurs because of the very close association of *Mycoplasma* when it is bound to a specific receptor site on the red blood cell. It has also been postulated that tracheal epithelial cell destruction may occur by the same mechanism.

EPIDEMIOLOGY AND PATHOGENESIS OF PAP. Primary atypical pneumonia (PAP) occurs most frequently where people live in close contact, as in military camps. Mycoplasmas are found in the respiratory tract of infected individuals, and the disease spreads via the respiratory route. The incubation period is two to three weeks; symptoms may vary from an inapparent or mild disease to a severe pneumonia characterized by headache, chills, fever, and general malaise. Chest X-rays usually show a patchy pneumonitis which frequently appears worse than anticipated from the physical examination. Major symptoms disappear between the third and tenth days of illness, but chest infiltration and coughing may continue for one to two months. The disease is rarely fatal.

LABORATORY DIAGNOSIS OF PAP. Prior to the discovery that PAP was caused by a mycoplasma, diagnosis was based on the clinical picture, chest X-rays, and two laboratory findings: (1) the development of cold hemagglutinins (antibodies that will agglutinate human type-O erythrocytes when incubated at 0–4°C, but not at 37°C), and (2) the presence of antibodies to a bacterium named streptococcus MG. Why these unusual antibodies develop during PAP is not known.

*Mycoplasma pneumoniae* can be grown in a medium containing serum, with penicillin added to inhibit the growth of contaminants. Conclusive identification is obtained by staining the organisms with a specific fluorescently-labeled antibody or by growth inhibition in the presence of specific antibody.

TREATMENT AND CONTROL OF PAP. Erythromycin or the tetracyclines are effective for the treatment of PAP. Experimental formalin-inactivated vaccines have been shown to prevent clinical illness in volunteers who were challenged with the virulent organisms, but no commercial vaccine is available.

### Mycoplasma hominis

*Mycoplasma hominis* can be isolated from the genital tract of 30–50% of asymptomatic humans, and the species has also been isolated from a variety of pelvic abscesses. As a result, there has been a great deal of controversy concerning the disease-producing potential of this organism.

**Figure 27-3.** This micrograph nicely demonstrates the size difference between colonies of the T-strain mycoplasma *Ureaplasma urealyticum* (small, dark colonies) and the "fried-egg" colonies of the classical large-colony *Mycoplasma hominis* ($\times$ 195). This is a standard agar culture on which the direct spot test for urease was applied: the dark (golden-brown) urease-positive T-strain colonies show the specific development of manganese reaction product, which positively identifies them as those of *Ureaplasma*. The larger, lighter, urease-negative *M. hominis* colonies have been counterstained with a blue dye.

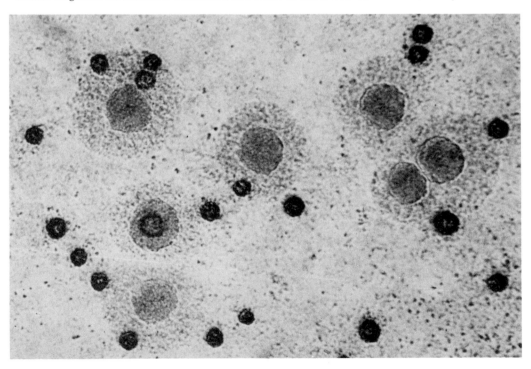

Current opinions can be summarized as follows: (1) *M. hominis* probably does cause occasional pelvic abscess, but, in all likelihood, is rarely (or never) involved in lower genital-tract infections such as cervicitis, vaginitis, or urethritis; and (2) in the majority of instances, *M. hominis* exists in the genital tract as a nonpathogenic parasite.

## T-STRAIN MYCOPLASMAS (*UREAPLASMA*)

T strains of mycoplasma are so named because they grow as exceptionally small, tiny colonies, usually 10 to 20 $\mu$m in diameter. Such colonies cannot be seen with the naked eye, and (as shown in Figure 27-3) they are much smaller than normal mycoplasma colonies and barely visible with the light microscope using 10$\times$ magnification.

T strains require both cholesterol and urea for growth, and the incorporation of 10% horse serum into a medium will supply both requirements. The organisms contain a urease that hydrolyzes urea to ammonia and carbon dioxide. Because of this absolute requirement for urea, the generic name of *Ureaplasma* has been suggested.

The question of T-strain mycoplasma pathogenicity has been debated for two decades, and the answer remains equivocal. As mentioned previously, these organisms can be isolated from the genital tract of up to 50% of asymptomatic persons, and they can also be found in 50–80% of individuals with nongonococcal urethritis. There have been a number of claims that mycoplasmas, particularly T strains, can be isolated from the joints of patients with arthritis, but other scientists have been unsuccessful in attempts to repeat such isolations. Thus the status of T-strain mycoplasma virulence is still unresolved. However, there seems to be a general consensus that they can definitely exist as parasites in the genital tract without causing illness, but, in some cases, they may be the etiologic agents of a nongonococcal urethritis.

The position of T strains with respect to arthritis in humans is even more insecure. The fact that some mycoplasmas are known to cause arthritis in other animals and reports that they have been occasionally isolated from human joint fluid and synovial tissue provide circumstantial evidence for their involvement in the human disorder. However, the inability of qualified investigators to routinely isolate mycoplasmas from arthritic patients casts doubt on their role in this disease.

## L-FORMS OF BACTERIA (CELL-WALL DEFECTIVE ORGANISMS)

L-forms are bacterial variant growth forms that no longer produce rigid peptidoglycan cell walls. Thus, they are in many ways analogous to mycoplasmas (see Figure 27-4).

The first isolation of a naturally occurring L-form took place at the Lister Institute (hence, the "L"), and it was later characterized by Louis Dienes. He found that L-forms (which produced tiny colonies on solid media) arose spontaneously from the bacterium *Streptobacillus moniliformis,* and that after prolonged incubation in broth, some of the L-forms would revert to the parent bacterium. Subsequently, L-forms were

**Figure 27-4.** L$_1$ phase variant of *Streptobacillus moniliformis* ($\times$ 2250); note the pleomorphism and the rounded appearance of individual cells, which lack peptidoglycan cell walls.

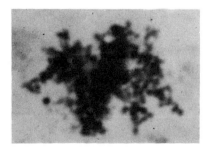

isolated from various sources by studying freshly isolated cultures of bacteria from pathological specimens. Still later, it was discovered that growth in the presence of penicillin could be used to select or induce the appearance of L-forms, and, under appropriate conditions, some strains in almost all studied species of bacteria can develop into L-forms. The terms protoplast, spheroplast, and L-form might be confusing, but one can define an L-form as any bacterium that has lost its ability to synthesize peptidoglycan but can still multiply.

The similarities between L-forms and mycoplasmas have prompted extensive speculation as to whether or not mycoplasmas might represent stable L-forms of bacteria, since they form structurally similar colonies and appear to reproduce in a similar manner. However, after much discussion, immunological studies, and studies of nucleic acid homology, the general consensus is that mycoplasmas are not related to L-forms. If mycoplasmas arose originally from bacteria, their origin must have occurred long ago on the evolutionary scale.

No actual situation is known where an L-form, by itself, can produce disease. *Streptobacillus moniliformis,* an organism that spontaneously forms L-forms, is the etiologic agent of rat-bite fever, but there is no evidence that the L-form is involved in the disease process.

There is, perhaps, a much more impoitant potential role for L-forms; they might function as antibiotic-resistant cells during treatment of a disease with antibiotics that inhibit cell wall synthesis. The isolation of L-forms following penicillin therapy has been reported. Thus, though speculative, L-forms could perhaps resist antibiotic therapy and later revert to the original bacterial form, resulting in relapse of disease.

## REFERENCES

Bradbury, J. M., C. A. Oriel, and F. T. W. Jordan. 1976. Simple method for immunofluorescent identification of *Mycoplasma* colonies. *J. Clin. Microbiol.* **3**:449–452.

Clyde, W. A. 1964. *Mycoplasma* species identification based upon growth inhibition by specific antisera. *J. Immunol.* **92**:958–965.

Furness, G. 1975. T-Mycoplasmas: Growth patterns and physical characteristics of some human strains. *J. Infect. Dis.* **132**:592–596.

Lin, J. S., and E. H. Kass. 1973. Serotypic heterogeneity in isolates of human genital T-mycoplasmas. *Infect. Immun.* **7**:499–500.

Maniloff, J., and H. J. Morowitz. 1972. Cell biology of the mycoplasmas. *Bacteriol. Rev.* **36**:263–290.

Maramorosch, K., ed. 1973. *Mycoplasma* and mycoplasma-like agents of human, animal and plant diseases. *Ann. New York Acad. Sci.* **255**.

McCormack, W. M., P. Braun, Y. Lee, J. O. Klein, and E. H. Kass. 1973. The genital mycoplasmas. *New Engl. J. Med.* **288**:78–89.

Razin, S. 1973. Physiology of mycoplasmas. *Adv. Microbiol. Phys.* **10**:2–80.

Razin, S., and J. G. Tully. 1970. Cholesterol requirement of mycoplasma. *J. Bacteriol.* **102**:306–310.

Robertson, J., M. Gomersall, and P. Gill. 1975. *Mycoplasma hominis:* Growth, reproduction and isolation of small viable cells. *J. Bacteriol.* **124**:1007–1018.

Shepard, M. C. 1967. Cultivation and properties of *Mycoplasma* associated with nongonococcal urethritis. *Ann. New York Acad. Sci.* **143**:505–514.

Shepard, M. C. 1973. Differential methods for the identification of T-mycoplasmas based on demonstration of urease. *J. Infect. Dis.* **127**:S22–S25.

Shurin, P. A., S. Alpert, B. Rosner, S. G. Driscoll, Y. Lee, W. M. McCormack, B. A. G. Santamarina, and E. H. Kass. 1975. Chorioamnionitis and colonization of the newborn infant with genital mycoplasmas. *New Engl. J. Med.* **293**:5–8.

Stanbridge, E. J. 1976. A re-evaluation of the role of mycoplasmas in human disease. *Annu. Rev. Microbiol.* **30**:169–187.

Tarr, P. I., Y. Lee, S. Alpert, J. R. Schumacher, S. H. Zinner, and W. M. McCormack. 1976. Comparison of methods for the isolation of genital mycoplasmas from men. *J. Infect. Dis.* **133**:419–423.

# 28

# Rickettsiae and Chlamydiae

## Rickettsiae

The rickettsiae are smaller than most other bacteria. In fact, most rickettsiae are just barely within the range of visibility of the ordinary light microscope. But, it is not size that sets them apart from other bacteria, but rather that (with one exception, *Rochalimaea quintana*) they grow only inside animal cells; in other words, they are obligate intracellular parasites. Thus, rickettsiae cannot be grown in the laboratory on artificial media, as can most bacteria, but require living cells for growth. Moreover, with the one exception of Q fever, all rickettsial diseases are transmitted from animal to animal (humans included) by the bite of an infected arthropod vector.

Rickettsiae appear to be closely related to the gram-negative bacteria. Typically, they are rod-shaped with average dimensions of 0.3 to 0.7 $\mu$m by 1.5 to 2.0 $\mu$m (see Figure 28-1). Electron microscopy reveals a cell wall consisting of an inner membrane and an outer membrane, a structure characteristic of gram-negative cells. Furthermore, when stained with the gram stain, they appear as gram-negative bacteria. Rickettsiae have also been shown to contain muramic acid (a substance existing only in bacteria and blue-green algae) and diaminopimelic acid (a compound found only in the cell walls of gram-negative bacteria). Thus, it seems that rickettsiae are really a unique type of gram-negative bacteria.

One might wonder, then, why rickettsiae are obligate intracellular parasites. If they originally descended from gram-negative bacteria, what have they lost that would allow them to grow extracellularly? Not all of the answers to these questions are known, and various theories propose to explain this restricted growth. Rickettsiae appear able to synthesize their own proteins, nucleic acids, and any other macromolecules necessary for their structural components. Moreover, they are able to oxidize glutamic acid, as well as a number of intermediates of the citric acid cycle, and are able to trap the energy released by these oxidations as ATP. However, rickettsiae are not able to metabolize glucose as a substrate.

Recent information makes it possible to speculate about their parasitic intracellular

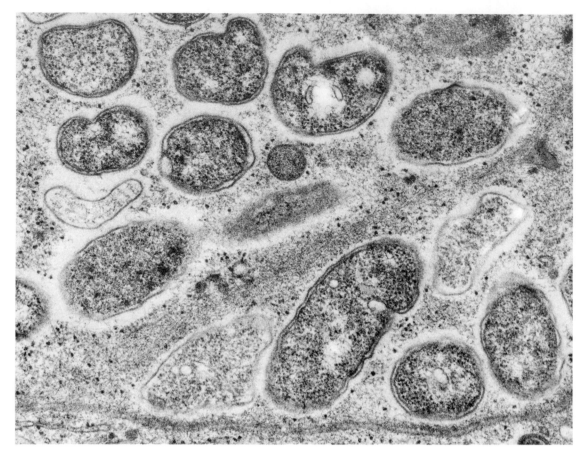

**Figure 28-1.** *Rickettsia prowazeki* in experimentally infected tick tissue (×45,000). Note the double-layered cell wall similar to that of gram-negative bacteria.

life style. When rickettsiae are removed from an intracellular environment, most of them rapidly lose viability and infectivity. This seems to be correlated with the loss of RNA and other intracellular metabolites. The organisms can be stabilized, or even restored to infectivity, by the addition of such metabolites as NAD, coenzyme A, ATP, and inorganic ions such as $K^+$ and $Mg^{++}$. The unexpected aspect of these observations is that substances such as NAD, coenzyme A, and ATP usually cannot enter a normal cell. That these metabolites can stabilize or restore infectivity to the rickettsiae certainly indicates that they do enter the cell, and recent publications indicate that rickettsiae do possess specific transport systems for these molecules. However, we are still left with the postulate that the unusual permeability of the rickettsial cell membrane may account, in large part, for its obligate intracellular habitat.

## TECHNIQUES FOR THE CULTURE OF RICKETTSIAE

In view of the above characteristics, how can we propagate rickettsiae in the laboratory? One way is to infect susceptible animals such as guinea pigs; rickettsiae can also be grown in cultures of living animal cells in test tubes. The most common method during the past several decades starts with the inoculation of rickettsiae into the yolk sac of a chick embryo. For this purpose, fertile hen eggs are incubated for seven to ten days, when the chick embryo is well along in its development. The rickettsiae are then injected into the yolk sac where they grow in the cells of the membrane surrounding the yolk. After an additional four or five days of incubation, the egg is opened and the yolk sac membrane is removed. The rickettsiae can then be partially purified by several techniques that usually involve disruption of the membrane cells followed by differential centrifugation.

## ANTIGENIC CHARACTERISTICS OF THE RICKETTSIAE

All rickettsiae produce soluble group antigens that are released into the surrounding environment. These antigens are characteristic for each group of rickettsial infections —those from the typhus group can be differentiated from the group antigens produced by the spotted fever group or the scrub typhus group, and so forth. In addition, each strain of Rickettsia produces a type-specific antigen which is attached to the cell wall and can be used to distinguish both species and strains within a species. Both the group-specific and type-specific antigens give rise to antibodies which can be measured using complement fixation tests.

A simpler and more general serological test for certain rickettsial diseases is called the Weil-Felix test. Here, the patient's antibodies are measured (preferably during acute illness and again after convalescence) for the ability to agglutinate certain strains of a gram-negative rod in the genus Proteus. Proteus organisms have nothing whatsoever to do with causing rickettsial diseases, but certain strains of these bacteria have an antigen on their cells that is also present in the rickettsiae. Three different strains of Proteus, designated Proteus OX-2, Proteus OX-19, and Proteus OX-K, have been used in

**Table 28-1. Weil-Felix Agglutination Reactions Arising During Various Rickettsial Infections**

| Disease | OX-19 | OX-2 | OX-K |
|---|---|---|---|
| Epidemic typhus | + + + + | + | 0 |
| Endemic typhus | + + + + | + | 0 |
| Brill-Zinsser disease | Variable, often negative | | 0 |
| Scrub typhus | 0 | 0 | + + + |
| Spotted fever group | { + + + +<br>{ + | { +<br>{ + + + | 0<br>0 |
| Q fever | 0 | 0 | 0 |
| Rickettsialpox | 0 | 0 | 0 |

this test. As seen in Table 28-1, not all rickettsial diseases induce a positive Weil-Felix test, nor is the test specific for those infections that do cause a positive reaction. However, when interpreted in conjunction with the clinical illness and history, the Weil-Felix test can be a valuable aid in diagnosis.

## SPOTTED FEVER GROUP

Diseases of the spotted fever group have, for the most part, received common names from the areas of the world where they are found. A few examples of rickettsial diseases in the spotted fever group are Rocky Mountain spotted fever, Queensland tick spotted fever, Boutonneuse spotted fever, and rickettsialpox. Organisms in the spotted fever group grow in both the nucleus and the cytoplasm of infected cells. They share a common group antigen but induce the formation of type-specific, complement-fixing antibodies.

### Rocky Mountain Spotted Fever

Rocky Mountain spotted fever (RMSF) was first recognized in the Rocky Mountain area, but the disease has now been reported in almost every one of the United States. The causative organism, Rickettsia rickettsii, is named for Howard Taylor Ricketts, an early pioneer in the study of rickettsial diseases who died as a result of his investigations of typhus.

EPIDEMIOLOGY AND PATHOGENESIS OF RMSF. Humans invariably contract RMSF from the bite of an infected tick. In the western United States the wood tick, *Dermacentor andersoni*, carries the disease, whereas the dog tick, *Dermacentor variabilis*, serves as the vector in the eastern United States (see Figure 28-2).

Rocky Mountain spotted fever is characterized by fever, severe headache, and a maculopapular rash (discolored spots—some may be elevated above the skin and others not) that usually appears first on the palms and soles. If untreated, the patient may die (usually during the second week of illness), or recovery will occur after an illness of about three weeks.

The organisms are widespread in the wild mammalian population as well as in the ticks themselves. A tick may become infected either as a result of a blood meal from an infected animal or by the transovarial passage of rickettsiae from mother to offspring. The disease does not harm ticks, and it has been estimated that approximately 3% of ticks are infected (although this figure varies greatly from one geographic area to another). It is interesting to note that the average mortality from untreated cases of Rocky Mountain spotted fever varies from 90% in areas of Montana to as low as 5% in eastern parts of the United States. This variation in severity is probably the result of different strains of the etiologic agent in separate geographical areas. The incubation period ranges from three to twelve days.

LABORATORY DIAGNOSIS OF RMSF. The diagnosis of RMSF is usually made on the basis of the clinical picture and a history of a tick bite. This is confirmed by use of the Weil-Felix test demonstrating a rise in titer to *Proteus* OX-19 organisms. The rickettsiae

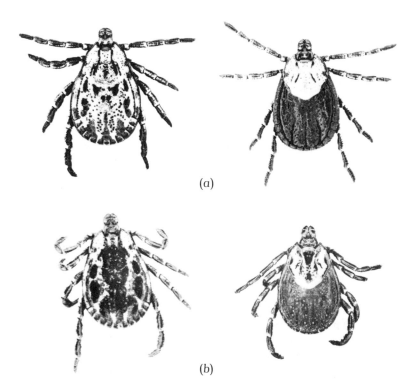

(a)

(b)

Figure 28-2 Tick vectors of Rocky Mountain spotted fever. *a. Dermacentor andersoni;* on the left is the male and on the right the female. *b. Dermacentor variabilis;* the male is to the left, female to the right.

can be grown in the yolk sac of embryonated hen eggs, and specific complement-fixation tests are then carried out using the washed rickettsial organisms.

TREATMENT AND CONTROL OF RMSF. Control of RMSF is possible, in part, by frequent examination of one's body for the presence of ticks when in geographical areas where ticks are likely to be found. Fortunately, a tick is unable to infect a person until approximately four hours after it has attached itself for a blood meal; this period is sometimes referred to as the rejuvenation period. Thus, a periodic removal of ticks, even though they may be infected with rickettsiae, is effective in preventing the disease.

A vaccine composed of killed *Rickettsia rickettsii* organisms seems to be reasonably effective for at least one year. However, since most of us are unlikely to come into contact with infected ticks, the vaccine is restricted to individuals whose occupations subject them to tick-infested environments.

Specific treatment with chloramphenicol or tetracyclines is quite effective against RMSF, particularly if started early in the illness, and immunity after recovery appears to be permanent.

### Rickettsialpox

Rickettsialpox was first described in 1946 after an epidemic in apartment houses in New York City. Subsequently, the causative organism, *Rickettsia akari,* has been found to have virtually worldwide distribution.

EPIDEMIOLOGY AND PATHOGENESIS OF RICKETTSIALPOX. The reservoir of *R. akari* is the common house mouse, and humans become infected from the bite of infected mites from mice. The infection varies considerably in severity from one person to another, but for the most part it is a mild disease. A primary lesion, similar to that seen in scrub typhus, develops at the location of the bite of the mite. After an incubation period of 10–24 days, fever and chills occur, and about three or four days later a rash not unlike the rash in chickenpox appears. The illness lasts 10–14 days, after which time recovery is routine.

LABORATORY DIAGNOSIS, TREATMENT, AND CONTROL OF RICKETTSIALPOX. The diagnosis may be based primarily on the clinical symptoms and history; however, the organisms can be readily isolated by inoculation of acute phase blood into mice, guinea pigs, or the yolk sac of a chick embryo. Organisms can be identified by the complement-fixation test using known serum.

Tetracycline and chloramphenicol are used for specific treatment, while control is directed toward elimination of rodents from areas proximal to humans.

## TYPHUS GROUP

There are two major diseases in the typhus group, epidemic typhus and endemic typhus. The etiologic agents for both infections share a common group antigen, but they can be differentiated on the basis of a specific complement-fixing antigen and on the basis of the epidemiology of the respective diseases.

### Epidemic Typhus

*Rickettsia prowazeki* is the causative agent of epidemic louse-borne typhus fever. Epidemic typhus has probably been more important than any other disease in shaping world history. The disease is one of filth, and no major war has escaped its ravages. Supposedly, Napoleon's retreat from Russia was started by a louse, and his was not the first army to suffer such an ignominious defeat.

EPIDEMIOLOGY AND PATHOGENESIS OF EPIDEMIC TYPHUS. Epidemic typhus is essentially a disease of substandard living conditions and poor sanitation. Humans are the sole reservoir for this organism, and the human body louse serves as the arthropod vector (see

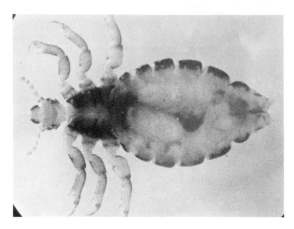

**Figure 28-3.** Micrograph of *Pediculus humanus,* the human louse that is the vector for epidemic typhus.

Figure 28-3). The rickettsiae are present in the alimentary canal of the infected louse and may be introduced when it bites a human. The organisms can also be introduced by feces, vomitus, or a crushed louse that is scratched into the skin.

The incubation period is usually about 12 days, but it may vary from 6 to 15 days. Interestingly, the rickettsiae are not passed transovarily in the louse as they are in the tick, and a louse dies several weeks after becoming infected. Thus, with the human as the sole reservoir and a susceptible louse as the sole vector, it is obvious that crowded and unsanitary conditions are essential to sustain a widespread epidemic.

The manifestations of epidemic typhus are the result of an overwhelming bacteremia with growth of the rickettsiae in the endothelial cells of the blood vessels. The patient's temperature rises to about 40°C (104°F), and after the fifth or sixth day of illness, a macular rash erupts on the trunk of the body and spreads to the extremities. Neurological changes characterized by delirium and stupor may also occur. In cold weather, gangrene of feet and fingers may be seen. Other symptoms include headache, chills, fever, malaise, and general aches and pains. Recovery or death occurs within two to three weeks after the initial symptoms.

LABORATORY DIAGNOSIS OF EPIDEMIC TYPHUS. Diagnosis is usually not difficult because the disease occurs in epidemics. Complement-fixing antibodies to both group and specific antigens become positive about one week after initial symptoms, as does the Weil-Felix test (as measured by agglutinins to *Proteus* OX-19).

TREATMENT AND CONTROL OF EPIDEMIC TYPHUS. Control is directed toward sanitation and the eradication of human lice. Impressive results were obtained during World War II, when epidemics were controlled immediately by spraying a susceptible population with DDT to kill human lice. Vaccines were originally prepared using rickettsiae obtained by washing out the intestines of infected lice, but they are now prepared from organisms grown in the yolk sac of chick embryos. The Cox vaccine, containing formalin-inactivated *Rickettsia prowazeki,* was effectively used during World War II; however, a newer living attenuated vaccine grown in yolk sacs appears to provide a longer, more solid immunity.

Both the tetracyclines and chloramphenicol are effective for the treatment of epidemic typhus.

### Brill-Zinsser Disease

Brill's disease occurs rarely, but it demonstrates an important property of the rickettsiae which cause epidemic typhus. It was first observed in the United States in 1898 in immigrants from eastern Europe. The disease was moderately mild, and, since these people were not infested with lice, it was originally thought to be endemic (flea-borne) typhus. However, subsequent work by Brill established that the infections were identical with the louse-borne epidemic typhus. Zinsser correctly postulated that these illnesses occurred in persons who had recovered from epidemic typhus many years before their current disease, but who had carried the virulent rickettsiae in their bodies in a latent state. Under conditions which are not understood, the organisms may break latency, multiply, and produce overt disease. However, as one might expect, cases of Brill's disease are usually quite mild because the individual already possesses a partial immunity and responds with an anamnestic immunological response. The most important aspect of Brill's disease is that these individuals provide the reservoir for epidemic typhus during interepidemic periods.

### Endemic Typhus

*Rickettsia typhi* is the etiologic agent of endemic flea-borne typhus. This disease, which is also called murine typhus, occurs sporadically, not in epidemics like the louse-borne type.

EPIDEMIOLOGY AND PATHOGENESIS OF ENDEMIC TYPHUS. *Rickettsia typhi* is closely related to the etiologic agent of epidemic typhus, and either disease confers immunity to both. The infection is considerably less severe than the epidemic form, but in other details it is clinically indistinguishable from epidemic typhus. The rat serves as the primary reser-

voir for *R. typhi,* although in the southwestern United States other wild rodents, such as ground squirrels, also may carry the disease. In the normal sequence of events, the disease is transmitted from rat to rat by the rat flea *Xenopsylla cheopis,* (see Figure 28-4). Only when a person accidentally interrupts this cycle by being bitten by the infected rat flea is this disease acquired. Because neither the rat nor the rat flea becomes ill as a result of the infection (in contrast to the death of the louse in epidemic typhus caused by *Rickettsia prowazeki*), they constitute the reservoir and vector, respectively, for endemic typhus.

LABORATORY DIAGNOSIS OF ENDEMIC TYPHUS. The diagnosis of endemic typhus makes use of the Weil-Felix test, as measured by an increase in agglutinins to *Proteus* OX-19. In addition, the more specific complement-fixation test can be used to distinguish between these organisms and the etiologic agent of epidemic typhus. Intraperitoneal inoculation of male guinea pigs with *R. typhi* causes severe scrotal swelling and testicular lesions, whereas *R. prowazeki* causes only a mild disease with no testicular involvement.

TREATMENT AND CONTROL OF ENDEMIC TYPHUS. Broad-spectrum antibiotics, particularly the tetracyclines and chloramphenicol, are effective for the treatment of endemic typhus.

Control measures are directed against both the rodent and the flea population in an endemic area. DDT has been very effective in reducing the flea population in rat-infested areas, and even though the use of DDT is now markedly curtailed by law, it would probably be used following a cluster of sporadic cases of endemic typhus. However, as is true in plague-infected rats, it is important to use DDT before attempting to exterminate the rat population to preclude the infected fleas from leaving dead rats to bite people.

Because of the sporadic nature of endemic typhus, vaccines are used only for those

**Figure 28-4.** Micrograph of *Xenopsylla cheopis* (female), the rat flea that acts as the arthropod vector for endemic typhus.

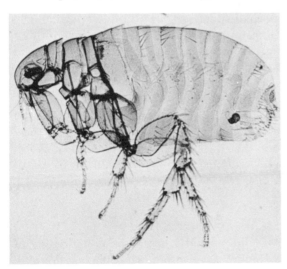

individuals (such as laboratory workers) who run a particularly high risk of becoming infected.

## OTHER RICKETTSIAL DISEASES

### Tsutsugamushi Fever (Scrub Typhus)

*Rickettsia tsutsugamushi* is the causative agent of scrub typhus, a disease found in Asia and the Southwest Pacific. It achieved particular importance for the United States during World War II and in Viet Nam, when large numbers of Allied troops were infected by these organisms. The death rate varied according to the prevalent strain of the organism, covering a range of from 0.6 to 35%.

EPIDEMIOLOGY AND PATHOGENESIS OF SCRUB TYPHUS. Scrub typhus normally occurs in rodents and is transmitted from rodent to rodent by a mite. Since the mite can pass the infection to its offspring, it acts both as a vector and as a reservoir for the rickettsiae.

Humans acquire the disease from the bite of an infected mite. Initial symptoms, 7–14 days after being bitten, include severe headache, chills, and fever; the disease is characterized by a primary lesion, called an eschar, which occurs at the location of the bite of the mite. Within a few days, a dull maculopapular rash appears; this may be accompanied by stupor and prostration. Recovery begins about three weeks after the initial symptoms, but convalescence may endure for several months.

LABORATORY DIAGNOSIS OF SCRUB TYPHUS. Agglutinins to *Proteus* OX-K, but not to OX-19 or OX-2, can be measured during the second week of illness. Isolation of the rickettsiae by inoculation of infected blood into white mice will result in death of the mice within two weeks, at which time the rickettsia can be observed as intracytoplasmic organisms in the mouse spleen cells.

TREATMENT AND CONTROL OF SCRUB TYPHUS. Both tetracyclines and chloramphenicol are highly effective for the treatment of scrub typhus. However, since rickettsiae in general appear to cause latent infections (as in Brill's disease), relapses are common unless treatment is prolonged.

Control is directed against the mite. During World War II, a mitocide was used quite effectively both as a repellent on clothing and to kill mites within a given geographical area.

Vaccines have not been successful due to the large number of immunologically different strains of *R. tsutsugamushi*.

### Trench Fever

Trench fever was first described in men engaged in trench warfare in Europe during World War I. The disease is spread from human to human by the body louse, and the etiologic agent, *Rochalimaea quintana,* is classified in a separate genus because it is the only rickettsia that can be grown on artificial media in the absence of living host cells.

The disease is one of filth and poor sanitation and seems to occur only during periods of war. Prominent symptoms are fever, headache, exhaustion, and a roseolar rash. Recovery is frequently followed by relapses occurring at five-day intervals (hence, the species name, *quintana*). Fatalities are rare, but recovery is slow.

Broad-spectrum antibiotics, particularly chloramphenicol, are effective in eliminating the symptoms of the disease, but prolonged therapy is required to eliminate the carrier state in humans.

Control is obviously directed at the louse, and since the disease seems to reappear only in unsanitary situations prevalent in warfare, the most effective but probably excessively idealistic control would be to eliminate wars.

### Q Fever

*Coxiella burnetii* is the etiologic agent of Q fever. Like other rickettsiae, *Coxiella* requires living cells for growth, but unlike other rickettsiae, an arthropod vector is not essential for transmission of the disease to humans. Moreover, *Coxiella* organisms are exceptionally stable outside host cells and can maintain their viability in dried excretions for extended periods of time. Their stability presents a paradox to the supporters of the leaky-membrane theory explaining the obligate intracellular growth of rickettsiae. In addition, *Coxiella* is heat resistant, being able to survive a temperature of 60°C for one hour. Since the organisms may occur in cows' milk, pasteurization temperatures are routinely being raised to 62.9°C to inactivate this organism.

EPIDEMIOLOGY AND PATHOGENESIS OF Q FEVER. While ticks serve as both vector and reservoir, they are not usually the direct source of human Q fever infections. Most human infections originate from animal carcasses, and it is thought that the inhalation of dried tick feces from cattle hides is the major mechanism of infection for slaughterhouse workers. Many dairy herds are infected with *C. burnetii,* and it is estimated, for example, that 10% of such herds in the Los Angeles area shed these organisms in their milk. However, even though the organism seems highly virulent when inhaled, the ingestion of contaminated milk does not often cause the disease.

Among the symptoms in humans are chills, headache, malaise, weakness, and severe sweats. Pneumonia, with a mild cough, occurs in most cases, and the condition is in many ways clinically similar to primary atypical pneumonia. The incubation period is usually two to three weeks.

LABORATORY DIAGNOSIS OF Q FEVER. Since the clinical symptoms are similar to many other infectious diseases, an unequivocal diagnosis requires the isolation and identification of the causative agent or a demonstration of a rise in specific complement-fixing antibodies during the patient's convalescence. The organisms can be grown in the yolk sac of embryonated eggs or in tissue cultures of mouse fibroblasts and are identified by direct immunofluorescent antibody staining. Inoculation of blood or sputum into hamsters is also an effective method for isolation of the organisms.

TREATMENT AND CONTROL OF Q FEVER. Broad-spectrum antibiotics such as the tetracyclines are effective, and relapses following adequate therapy are rare.

Control lies primarily in the pasteurization of milk. Also, there is a killed rickettsial vaccine that can be administered to persons, such as laboratory personnel and stockyard employees, whose occupations bring them into contact with the agent.

# Chlamydiae

The chlamydiae, like the rickettsiae, comprise a group of obligately intracellular procaryotic parasites which, prior to 1952, were referred to as large viruses or as the psittacosis-lymphogranuloma venereum-trachoma group of agents. We now know that the chlamydiae are not viruses but are, in all likelihood, distantly related to the gram-negative bacteria.

## MULTIPLICATION OF CHLAMYDIAL AGENTS

The characteristic which most delineates the chlamydiae as a distinct group of organisms is their complex method of reproduction. The developmental cycle occurs as follows: (1) a small dense cell about 0.3 μm in diameter, called an elementary body (see Figure

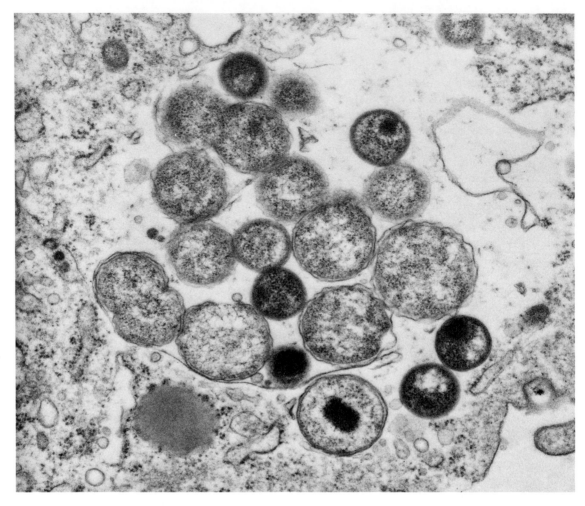

**Figure 28-5.** Microcolony of *Chlamydia psittaci* in a McCoy cell (about ×34,000). In this electron micrograph both small, dense, infectious elementary bodies (two are at the lower right) and larger, thin-walled, noninfectious initial bodies are shown. The initial body on the left is dividing.

28-5), is taken into a host cell by phagocytosis; (2) during the next eight hours, the elementary body undergoes a "reorganization" into a large, less dense cell called an initial or reticulate body; (3) the initial body, approximately 1.0 μm in diameter, grows in size and divides by binary fission; (4) after 24 to 48 hours, the initial bodies (which, by themselves, are noninfectious) reorganize into small, dense elementary bodies, and the developmental cycle is completed when the host cell bursts and liberates the small, dense, infectious cells. It is not known what triggers the reorganization of the large cells back into small cells, but it is known, however, that this reduction in size is accompanied by the loss of a great deal of RNA from the large cell (the RNA to DNA ratio in the small elementary body is approximately 1:1, while that of the large, initial body is about 4:1). The high content of RNA in the dividing large cells is undoubtedly responsible for the high rate of reproduction of the initial bodies—and, hence, protein synthesis—taking place in the large cells. Since the small cells do not divide, a high concentration of RNA is not necessary for their maintenance.

In spite of their rather complex method of reproduction, the chlamydiae are probably distant descendants of the gram-negative bacteria. Their cell walls appear to contain muramic acid; they reproduce by binary fission; they contain both RNA and DNA; and their DNA is not surrounded by a nuclear envelope. We are faced, however, with the question of why these organisms can grow only inside host cells. They are able to metabolize a few intermediates of the tricarboxylic acid cycle and can metabolize glucose through a portion of the pentose cycle to pyruvic acid. Cytochromes and flavoproteins have not been demonstrated, so it appears that the chlamydiae grow as anaerobic organisms.

Chlamydiae are also able to arrest the host-cell cycle in the G-1 phase of division, inhibiting host-cell synthesis of macromolecules. They can synthesize their own proteins, lipids, and macromolecules; but these syntheses require energy, and the chlamydiae seem to be metabolically defective in that they have no mechanism for the production or trapping of energy. Thus, they are energy parasites, unable to synthesize their own ATP. Moreover, it appears they have a leaky membrane—at least, during the reproductive step of their developmental cycle—since they are able to take up highly-charged compounds such as ATP, NADP, and glucose-6-phosphate as well as entire enzyme molecules such as hexokinase or trypsin. Quite obviously, these organisms would find it impossible to survive the chemical onslaught of extracellular life.

## CLASSIFICATION AND ANTIGENIC STRUCTURE OF CHLAMYDIAE

During the past several decades, there have been numerous attempts to classify this very complex group of organisms. Early schemes assumed the chlamydiae were large viruses, and classification was, for the most part, restricted to a clinical description of the disease syndrome. Later, taxonomists tended to group the chlamydiae with the rickettsiae, since both groups are made up of procaryotic organisms that are obligately intracellular parasites. However, it is now apparent that the complex developmental cycle of the chlamydiae clearly separates this group of organisms from all other procaryotic cells; no other bacterial organisms produce daughter cells that must undergo a morphological reorganization before they are able to infect a host cell.

## Morphological and Chemical Differentiation of the Chlamydiae

The chlamydiae are divided into two subgroups based on the morphological appearance of their intracellular inclusion bodies, the presence or absence of glycogen in the inclusion, their sensitivity to sulfonamides, and the extent of DNA homology between related organisms. Organisms in group A, which contains the etiologic agents of trachoma, inclusion conjunctivitis, and lymphogranuloma venereum, have been placed by many investigators into a single species named *Chlamydia trachomatis*. These organisms form compact inclusion bodies containing glycogen (see Figure 28-6) and are inhibited by sodium sulfadiazine. Group B, which has been named *Chlamydia psittaci,* produces a diffuse inclusion body that does not contain glycogen and, since it requires preformed folic acid, is resistant to the presence of sulfonamides. Moreover, there is considerable DNA homology within each species but very little interspecies homology.

### Antigenic Characteristics of Chlamydiae

All chlamydiae possess heat-stable group-specific antigens that can be detected by complement fixation, agglutination, hemagglutination inhibition, and intradermal

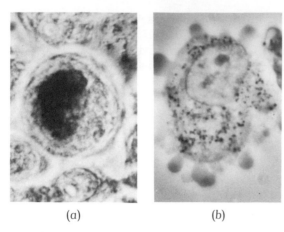

(a)                              (b)

**Figure 28-6.** *a*. Compact inclusion body of *Chlamydia trachomatis* in a McCoy cell. The glycogen-containing inclusion appears dark after staining with 5% I-KI. *b*. Diffuse inclusion of *Chlamydia psittaci* in a mononuclear mouse cell. The chlamydiae are the small dark bodies distributed about the cytoplasm in this phase-contrast micrograph of a fresh wet mount.

tests. These group-specific antigens apparently contain carbohydrate, inasmuch as they are readily destroyed by periodate oxidation. Most group-specific antigens are assumed to be associated with the cell wall structure.

Species-specific antigens stimulate the formation of infectivity-neutralizing antibodies. These antigens are resistant to periodate oxidation and are, for the most part, heat labile. Antibodies directed against species-specific antigens react only with the homologous or closely related strains of chlamydiae, and on the basis of species-specific antigens, the chlamydiae have been subdivided into a series of subgroups. Curiously, antibodies to these cell-wall type-specific antigens seem to prevent infection of host cells but have little effect on chlamydiae that have already established an intracellular existence. In fact, as we shall see, many of the chlamydial diseases can remain chronic for long periods of time, and the existence of a detectable immune response may not always be effective in eliminating the chlamydiae from the host.

A hemagglutinin has been found associated with many chlamydial strains. It is soluble and can readily be disassociated from the elementary bodies during centrifugation. Based on antigenic specificity, the hemagglutinin seems to be related to the group-specific antigens.

## CHLAMYDIA TRACHOMATIS (GROUP A)

*Chlamydia trachomatis* is the specific name for the etiologic agents of trachoma, inclusion conjunctivitis, and lymphogranuloma venereum. With the exception of an aberrant strain causing pneumonitis in mice, all of the chlamydiae classified as *C. trachomatis* are solely human pathogens. However, this name does not imply a single organism, and various diseases may be caused by different strains of *C. trachomatis*.

### Trachoma

This clinical disease has been known for over 3000 years, and it was at one time listed as one of the three most important diseases of humans. The World Health Organization estimates that approximately 400 million persons are infected with trachoma, and six to ten million of these are totally blind as a result of this disease.

EPIDEMIOLOGY AND PATHOGENESIS OF TRACHOMA. Trachoma occurs only in humans, where it grows exclusively in the conjunctival cells. It is transmitted by direct contact with fingers or contaminated towels and clothing, and in many areas of the world (for example Egypt and the Middle East) it is so prevalent that children routinely become infected during early childhood. There are three immunological variants of trachoma, designated A, B, and C, and all three serotypes may be endemic within a given geographical area. The infections occur primarily in geographical areas were poor hygienic practices are common. In the United States the American Indians and stonecutters have probably been the most frequent victims.

The overt disease may begin suddenly with an inflammation of the conjunctiva. Leukocytes enter the area and form follicles under the conjunctiva. As vascularization and infiltration of the cornea continues, the resulting scarring of the conjunctiva may cause partial or complete blindness. Simultaneous bacterial infection is common and also contributes to the inflammation and scarring.

LABORATORY DIAGNOSIS OF TRACHOMA. Trachoma is usually diagnosed on the basis of the pathological findings associated with the disease. However, the agent may be grown by the inoculation of conjunctival scrapings into cell cultures or the yolk sacs of chick embryos, or it may be identified by staining the characteristic inclusion bodies with flourescein-labeled antibody.

TREATMENT AND CONTROL OF TRACHOMA. Treatment of trachoma with both systemic and topical sulfonamides and tetracycline is usually effective in alleviating the overt signs of the disease. However, advanced or chronic infections may be difficult to cure, and relapses are not uncommon.

In endemic regions most infected persons recover spontaneously, probably as a result of IgA antibody and a cellular immune response. Immunity does not appear to be long-lasting, since reinfection or relapses may occur; however, chlamydiae characteristically produce latent infections, so it also seems possible that relapses may result from a reactivation of the latent state.

## Inclusion Conjunctivitis

The etiologic agent of this disease is so similar to trachoma that the two organisms are frequently called the TRIC (trachoma-inclusion conjunctivitis) agents. However, the pathogenesis of infection and the pathology of the conjunctivitis is considerably different from that of trachoma.

EPIDEMIOLOGY AND PATHOGENESIS OF INCLUSION CONJUNCTIVITIS. The agent of inclusion conjunctivitis is most commonly found in the human genitourinary tract, from which it is passed from human to human by sexual contact. As a venereal disease, the organisms grow in the epithelial cells of the female cervix or in the lining of the urethra of both sexes. The genital symptoms are usually very mild or absent, and by far the majority of cases of venereal inclusion conjunctivitis are undiagnosed.

However, as the name of the agent implies, infections of the conjunctiva are not so benign. They are seen most frequently in the newborn approximately 5–12 days after birth. In such cases the infection is acquired from the mother by the infant as it moves through the birth canal. The symptoms usually begin with an acute purulent conjunctivitis, which starts to subside after several weeks and spontaneously disappears in a few months. Inclusion conjunctivitis does not result in blindness.

Adult infections of the conjunctiva also may occur, and prior to the use of chlorine in swimming pools, such infections were often called "swimming-pool conjunctivitis." Now, most conjunctival infections of adults occur by contamination with fingers or towels.

LABORATORY DIAGNOSIS, TREATMENT, AND CONTROL OF INCLUSION CONJUNCTIVITIS. Diagnosis of inclusion conjunctivitis may rely heavily on the history and clinical findings. However, laboratory confirmation requires the isolation of the agent or the demonstration of cellular inclusions that will stain with fluorescently-labeled specific antibody.

Both the conjunctivitis and the genital infection respond to treatment with tetracycline and sulfonamides. Nevertheless, reinfections can occur, and it is not clear whether specific immunity is ineffective or subsequent infections are caused by a different one of the six specific serotypes of inclusion conjunctivitis.

## Lymphogranuloma Venereum

The etiologic agent of lymphogranuloma venereum is closely related to the TRIC agents, but the pathogenesis of infection is, again, considerably different. This disease is strictly a venereal infection, thought to be spread only through sexual contact. It is most prevalent in the tropics but is seen also in the United States—particularly in the South.

EPIDEMIOLOGY AND PATHOGENESIS OF LYMPHO-GRANULOMA VENEREUM. Approximately 7–12 days after sexual contact the infection becomes manifest by the appearance of a small erosion or painless papule in the genital area. The organisms migrate to the regional lymph nodes, and most symptoms result from this lymph-node involvement. The original papule soon heals, but after one to two months the regional lymph nodes become enlarged and tender and may break open and drain. These enlarged lymph nodes are called buboes, and as they enlarge, the draining lymph channel may be completely obstructed. Such restriction can cause a tremendous enlargement (elephantiasis) of the genitalia, and rectal strictures may occur as an effect of perirectal scarring.

LABORATORY DIAGNOSIS OF LYMPHOGRANU-LOMA VENEREUM. The diagnosis is made on the clinical picture, history, complement-fixation test for antibodies, biopsy of infected nodes for isolation of the organisms, and the Frei skin test. The Frei test is conducted by injecting the killed organisms into the skin and observing for a delayed-type skin reaction similar to the tuberculin reaction. But, the Frei test is not specific and will give positive results in persons with psittacosis.

TREATMENT AND CONTROL OF LYMPHOGRANU-LOMA VENEREUM. Control measures are, in general, the same as for other venereal diseases. It is not known whether or not infection induces a lasting immunity, but, like syphilis, there appears to be an infection immunity which will prevent lymph-node involvement from a second contact in an already infected person. Moreover, the frequency of relapses and the usual lifelong delayed-type hypersensitivity to the organism has led to the postulation that in many individuals a spontaneous "cure" may represent only a latent state of the infection.

Both tetracycline and sulfonamides are effective for the treatment of lymphogranuloma venereum.

## CHLAMYDIA PSITTACI (GROUP B)

In the early 1900's, reports described a disease acquired from contact with parrots and other psittacine birds. This infection, called psittacosis, has since been found to exist in at least 130 species of birds, and the trend is toward changing the name to ornithosis. Another proposal, which has not yet gained wide acceptance, is to call the disease chlamydiosis.

## Psittacosis-Ornithosis

One of the characteristics of the avian disease is its propensity to exist as an asymptomatic latent infection that can become overt following stresses such as crowding, unsanitary conditions, and bacterial infections—all of which are likely to occur during shipment of birds. Once activated, the chlamydiae cause a generalized infection in which the organisms can be found in essentially every organ of the bird. Fecal excretions contain many organisms and provide the major source of infection for humans and other birds.

EPIDEMIOLOGY AND PATHOGENESIS OF ORNI-THOSIS. Humans usually acquire the infection by the inhalation of dried infected feces, and, as in birds, the disease in humans may be asymptomatic or mild. However, in many cases a severe and frequently fatal pneumonia develops after an incubation period of one to three weeks. In severe cases, organs other than the lungs may be involved, occasionally resulting in jaundice and acute thyroiditis. Meningitis accompanied by delirium may occur, and in the terminal stages, death may result from pulmonary insufficiency and a generalized toxemia.

LABORATORY DIAGNOSIS OF ORNITHOSIS. Diagnosis requires the isolation of the etiologic agent. Injection of acute-stage blood or sputum into cell cultures or embryonated eggs is followed by identification with fluorescently-labeled specific antibody, complement-fixation tests, or neutralization of infectivity by the use of specific antibody.

TREATMENT AND CONTROL OF ORNITHOSIS. Tetracycline is the drug of choice for psittacosis-ornithosis, and adequate therapy with this antibiotic seems to produce a rapid and permanent cure.

Control is difficult since the disease prevails so widely as a latent infection of birds. Infection is an occupational hazard for workers in poultry slaughterhouses, particularly turkey abattoirs, although ducks and pigeons also provide a reservoir for ornithosis. Obviously, exclusion of parakeets as pets would also reduce sources of infection.

## POTENTIAL CHLAMYDIAL INFECTIONS OF HUMANS

Chlamydial infections of animals are widespread. For example, C. psittaci causes pneumonitis and conjunctivitis in cats, dogs, goats, calves, lambs, horses, rabbits, and swine; fatal enteritis in cattle and wild hares; polyarthritis in calves, lambs, and piglets; and placentitis leading to abortion in cattle and sheep. Much of the premise that chlamydiae can produce any of these symptoms in humans is either preliminary or circumstantial. However, chlamydial agents have been isolated from the aborted conceptuses of women in California and France, and the isolation of chlamydiae from the joints of patients with Reiter's syndrome (which is character-

ized by polyarthritis, conjunctivitis, and urethritis) has been reported. It must be emphasized that even though such isolations undoubtedly occurred, any cause or relationship is purely circumstantial. Nevertheless, the similarity of human and animal symptoms makes it tempting to incriminate chlamydiae in these human disorders.

## REFERENCES

Anacker, R. L., R. K. Gerloff, L. A. Thomas, R. E. Mann, and W. D. Bickel. 1975. Immunological properties of Rickettsia rickettsii purified by zonal centrifugation. Infect. Immun. 11:1203–1209.

Brill, N. E. 1910. An acute infectious disease of unknown origin. A clinical study based on 221 cases. Amer. J. Med. Sci. 139:484–502.

Bulla, L. A., and T. C. Cheng, eds. 1975. Pathobiology of inverterbrate vectors of disease. Ann. New York Acad. Sci. 266.

Durfce, P. T. 1975. Psittacosis in humans in the United States. 1974. J. Infect. Dis. 132:604–605.

Grayson, J. T., and S. P. Wang. 1975. New knowledge of chlamydiae and the diseases they cause. J. Infect. Dis. 132:87–105.

Nichols, R. L., ed. 1971. Trachoma and Related Diseases Caused by Chlamydial Agents. Proceedings of a Symposium held in Boston, Mass. 17–20 Aug. 1970. Excerpta Medica.

Ormsbee, R. A. 1969. Rickettsiae (as organisms). Annu. Rev. Microbiol. 23:275–292.

Philip, R. N., E. A. Casper, R. A. Ormsbee, M. G. Peacock, and W. Burgdorfer. 1976. Microimmunofluorescence test for the serological study of Rocky Mountain spotted fever and typhus. J. Clin. Microbiol. 3:51–61.

Schachter, J., L. Hanna, E. C. Hill, S. Massad, C. W. Sheppard, J. E. Conte, S. N. Cohen, and K. F. Meyer. 1975. Are chlamydial infections the most prevalent venereal disease? JAMA 231:1252–1255.

Storz, J. 1971. Chlamydia and Chlamydia-Induced Diseases. Charles C. Thomas, Springfield, Illinois.

Wang, S. P., and J. T. Grayston. 1970. Immunologic relationship between genital TRIC, lymphogranuloma venereum, and related organisms in a new microtiter indirect immunofluorescence test. *Amer. J. Ophthalmol.* **70:**367–374. **70:**367–374.

Weiss, E. 1973. Growth and physiology of rickettsiae. *Bacteriol. Rev.* **37:**259–283.

Winkler, H. H. 1976. Rickettsial permeability: An ADP-ATP transport system. *J. Bacteriol.* **251:**389–396.

Wisseman, C. L., and A. D. Waddell. 1975. *In vitro* studies on rickettsia-host cell interactions: Intracellular growth cycle of virulent and attenuated *Rickettsia prowazeki* in chicken embryo cells in slide chamber cultures. *Infect. Immun.* **11:**1391–1401.

Woodward, T. E. 1973. A historical account of the rickettsial diseases with a discussion of unsolved problems. *J. Infect. Dis.* **127:**583–594.

Zinsser, H. 1934. Varieties of typhus virus and the epidemiology of the American form of European typhus fever (Brill's disease). *Amer. J. Hyg.* **20:**513–532.

Zinsser, H. 1935. *Rats, Lice and History.* Little, Brown and Co., Boston.

# 29

# Medical Mycology

Mycology is defined as the study of fungi (commonly called yeasts and molds), and medical mycology concerns itself with those fungi that cause disease in humans and other animals. The fungi discussed in this chapter are eucaryotic organisms unrelated to bacteria. We shall first discuss a large group of procaryotic organisms that are smaller but morphologically similar to fungi. These organisms are termed the actinomycetes.

## Actinomycetes

Actinomycetes is the collective name for eight different families of bacteria which grow as frequently-branched long or short filaments of cells (hyphae-unbranched; mycelia-branched). They divide by binary fission and may or may not produce external spores. By far, the majority of these organisms are soil and water saprophytes (organisms living on decaying organic matter) and are exceedingly important for their roles in the cycles of nature, such as the decomposition of organic material and the fixation of nitrogen.

Although mold-like in outward appearance, actinomycetes are truly bacteria, as judged by all the criteria for a procaryotic cell (see Figure 29-1). They contain muramic acid in their cell walls, they lack mitochrondria, they contain 70S ribosomes, they lack a nuclear envelope, the diameter of their cells ranges from 0.5–2.0 $\mu$m, and they are killed or inhibited by many antibacterial antibiotics. As a result, it is difficult to imagine a direct phylogenetic link between the procaryotic actinomycetes and the eucaryotic fungi.

Of the many different genera which are currently classified in the order Actinomycetales, only a few produce disease in humans, and we shall confine our discussion to those medically important actinomycetes.

### ACTINOMYCES

The genus *Actinomyces* contains obligately anaerobic or microaerophilic gram-positive organisms that grow in a mass of vegetative mycelium which readily breaks up into

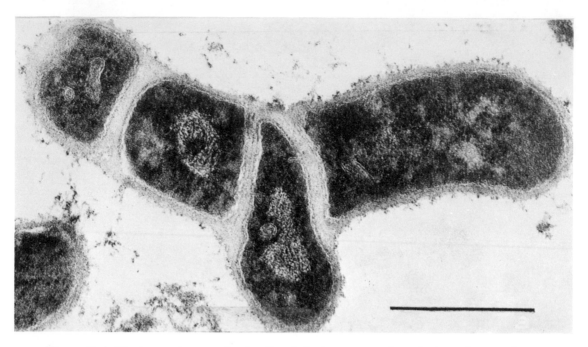

**Figure 29-1.** Electron micrograph of cells of *Actinomyces odontolyticus* showing basic procaryotic features (scale = 0.5μm); the downward-pointing cell is budding.

bacillary and coccoid forms. They do not form spores, and only two species are of major medical importance. Both—*Actinomyces bovis,* the causative agent of lumpy jaw, and *Actinomyces israelii,* the etiologic agent of actinomycosis in humans—cause similar types of infections. In addition *Actinomyces naeslundii* (which may be a variant of *A. israelii*) and *Actinomyces eriksonii* (also called *Bifidobacterium eriksonii*) have been reported to cause occasional infections in humans.

### Epidemiology and Pathogenesis of Human Actinomycoses

*Actinomyces israelii* occurs as part of the normal flora in the crypts of the tonsils, in dental caries, and occasionally in the intestinal tract or the lungs. Thus, infections caused by this organism originate from an endogenous source, and the initial lesions, which usually contain a mixture of actinomycetes with other endogenous bacteria, occur in the cervicofacial, abdominal, or lung tissue.

CERVICOFACIAL ACTINOMYCOSIS. Infection may occur as a result of trauma to the mucous membranes of the mouth or tonsils or begin as a dental abscess caused by poor oral hygiene. Initial symptoms include minor pain together with a hard nodular or lumpy swelling of the jaw. Later, the swelling softens, and the organisms spread and eventually extend through the skin, forming multiple draining abscesses. Advanced cases show considerable bone destruction, and in rare instances the organisms may penetrate the cranium, causing fatal brain lesions.

The skin abscesses discharge a purulent material containing firm microcolonies of *Actinomyces israelii,* cellular debris, and associated microorganisms. Because of the yellow color of these granules, they are usually referred to as sulfur granules, and their appearance in a draining abscess provides good presumptive evidences for a diagnosis of actinomycosis.

ABDOMINAL ACTINOMYCOSIS. There is no general agreement on whether abdominal actinomycosis results from swallowing the etiologic agent, or whether *A. israelii* is also part of the normal flora of the caeco-appendicular regions. In either event, a diseased appendix or a perforated intestinal ulcer seems to provide the initial site for the actinomycotic lesion. The lesions may also extend to infect various internal organs, such as the viscera, liver, and the urinary system; involvement of the spinal column can cause destructive bone lesions. Penetration of the abdominal wall, yielding draining abscesses containing so-called sulfur granules, provides the means of diagnosis in the absence of a surgical exploration.

THORACIC ACTINOMYCOSIS. This variation of actinomycosis may occur as a primary lesion in the lung, or it may result from an extension of the disease from a cervicofacial infection. The lesions eventually spread through the thoracic wall, causing external draining abscesses. Rib destruction may occur in advanced cases.

### Diagnosis, Treatment, and Control of Actinomycoses

The presence of sulfur granules in a draining abscess provides reasonable evidence for the diagnosis of actinomycosis. Crushing and staining a granule on a microscope slide will show gram-positive filaments, as well as bacillary and coccoid forms of the organism (see Figure 29-2). The isolation and identification of the organisms provides an absolute diagnosis, but because of the associated microorganisms, it is somewhat difficult to obtain pure cultures. However, *A. israelii* can be grown anaerobically on a brain-heart infusion blood agar plate.

Penicillin is the drug of choice, but therapy must be continued for periods as long as 12–18 months, and surgical excision may be necessary in cases of advanced disease. Chlorotetracycline, chloramphenicol, streptomycin, sulfadiazine, and other sulfonamides may also be used to treat actinomycosis.

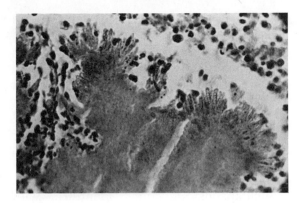

**Figure 29-2.** Hematoxylin and eosin stain of an *Actinomyces israelii* sulfur granule (about ×1900); note the peripheral "clubs."

Control is especially difficult since the etiologic agent is a part of the human normal flora. Good oral hygiene appears to lessen the possible occurrence of actinomycosis, although many cases occur in apparently healthy young adults.

### NOCARDIA

Members of the genus *Nocardia* are distributed worldwide in the soil. However, only two species, *Nocardia asteroides* and *Nocardia brasiliensis,* are considered valid pathogens for humans.

The organisms grow aerobically on simple media, forming long filaments that easily fragment into rather pleomorphic bacillary and coccoid-shaped cells. The pathogenic species are gram-positive and partially acid fast; as a result, the fragmented hyphae can be mistaken for tubercle bacilli.

### Epidemiology and Pathogenesis of Human Nocardiosis

Although species of *Nocardia* may occasionally be found in healthy individuals, they are not considered to be normal flora. Nocardiosis occurs most frequently as a pulmonary disease following the inhalation of the fragmented mycelium. In the usual course of events, one or more lung abscesses may develop and enlarge to form cavities similar to those seen in chronic tuberculosis. From the lung, the organisms may spread via the bloodstream potentially to establish lesions in any area of the body, particularly the brain and kidneys. Unlike actinomycosis, bone destruction is rare; however, both *Nocardia asteroides* and *Nocardia brasiliensis* may form mycetomas (chronic subcutaneous infections identified with fungi) in which the abscesses extend by the destruction of soft tissue and bone to eventually erupt through the skin.

### Diagnosis, Treatment, and Control of Nocardioses

Pulmonary nocardiosis can mimic many other infections, such as tuberculosis, carcinoma, actinomycosis, or fungal infections of the lung. Thus, a definitive diagnosis requires the visualization of long branching gram-positive filaments and fragmented bacillary bodies that are partially acid fast. The organisms are easily grown, and the classic wrinkled, frequently pigmented colonies of *Nocardia* are easily recognized (see Figure 29-3).

The drug of choice is sulfadiazine, but the prognosis of nocardiosis is poor—particularly if the organisms have metastasized to other organs of the body.

Because of the widespread occurrence of species of *Nocardia,* control is impossible. However, humans undoubtedly possess considerable resistance to infection by these forms because the majority of cases occur in debilitated or immunosuppressed patients.

### ACTINOMYCOTIC MYCETOMA

Actinomycetoma is a relatively painless, locally invasive indolent tumor-like process commonly occurring in the extremities. The actinomycetes that are most often isolated are *Actinomyces israelii* and *Nocardia as-*

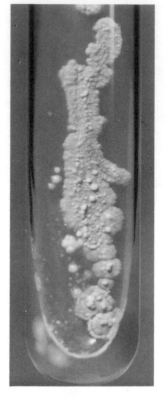
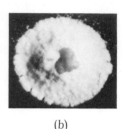

(b)

(a)

Figure 29-3. *a.* Colonies of *Nocardia asteroides* grown on Sabouraud's dextrose agar. *b.* Single colony of *N. asteroides* grown on an inorganic salts-yeast extract-glycerol agar medium in a humid atmosphere at 37°C.

*teroides,* but other species of *Nocardia* and one species of *Streptomyces* have also been isolated from draining abscesses. In addition, at least nine taxa of eucaryotic fungi are known to be occasional etiologic agents for these destructive lesions.

### *STREPTOMYCES*

The genus *Streptomyces* includes an extremely large group of organisms distributed worldwide. Like the other actinomycetes, they grow in long, branched filaments, but unlike members of the genera *Actinomyces* and *Nocardia,* they form long chains of aerial spores called conidia. Members of the genus *Streptomyces* are only rarely pathogenic, but occasional cases of actino-mycetoma have been attributed to these organisms.

Members of the genus *Streptomyces* have achieved prominence as a result of their ability to produce antibiotics. Streptomycin and actinomycin were the first to be isolated and characterized, but since 1940 over 500 different antibacterial compounds, including most of the antibiotics in use today, have been isolated and characterized from organisms classified as *Streptomyces*.

## Medically Important Fungi

The fungi, being eucaryotic organisms, differ from the actinomycetes in their cell-wall composition, nuclear structure, ribosome structure, and size. Included among the fungi are such macroscopic organisms as mushrooms, toadstools, and puffballs, as well as the microscopic organisms known as molds and yeasts.

It is estimated that over 100,000 different species of fungi participate in the cycles of nature, but, fortunately, only a few of these cause disease in humans.

### CHARACTERISTICS OF FUNGI

Fungi lack chlorophyll, are nonmotile (with the exception of certain spore forms), and may grow as single cells (yeasts), or as long branched, filamentous structures (mycelia) (see Figure 29-4). Most fungi produce both asexual and sexual spores, and their identification into classes is, for the most part, based on the type of spore and the method by which these spores are produced (see Table 29-1).

**Figure 29-4.** *a.* Yeast cells of *Pityrosporum furfur* among hyphae or pseudohyphae (×700). *b.* Mycelial strands of *Microsporum canis* (×250).

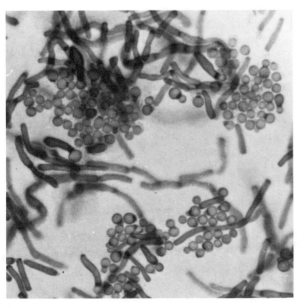

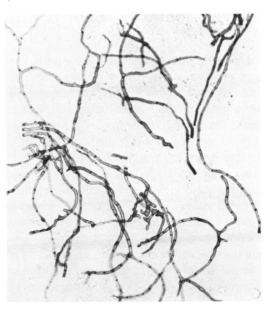

(a)                                                      (b)

### Table 29-1. Fungal Spore Types

| Name | Type | Fungal Groups | Morphological Characteristics |
|------|------|---------------|-------------------------------|
| Arthrospores | Asexual | *Geotrichum, Coccidioides* | Produced by fragmentation of septate hyphae into single, slightly thickened cells |
| Chlamydospores | Asexual | Found in all fungi | Thick-walled spores formed either within segments of hyphae or as terminal spores of a hyphal filament |
| Blastospores | Asexual | Found in all yeasts | Appear as buds on mother cell |
| Microconidia | Asexual | Found in most fungi except Zygomycetes | Produced by constriction of hypha—borne on a stalk (conidiophore) and may occur singly or in chains |
| Macroconidia | Asexual | Found in dermatophytes | Large multicelled spores borne on a stalk (conidiophore) |
| Sporangiospores | Asexual | Zygomycetes | Spores formed within a sac (sporangium) which is borne on a sporangiophore |
| Zoospores | Asexual | Zygomycetes | Same as sporangiospores except motile by means of a flagellum |
| Ascospores | Sexual | Ascomycetes | Spores that are formed within a sac-like structure called an ascus |
| Zygospores | Sexual | Zygomycetes | Resting spore resulting from the fusion of two morphologically similar cells |
| Basidiospores | Sexual | Basidiomycetes | Spores that are borne externally on a club-shaped cell called a basidium |

## CLASSIFICATION OF MEDICALLY IMPORTANT FUNGI

For many years, the fungi were divided into four major classes: Phycomycetes, Ascomycetes, Basidiomycetes, and the Deuteromycetes (also called the Fungi Imperfecti). Based on differences in their sexual and asexual spores, habitat, gross morphologic structure, and, to some extent, nutritional properties, the Phycomycetes are now additionally subdivided into the first six classes of fungi described in Table 29-2. These six classes of organisms normally lack regular septa (crosswalls) in their hyphal filaments (coenocytic hyphae), resulting in the presence of many nuclei in each cell filament. Members of these six classes include organisms that are infrequent causes of human disease—even though several genera in the class Zygomycetes do cause occasional

serious infections in debilitated or immunologically-compromised persons. The frequency of such infections is quite low.

Ascomycetes, or sac fungi, form one or more (usually eight) sexual spores within a sac-like cell called an ascus. The asexual spores produced by the Ascomycetes may be single- or multi-celled conidia. The single-celled conidia are frequently produced in long chains extending from an aerial hypha called a conidiophore (meaning "conidia-bearing"), whereas the multi-celled conidia are borne on short stalks as single structures.

The Ascomycetes produce regular septa which divide the mycelium into a large number of individual cells. Each septum, however, has a "hole" in it which permits the free flow of cytoplasmic and nuclear material between cells. Many grow only as single cells, and by far the best known yeast in this class is in the genus *Saccharomyces*, upon which both the baking and the alcoholic beverage industries are totally dependent.

Basidiomycetes form their sexual basidiospores externally on club-shaped cells called basidia. Asexual reproduction may occur by budding, conidia, or by fragmentation of the mycelium. The hyphae are usually septate. Very few human diseases are caused by members of Basidiomycetes, although organisms in this class do cause several plant diseases. Note that mushrooms, which may be highly toxic, also belong to this class.

**Table 29-2. Classes of Fungi**

| Name | Description | Name | Description |
|------|-------------|------|-------------|
| Chytridiomycetes | Mostly aquatic; asexual spores motile by means of a single posterior whiplash flagellum | | from the fusion of two similar cells to form a zygospore. Sporangiospores are nonmotile. Some are parasitic on insects, nematodes, protozoa, and plants. Human infections are routinely caused by opportunistic parasites that are normally saprophytic organisms |
| Hyphochytridiomycetes | Aquatic fungi; asexual spores motile by means of a tinsel flagellum on anterior end that pulls the cell through the water | | |
| Oomycetes | Most aquatic; some parasitize fish and some are major plant pathogens. Sexual spores result from the fusion of two cells of considerably different size. Asexual spores possess two oppositely directed flagella—one whiplash, the other tinsel | Ascomycetes | Produce sexual spores within a sac called an ascus. Yeasts are important for fermentation and baking. Some produce serious plant diseases (Dutch elm disease, rusts). Some cause human diseases |
| Plasmodiophoromycetes | Intracellular, parasitic slime molds of plants causing diseases such as clubroot of cabbage and powdery scab of potatoes. Motile asexual spores possess two anterior flagella, both whiplike | Basidiomycetes | Sexual spores are borne externally on a basidium. Some cause plant diseases such as rusts and smuts. Many mushrooms in this class are extremely toxic if ingested |
| Trichomycetes | All are parasites of arthropods, where they exist attached to the intestinal tract or cuticle | Deuteromycetes | Artificial class for which no sexual stage has been demonstrated; also called Fungi Imperfecti. Many human and animal pathogens are found in this class |
| Zygomycetes | Primarily terrestrial; sexual spores result | | |

Deuteromycetes, or Fungi Imperfecti, form a large group of fungi for which no sexual stage has been demonstrated. Some members have recently been shown to produce sexual spores when mixed with the correct mating type and, as a result, have acquired two names, one for the sexual classification as well as the older asexual name. Since many of the human fungal pathogens belong to Deuteromycetes, the tendency has been to retain the older name even though a sexual stage has been shown to exist. Most mycologists, however, believe the sexual-stage name is the preferred terminology and should eventually be the only name. Many species of this class produce conidia and chlamydospores, and many produce arthrospores and blastospores (see Table 29-2).

Diseases caused by the deuteromycetes include: (1) superficial infections that are of concern only because of their cosmetic appearance, (2) cutaneous infections caused by the dermatophytes, which are restricted to the keratinized tissues such as the nails, hair, and stratum corneum of the skin, and (3) the subcutaneous and deep-seated systemic infections that cause debilitating and fatal diseases.

Early concepts of many of the superficial and dermatophytic infections attributed these infections to insects. The Romans named these infections *tinea,* meaning small insect larva, and this prefix is still used as part of the clinical terminology for these diseases.

## SUPERFICIAL FUNGAL INFECTIONS

Superficial infections induce little or no pathology or symptoms and usually are seen by a physician because of their discoloring appearance.

### Tinea Versicolor

This is a mild infection of the superficial layers of the skin, causing discoloration or depigmentation. The etiologic agent is *Pityrosporum orbiculare,* although this organism may also be called *Pityrosporum furfur. Pityrosporum orbiculare* has been shown to be part of the normal human flora, but for reasons as yet unknown it only rarely produces recognizable disease.

The diagnosis is primarily a clinical one based on the color of the skin (which intensifies after exposure to sunlight) and on the appearance of the scaly lesions (see Figure 29-5a). A more definitive diagnosis can be obtained by observing a KOH preparation of skin scrapings for the characteristic yeast cells or by examining the affected area under an ultraviolet light (Wood's lamp) for a yellow fluorescence.

Infections caused by *P. orbiculare* are treated with one of several topical agents such as salicylic acid, mild fungicides, 2% sulfur in an ointment base, or 1% selenium sulfide in a water-miscible ointment or as a shampoo. Unfortunately, recurrences are common.

### Tinea Nigra

Tinea nigra, caused by *Cladosporium werneckii,* results in dark brown to black, painless, mottled areas on the skin, usually on the palms of the hands (see Figure 29-5b). The disease occurs primarily in the tropics but is now being seen with greater frequency in the United States.

Skin scrapings dispersed in 10% KOH reveal septate hyphal filaments, and these can be grown on Sabouraud's glucose agar. The organism is slow to grow and may require as long as three weeks incubation on a suitable medium before visible growth appears. The growth is at first yeast-like but later develops into a mycelium.

Treatment as described for *Pityrosporum orbiculare* is effective in eliminating the infection.

### Black Piedra and White Piedra

The agents responsible for these two superficial infections are unrelated and are

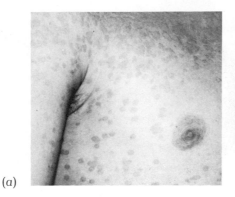

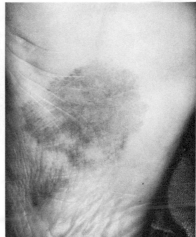

(a)

(b)

**Figure 29-5.** *a.* Hyperpigmented lesions of tinea versicolor on shoulder and chest. *b.* Tinea nigra on the sole of a patient's foot.

grouped together here only because they are restricted to growth in or on the hair.

Black piedra is characterized by hard, black nodules, which usually occur on the scalp hair and are composed of a hyphal mass cemented together by a capsule. The etiologic agent, *Piedraia hortae,* infects humans and other primates in the tropical areas of Asia, Africa, and South America.

White piedra, caused by *Trichosporon beigelii,* is seen less frequently than black piedra, but it occurs in both temperate and tropical areas of the world. This fungus may infect hairs on the face and genital areas in addition to those on the scalp.

Both infections weaken the hair shaft causing the hair to be easily broken. Diagnosis is based on the microscopic examination of infected hairs in a 10% potassium hydroxide solution. Shaving the head or cutting off the infected hair usually provides an effective cure, but daily shampooing with an antifungal agent is also recommended.

## DERMATOPHYTOSES

The etiologic agents of the dermatophytoses are closely related organisms which utilize keratin for growth. These organisms share antigenic and physiologic properties, and,

for the most part, cause similar types of infections, even though the same species of dermatophyte may cause different symptoms in varying anatomic sites. Thus, the major differentiation between the three genera of dermatophytes (*Trichophyton, Microsporum,* and *Epidermophyton*) is based on the kinds and the appearance of spores and hyphae (see Figure 29-6). In spite of the fact that the dermatophytes are usually considered to be members of the Deuteromycetes, sexual spores characteristic for Ascomycetes have been observed in about half of the known species of *Trichophyton* and *Microsporum.* As a result, sexual species of *Trichophyton* are also classified in the genus *Arthroderma,* while species of *Microsporum* known to produce sexual spores are additionally placed in the genus *Nannizzia.*

Dermatophytes invade only keratinized tissues, such as hair, nails, and the stratum corneum of the skin, causing an infection that does not extend into the subcutaneous areas of the body. In general, dermatophyte infections begin in the horny layer of the skin and spread in a centrifugal pattern showing a "ringworm" appearance.

The major clinical infections are termed: (1) tinea pedis (ringworm of the feet), (2) tinea corporis (ringworm of the smooth skin),

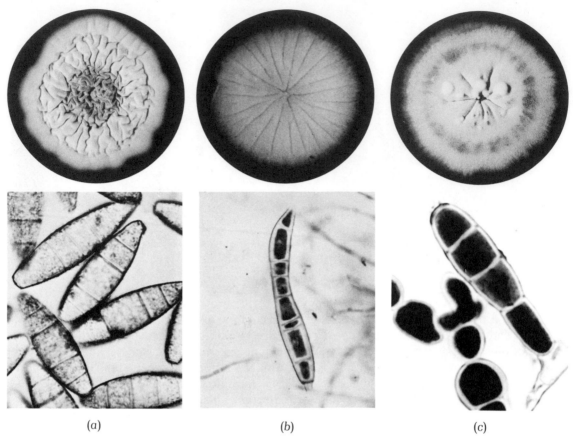

(a)                    (b)                    (c)

**Figure 29-6.** *a.* Colony and macronconidia of *Trichophyton gallinae. b.* Colony and macro-conidium of *Microsporum audouinii. c.* Colony and macroconidium of *Epidermophyton floccosum.*

(3) tinea capitis (ringworm of the scalp), and (4) tinea unguium (ringworm of the nails). In addition, a further breakdown can be used which includes: (1) tinea cruris (ring-worm of the groin), (2) tinea barbae (ring-worm of the beard), and (3) tinea manuum (ringworm of the hand). All genera of der-matophytes may cause any of these clinical entities. However, species of *Microsporum* usually invade the hair and skin but not the nails; *Epidermophyton floccosum* invades the skin and nails but not the hair; and spe-cies of *Trichophyton* infect the hair, skin, and the nails.

### Tinea Pedis

This infection, also known as athlete's foot, is a common fungal disease of humans. The majority of cases are caused by *T. rubrum, T. mentagrophytes,* and *E. floccosum;* and since the infection appears to require warmth and moisture to progress, the disease is usually found primarily in individuals who wear shoes.

It is estimated that 30–70% of the popula-tion of the Western World is infected; however, the majority of such cases exist subclinically. The infection usually begins between the toes, and symptoms may vary from a chronic disease with peeling and cracking of the skin to an acute ulcerative form of the infection. It is thought that initial contact with the organisms probably occurs in such places as common shower stalls and bathing facilities and that genetic factors may provide predisposing conditions for overt infections.

Chronically infected persons frequently develop a hypersensitivity to the fungus which may cause an allergic response. This is called a dermophytid (usually abbreviated "id") reaction and is manifested by the appearance of vesicles, usually on the hands. Such individuals will also strongly react to an extract of the fungus (called trichophytin) to give a delayed-type skin reaction.

### Tinea Corporis

Ringworm of the body may be produced by any of the species of dermatophytes, although *T. rubrum* and *T. mentagrophytes* are the most common etiologic agents. Invasion of the horny layer of the skin is followed by the centrifugal spread of the organism, causing characteristic rings of inflammation (see Figure 29-7). Healing begins in the center of the ring. In the usual course of events, such infections will spontaneously clear within a few months.

### Tinea Capitis

This infection appears as scaly red lesions. Hair loss (alopecia) can also occur on the scalp, eyebrows, and eyelids. The most common etiologic agents in the United States are *M. canis, M. audouinii* and *T. tonsurans*. Other geographical areas of the world may have different organisms as the prevalent cause of tinea capitis. Infections appear as expanding rings on the scalp with organisms growing in and on the hair. Inflammatory reactions may cause deep ulcers, which heal with scarring and permanent loss of hair.

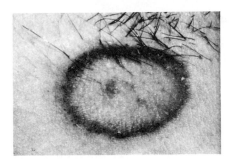

**Figure 29-7.** Tinea corporis (ringworm of the body), showing characteristic ring of inflammation.

It was formerly believed that healing occurred only at puberty, but it is now apparent that spontaneous healing can occur after less than one year and well before the age of puberty. Obviously, some mechanism other than pubescent change is operative.

### Tinea Unguium

Infection of the nails is commonly associated with dermatophyte infections of other areas of the body. Almost all species of dermatophytes have been involved as etiologic agents, but *T. rubrum* is found most commonly. The disease is characterized by thickened, discolored, brittle nails and may continue for years as a chronic infection (see Figure 29-8).

**Figure 29-8.** Tinea unguium (ringworm of the nails, or onychomycosis) in the toenails of a 61-year-old male.

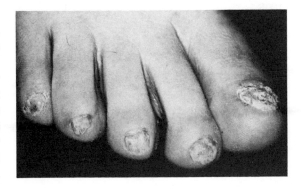

## Epidemiology of the Dermatophytoses

The course of infection for the dermatophytes may be human to human (anthropophilic), animal to human (zoophilic), or soil to human (geophilic). It is believed that tinea pedis and tinea capitis are spread from human to human indirectly through contaminated floors, towels, combs, theater seats, bed linens, and similar objects coming into contact with infected areas of the body. Other types of dermatophytoses appear to arise most frequently from human contact, but animal sources may be involved. Soil abounds with keratinophilic fungi with the potential to infect humans, but infections of geophilic origin are infrequent.

## Treatment of the Dermatophytoses

Topical applications of long-chain fatty acids, salicylic acid, selenium sulfide, sulfur in ointment, and many other compounds have for years been used to treat the dermatophytic fungal infections. Currently, the treatment of choice is griseofulvin, an antibiotic produced by a mold belonging to the genus *Penicillium*. Griseofulvin, given orally, becomes incorporated into newly synthesized keratin layers, rendering them resistant to fungal infection, but has little effect on keratin structures that are already infected. Thus, depending on the site of the body involved and the causal organism, therapy can consist of a single dose of griseofulvin (for tinea capitis caused by *M. audouinii*) to use for many months (for nail infections caused by *T. rubrum*).

## PATHOGENIC YEASTS

It is perhaps a bit of a misnomer to set aside a section entitled pathogenic yeasts, since the separation of yeasts from the filamentous fungi is frequently based on conditions of growth. Many pathogenic fungi will grow as single-celled yeasts under one circumstance and as long filamentous hyphae when growth conditions are changed. (This ability to grow as two distinct forms—either yeast cells or as filamentous fungi—is an example of the phenomenon known as dimorphism.) This section will be concerned with those pathogenic fungi that appear only as yeasts, or only rarely form a true mycelium.

### Candida

Although the genus *Candida* contains a number of species, *Candida albicans* is by far the most frequent species encountered in candidiasis (infections caused by *Candida*; synonyms: moniliasis and candidosis). Under normal conditions, members of *Candida* occur in small numbers in the alimentary tract, mouth, and vaginal area, and disease results only when a major change in other normal flora or a disturbance of the normal immune response occurs. Under such conditions, candidiasis may present any one of many forms.

*Candida albicans* usually appears as oval yeast-like cells that reproduce by budding (see Figure 29-9); however, in infected areas filamentous hyphae plus pseudohyphae (which consist of elongated yeast cells that remain attached to each other) may also be seen. The yeast is easily grown at 25–37°C on Sabouraud's glucose agar, and if grown on cornmeal agar at 25°C, the organisms can produce many characteristic thick-walled chlamydospores.

ORAL CANDIDIASIS.   This type of candidiasis (also called thrush) occurs most frequently in the newborn and is probably acquired during passage through an infected vagina. The yeast appears as a creamy, gray membrane covering the tongue and appears able to produce disease only because of the absence of other resident normal flora. If thrush has not occurred by the third day of life, it is unlikely that it will appear, but if it should occur, it will usually disappear without treatment as other members of the normal flora are acquired.

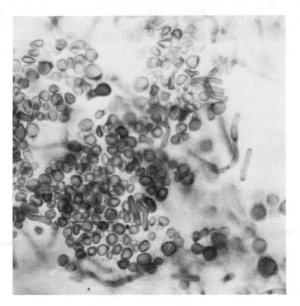

**Figure 29-9.** Yeast cells and pseudohyphae of *Candida albicans* on a skin scale (about ×675).

Oral thrush in older children or adults may occur as a result of endocrine disturbances, avitaminosis (particularly riboflavin), a complication of diabetes, poor oral hygiene, or following the administration of corticosteroids or antibiotics.

VAGINITIS. Vaginal candidiasis is usually seen by the physician when the patient complains of a yellow, milky, vaginal discharge. Yeast cells and pseudomycelium can be found on the mucous membranes, and the organisms may produce an intense inflammation of the entire inguinal area.

ALIMENTARY CANDIDIASIS. This disease may follow essentially any of the predisposing conditions listed for adult oral thrush; however, the majority of cases occur as a result of prolonged, broad-spectrum antibiotic therapy which destroys a large part of the normal flora of the intestine. The organisms may also cause intense inflammation of the perianal (around the anus) region and may spread to the buttocks and thighs.

CUTANEOUS AND SYSTEMIC CANDIDIASIS. Infection of the skin by *Candida* usually occurs in individuals with metabolic disorders, obesity resulting in continuously moist folds of skin, or in individuals with parts of the body kept moist under surgical dressings.

Systemic candidiasis is extremely rare, but in debilitated persons or those receiving immunosuppressive drugs, *Candida albicans* can cause urinary tract infections, endocarditis, and meningitis.

THERAPY FOR INFECTIONS DUE TO CANDIDA. Oral and cutaneous candidiasis respond best to a 1% solution of crystal violet. Nystatin is also effective when applied topically, but amphotericin B is the only effective therapeutic agent for systemic infections caused by species of *Candida*.

### Cryptococcosis

Cryptococcosis (also called European blastomycosis) is caused by *Cryptococcus neoformans*. This species is distributed worldwide in soil, but most human infections are thought to be acquired by the inhalation of dried, infected pigeon feces. Curiously, this mycosis is reported more often in males than in females, but it is not known whether this is a function of exposure or a matter of hormonal differences. Pigeon breeders have a higher than normal occurrence of antibody to cryptococci but no greater rate of overt infection.

CLINICAL CRYPTOCOCCOSIS. Since the organisms are acquired by inhalation, primary infection occurs in the lungs. Most infections are either asymptomatic or undiagnosed, and the resolution of the primary lesions usually occurs spontaneously. Fulminating (intense or sudden) pneumonia may result in spread of the organisms via the bloodstream, causing infections in many areas of the body, but the most frequent complication is involvement of the brain and meninges.

DIAGNOSIS AND TREATMENT OF CRYPTOCOC-
CUS INFECTIONS. *Cryptococcus neoformans*
grows primarily as a yeast that produces
a large capsule, but several strains are now
known than can form a mycelium. An India-
ink wet mount provides an easy method to
visualize this encapsulated yeast (see Figure
29-10), and the presence of characteristic
organisms in such a preparation provides a
tentative diagnosis. The organisms can be
readily grown but are sensitive to cyclohexa-
mide, which is frequently incorporated into
fungal media. Specific identification of *C.
neoformans* requires physiological tests,
growth at 37°C, and observed pathogenicity
for mice.

Untreated meningitis due to *C. neoformans*
is invariably fatal; however, amphotericin
B is usually effective and is currently the
therapy of choice.

### Miscellaneous Yeast Infections

*Torulopsis glabrata,* a member of the human
normal flora, only rarely causes toruloposis
in persons receiving long-term antibiotics,
cortisone, or immunosuppressive drugs.
The most common site of infection is the
genitourinary tract, although infections of
the mouth, lungs, and kidneys have been
reported.

*Rhodotorula rubra,* also, has been occasionally isolated from the lungs, kidney,

**Figure 29-10.** India-ink wet mount of *Cryptococcus neoformans* demonstrating the
capsule around a yeast cell.

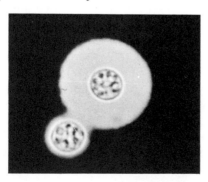

and central nervous system of debilitated
patients. The yeast is a common contaminant
of skin and feces and has been isolated from
soil and a number of food sources. Infections
are frequently caused by contaminated
catheters, heart-lung machines, and other
intimate medical devices, and usually spontaneously resolve when the source of infection is removed.

Treatment with amphotericin B is effective
for infections caused by both *Torulopsis
glabrata* and *Rhodotorula rubra.*

## SUBCUTANEOUS MYCOSES

Subcutaneous mycoses are mycotic infections that gain entrance to the body as a result
of trauma to the skin. Once established, these
mycoses generally remain localized in the
traumatized area but may extend via draining lymph channels to regional lymph nodes.
Fungi involved in subcutaneous types of
mycoses are normal soil inhabitants whose
localized infection and slow progression
cause them to be considered organisms of
low virulence.

### Sporotrichosis

*Sporothrix schenckii,* the etiologic agent of
sporotrichosis, is found in soil and plants in
a worldwide but sporadic distribution. It
also occurs in wood and moss, and infections frequently result from inoculation by
splinters, thorn pricks, sphagnum moss,
grasses, or garden soil. Thus, infection is an
occupational hazard for gardeners and green-
house workers. It is frequently seen in South
America in persons gathering grass or culti-
vating house plants. Curiously, endemic
areas have shifted over the years, and it has
been proposed that nutritional deficiencies
might explain the high incidence of sporotrichosis in areas of rural South America.

EPIDEMIOLOGY AND PATHOGENESIS OF SPORO-
TRICHOSIS. Sporotrichosis is usually a localized infection of the skin, subcutaneous

tissues, and regional lymphatics, gaining entrance to the body following trauma or through open wounds. After an incubation period varying from a week to six months, a subcutaneous nodule appears and develops into a necrotic ulcer. The initial lesions heal as new ulcers appear in adjacent areas. Lymphatics in the area develop nodules and ulcers along the lymph channels and these may persist for months or years.

In highly endemic areas, many persons develop a cellular immunity to the organism; this can be demonstrated as a delayed-type skin reaction to sporotrichin. Such individuals appear able to localize the initial infection to the original site of invasion. Rarely, *Sporothrix schenckii* may invade the blood and spread to various organs of the body; occasionally, the fungi may enter the host via the respiratory tract, resulting in a primary pulmonary sporotrichosis.

LABORATORY DIAGNOSIS AND TREATMENT OF SPOROTRICHOSIS. *Sporothrix schenckii* is a dimorphic fungus that grows in culture, soil, or plant material, as septate branching hyphae with clusters of pear-shaped conidia at the ends of the branches. In contrast, the organisms appear in infected tissues as cigar-shaped yeast cells that reproduce by budding (see Figure 29-11).

**Figure 29-11.** Gram stain of yeast cells in pus from a mouse infected with *Sporothrix schenckii.*

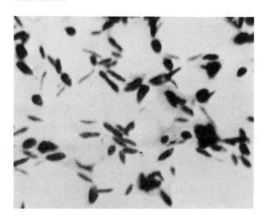

A definitive diagnosis requires the growth and identification of the infecting organism, even though lymphocutaneous sporotrichosis with lymph channel ulceration can be diagnosed clinically with reasonable confidence. Few organisms are present in the lesions, so a histologic examination frequently may be negative. The mycelial form from a Sabouraud's glucose agar medium grown at 25°C can be transformed to the yeast phase by growth in moist blood agar tubes at 37°C.

Oral potassium iodide administered over a period of weeks is the most common treatment for localized sporotrichosis; however, amphotericin B is used for relapsing cases as well as for pulmonary and disseminated sporotrichosis.

### Chromomycosis

Chromomycosis (also known as chromoblastomycosis and verrucous dermatitis) is a term applied to a clinical infection that may be caused by any one of several different fungi. The taxonomy of this group of agents is not yet firm, but the principal genera involved in chromomycosis are *Fonsecaea, Phialophora,* and *Cladosporium.*

EPIDEMIOLOGY AND PATHOGENESIS OF CHROMOMYCOSIS. The causative agents of chromomycosis are soil saprophytes found in decaying vegetative matter and rotting wood. Most infections appear to originate from puncture wounds, and by far the majority of these occur in the tropics, particularly in Mexico and South America.

Most infections occur on the feet and legs in rural areas where shoes are rarely worn. The original lesion appears as a small, raised, violet papule, and over a period of months to years additional lesions appear in adjacent areas. The lesions are hard, dry, and usually raised 1–3 mm above the skin surface; clusters of such growths resemble florets of cauliflower.

The infection generally remains localized

without involving bone or muscle or even causing particular discomfort to the patient. Lesions may become secondarily infected with bacteria resulting in a purulent exudate. Rare spreading may occur via the bloodstream to involve other areas of the body, including various organs such as lungs and brain; occasional blockage of lymph channels may result in elephantiasis.

DIAGNOSIS AND TREATMENT OF CHROMOMYCOSIS. Skin scrapings mounted in KOH show brown branching hyphae and brown chlamydospores which can be easily cultured on Sabouraud's glucose agar; however, the specific identification of the etiologic agent usually requires considerable taxonomic knowledge.

Potassium iodide given orally over a period of years has been a standard treatment for chromomycosis. More recently, topical and intravenous amphotericin B has been successfully employed; newer drugs include thiabendazole and 5-fluorocytosine. Surgical excision of the lesion, particularly during the early stages of the disease, has also proven effective.

## THE SYSTEMIC MYCOSES

The fungi causing systemic diseases (also called the deep mycoses) are all dimorphic—they exist as filamentous organisms in nature and as yeast cells in infected tissue. Moreover, their distribution is extremely limited, occurring mostly within limited geographic areas. The diseases begin as lower respiratory infections resulting from the inhalation of fungal spores. It appears that the majority of such cases are asymptomatic or undiagnosed, and only a small percentage progress to serious systemic manifestations.

### Blastomycosis

Blastomycosis (also called North American blastomycosis or Gilchrist's disease) is caused by a single organism, *Blastomyces*

*dermatitidis*. The disease appears to be endemic in the eastern part of the United States, but cases have been reported in Mexico and Africa. A sexual stage for the organism, described in 1967, technically classifies the fungus in the Ascomycetes as *Ajellomyces dermatitidis*.

EPIDEMIOLOGY AND PATHOGENESIS OF BLASTOMYCOSIS. Although all evidence indicates that the human disease is initiated by inhalation of the fungal spores, attempts to isolate the etiologic agent from its natural habitat have failed. Rare, successful isolations from soil are usually followed by failure when subsequent samples are cultured from identical sites, and this has led to the postulate that the organism may be dormant except under specific environmental conditions.

Blastomycosis has been divided into pulmonary, cutaneous, and systemic conditions, but it is now generally believed that all three types originate in the lung from a primary pulmonary blastomycosis. The pulmonary lesions are not unlike those of tuberculosis, carcinoma, or histoplasmosis, and misdiagnoses based on X-ray findings are not unusual. Unresolved pulmonary infections progress to acute lobar pneumonia accompanied by spread of the organisms via the bloodstream to other internal organs, bone, and skin.

Skin lesions, which eventually evolve into ulcerated granulomas, are the most common symptom of the disease. Such lesions may progress over a period of years, eventually involving large areas of the body. Bone invasion, causing arthritis and bone destruction, occurs in 25–50% of reported cases. Multiple internal organs may become infected, with those of the genitourinary system being most common and those of the central nervous system rare.

DIAGNOSIS AND TREATMENT OF BLASTOMYCOSIS. There is no specific serological test for blastomycosis. Blastomycin, a filtrate extracted from *B. dermatitidis* grown on a liquid medium, cross-reacts so strongly with histoplasmin and coccidioidin that skin tests are of little value. A specific flourescently-labeled antibody has been prepared that will react with the yeast cells in histological tissue sections. Definitive laboratory diagnosis, however, is best accomplished by the growth and identification of the etiologic agent.

When cultured on Sabouraud's glucose agar at 25°C, the organism grows as a white fungus that darkens with age and bears spherical conidia from the sides of the hyphae. The conidia are the infectious elements of this organism. Specific identification requires growth at 37°C, which converts the hyphal form of the organism to the yeast phase. The yeast cells are large, thick-walled, spherical cells which can be readily identified by the single buds which arise from the parent cell on a very broad base (see Figure 29-12).

Intravenous amphotericin B is the treatment of choice for all forms of blastomycosis, and relapses occur only following inadequate therapy. However, the doses of amphotericin B used are usually quite toxic, and additional drugs to control nausea, pain, and headache may be required.

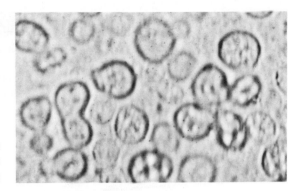

**Figure 29-12.** Yeast cells, many with buds, of *Blastomyces dermatitidis* in a culture of sputum.

### Histoplasmosis

*Histoplasma capsulatum,* the etiologic agent of histoplasmosis, is distributed worldwide, although certain areas such as the central and mid-eastern United States appear to be the most heavily contaminated with this fungus. It is certainly one of the more common mycoses in humans; it has been estimated that 40 million persons in the United States have been infected and that 200,000 new cases occur annually. The dimorphic organism has recently been shown to have a sexual stage and as a result has also been classified with the Ascomycetes and given the additional name of *Emmonsiella capsulata.*

EPIDEMIOLOGY AND PATHOGENESIS OF HISTO-PLASMOSIS. *Histoplasma capsulatum* is widely distributed in soil and preferentially grows in association with bird and bat feces. Thus, highly infectious areas may be found in chicken coops, bat caves, bird roosts, or any environment extensively inhabited by birds. It has even been proposed that there may be a correlation between the highly endemic places of the United States and the enormous numbers of starlings that inhabit these areas. When growing in soil, *H. capsulatum* is found only as branched hyphal filaments which form small single conidia and larger spiny spores referred to as tuberculated chlamydospores (Figure 29-13a). Infection follows inhalation of the small microconidia into the lung where they germinate and are transformed into budding yeast cells.

The yeast cells are distributed from the lungs throughout the internal organs via the bloodstream, and in the vast majority of cases the organisms are destroyed or sequestered by the host's immune responses. The lung lesions heal, followed by a fibrosis and calcification similar to healed calcified tuberculous lesions. If the initial exposure is large, the symptoms may be acute with high fever and severe pneumonia. However, even in severe epidemics of histoplasmosis, the mortality rate is only about 1% while most of the remaining cases are resolved.

A small percentage of infected individuals develop a chronic form of histoplasmosis

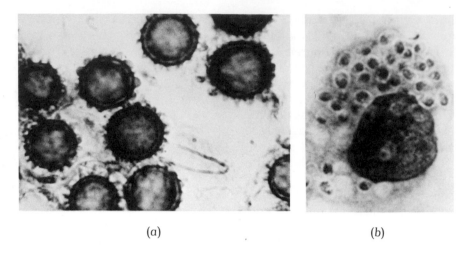

(a)                     (b)

**Figure 29-13.** *a.* Tuberculated chlamydospores (more properly macroaleuriospores) of *Histoplasma capsulatum. b.* Yeast cells of *H. capsulatum* in a macrophage are shown in this example from a Giemsa-stained tissue smear (human case).

which is pathologically similar to the cavitation of chronic tuberculosis. These patients usually have a productive cough accompanied by fever and weakness, and the organisms frequently become disseminated throughout the host causing a progressive, fatal disease not unlike miliary tuberculosis.

Recently, reactivation histoplasmosis has been commonly recognized in endemic areas where the highest disease rates are seen in infancy and during the fifth and sixth decades of life. Such endogenous reactivation is identical to that seen for tuberculosis, and, not infrequently, it may coexist with tuberculosis. Thus, it appears that the calcified, healed lesions of histoplasmosis contain dormant, but viable, yeast cells.

DIAGNOSIS AND TREATMENT OF HISTOPLASMOSIS. Histoplasmosis is an intracellular disease in which the yeast cells generally exist and grow within the reticuloendothelial system and macrophages. Histological examination of the buffy coat (containing the white blood cells) of centrifuged blood samples, or biopsy material from lesions, particularly during the acute disease, may reveal many yeast cells within the macro-

phages (see Figure 29-13b). Such material, as well as sputum, can be readily cultured on Sabouraud's and blood agar. Colonies of *H. capsulatum* showing hyphal growth at 25°C produce characteristic tuberculated chlamydospores which should be seen within 4 to 6 weeks. Growth of these organisms on blood agar at 37°C will produce ovoid budding yeast cells.

Concentration of the filtrates of broth cultures of *H. capsulatum* yields a material called histoplasmin, analogous to tuberculin. Injection of dilutions of histoplasmin (usually 1:100 or 1:1000) intradermally will cause a delayed-type skin reaction in individuals who have developed a cellular type immunity to the organisms. However, a positive skin test is of little actual diagnostic value since it may represent only a past contact with the organism. Skin testing with histoplasmin has limited diagnostic value and may interfere with the complement-fixation tests for histoplasmosis and coccidioidomycosis. Histoplasmin should not, therefore, be used for the general screening of individuals.

Other serological tests used for the diagnosis of histoplasmosis include complement fixation, immunodiffusion using histoplasmin as the antigen, and latex particle agglutination in which the latex particles are coated with histoplasmin and mixed with dilutions of serum. Specific fluorescently labeled antibody has also been used as a diagnostic aid in the absence of cultures.

By far, the vast majority of cases of histoplasmosis are undiagnosed, and recovery is spontaneous. Even moderately severe cases of primary histoplasmosis can be adequately treated with bed rest. However, disseminated or systemic disease requires antimicrobial therapy. Amphotericin B is effective and recovery is rapid.

### Coccidioidomycosis

*Coccidioides immitis,* the etiologic agent of coccidioidomycosis, is found in soil only in arid regions, and one of the most highly endemic areas includes the southwestern United States and northern Mexico. Endemic areas exist also in Central and South America.

EPIDEMIOLOGY AND PATHOGENESIS OF COCCIDIOIDOMYCOSIS. *Coccidioides immitis* grows in soil as a septated filamentous fungus that characteristically produces thick-walled arthrospores in alternating cells of a hyphal filament. The mature hyphae easily fragment, and the liberated arthrospores are readily carried on surrounding dust particles.

Human infection follows inhalation of the arthrospores and, like histoplasmosis, it may result in an asymptomatic or mild to severe respiratory infection. Infection may also produce either a chronic progressive disease or an acute disseminated infection. Epidemiological studies have led to the conclusion that approximately 60% of all primary infections are asymptomatic, about 40% produce a mild to severe pulmonary disease, and 0.2–0.5% result in chronic or acute disseminated infections.

Following inhalation, the arthrospore differentiates into a large, round, thick-walled structure, 30–60 $\mu$m in diameter,

which becomes multinucleate and, eventually, forms several hundred uninucleated endospores that are 2 to 5 $\mu$m in diameter (see Figure 29-14). This rounded structure, called a spherule, breaks open when mature, liberating the enclosed endospores. The morphologic events of spherule and endospore formation are now recognized to be analogous to sporangium and sporangiospore production. As a result, *Coccidioides* is currently classified with the Zygomycetes. In the majority of cases the liberated spores are phagocytosed and killed, and in the absence of a positive coccidioidin skin test (analogous to histoplasmin) there would be no evidence that an infection had occurred.

Symptomatic pulmonary infections are characterized by fever, chest pain, a mild cough, headache, and loss of appetite. X-rays show small nodules in the lung not unlike those seen in primary tuberculosis. Such lesions may form cavities which usually become fibrotic and later calcify. Curiously, in about 5–10% of such cases allergic reactions (as manifested by sterile, erythematous

**Figure 29-14.** Endospore-filled spherule from a case of coccidioidomycosis.

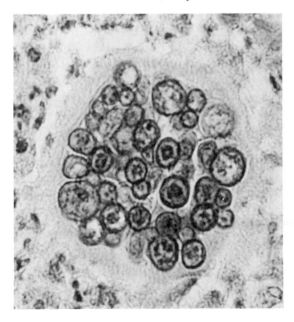

lesions and nodules) may appear, usually on the legs, within a few days after the beginning of the initial symptoms. These lesions ordinarily disappear in about a week, but in endemic areas of coccidioidomycosis, their occurrence is strongly suggestive of this disease.

Coccidioidomycosis may also take the form of a benign chronic disease in which the organisms remain localized in the lung, causing enlarged cavities which are usually filled with spherules of *C. immitis*. Such cavities may fibrose (grow white fibrous connective tissue) and calcify, or may require surgical removal. This condition may remain chronic for years.

The disseminated form of the disease may occur soon after the primary infection, particularly in dark-skinned individuals, or it may occur after years of chronic pulmonary disease. Disseminated coccidioidomycosis may produce an acute or chronic meningitis, or a generalized disease which is characterized by lesions in many internal organs may result. Cutaneous lesions appear as granulomas which may eventually heal or, in advanced disease, form draining ulcers.

DIAGNOSIS AND TREATMENT OF COCCIDIOIDOMYCOSIS. Direct examination of sputum, pus, or gastric washings will frequently reveal the presence of mature spherules. Culture of the organisms is dangerous and should be done only by experienced personnel using special precautions, since the arthrospores produced are extremely infectious. The organism is, however, readily grown on Sabouraud's medium, and the presence of typical arthrospores (in a formalized preparation) is indicative of *C. immitis*. Spherule formation has been accomplished *in vitro* under special conditions, but it is most easily demonstrated by injection of the organisms into mice.

Coccidioidin is the most useful of the skin test materials. It can be used as a diagnostic aid and as a screening test. Immunodiffusion tests and latex particle agglutination assays have proved useful as a serologic aid in the diagnosis of the disease.

A primary infection, even though asymptomatic, induces a solid immunity to reinfection. As in other mycotic infections, amphotericin B is the therapy of choice for chronic pulmonary or disseminated disease; however, surgical removal of lung cavities may be required in cases of advanced pulmonary disease.

## Paracoccidioidomycosis

Paracoccidioidomycosis (synonym: South American blastomycosis) is caused by *Paracoccidioides brasiliensis*. (An older name is *Blastomyces brasiliensis*.) The disease is found only in Central and South America.

EPIDEMIOLOGY AND PATHOGENESIS OF PARACOCCIDIOIDOMYCOSIS. Despite the restricted geographical location of paracoccidioidomycosis, the natural habitat of the etiologic agent is not evident, although it has on rare occasions been isolated from soil samples in endemic areas.

*Paracoccidioides brasiliensis* is a dimorphic organism that exists in soil as a filamentous fungus, producing a variety of spore types—single microconidia, chlamydospores, and arthrospores. Primary infection was long believed to result from the direct implantation of the organisms into the oral mucosa, but it is now apparent that, like the other systemic mycoses, paracoccidioidomycosis originates as a pulmonary infection.

Initial infection probably results from the inhalation of spores of *P. brasiliensis* that subsequently differentiate into the yeast form of the organism. Skin testing in endemic areas of the disease indicates that the majority of infections occur as asymptomatic or undiagnosed cases and that progressive pulmonary disease and secondary lesions from disseminated infections are rare. Primary infections usually resolve spontaneously and may or may not result in the occurrence of calcified pulmonary lesions. When chronic, progressive pulmonary disease does occur, considerable areas of the lung may become fibrosed.

More commonly, the pulmonary involvement is subclinical, and the invading yeast cells are disseminated (possibly by macrophages) to the oropharyngeal mucosa. The characteristic ulcerative lesions occurring in the mouth and nose are frequently the first symptom, so it is understandable that the initial pulmonary aspect of this infection was not appreciated until recently. Lymph nodes may become infected, ulcerate, and drain.

Disseminated organisms may also infect other organs such as the spleen, liver, and adrenals, resulting in a spread of the lesions and a corresponding involvement of the regional lymph nodes.

DIAGNOSIS AND TREATMENT OF PARACOCCIDIOIDOMYCOSIS. Direct examination of sputum, draining lymph nodes, or biopsy material reveals large, round yeast cells that may possess from 1–12 buds surrounding the parent yeast (see Figure 29-15). These cells can be readily differentiated from *Blastomyces dermatitidis* which forms a single bud on a broad base.

Culture at 25°C yields the mycelial form,

**Figure 29-15.** Yeast cells of *Paracoccidioides brasiliensis* with multiple buds.

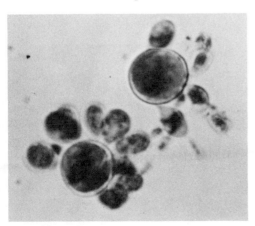

which is difficult to identify; however, incubation at 37°C on blood agar converts the organism to the typical yeast morphology.

A skin-testing antigen, termed paracoccidioidin, can be used to evaluate total infections in an endemic area, but a positive skin reaction does not necessarily indicate active disease. Complement fixation, immunodiffusion, and fluorescently labeled antibody have all been used with varying success.

Sulfonamide therapy will result in the remission of symptoms, but the effect is temporary and cessation of therapy results in relapse. Amphotericin B remains the only effective chemotherapeutic agent for paracoccidioidomycosis.

### Geotrichosis

*Geotrichum candidum,* the etiologic agent of geotrichosis, appears to be one of the more ubiquitous of the fungi that occasionally infect humans. It has been isolated from the stools, urine, and vaginal secretions of approximately one-third of all individuals checked, having caused no apparent disease. It has also been found in decaying plant material, dairy products, and on normal skin.

EPIDEMIOLOGY AND PATHOGENESIS OF GEOTRICHOSIS. As can be seen from the widespread occurrence of *Geotrichum candidum,* human contact with this fungus must occur frequently. The fact that it only rarely causes disease indicates that it possesses little virulence for animals or humans. Diagnosed infections are most frequently pulmonary and may be secondary infections to tuberculosis. Oral infections, clinically identical to thrush caused by *Candida albicans,* also may occur.

LABORATORY DIAGNOSIS AND TREATMENT OF GEOTRICHOSIS. The diagnosis of *Geotrichum candidum* as the etiologic agent of disease is difficult because of its ubiquity. One should find the organism frequently

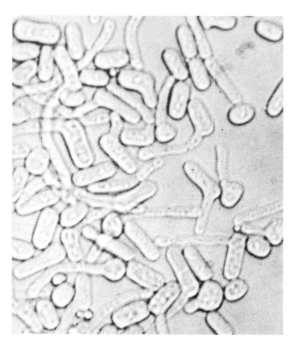

**Figure 29-16.** Arthrospores of *Geotrichum candidum.*

and in large numbers in sputum or in oral lesions to support the diagnosis. Growth and the demonstration of characteristic rectangular arthrospores (Figure 29-16) are required for a culture confirmation of geotrichosis. Treatment may include iodides, aerosol nystatin, or amphotericin B.

## OPPORTUNISTIC FUNGI

Many of the mycotic agents that have been discussed in this chapter could be considered as opportunistic fungi, since they may commonly occur in endemic areas and yet rarely produce progressive disease. However, the fungi considered briefly here are of world-wide distribution and under normal circumstances do not usually cause even asymptomatic infections in humans. However, they may cause serious disease in debilitated persons, in diabetics, in patients with leukemia or lymphoma, in immunosuppressed individuals, or in persons who are heavily exposed to large numbers of spores.

### Aspergillosis

Individuals who are heavily exposed to spores from the genus *Aspergillus* may develop IgE and IgG antibodies, as well as a delayed-type hypersensitivity, and much of the resulting pulmonary disease may produce an asthmatic allergy to the fungus. In progressive disease, the growth of the hyphae may seriously interfere with normal gas exchange.

*Aspergillus* "balls" may also develop in tuberculous cavities and partially fill them with tangled masses of mycelia. Hyphae may

**Figure 29-17.** Conidiophores of *Aspergillus fumigatus.*

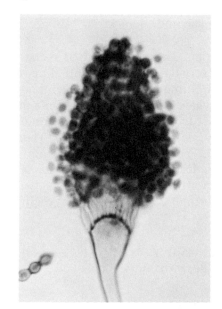

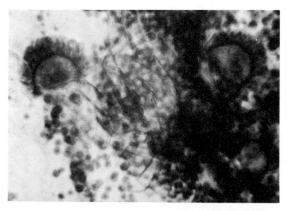

invade the adjacent blood vessels causing the production of bloody sputum. Rarely, species of *Aspergillus* may infect the nasal sinuses, or become widely disseminated, infecting multiple organs; however, such manifestations may follow corticosteroid therapy.

The diagnosis is difficult because of the very universality of species of *Aspergillus*. Direct examination of sputum should show branching hyphal filaments in a characteristic "Y" shape, and may show the conidiophores still attached to the spore head (see Figure 29-17). *Aspergillus fumigatus*, the most common pathogen, is somewhat thermophilic and will readily grow at 45°C.

Certain types of infections caused by members of the genus *Aspergillus* may remain chronic for years, but invasive aspergillosis is normally fatal if untreated. Prednisone has proved of value for the treatment of allergic aspergillosis, but pulmonary cavities filled with mycelia must frequently be surgically removed. Nystatin and natamycin appear to be the most effective chemotherapeutic agents.

### Mucormycosis

Mucormycosis (also called phycomycosis) is caused by members of the class Zygomycetes and occurs in the diseased and debilitated individual. Human disease is most frequently caused by species of *Rhizopus*, but the genera *Mucor* and *Absidia* are also involved.

As a result of the usual poor physical condition of the patient, infection with these agents is frequently a fulminating and fatal disease. The spectrum of disease types will depend upon the condition of the patient but frequently involves the rhinocerebral area, lungs, central nervous system, and viscera.

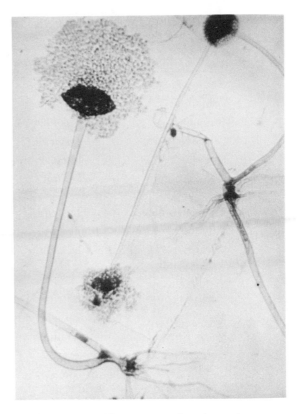

**Figure 29-18.** Two ruptured and one intact sporangia and nonseptate hyphae are shown in this micrograph of *Rhizopus arrhizus*.

The organism is easily visualized in infected tissues as it extends through contiguous cells and blood vessels. Identification of the fungi can be done by staining with hematoxylin-eosin and observing the large nonseptate hyphae (see Figure 29-18).

Mortality is usually high because of the debilitated condition of the patient. However, amphotericin B has been used with some success.

## Mycotoxicosis

Mycotoxicosis is any disease that is induced by the consumption of food that has been made toxic by fungal toxins. These toxins, called mycotoxins, are found in a wide variety of foodstuffs consumed by humans and animals, and in all likelihood the diseases resulting from the ingestion of mycotoxin-contaminated food are consid-

Table 29-3. Partial List of Mycotoxins and
Mycotoxin-Producing Fungi

| Mycotoxin | Mycotoxin-Producing Fungi |
|---|---|
| Aflatoxin | A. flavus, A. parsiticus, etc. |
| Ascladiol | A. clavatus |
| Butenolide | F. tricinctum, F. nivale, F. equiseti |
| Citreoviridin | P. citreo-viride, P. ochrosalmoneum |
| Citrinin | P. citrinum, P. implicatum, P. citreo-viride, A. terreus, etc. |
| Cyclopiazonic acid | P. cyclopium |
| Ergot alkaloid | Claviceps spp. |
| Fumigatin | A. fumigatus |
| Chlorine-containing peptide | P. islandicum |
| Luteoskyrin | P. islandicum, Mycelia sterilia |
| Maltoryzine | A. oryzae var. microsporus |
| Muscarine, etc. | Amanita muscaria, etc. |
| Ochratoxin A | A. ochraceus |
| Patulin | P. urticae, A. clavatus, P. claviforme, P. expansum, A. giganteus, etc. |
| Penicillic acid | P. puberulum, P. cyclopium, P. thomii, etc. |
| Phalloidine | Amanita phalloides |
| Psilocybine | Psilocybe spp. |
| Psoralens | Sclerotinia sclerotiorum |
| Rubratoxin B | P. rubrum, P. purpurogenum |
| Regulosin | P. rugulosum, P. brunneum, P. tardum, P. variabile, etc. |
| Scirpenols (nivalenol, fusarenon) | F. nivale, F. tricinctum |
| Sporidesmolides | Pithomyces chartarum |
| Sterigmatocystin | A. versicolor, A. flavus (O-methyl-) |
| Xanthocillin X | A. chevalieri |

A. = Aspergillis; F. = Fusarium; P. = Penicillium

erably more serious than are the fungal infections discussed earlier in this chapter. Table 29-3 shows a partial list of known mycotoxins; any detailed discussion of the chemical structure and the biological action of mycotoxins is far beyond the scope of this text. Nevertheless, a few highlights deserve mention.

## AFLATOXIN

The discovery of aflatoxin in 1960 occurred as a result of a fatal disease in turkeys, which was tentatively named "turkey X" disease. Autopsies revealed severe liver necrosis resembling alkaloid poisoning. Examination of turkey feed failed to show alkaloids but did show the toxic material to be present in a Brazilian groundnut meal in the feed. Subsequent studies reported that ingestion of the meal for a few days caused liver necrosis in ducklings and liver cancer in rats and trout. In 1961, it was found that the toxic material in the groundnut meal was produced by the saprophytic mold *Aspergillus flavus,* and for that reason the toxin was named aflatoxin. Research in the following decade led to the isolation and chemical characterization of a family of 16 different aflatoxins.

### Biologic Effect of Aflatoxins

The ability of aflatoxins to cause liver damage has been demonstrated in many mammals, fish, and birds, and initiation of liver carcinoma by aflatoxin is known to occur in ducklings, trout, rats, and ferrets. The role of aflatoxins in human disease is mostly circumstantial, but the fact that many foods consumed by humans are contaminated with *Aspergillus flavus* is cause for grave concern. Peanuts and peanut butter are one of the main sources of aflatoxins for humans, but these toxins have also been found in rice, cereal grains, beans, dried sweet potatoes, African beers, and cow's milk. The fact that half of all cancers occurring in Africa south of the Sahara are liver tumors may be correlated with a report that 40% of the foods screened in Uganda contained measurable quantities of aflatoxin. The considerably higher incidence of childhood liver cirrhosis in tropical countries (where the warm, moist climate provides ideal conditions for the growth of *Aspergillus flavus* over that seen in northern, drier areas) can also be correlated with the presence of aflatoxins in foods such as breast milk. Moreover, out of 50 urine samples taken from children with liver cirrhosis, 18 were shown by thin-layer chromatography to contain aflatoxins.

The data linking aflatoxins with human liver disease is still circumstantial, but the fact that these toxins produce liver damage in essentially all experimental animals certainly makes them highly suspect. The most frustrating aspect of this problem is that it has no current solution. The ingestion of moldy foods in areas where poverty, starvation, and malnutrition are routine will undoubtedly continue. The long-term answer lies in increased economic and educational efforts in behalf of the underprivileged peoples in the world.

### OCHRATOXINS

Two mycotoxins, ochratoxin A and B, are produced by *Aspergillus ochraceus.* These toxins occur in corn, grains, peanuts, Brazil nuts, fermented fish, and cottonseed meal as well as in many other human and animal foods.

In ducklings, the $LD_{50}$ (the amount that comprises a lethal dose for 50% of the test animals) for ochratoxin A is 25 $\mu$g while that for ochratoxin B is about 150 $\mu$g. Both mycotoxins produce liver necrosis, but neither appears to be carcinogenic. There is no proven evidence that the ochratoxins contribute to human disease, but their hepatotoxic (toxic to the liver) properties in other animals and their widespread occurrence in moldy food products make it likely that they are involved in human disease.

### MISCELLANEOUS MYCOTOXINS

There are a number of mycotoxin-producing species of *Penicillium* that often are found on moldy rice. Two mycotoxins, luteoskyrin and cyclochlorotine, have been isolated as a metabolite of *Penicillium islandicum.* In experimental animals both toxins produce severe liver damage varying from cirrhosis to liver carcinoma.

Some mycotoxins produce effects beyond liver damage. The injection of crude extracts from moldy rice on which *Penicillium toxicarium* is growing causes paralysis, blindness, and death in experimental animals. Animals fed corn infected with *Penicillium rubrum* showed intense inflammation of the stomach, large and small intestines, and the liver. Another mycotoxin (produced by the mold *Fusarium graminearum*) is an estrogen. Female animals ingesting food contaminated with this mold experience a severe inflammation of the vulva and vagina, an increase in the size of the uterus, and growth and lactation of the mammary glands. The effect in young males is a feminizing one with atrophy of the testes and an enlargement of the mammary glands.

There are many other mycotoxins but the last one we shall discuss causes a disease known as alimentary toxic aleukia (ATA). This disease has occurred in Russia and Siberia in endemic forms. The symptoms of ATA include fever, bleeding from the nose, throat, and gums, a hemorrhagic rash, and a marked reduction in the number of circulating leukocytes. Mortality may run as high as 60%, and frequently whole families and villages have been affected. The etiology of ATA is a mycotoxicosis caused by eating grains that have overwintered under snow. The disease was particularly severe during the 1940's when famine forced many persons to collect and eat such overwintered grain. There are several genera of fungi implicated in the production of this particular mycotoxin, of which *Fusarium* and *Cladosporium* are noted most frequently. Like all other mycotoxicoses, prevention is accomplished only through education.

## REFERENCES

Ainsworth, G. C., and G. R. Bisby. 1961. *Dictionary of Fungi*, 5th ed. Commonwealth Mycological Institute, Kew, Surrey, England.

Applegate, K. L., and J. R. Chipley. 1976. Production of ochratoxin A by *Aspergillis ochraceus* NRRL-3174 before and after exposures to $^{60}$Co irradiation. *J. Appl. Microbiol.* **31**:349–353.

Baker, R. D. 1971. *Human Infection with Fungi, Actinomycetes and Algae*. Springer-Verlag, New York.

Ciegler, A., S. Kadis, and S. J. Ajl, eds. 1971. *Microbial Toxins*, Vol. VI. Academic Press, New York.

Conant, N. F., D. T. Smith, R. D. Baker, and J. L. Callaway. 1971. *Manual of Clinical Mycology*, 3rd ed. W. B. Saunders Co., Philadelphia.

Emmons, C. W., C. H. Binford, J. P. Utz, and K. J. Kwon-Chung. 1970. Medical Mycology, 3rd ed. Lea and Febiger, Philadelphia.

Grappel, S. F., C. T. Bishop, and F. Blank. 1974. Immunology of dermatophytes and dermatophytosis. *Bacteriol. Rev.* **38**:222–250.

Hazen, E. S., M. A. Gordon, and F. C. Reed. 1970. *Laboratory Identification of Pathogenic Fungi Simplified*, 3rd ed. Charles C. Thomas, Springfield, Ill.

Howarth, B., Jr., and R. D. Wyatt. 1976. Effect of dietary aflatoxin on fertility, hatchability and progeny performance of broiler breeder hens. *J. Appl. Microbiol.* **31**:680–684.

Kadis, S., A. Ciegler, and S. J. Ajl, eds. 1971. *Microbial Toxins*, Vol. VII. Academic Press, New York.

Kalakoutskii, L. V., and N. S. Agre. 1976. Comparative aspects of development and differentiation in actinomycetes. *Bacteriol. Rev.* **40**:469–524.

Krick, J. A., E. B. Stinson, and J. S. Remington. 1975. Nocardia infections in heart transplants. *Ann. Internal Med.* **82**:18–26.

Landcaster, M. C., F. P. Jenkins, and J. McL. Phelp. 1961. Toxicity associated with certain samples of groundnuts. *Nature* **192**:1095–1096.

Lillehoj, E. B., and A. Ciegler. 1975. Mycotoxin synergism. In David Schlessinger, ed., *Microbiology 1975*. Amer. Soc. Microbiol., Washington, D. C.

Rippon, J. W. 1974. *Medical Mycology: The Pathogenic Fungi and the Pathogenic Actinomycetes*. W. B. Saunders Co., Philadelphia.

Sinski, J. T. 1974. *Dermatophytes in Human Skin, Hair and Nails*. Charles C. Thomas, Springfield, Ill.

Smith, R. B., Jr., J. M. Griffin, and P. B. Hamilton. 1976. Survey of aflatoxicosis in farm animals. *J. Appl. Microbiol.* **31**:385–388.

Waksman, S. 1967. *The Actinomycetes*. Ronald Press, New York.

Webster, J. 1970. *Introduction to Fungi*. Cambridge University Press, New York.

# 30

# Diagnostic Bacteriology

The most important aspects of diagnostic bacteriology are (1) the collection of an adequate amount of the correct specimen and (2) communication between the physician and the microbiologist, outlining the clinical diagnosis and suggesting a limited range of organisms that could be the causative agent of the disease in question. Provided with a specimen and the clinical evaluation of the disease, it is the job of the microbiologist to isolate the etiologic agent of the disease, supply a profile of antibiotic sensitivities for the physician, and, insofar as possible, quickly identify the organism. However, even after the isolation and identification of organisms present in a laboratory specimen, one cannot always be positive that such organisms are the etiologic agents of the disease in question, inasmuch as they may be merely contaminants from the normal flora. As shown in Table 30-1, there are many organisms that may be present without causing disease or symptoms of any kind but can, under special conditions, produce serious infections.

We do not always know why an organism sometimes causes disease and sometimes not, but we do know that organisms of the genera *Fusobacterium* and *Bacteroides* rarely cause disease when confined to their normal habitat in the large intestine but cause severe abscesses when introduced into wounds. *Staphylococcus aureus* causes its most severe infections as a secondary invader following a viral infection or when other normal flora have been destroyed by antibiotic therapy. This chapter can do little about this question beyond emphasizing its existence. Rather, this section is designed to furnish a brief outline of the steps in the isolation and identification of the organisms causing bacterial infections.

## Collection and Culturing of Specimens

Needless to say, the collection of an adequate specimen is useless if the time between collection and culturing allows the disease-producing organism to die or to be overgrown by normal flora that may contaminate the specimen. It is of utmost importance that

413

**Table 30-1. Bacteria Frequently Present as Normal Flora, Occasionally Causing Overt Disease**

| Organisms | Usual Locale | Infectious Disease Process |
|---|---|---|
| *Staphylococcus aureus* | Nose, skin | In all areas of the body, nosocomial diseases, food poisoning |
| *Staphylococcus epidermidis* | Skin, nose, vagina | Endocarditis, nosocomial phlebitis; acne |
| Enterococci | Feces | Blood, wounds, urinary tract, endocarditis |
| Viridans streptococci | Saliva | Endocarditis |
| *Peptostreptococcus* sp. | Mouth, feces, vagina | Abscess formation, gangrene |
| *Neisseria* sp. | Throat, mouth, nose | Rarely meningitis |
| *Veillonella* sp. | Mouth (saliva) | Bacterial endocarditis |
| *Lactobacillus* sp. | Mouth, feces, vagina | Bacterial endocarditis (very rare), lung abscess (1 report) |
| *Nocardia* sp. | Mouth, nasopharynx, foods | Nocardiosis |
| *Corynebacterium* sp. | Nasopharynx, skin, vagina | Bacterial endocarditis |
| *Mycobacterium* | Prepuce, clitoris, lung, feces, tonsils, food, skin | Suspected in some infectious disease processes |
| *Clostridium* sp. | Feces, skin, environment including food, vagina | Clostridial myositis, cellulitis, food poisoning |
| Enterobacteriaceae | Feces, vagina, mouth, urethra | Urinary tract, wounds, pneumonia, nosocomial enteritis, abscesses, meningitis, blood, peritonitis, abcesses, etc. |
| *Moraxella* sp. | Nose, genitourinary tract | Conjunctivitis |
| *Achromobacter* sp. | Nose, genitourinary tract, skin | Meningitis, blood, urethritis, burns |
| *Pseudomonas* sp. | Feces, skin | Blood, burns, wounds, urinary tract, respiratory tract, meningitis |
| *Alcaligenes fecalis* | Feces | Blood, urinary tract, conjunctiva, respiratory tract, meningitis |
| *Haemophilus* sp. | Nasopharynx, conjunctiva, vagina | Laryngotracheobronchitis, meningitis, pyarthrosis, conjunctivitis, genitourinary tract |
| *Fusobacterium* sp. | Mouth, saliva, feces | Infected human bites, gangrene |
| *Bacteroides* sp. | Feces, mouth, throat | Bacterial endocarditis, abscesses, mixed infections |

specimens be transported quickly to the diagnostic laboratory where they can be promptly processed to ensure the best possible chance of growth, isolation, and identification. In some situations, it is recommended that the growth medium be inoculated immediately after obtaining the specimen from the patient and that the inoculated medium then be taken to the laboratory to be grown and the bacteria identified. In other cases, material should be first dispersed in a nutrient broth or buffered transport medium and then transported to the laboratory to be grown. In all cases, quick processing of specimens aids in providing the fastest and most reliable identification of the disease-producing organism.

## BLOOD

Bacteremia, bacteria in the blood, is frequently accompanied by the onset of chills and fever, an increase in pulse rate, and a drop in blood pressure. Even in infections in which bacteremia is a major aspect of the disease, the organisms in the bloodstream are not always constantly present in sufficient numbers to be grown from a single blood specimen. Such patients may be required to give several blood specimens before the causative agent can be isolated. When an intermittent bacteremia is suspected, it is routine to obtain three 10 ml blood samples over a 24-hour period to maximize chances for isolation of the organism.

### Collection of a Blood Specimen

In taking a blood specimen for culture, one should be aware that, although blood is normally sterile, the skin that must be penetrated is not sterile. Routinely, the skin should be first cleansed with 70–95% alcohol to remove dirt, lipids, and fatty acids. The site should then be scrubbed with a circular, concentric motion (working out from the starting point) using a sterile gauze pad soaked in 2% iodine. The iodine should be allowed to remain on the skin for at least one minute before it is removed by wiping with a sterile gauze pad soaked with 70–95% alcohol. It must be emphasized, however, that all this will be useless if the person drawing the blood palpates the vein after the cleaning process, thereby contaminating the very site that had been cleaned.

After cleansing the penetration site, the blood may be withdrawn using either a sterile needle and syringe or a commercially available, evacuated blood-collection tube. These tubes routinely contain a small amount of a nonsterile anticoagulant, and, even though the tubes contain only 0.1 atmosphere of gas pressure as $CO_2$, backflow has been shown to cause nosocomial infections. When using evacuated blood-collection tubes, therefore, it is recommended that containers be held below the level of the venipuncture and that care be taken not to move the patient's arm during sampling, since this may cause a lowering of venous pressure and allow backflow.

### Media Inoculated with Blood Specimens

Blood should always be inoculated into the appropriate medium at the bedside. Partially-evacuated, commercially available, blood-culture bottles, which contain 50 to 100 ml of a rich, liquid medium such as brain-heart infusion or Trypticase soy broth, are routinely employed. It is important that such a blood medium contain an anticoagulant to prevent any bacteria from becoming entrapped in small clots, thus going undetected or requiring a longer time for their detection. Many anticoagulants show toxicity for all or selective bacteria—ammonium oxalate for most bacteria and sodium citrate for staphylococci. Most blood media now incorporate 0.025% sodium polyanethol sulfonate (SPS) into the medium to which the blood will be added. SPS is a heat-stable, nontoxic anticoagulant, and a number of studies have shown that media containing SPS provide a better recovery of organisms than does plain thioglycollate or thiocitrate media. This is

**Table 30-2. Growth Characteristics of Frequently Isolated Bacteria from Blood on Some Commonly Used Agar Media**

| | Selective Entero-coccus Agar | Staphylococcus 110 Agar | Mannitol, Salt | Mitis-Salivarius Agar | Chocolate Agar | Thayer Martin |
|---|---|---|---|---|---|---|
| Enterococci | Translucent to whitish colonies surrounded by dark-brown to black zones | Mostly inhibited | Mostly inhibited | Blue-black, shiny center, clear periphery | White to gray | |
| Listeria | Pin-point colonies with reddish to black-brown zones | Inhibited | Inhibited | Inhibited | Gray | |
| Neisseria sp. | | | | | Opaque, grayish white | Mostly inhibited |
| N. gonorrhoeae | | | | | Opaque, grayish white | Gray |
| N. meningitidis | | | | | Opaque, grayish white | Gray |
| Staphylococcus | Small, white-gray colonies | White; orange to yellow | Colonies with yellow zones (mannitol fermenters); colonies with red or purple zones (mannitol not fermented) | Mostly inhibited | White to gray | White to gray, mostly inhibited |
| Streptococci Beta-hemolytic Alpha-hemolytic Nonhemolytic S. salivarius | Tiny colonies Tiny colonies | Mostly inhibited | Mostly inhibited | Small blue colonies Blue gum drop colonies | | White to gray |
| S. mitis | | | | Small blue colonies | | |

possibly due to the fact that SPS is anticomplementary, kills leukocytes, and inactivates certain aminoglycoside and polypeptide antibiotics.

If possible, 10 to 20 ml of blood should be taken from the patient and inoculated into an approximately ten-fold excess of the blood-culture medium. The commercially available bottles are provided with a venipuncture set which allows the blood to be injected directly into the medium. When possible, two such bottles should be inoculated. One is vented to permit the growth of aerobic bacteria (by inserting a sterile, cotton-plugged needle through the rubber stopper until the bottle has filled with air), while the other is not vented to allow the growth of anaerobic organisms.

### Identification of Blood Isolates

Cultures are incubated at 35°C and observed daily for at least a week for evidence of turbidity or hemolysis. Gram stains, streak plates, and antibiotic sensitivities (see Chapter 10) should be carried out as quickly as possible after the observation of visible growth in the original broth culture. In the absence of obvious growth in one or two days, blind subcultures on chocolate blood-agar plates may speed the appearance of obligately aerobic organisms. Commercially available penicillinase may be added to blood cultures obtained from patients who have been on penicillin therapy. Penicillinase preparations should be periodically checked for sterility to eliminate them as a potential source of contamination.

Once a Gram stain has provided some information concerning the type of organism involved, special supplementary or differential media should be inoculated. MacConkey or eosin methylene-blue plates should be streaked if gram-negative rods are present, and prereduced media containing 0.05% cysteine should be inoculated if obligate anaerobes such as Bacteroides or Fusobacterium are suspected. Table 30-2 lists a few of the more common organisms that could be isolated from blood, with their colonial appearance on certain specialized media.

The finding of organisms that constitute the normal flora or are frequent inhabitants of the skin (diphtheroids, Staph. epidermidis, Bacillus sp.) is usually viewed with suspicion unless the frequency of isolation indicates they did not arrive as contamination during the collection of the blood.

## RESPIRATORY TRACT AND MOUTH

Because of the myriad normal resident flora in the upper respiratory tract, the isolation of lower respiratory tract infectious agents can be difficult and confusing. This is further complicated by the presence of potential pathogens such as pneumococci, meningococci, streptococci, Staphylococcus aureus, Haemophilus influenzae, or enterics that are indigenous to the upper respiratory tract.

### Specimen Collection from the Respiratory Tract

One must be certain that lower respiratory specimens represent sputum that has been brought up by a deep cough. It may not be possible, however, to obtain a good sputum sample from a very young child, a debilitated older individual, or someone who is comatose. In such situations other procedures must be carried out to obtain a specimen from the lower respiratory tract. One commonly employed technique is transtracheal aspiration, which, as shown diagramatically in Figure 30-1, employs a needle and tube about 30 cm long inserted through the trachea into the lung. This technique also overcomes the problem of oropharynx contamination. On some occasions sterile saline is injected through the tube into the lung before aspiration if it is impossible to obtain material directly from the lung with a syringe.

Organisms causing upper respiratory infections that appear as vesicles or ulcers in the throat should be obtained with a cotton

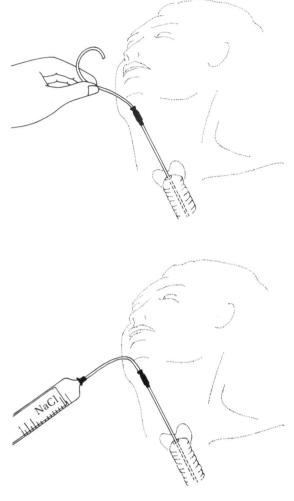

**Figure 30-1.** Transtracheal aspiration. A pillow should be placed beneath the neck to permit maximum extension of the neck. After cleansing the skin, a 14 gauge needle is inserted into the trachea and a polyethylene tube is passed through the needle into the lung. The needle is withdrawn and the tube is connected to a syringe containing three to four ml of physiological saline. The saline is injected into the lung and immediately withdrawn for culture.

ing the tongue and oropharynx. Nasopharyngeal cultures are especially important for detecting carrier states for meningococci, *Corynebacterium diphtheriae*, group A beta-hemolytic streptococci, and *Haemophilus influenzae*. The latter organism may also cause an acute epiglottitis, but initial treatment for that infection is based on clinical evaluation and Gram stains and must be initiated before laboratory isolation would be possible.

### Media Inoculated with Respiratory Tract Specimens

All throat swabs should be streaked immediately on a sheep's blood agar plate and the swab immersed in nutrient broth, both to be delivered to the laboratory. Special media are used for the isolation of specific pathogens, and the laboratory should be informed by the clinician what range of pathogens is possible. For instance, sheep's blood agar plates are sufficient for the isolation of a beta-hemolytic streptococcus, *Streptococcus pneumoniae*, *Neisseria meningitidis*, and *Staphylococcus aureus*. A suspected *Corynebacterium diphtheriae* would be additionally inoculated on a Loeffler's coagulated-serum slant and a potassium tellurite agar plate. To isolate and identify *Bordetella pertussis* from a suspected case of whooping cough, a Bordet-Gengou plate would be inoculated from a swab or by having the patient cough directly onto the exposed plate. A swab containing a possible *Haemophilus influenzae* would be streaked on a chocolate blood agar plate, and discs containing X and Y factors (hematin and NAD) would be laid on top of the inoculated plate. Thick sputum which is to be cultured for *Mycobacterium tuberculosis* is usually thinned by digestion in 4% NaOH at 37°C for one hour, followed by high-speed centrifugation (2000 times gravity for 30 minutes). Other digestion procedures using 5% oxalic acid have also been reported. These procedures result in concentration of the tubercle bacilli and destruction of most contaminating

swab and streaked on a blood-agar plate as soon as possible. Nasopharyngeal cultures are usually obtained with a cotton swab on a bent wire which can be passed either through the nose or via the mouth, carefully bypass-

organisms. It should be recognized that these digestion procedures also destroy the tubercle bacilli, and the time and temperature should not be extended beyond the recommended limits. Following centrifugation, sedimented material can be used to inoculate media, such as Lowenstein-Jensen medium, and to inoculate a guinea pig.

**Identification of Respiratory Tract Isolates**

The appearance of the colony on sheep's blood agar and the use of the Gram stain are the most powerful tools available for a tentative identification of a potential pathogen. If tuberculosis is suspected, acid-fast stains should be made on the centrifuged sediment obtained from the sputum digestion procedure described above.

There are many other specialized procedures, and the choice will depend upon information received from the clinician and upon the appearance of the initial isolate. Fluorescently-labeled antibody directed against group A streptococci provides rapid identification of these organisms. Counterimmunoelectrophoresis (see Chapter 13) is used to identify a number of organisms—especially the meningococci and group B streptococci. This procedure uses known antiserum and a group-specific antigen extracted from the isolated organisms; these are moved toward each other in an electric field while embedded in agar on a microscope slide. A specific reaction is seen as a precipitin line. Table 30-3 lists some common isolates from the respiratory tract with a few of the special procedures that aid in their identification.

**CEREBROSPINAL FLUID**

The usual clinical signs of meningitis are headache, fever, vomiting, and a stiff neck; however, many of these signs may be absent in infants. As discussed in earlier chapters of this unit, there are several specific organisms which are frequent causes of meningitis, namely *Neisseria meningitidis* and *Haemophilus influenzae*. In addition, other organ-

**Table 30-3. Organisms Commonly Isolated from Respiratory Tract Samples and Specialized Procedures Used for Their Identification**

| Organism | Special Procedures |
|---|---|
| Streptococcus group A, beta-hemolytic | Sensitive to commercially available bacitracin discs; catalase negative; fluorescently-labeled antibody |
| Streptococcus pneumoniae alpha-hemolytic | Sensitive to optochin discs; lethal for mouse in 18 hours |
| Staphylococcus aureus | Vogel Johnson medium; ferments mannitol; coagulase-positive |
| Haemophilus influenzae | Streak blood plate and check for hematin and NAD requirement; do quellung test with specific antiserum |
| Neisseria meningitidis | Grow in Thayer-Martin medium; do quellung test with specific antiserum |
| Bordetella pertussis | Bordet-Gengou agar plates |
| Corynebacterium diphtheriae | Loeffler's coagulated serum and potassium tellurite plates |

isms such as *Streptococcus pneumoniae, Mycobacterium tuberculosis,* and *Cryptococcus neoformans* infrequently cause meningitis. One important concept concerning meningitis is that essentially any organism gaining entrance to the fluid surrounding the brain and spinal cord may grow and cause an inflammation of the meninges. Such infections are frequently severe and, unless promptly and adequately treated, may result in the death of the patient in a matter of hours.

**Specimen Collection of Cerebrospinal Fluid**

Cerebrospinal fluid (CSF) is obtained by a puncture into the lumbar region of the lower spinal cord. It is of utmost importance that the puncture site be disinfected in the manner described previously for venipunctures to ensure that no contaminating organisms are mechanically injected into the CSF. The collected specimen should be placed into a sterile screw-cap tube and delivered immediately to the diagnostic laboratory.

### Media Inoculated with Cerebrospinal Fluid

A diagnosis of meningitis is usually based upon both the microbiological findings in the CSF and a chemical determination for the total protein and glucose present in the fluid. Since the total specimen is frequently only 1 to 2 ml, the sample must suffice for both the chemistry and the microbiological findings. The CSF is, therefore, routinely centrifuged for ten minutes at 1200 times gravity; part of the supernatant is used for the chemical assays while the sediment is the source for the bacteriologic evaluation.

The sediment from the centrifuged sample is inoculated onto two blood agar plates. One is incubated aerobically at 35°C and discs of hematin and NAD are added to enrich the growth of Haemophilus influenzae. Another method of providing these required factors is to make a single streak of Staphylococcus aureus across the plate. The staphylococci release these factors by lysis of the red blood cells in the agar and Haemophilus influenzae will be found growing only as satellite colonies adjacent to the growth of the staphylococci. A second blood agar plate is incubated under an atmosphere of 10% $CO_2$. Both thioglycollate broth, for the growth of anaerobes, and nutrient broth should be inoculated with the CSF sediment. All cultures should be inspected daily, and in the event of growth broth media should be subcultured onto an appropriate agar medium.

### Identification of Isolates from Cerebrospinal Fluid

Since meningitis frequently presents an emergency situation, it is imperative that a tentative diagnosis be made as soon as pos-

sible. It is mandatory that the sediment from the centrifuged CSF be Gram-stained and examined microscopically; because the number of organisms is often small, it is recommended that at least thirty minutes be spent for such an examination. If organisms are seen, additional procedures can sometimes be used to immediately substantiate a tentative identification. The most common of these would be to carry out a quellung reaction with known specific antiserum or to stain with specific, fluorescently-labeled antiserum. Spinal fluid from a possible case of tuberculosis meningitis should be stained for acid-fast organisms, and a possible infection by Cryptococcus neoformans can be tentatively diagnosed using wet mounts of spinal fluid sediment mixed with India ink or nigrosin to demonstrate the large capsules surrounding the yeast cells.

An evaluation of a patient's inflammatory response may also aid in the diagnosis of a meningeal infection. In general, one finds predominately polymorphonuclear leukocytes in the CSF in acute bacterial infections, whereas meningitis resulting from fungi, leptospira, or Mycobacterium tuberculosis is characterized by the presence of lymphocytes.

## WOUNDS AND ABSCESSES

Pus and exudate from an infected wound, draining ulcer, or open abscess would be expected to contain the etiologic agent of the infection. In open wounds, however, one almost invariably finds skin and soil contaminants which could, under appropriate growth conditions, outgrow the true infectious organism, resulting in an incomplete laboratory report.

### Collection of Specimens from Wounds and Abscesses

Whenever possible, a sterile syringe and needle should be used to collect specimens. The use of a swab is routinely unsatisfactory because of the limited amount of material collected by this method and because many organisms die as the swab dries, making it difficult or impossible to isolate the etiologic agent or agents. It is important to remember, also, that wounds and abscesses are commonly infected with obligately anaerobic bacteria which quickly die on a swab that is exposed to the atmosphere. Therefore, all aspirates should be transported to the laboratory in special bottles containing oxygen-free gas. Such bottles, which can be obtained commercially, usually contain a few drops of 0.0003% resazurin, an oxidation-reduction indicator that turns pink if air contaminates the bottle. Table 30-4 lists some of the more common types of infections in which the obligate anaerobes are involved.

Burns often are infected with opportunists such as *Pseudomonas aeruginosa,* enterics, staphylococci, and yeast, and the isolation of the definitive infectious agent may be extremely difficult. Specimens of burned tissue and any drainage material should be sent to the laboratory for culture and evaluation.

## Media Inoculated with Wound and Abscess Specimens

Because the array of organisms that may infect a wound is so great, the choice of inoculation media can be difficult. In general, obligate anaerobes, such as those in the genera *Clostridium, Bacteroides, Eubacterium, Fusobacterium,* and *Actinomyces,* must be considered. Table 30-5 lists a few of the features that would suggest the involvement of one of these anaerobes.

There are numerous specialized media that may be successfully used for the growth of the obligate anaerobes. Most contain whole or lysed blood from sheep, complex infusions such as brain-heart infusion or chopped meat, vitamin supplements such as yeast extract and additional vitamin K, and, if a broth, a reducing agent such as thioglycolate, cysteine, ascorbic acid, sodium formaldehyde sulfoxyalate, or thiomalic acid with 0.1% agar added to reduce convection currents.

**Table 30-4. Infections in which Anaerobes Are the Predominant Pathogens or Are Commonly Present**

| Region | Type of Infection |
|---|---|
| Head and Neck | Brain abscess |
| | Otogenic meningitis, extradural or subdural empyema |
| | Chronic otitis media |
| | Dental infection |
| Pleuropulmonary | Pneumonia secondary to obstructive process |
| | Aspiration pneumonia |
| | Lung abscess |
| | Bronchietasis |
| | Thoracic empyema |
| Intra-abdominal | Liver abscess |
| | Pylephlebitis |
| | Peritonitis |
| | Appendicitis |
| | Subphrenic abscess |
| | Other intra-abdominal abscess |
| | Wound infection following bowel surgery or trauma |
| Female Genital | Puerperal sepsis |
| | Postabortal sepsis |
| | Endometritis |
| | Tubo-ovarian abscess |
| | Other gynecologic infection |
| Other | Perirectal abscess |
| | Gas-forming cellulitis |
| | Gas gangrene |
| | Breast abscess |

Because most wound infections or abscesses contain multiple organisms, the use of liquid media alone is not satisfactory. In fact, if isolated colonies are obtained on agar plates, little is gained by the examination of broth cultures. Agar plates must be incubated, however, in an anaerobic jar from which all oxygen has been removed.

Blood agar plates and differential media for the growth of the enterics, such as eosin methylene blue or MacConkey, also must be inoculated and then incubated aerobically at 35°C.

**Table 30-5. Clinical and Bacteriologic Features Suggesting Possible Infection with Anaerobes**

| Clinical | Bacteriologic |
|---|---|
| Foul-smelling discharge | Unique morphology on Gram stain |
| Location of infection in proximity to a mucosal surface | Failure to grow aerobically; organisms seen on Gram stain of original exudate. Furthermore, failure to obtain growth in fluid thioglycollate medium is not adequate assurance that anaerobes were not present |
| Necrotic tissue, gangrene; pseudomembrane formation | |
| Gas in tissues or discharges | |
| Endocarditis with negative routine blood cultures | Growth in anaerobic zone of fluid media or of agar deeps |
| Infection associated with malignancy or other process producing tissue destruction | Growth anaerobically on media containing 100 μg/ml of kanamycin, neomycin, or paromomycin (or medium also containing 7.5 μg ml of vancomycin for gram-negative anaerobic bacilli) |
| Infection related to the use of aminoglycosides (oral, parenteral, or topical) | |
| Septic thrombophlebitis | Gas and foul odor in specimen or culture |
| Bacteremic features with jaundice | Characteristic colonies on agar plates anaerobically |
| Infection following human or other bites | |
| Black discoloration of blood-containing exudates; these exudates may fluoresce red under ultraviolet light (*Bacteroides melaninogenicus* infections) | Young colonies of *Bacteroides melaninogenicus* may fluoresce red under ultraviolet light |
| "Sulfur granules" in discharges (actinomycosis) | |
| Classic clinical features of gas gangrene | |

**Identification of Wound Isolates**

The multiplicity of genera that may be in an open wound makes it difficult to list firm rules for their identification. One should first observe a Gram stain of all specimens. The results of microscopic examination may provide information which will aid in a decision as to which media to inoculate and under what conditions the culture should be incubated. This discussion should indicate that it is no simple affair to differentiate between the true etiologic agents of wounds and abscess infections and contaminants that go along for the ride.

**FECES**

Gastrointestinal illnesses are usually characterized by diarrhea or the presence of blood and mucus in voided stools. Many such disturbances are cases of food poisoning resulting from the ingestion of a preformed toxin. Symptoms of such intoxication rarely last beyond 24 hours, and treatment is usually confined to the intravenous replacement of lost fluids and electrolytes.

A bacteriologic examination of food suspected of causing an illness would be more likely to yield informative data concerning the etiology of an intoxication than would an examination of a fecal specimen. For example, a Gram stain revealing large numbers of staphylococci—together with a history and the clinical symptoms of staphylococcal food poisoning (see Chapter 18)—would provide strong circumstantial evidence that the gastroenteritis was due to the ingestion of food contaminated with staphylococcal enterotoxin. A similar situation would be true for food poisoning due to *Clostridium perfringens* (see Chapter 23). In both cases, the organisms would be present in large numbers in the contaminated food; however, because the staphylococcal enterotoxin is more stable to heat inactivation than are the staphylococci themselves, it would not be unusual to see large numbers of staphylococci in a Gram stain (of a heated cream soup, for example) and yet not be able to culture significant numbers of organisms from the suspected food. On the other hand, because the *Clostridium perfringens* enterotoxin is produced only during sporulation, one might find large numbers of viable organisms in a similar situation. It is likely that many cases of gastroenteritis are of viral origin, and some of these agents are discussed in Unit Four. With the above qualifications as a preface, we may turn to the laboratory diagnosis of gastrointestinal infections that result from the presence of the etiologic agent in the intestinal contents.

### Specimens from Intestinal Contents

When one wishes to culture intestinal contents, there is no wide choice as to the material to be taken from the patient, although best results will be obtained if the fecal specimen is collected during the acute stage of an episode of diarrhea. If a specimen contains blood or mucus, these should be included in material to be sent to the laboratory. When a sterile swab is used instead of a fecal specimen, the swab must be inserted past the anal sphincter and rotated several times before being withdrawn.

It is a common misconception that the microorganisms found in feces are rather hearty and that special precautions to preserve the viability of suspected pathogens are not required. Nothing could be farther from the truth. Unless fecal specimens can be taken directly to the laboratory for culturing, they must be placed in a stool preservative containing a buffer that will maintain the pH near neutrality. One such preservative uses approximately equal parts of sterile glycerol (containing 0.033 M phosphate buffer, pH 7.4)

and feces. A pH indicator may also be included to assure that a pH drop will not go unnoticed. Failure to use a preservative will result in the death of many of the enteric pathogens—especially the shigellae and, to a lesser extent, the salmonellae. Fecal specimens of 1–2 grams are adequate for bacteriologic procedures. When rectal swabs are used, they should be immersed in a commercially available, gram-negative enrichment broth (GN broth) until they can be inoculated onto appropriate media.

### Media Inoculated with Intestinal Specimens

As discussed in Chapter 20, the major intestinal flora consists of obligately anaerobic gram-negative rods, including organisms in the genera *Bacteroides*, *Fusobacterium*, *Eubacterium*, and *Clostridium*. All of these can cause serious abscesses but, with the exception of the enterotoxin from *Clostridium perfringens*, none of the obligate anaerobes has been implicated in gastrointestinal disease characterized by diarrhea. Therefore, unlike the processing of blood or abscess specimens, it is not usual to culture fecal specimens under anaerobic conditions.

When species of either *Salmonella* or *Shigella* are the possible pathogens, it is advisable to inoculate an enrichment medium that will selectively permit the growth of these organisms over that of the normal gram-negative flora. There are many such media available, and it is probable that some diagnostic laboratories use various modifications of these media. Two of the more common enrichment media are a tetrathionate and a selenite F medium—both of which are commercially available. After incubation of the inoculated enrichment medium for 12–16 hours at 35–37°C, it should be streaked on standard, differential media such as MacConkey's, eosin methylene blue, or deoxycholate agar plates. Hektoen's enteric and xylose-lysine deoxycholate (XLD) plates also may be used—particularly if the specimen has not been previously cultured in one of the enrichment media just described. There are many other differential and selective media which may be used for the isolation of the pathogenic Enterobacteriaceae, and it is likely that diagnostic laboratories will vary somewhat in their preference of one medium over another.

In cases of suspected cholera, fecal specimens or rectal swabs should be plated directly on nonselective media such as taurocholate gelatin agar and on nutrient agar. In addition, selective agar plates containing thiosulfate-citrate-bile salts or tellurite-taurocholate gelatin should be heavily streaked. Because *Vibrio cholerae* will grow at a more alkaline pH than most enteric organisms, an enrichment peptone broth, pH 8.5, should be inoculated. All enrichment cultures should be streaked on nonselective media after 8–18 hours of incubation at 35°C.

*Vibrio parahemolyticus,* a major source of food poisoning acquired from eating undercooked seafood, is a halophilic (salt-loving) organism that can be enriched by growth in a medium containing excess NaCl. Thus, the inoculation of a fecal specimen into a 1% peptone broth (pH 7.1) containing 3% NaCl will greatly increase the chances of isolation of this organism. The enrichment broth can then be streaked on any of several nonselective agar plates (such as described for *V. cholerae*) for final isolation.

In addition to staphylococcal food poisoning resulting from the ingestion of preformed enterotoxin, *Staphylococcus aureus* may on rare occasions cause an ulcerative enteritis as a consequence of the actual invasion of the bowel wall. In such cases, blood or mucus present in the stool should be plated on a blood agar medium and a selective medium such as mannitol-salt agar.

### Identification of Fecal Isolates

Because of the large numbers of facultative, gram-negative rods that make up the normal intestinal flora, the isolation and identification of the morphologically similar shigellae and salmonellae require the use of selective

and differential media as well as considerable experience in working with these organisms. Table 30-6 lists a few of the enteric organisms for a number of the media commonly used to culture these organisms. One or two representative colonies that are characteristic for these enteric pathogens are picked and transferred to a Kligler's-iron or triple-sugar-iron slant. If subsequent growth shows a slow or nonlactose-fermenting gram-negative rod, the organism can be identified by the biochemical and serologic tests described in Chapter 20. If the etiologic agent of the gastroenteritis is a rapid, lactose-fermenting enteric such as the enteropathic *E. coli* or *Enterobacter,* the process of establishing the etiology is considerably more complex. Several colonies can be grown in a broth which is subsequently assayed for enterotoxin using a ligated ileal loop or Chinese hamster ovary cells (see Chapter 20). Those *E. coli* that produce disease in a manner similar to the shigellae by direct invasion of the bowel wall would be implicated as disease agents only from biopsy material demonstrating intestinal wall invasion.

By their curved shape and rapid motility, vibrios can sometimes be observed by a direct, dark-field examination of the stool specimen. However, it is more usual that these organisms are identified by Gram stains and dark-field examination of isolated colonies from enrichment media, such as a medium with a high pH to grow *V. cholerae* and one with a high salt concentration for *V. parahemolyticus.*

The identification of staphylococci from a fecal specimen is a moderately easy task if the laboratory has been instructed that the clinical symptoms are compatible with those of a staphylococcal enteritis. Large colonies showing beta-hemolysis and grapelike clusters of gram-positive cocci should be additionally tested for coagulase production, phage type, and, if specific antiserum is available, for the production of enterotoxin.

Intestinal infections by yeast, such as species of *Candida,* or any of the many parasitic protozoa or worms are diagnosed by the direct microscopic examination of a fecal specimen. Additional details concerning these agents are discussed in Chapter 29 and Unit 5.

## URINE

Most urinary tract infections are initiated by organisms that gain entrance to the bladder by ascending through the urethra, and they are more common in females than in males. In the male, however, a chronic infection of the prostrate gland may also be the source for a bladder infection (cystitis) or a kidney infection (pyelonephritis). In both sexes, the majority of all urinary tract infection are caused by normal-flora enterics, among which may be species of *Escherichia, Klebsiella, Enterobacter, Proteus,* and *Pseudomonas.*

### Collection of Urinary Specimens

Urethral catheterization may yield samples with minimal contamination, but the danger of introducing organisms from the urethra into the bladder provides some risk to this procedure. Moreover, microbial flora in the urethra, particularly in the male, may contaminate the specimen, leading the microbiologist to an erroneous conclusion. As a result, catheterization is not routinely performed for the collection of urine samples. Instead, voided samples are obtained after careful cleansing of the external genitalia. The following considerations must, however, be strictly adhered to if bacteriological reports on voided urine samples are to be meaningful. First, all voided urine samples will contain some bacteria, and, therefore, a quantitative assay for the number of bacteria present must be carried out. Second, this number will be grossly misleading unless the exterior genitalia are carefully cleaned to remove contaminating bacteria from the female vulva and perineal area and the male urethral meatus. The patient must be carefully instructed in how to wash these areas with soap and water, to be followed by a thorough rinsing with sterile water to remove any residual soap. The female must be instructed to keep the labia continuously apart during the washing, rinsing, and voiding of urine. Urine from both sexes should be collected in a sterile cup only after the first 20–25 ml of urine has been voided, because the flushing action of the initial flow will remove many of the organisms present in the urethra.

On rare occasions it may be necessary to collect the urine directly from the bladder with a needle and syringe. This procedure is done by a puncture of the abdominal wall directly into the bladder. In other cases a urine sample may be required from an individual having an indwelling catheter in place. In such situations, the urine should be collected with a needle and syringe directly from the catheter tubing and never from the drainage bag because considerable bacterial growth may have occurred in the urine receptacle.

### Media Inoculated with Urinary Specimens

It must be remembered that all voided urine samples, as well as most samples collected by catheterization, contain some bacteria and that the clinical diagnosis of an infection, therefore, is based entirely on the numbers of bacteria in the urine. Considerable experimental data has resulted in the formulation of the following rules: (1) $10^5$ bacteria or more per ml from a clean, voided specimen indicate a urinary tract infection; (2) a value of $10^3$ to $10^4$ bacteria per ml should be repeated; and (3) $10^3$ or less bacteria per ml are not considered significant in a voided sample. Single samples cannot be considered to be 100% accurate, and it is frequently advisable that duplicate samples collected at different times be sent to the diagnostic laboratory.

Because of the necessity for quantitating the bacteria present in a sample of urine, a number of different techniques have been devised to accomplish enumeration as rapidly as possible. An old and still used procedure is to add 0.1 ml of the urine to 9.9 ml of sterile water and then to prepare a pour plate by mixing 10 to 20 ml of nutrient agar

**Table 30-6. Growth Characteristics on Some Commonly Used Agar Media of Bacteria Frequently Isolated from Feces**

| Organism | Eosin Methylene Blue Agar | MacConkey | Hektoen Enteric Agar | Salmonella-Shigella Agar | Bismuth Sulfite Agar | Xylose-lysine-deoxycholate Agar | Selective Enterococcus Agar |
|---|---|---|---|---|---|---|---|
| Arizona | Translucent, colorless | Uncolored, transparent; red (LF) | Similar to Salmonella | Black centered, clear periphery | Black; green brown (LF) | Black-centered red colonies | Inhibited |
| Citrobacter | Translucent colonies, greenish metallic sheen (LF) | Uncolored, transparent; red (LF) | Usually inhibited; when present, colonies are small and bluish-green | Similar to Arizona | Black; green-brown | Opaque, yellow | Inhibited |
| Enterobacter Serratia | Metallic sheen, similar to E. coli but somewhat larger | Red-pink | Green centers with yellow to brown periphery | White or cream colored, opaque, mucoid | Raised mucoid colonies, silvery sheen | Opaque, yellow | Inhibited |
| Escherichia coli (rapid lactose fermenters) | Dark center; greenish metallic sheen | Red or pink, may be surrounded by a zone of precipitated bile | Moderately inhibited; orange to salmon-pink | Red to pink; colorless with a pink center | Mostly inhibited; black-brown greenish surface; no metallic sheen | Opaque, yellow | Inhibited |
| Klebsiella | Larger than E. coli. mucoid, brownish, tend to coalesce, often convex | Pink, mucoid | Yellow centers, periphery orange | Red to pink; colorless with a pink center | Mostly inhibited | Opaque, yellow | Inhibited |

**Table 30-6. Growth Characteristics on Some Commonly Used Agar Media of Bacteria Frequently Isolated from Feces (continued)**

| Organism | Eosin Methylene Blue Agar | MacConkey | Hektoen Enteric Agar | Salmonella-Shigella Agar | Bismuth Sulfite Agar | Xylose-lysine-deoxycholate Agar | Selective Entero-coccus Agar |
|---|---|---|---|---|---|---|---|
| Proteus | Translucent, colorless | Uncolored, transparent | Most strains are inhibited; dark centered, greenish ($H_2S$ producers), similar to Salmonella | Black centered, clear periphery | Green; black ($H_2S$ producers), mostly inhibited | Opaque, yellow (P. mirabilis, P. vulgaris), red (P. rettgerii, P. morganii) | Small grey colonies (few) |
| Pseudomonas | Translucent, colorless; amber | Uncolored, transparent | Most strains are inhibited; colonies are small, flat and green to brown | Mostly inhibited, transparent, colorless colonies | Inhibited | Sometimes red colonies | Inhibited |
| Salmonella | Translucent amber colonies; colorless | Uncolored, transparent | Blue to blue-green; most colonies have black centers, ($H_2S$ producers) | Opaque; transparent; uncolored; black centered, clear periphery | S. typhi black with sheen or dotted black or greenish-gray; other Salmonella are black or green | Black-centered red ($H_2S$ producers); red color (no $H_2S$) | Inhibited |
| Shigella | Translucent, amber colonies; colorless | Uncolored, transparent | Blue to blue-green, periphery of colonies lighter than center portion | Opaque, transparent | Mostly, inhibited; S. flexneri and S. sonnei are brown, raised, and crater-like | Red | Inhibited |

LF = lactose fermenter.

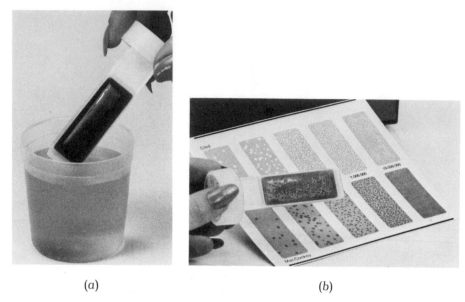

(a)                              (b)

**Figure 30-2.** Uricult provides one method for screening urine samples. *a.* An agar-coated paddle is dipped in the urine sample. *b.* After incubation the colony count may be quickly (and roughly) determined by comparison of growth on the paddle with a chart for the appropriate type of agar medium.

with 0.1 ml of the urine dilution. Because this represents an overall dilution of $10^{-3}$, each colony appearing on the pour plate after incubation would represent 1000 microorganisms in the original urine sample.

A standard platinum dilution loop (commercially available) will hold approximately 0.001 ml of liquid. Such a loop can be used to streak a urine specimen directly on a nutrient agar plate. If the loop is calibrated monthly by comparison with counts obtained by the pour-plate method, the over-all accuracy of the calibrated loop technique is equivalent to that of a pour plate.

There are a variety of screening kits available commercially for suspected urinary tract infections. One, called a paddle or dipslide type, has a selective agar medium coated on one side and a nonselective agar medium on the other side. The paddle is merely dipped into the urine specimen, reinserted into its sterile container, and incubated at

35°C for 18–24 hours before counting the colonies (see Figure 30-2). The amount of urine adhering to a paddle has been experimentally determined by the manufacturer, and this is reported to be about 95% as accurate as the pour-plate procedure. A number of other kits are available, and it is likely that each laboratory has its preferred method for enumerating the microorganisms present in a urine specimen.

### Identification of Urine Isolates

It is recommended that a Gram stain of the uncentrifuged urine specimen be examined—primarily because if one drop is allowed to dry on a slide without spreading, the appearance of one or more bacteria per oil-immersion field (sometimes with leukocytes present) is indicative of a total bacterial count greater than $10^5$ organisms per ml of urine.

Blood agar plates, as well as MacConkey and eosin methylene blue plates, should be streaked with the urine specimen. Because members of the Enterobacteriaceae are, by far, the most frequent causes of urinary tract infections, the final identification of the organism is done as outlined in Chapter 20.

# Serological Techniques

The measurement of antibodies arising in response to an infectious agent can aid in the diagnosis of some infections. In the case of syphilis, for example, a diagnosis is usually dependent upon showing the presence of antibodies that were formed in response to the infection. These tests are discussed in detail in Chapter 26, however, and will not be repeated in this section.

Examples of other diseases for which the patient's antibody response can be used as an aid in making a diagnosis include typhoid fever, brucellosis, listeriosis, and tularemia. In these cases antibody is measured by determining the agglutination titer of the patient's serum against the known organisms. Such tests, however, are not a substitute for the isolation and identification of the etiologic agent and should be used only to support culture techniques or to provide a retrospective diagnosis when attempts to isolate the disease-producing agent have failed. Moreover, the mere presence of specific antibodies cannot be used to support a serologic diagnosis for a disease because such information does not show when the antibody formation occurred. It is necessary to show that a rise in antibody titer occurred during the course of the illness. This is accomplished by using paired sera—an acute phase serum taken early in the illness, and a convalescent phase serum taken one or two weeks later. The usual rule of thumb is that for data to be significant, there should be at least a four-fold rise in antibody titer in these paired sera.

For some diseases such as leptospirosis, mycoplasma pneumonia, toxoplasmosis (see Chapter 43), and rickettsial infections, it can sometimes be difficult to isolate or visualize the causative agent, and an increase in antibody may provide the only information for a diagnosis. Other diseases such as the late sequelae that may follow a group A streptococcal infection (for example rheumatic fever or acute glomerulonephritis) occur after recovery from the bacterial infection and the causative organisms are no longer present. In these cases, the occurrence of a recent streptococcal infection can be established only by showing the presence of antibodies to a group A streptococcal antigen such as streptolysin O (see anti-streptolysin O Chapter 18).

## FLUORESCEIN-LABELED ANTIBODY

Fluorescently-labeled antibodies facilitate a procedure for rapidly determining the presence of specific antibodies. As illustrated in Figure 30-3, the indirect method can be used to detect the presence of antibodies to any bacterium. One requires only known bacteria, the patient's serum, and some fluorescein-labeled, anti-human gamma globulin.

The direct method, also illustrated in Figure 30-3, can be used to confirm a tentative identification of an isolated organism. In this case, however, one is limited by the availability of fluorescein-labeled specific antibody.

## QUELLUNG REACTIONS

Before antibiotics, it was imperative that organisms such as the pneumococcus, meningococcus, and *Haemophilus influ-*

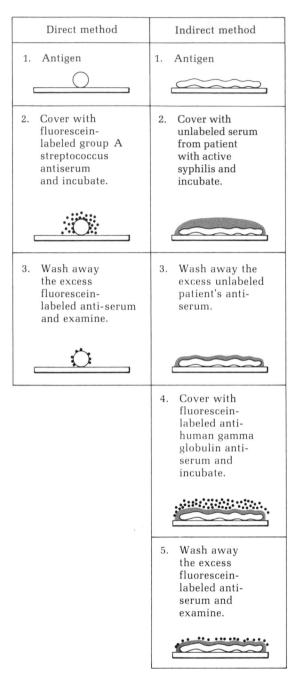

| Direct method | Indirect method |
|---|---|
| 1. Antigen | 1. Antigen |
| 2. Cover with fluorescein-labeled group A streptococcus antiserum and incubate. | 2. Cover with unlabeled serum from patient with active syphilis and incubate. |
| 3. Wash away the excess fluorescein-labeled anti-serum and examine. | 3. Wash away the excess unlabeled patient's anti-serum. |
| | 4. Cover with fluorescein-labeled anti-human gamma globulin anti-serum and incubate. |
| | 5. Wash away the excess fluorescein-labeled anti-serum and examine. |

**Figure 30-3.** Fluorescein-labeled antibody test methods. Note that one must have fluorescein-labeled antibody that is specific for the organism in question in order to use the direct method; however, the indirect method can be adapted to any organism using fluorescein-labeled anti-human gamma globulin as the only labeled antiserum.

*enzae* be typed so that the proper specific serum therapy could be started. Currently, quellung reactions are valuable for the rapid identification of organisms present in the cerebrospinal fluid of patients with meningitis. A quellung reaction can be used to confirm a tentative identification from a Gram stain.

## REFERENCES

Balows, A. 1975. *Clinical Microbiology: How to Start and When to Stop.* Charles C. Thomas, Springfield, Illinois.

Barry, A. L., P. B. Smith, and M. Turck. (T. L. Gavan, coordinating editor.) 1975. *Laboratory Diagnosis of Urinary Tract Infections.* Cumitech 2. Amer. Soc. Microbiol., Washington, D. C.

Bartlett, R. C., P. D. Ellner, and J. A. Washington II. (J. C. Sherris, coordinating editor.) 1974. *Blood Cultures.* Cumitech 1. Amer. Soc. Microbiol., Washington, D. C.

Blazevic, D. J., and G. M. Ederer. 1975. *Principles of Biochemical Tests in Diagnostic Microbiology.* John Wiley and Sons, New York.

Blundell, G. P. 1970. Fluorescent antibody techniques. In M. Stefanini, ed., *Progress in Clinical Pathology,* Vol. III. Grune and Stratton, New York.

Bondi, A., J. Bortola, and J. E. Prier, eds. 1977. *The Clinical Laboratory as an Aid in Chemotherapy of Infectious Disease.* University Park Press, Baltimore.

Chow, A. W., P. J. Cunningham, and L. B. Guze. 1976. Survival of anaerobic and aerobic bacteria in a nonsupportive gassed transport system. *J. Clin. Microbiol.* **3:**128–132.

Cowan, S. T. 1974. *Manual for the Identification of Medical Bacteria.* Cambridge University Press, New York.

Hill, H. R. 1975. Rapid detection and specific identification of infections due to group B streptococci by counterimmunoelectrophoresis. In David Schlessinger, ed. *Microbiology 1975.* Amer. Soc. Microbiol., Washington, D. C.

Isenberg, H. D., and J. I. Berkman. 1966. Recent practices in diagnostic bacteriology. In M. Stefanini, ed., *Progress in Clinical Pathology,* Vol. I. Grune and Stratton, New York.

Isenberg, H. D., and J. D. MacLowry. 1976. Automated methods and data handling in bacteriology. *Annu. Rev. Microbiol.* **30:**483–505.

Nagel, J. G., C. U. Tuazon, T. A. Cardella, and J. N. Sheagren. 1975. Teichoic acid serologic diagnosis of staphylococcal endocarditis. *Ann. Internal Med.* **82:**13–17.

Prier, J. E., J. T. Bartola, and H. Friedman, eds. 1976. *Modern Methods in Medical Microbiology: Systems and Trends.* University Park Press, Baltimore.

Sielaff, B. H., E. A. Johnson, and J. M. Matsen. 1976. Computer-assisted bacterial identification utilizing antimicrobial susceptibility profiles generated by Autobac 1. *J. Clin. Microbiol.* **3:**105–109.

Sutter, V. L., and S. M. Finegold. 1973. Anaerobic bacteria: Their recognition and significance in the clinical laboratory. In M. Stefanini, ed., *Progress in Clinical Pathology.* Grune and Stratton, New York.

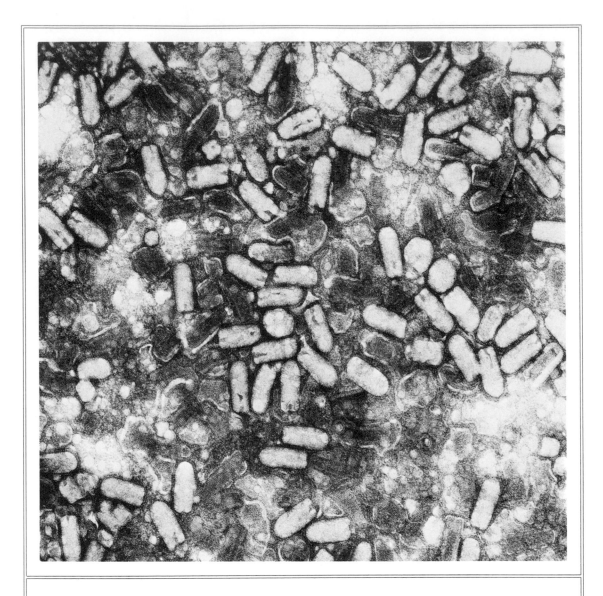

## UNIT FOUR

# Viruses

As we begin our study of viruses, we leave much of the familiar world of both the eucaryotic and the procaryotic cell. We shall be concerned with biological entities which do not by themselves possess life, since viruses manifest life, as measured by reproduction, only when a virus has entered a susceptible host cell. Thus viruses exist in the fuzzy semantical area between "living" and "nonliving," their status changing with each stage of the infectious cycle.

There are probably few cells, eucaryotic or procaryotic, that cannot be infected by a virus. In addition to the bacteriophages previously described, viruses can infect other procaryotic cells such as actinomycetes (actinophages), blue-green algae (cyanophages), and even free-living mycoplasmas. Among the invaders of eucaryotic cells, viruses have been described which infect fungi, protozoa, invertebrates, and probably every higher animal in existence.

There has been much scientific speculation about the origin of viruses. Since viruses require host cells for their replication, they are most likely younger on the evolutionary scale than their more complex host cells. This suggests two major possibilities: (1) they are the result of a retrograde evolution of procaryotic or eucaryotic cells, or (2) they originated from genetic material in host cells which mutated in such a manner that it could not only reproduce independently within a host cell, but could exist extracellularly and still maintain its ability to subsequently infect other cells. There is no absolute answer as to which of these theories of viral origins is correct, but most virologists believe that the latter is the more probable explanation.

Major changes occur in a host cell once it is infected by a virus. If the virus is to be replicated within the cell, the host cell would not usually continue to function as a normal uninfected cell. In fact, death probably is the most common fate of an infected cell. This is most dramatically illustrated when nonregenerating nervous tissue is infected with viruses such as those that cause polio or rabies; the destruction of the infected nerve cell results in either permanent disability or death of the entire host organism.

Other viruses may cause the proliferation of infected cells, resulting in such manifestations as warts. Yet others may cause membrane changes that result in the fusion of adjacent cells, creating new multinucleated cells. Viruses causing such cell fusions are being used in research laboratories to determine the location of specific genes on human chromosomes. This is accomplished by creating human-mouse cell hybrids, which tend to lose their human chromosomes when maintained over many transfers. By associating the loss of a specific cell function with the loss of a specific human chromosome one can assign genes to specific chromosomes.

Still other viruses may cause changes that transform the normal cell into a cancer cell, no longer affected by the controls that regulate normal growth. These cells acquire new membrane antigens, as well as many other new properties specific for the virus that induced the change. In some cases, such transformed cells are recognized as foreign and are destroyed by the host organism's immunological system; in other cases, the transformed cells proliferate, resulting in the uncontrolled growth of the infected cells. In such a situation a local tumor may develop, or, if the cells spread throughout the host and supplant normal tissues, a cancer or malignancy may result.

Finally, it should be pointed out that some (perhaps many) viruses do not cause any noticeable damage to the infected cell. They appear to have reached the ultimate state of parasitism wherein both the virus and the host cell continue to replicate. In other instances the effect of a virus may be so subtle that one can only postulate the mechanism by which it can damage its host. Such a case is provided by the infection of women with German measles during their first trimester of pregnancy. When the virus infects the fetus, its major effect is to diminish cell growth and interfere with cell differentiation, resulting in either death of the fetus or a large variety of abnormalities. After cell differentiation is completed, however, infection of the fetus appears uneventful and is followed by complete recovery.

Before we can hope to understand what viruses do, however, we must learn what they are, how they replicate, and how they can be distinguished from each other. It is the purpose of this unit to answer these questions, as well as to characterize those animal viruses causing disease in humans.

## REFERENCES

Acton, J. D., L. S. Kucera, Q. N. Myrvik, and R. S. Weiser. 1974. *Fundamentals of Medical Virology.* Lea & Febiger, Philadelphia.

Andrewes, C., and H. G. Pereira. 1972. *Viruses of Vertebrates,* 3rd ed. Williams & Wilkins, Baltimore.

Burrows, W. 1973. *Textbook of Microbiology,* 20th ed. W. B. Saunders, Philadelphia.

Davis, B. D., R. Dulbecco, H. N. Eisen, H. S. Ginsberg, W. B. Wood, and M. McCarty. 1973. *Microbiology,* 2nd ed. Harper and Row, New York.

Fenner, F., B. R. McAusland, C. A. Mims, J. Sambrook, and D. O. White. 1974. *The Biology of Animal Viruses,* 2nd ed. Academic Press, New York.

Fenner, F., and D. O. White. 1976. *Medical Virology,* 2nd ed. Academic Press, New York.

Fox, C. F., and W. S. Robinson, eds. 1973. *Virus Research.* Second ICN-UCLA Symposium on Molecular Biology. Academic Press, New York.

Jawetz, E., J. L. Melnick, and E. A. Adelberg. 1976. *Review of Medical Microbiology,* 12th ed. Lange Medical Publications, Los Altos, Calif.

Joklik, W. K., and H. P. Willett, eds. 1976. *Zinsser Microbiology,* 16th ed. Appleton-Century-Crofts, New York.

Knight, C. A. 1974. *Molecular Virology.* McGraw-Hill, New York.

Lonberg-Holm, K., and L. Philipson. 1974. *Early Interaction between Animal Viruses and Cells.* Reprinted in J. L. Melnick, ed. *Monographs in Virology;* Vol. 9. Phiebig.

# 31

# Structure and Classification
# of Animal Viruses

Viruses are perhaps the simplest form of life known—simple, at least, when compared structurally with procaryotic and eucaryotic cells. They are able to exist and replicate despite their simple structure because, like several other groups of organisms previously discussed, they are obligate intracellular parasites. But here the comparison of the viruses with rickettsiae or chlamydiae ends. For example, someone may one day devise a nutrient medium which will sustain extracellular division of the rickettsiae. Such a thing is impossible in the case of viruses, because a virion (infectious virus particle) lacks certain components absolutely essential for its own replication and must depend on the host cell to provide these missing factors.

One component missing from all viruses is an ATP-generating system. Biological syntheses require energy, and this energy is provided by ATP in the form of high-energy phosphate bonds, broken to release energy for biosynthetic reactions. For independent life a cell must carry out oxidation to provide energy for the regeneration of those high-energy bonds. No virion possesses this regeneration system, forcing it to rely on the ATP-generating system present in the infected host cell.

A second class of components lacking in viruses are the structural sites of protein synthesis, ribosomes and associated membranes. The synthesis of any protein requires that a ribonucleic acid (messenger RNA) be attached to a ribosome so that the genetic code can be translated into an amino acid sequence to form a polypeptide chain. The virion carries its own genetic code in ribonucleic acid (RNA) or deoxyribonucleic acid (DNA), which can be transcribed into messenger RNA, but as far as is known, all viruses must use the ribosomes of the host cell for protein synthesis. One seeming contradiction to this statement is seen in a group of RNA viruses called the arenaviruses. These viruses do indeed appear to contain ribosomes, but there is a consensus that these are host-cell ribosomes incorporated into the virion during the assembly and budding of the virus from the host cell.

Another characteristic peculiar to viruses is that unlike all other forms of life that contain both RNA and DNA, viruses contain only one type of nucleic acid; in some cases it is RNA, and in others it is DNA, but never both. Minor exceptions to this statement may be seen in the very complex DNA-containing poxviruses that apparently contain very small amounts of their own RNA and in the RNA-containing retroviruses which may contain trace amounts of DNA. However, in both cases these trace amounts of "contaminating" nucleic acid are probably not necessary to the virus.

## SIZES OF VIRUSES

Viruses vary considerably in size, but in general they are well below the limit of visibility of the light microscope. In early literature they were often referred to as filterable viruses because they would go through filters that would not allow bacteria to pass. In fact, errors concerning the etiology of a disease have occurred when a virus was considered to be the causative agent merely because the infectious agent was filterable.

Virus sizes range from 20 to 250 nanometers (nm = $10^{-9}$ meter, or one-thousandth of a $\mu$m), although as you will see, such measurements can be misleading for helical-shaped viruses such as the rhabdoviruses. Three basic techniques are used to determine virus size: (1) filtration through graded collodion membranes for which the size of the pores in each membrane is known; (2) high speed centrifugation (greater than 100,000 times gravity), which provides data for the calculation of virus size based on the rate at which a particle of known shape will travel toward the bottom of the centrifuge tube at a known centrifugal force; and (3) direct observation using an electron microscope, often including objects of known size in the preparation for comparison.

## CHEMICAL COMPOSITION AND STRUCTURE

One can think of a virus in its simplest form as nothing more than nucleic acid (either DNA or RNA) surrounded by a protein overcoat called a capsid. Many viruses, however, are more complex, in that they may contain enzymes such as RNA polymerase or DNA polymerase. Also, some may have carbo-

hydrates bound to their coat proteins (glycoproteins), and others may be enclosed in a membrane that is composed of virally coded proteins and host-cell lipids. We shall begin our discussion of virus structure with the function and structure of the viral capsid.

### Viral Capsids

In essence, the viral capsid protects the enclosed nucleic acid from both physical destruction and enzymatic hydrolysis by nucleases. It also possesses binding sites that enable the virus to attach to specific receptor sites on the host cell. Finally, the capsid is responsible for the ultimate shape of the virion. Electron microscopy has revealed that, with the exception of the relatively complex poxviruses, all animal viruses are either isometric or helical in shape. All DNA-containing animal viruses are icosahedrons, again with the exception of the brick-shaped poxviruses; RNA-containing animal viruses may exist as icosahedrons or as helical viruses. We shall examine the isometric viruses first.

Isometric viruses appear to be in the shape of an icosahedron. This particle has 20 facets, each an equilateral triangle. These facets come together to form 12 vertices of 5 facets each. Schematic and electron microscopic views of such a virus are shown in Figure 31-1. As depicted in this figure, the completed capsid is made up of repeating morphological units called capsomers. These capsomers are visible by electron microscopy as small protein structures. For some viruses, each capsomer may be composed of only a single repeating polypeptide, while in other viruses each capsomer may consist of several different polypeptide molecules held together by noncovalent bonds to form the completed capsomer. Examination of Figure 31-1 will show that the capsomer at each of the 12 vertices is surrounded by only five other capsomers, whereas all other capsomers are adjacent to six other capsomers. The capsomers at the vertices are called pentons, or

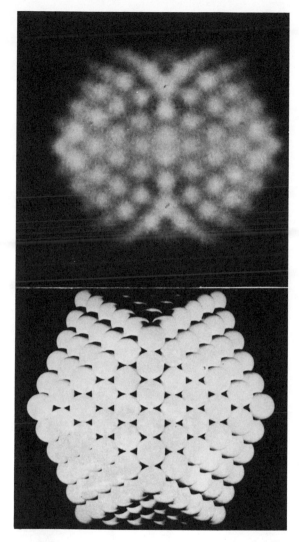

**Figure 31-1.** *Top:* electron micrograph of a negatively-stained adenovirus virion. *Bottom:* model of the same virion showing 252 spheres in icosahedral symmetry.

One means of classifying viruses is based on the number of capsomers present in the viral capsid. This number can be calculated for many isometric virions by using the formula $N = 10(n - 1)^2 + 2$, where $n$ is the number of capsomers on one side of each equilateral triangle. Examples that fit this formula would include herpesvirus, with five capsomers on the side of each triangular surface and thus a total of 162 capsomers making up the intact capsid, and adenovirus, with six capsomers per side and a total of 252 capsomers per intact virion.

A second method of grouping viruses possessing icosahedral symmetry is by the use of their triangulation numbers. If a line is drawn joining all adjacent capsomers, one forms a number of small equilateral triangles on each facet. This number of new triangles per triangular facet is called the triangulation number. Figure 31-3 illustrates graphically the triangulation number ($T$) for the herpes-

**Figure 31-2.** Features of icosahedral symmetry. Depending upon the angle of observation, the icosahedron will show two, three, or five axes of symmetry. *a.* Thus, looking down on the edge between two triangular facets, one can rotate the icosahedron 180° and observe the same symmetry. *b.* Looking at the center of a triangular facet, one will observe an identical symmetry with each 120° of rotation—thus showing three axes of symmetry. *c.* However, looking directly down on a penton capsomer, five axes of symmetry will be observed by rotating the icosahedron in a series of 72° steps.

pentomers, while the remaining capsomers are referred to as hexons, or hexomers.

A special property of an icosahedral structure is its multiple axes of symmetry. One can see from Figure 31-2 that it is possible to see three different types of symmetry as one rotates the icosahedron, through the edges, faces, and vertices, resulting in what is referred to as 5:3:2 symmetry.

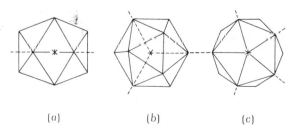

(a)                    (b)                    (c)

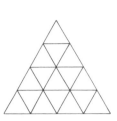
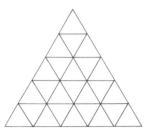

Herpesvirus          Adenovirus

**Figure 31-3.** A line drawn from the center of each capsomer to all adjacent capsomers will divide each facet into a number of smaller triangles. The number of triangles on a facet is the triangulation number, and it can be used to calculate the total number of capsomers in the icosahedron. Here are illustrated facets of a herpesvirus and an adenovirus, with triangulation numbers of 16 and 25 respectively.

virus group and the adenovirus group. Knowledge of the triangulation number enables one to calculate the total number of capsomers using the formula $N = 10T + 2$. Thus, for herpesvirus with a triangulation number of 16, there are 162 capsomers, and for adenovirus with a triangulation number of 25, there are a total of 252 capsomers per capsid. (Note the agreement with the calculations in the preceding paragraph.)

In the case of helical viruses the viral nucleic acid is closely associated with the protein capsid, forming a coil-shaped nucleocapsid that becomes enclosed in a membrane as it buds from the host cell. The exact nature of the nucleic acid interaction with the capsid is not well understood, but the protein protects the RNA from enzymatic degradation by RNase, while still allowing the RNA to be transcribed from the intact nucleoprotein. Figure 31-4 shows electron micrographs of rhabdovirus virions in which the striations of nucleic acid can be seen wound in a helical pattern in the interior of the particles.

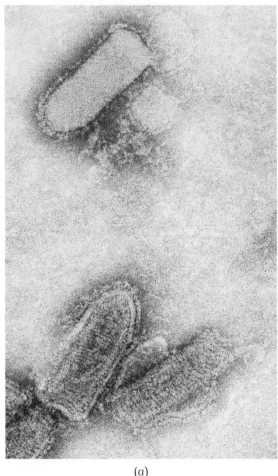

(a)

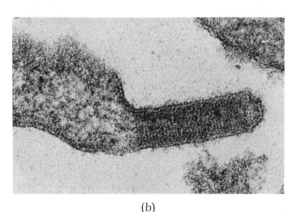

(b)

**Figure 31-4.** a. Virions of vesicular stomatitis virus (VSV); the helical nucleocapsid is visible as cross striations ($\times 207{,}000$). b. VSV budding from a cell ($\times 147{,}000$).

With the exception of the bullet-shaped rhabdoviruses, other helical animal viruses exist as spherical virions containing a helical-shaped nucleocapsid surrounded by a membrane.

### Viral Nucleic Acid

As mentioned in our initial characterization of viruses, each family of viruses possesses a nucleic acid that is characteristic for that group and which, along with the properties of the virion capsid, is used for the classification of the virus. As listed in Tables 31-1 and 31-2, viruses may possess double-stranded DNA (ds DNA), single-stranded DNA (ss DNA), ds RNA, or ss RNA. Furthermore, the amount of nucleic acid present may vary from enough to code for only three or four proteins (parvoviruses, picornaviruses), to that seen in the herpesviruses and poxviruses which can code for hundreds of proteins.

**Table. 31-1. Chemical and Physical Properties of Animal DNA Viruses**

| Families & Genera of DNA Viruses | Capsid Shape (symmetry) | Number of Capsomers | Presence of an Envelope | Triangulation Number | Mol. Wt. (in millions of daltons) of Virion Nucleic Acid[A] | Approx. Dia. of Virion (nm) |
|---|---|---|---|---|---|---|
| **ADENOVIRIDAE** | | | | | | |
| *Mastadenovirus* (infects mammals) | Icosahedral | 252 | Yes | 25 | 20–25 ds | 70 |
| *Aviadenovirus* (infects birds) | Icosahedral | 252 | Yes | 25 | | |
| **HERPETOVIRIDAE** | | | | | | |
| *Herpesvirus* (human herpes) | Icosahedral | 162 | Yes | 16 | 100 ds | 150[B] |
| **POXVIRIDEAE** | | | | | | |
| *Orthopoxvirus* (vaccinia and smallpox) | Very complex brick-shaped | Not applicable | Yes, but ether resistant | Not applicable | 100–200 ds | 300 × 240 |
| **PAPOVAVIRIDAE** | | | | | | |
| *Polyomavirus* (rodents and primates) | Icosahedral | 72 | No | 7 | 3 ds | 45 |
| *Papillomavirus* (produces papillomas) | Icosahedral | 72 | No | 7 | 5 ds | 55 |
| **PARVOVIRIDAE** | | | | | | |
| *Parvovirus* (infects vertebrate hosts) | Icosahedral | 32 | No | 3 | 1.2–1.8 ss | 20 |

[A]ds—double-stranded; ss—single-stranded
[B]Includes envelope—naked capsid is approximately 100 nm in diameter.

**Table 31-2. Chemical and Physical Properties of Animal RNA Viruses**

| Families & Genera of RNA Viruses | Capsid Symmetry | Number of Capsomers | Envelope | Triangulation Number | Mol. Wt. (in millions of daltons) & Physical Properties of Virion Nucleic Acid | Approx. Dia. of Virion (nm) |
|---|---|---|---|---|---|---|
| PICORNAVIRIDAE | | | | | | |
| *Enterovirus* (enteric) | Icosahedral | ?[A] | No | | 2.6 ss | 27 |
| *Rhinovirus* (respiratory) | Icosahedral | ?[A] | No | | 2.6 ss | 28 |
| *Calicivirus* (possible genus swine infection) | Icosahedral | 32 | No | 3 | | 35–40 |
| TOGAVIRIDAE | | | | | | |
| *Alphavirus*[B] (group A arboviruses) | Icosahedral[C] | 32 | Yes | 3 | 3 ss | 50–70 |
| *Flavivirus*[D] (group B arboviruses) | Icosahedral | 32 | Yes | 3 | 3 ss | 50 |
| *Rubivirus*[E] (rubella) | ? | | Yes | | 2.5–3 ss | 50–80 |
| ORTHOMYXOVIRIDAE | | | | | | |
| *Influenzavirus* (influenza) | Helical | | Yes | | 5[F] ss | 100 |
| PARAMYXOVIRIDAE | | | | | | |
| *Paramyxovirus* (Newcastle disease) | Helical | | Yes | | 6.5–7.5 | 150–300 |
| *Morbillivirus* (measles) | Helical | | Yes | | | |
| *Pneumovirus* (respiratory syncytial) | | | Yes | | | |
| RHABDOVIRIDAE | | | | | | |
| *Lyssavirus* (rabies group) | Helical | | Yes | | 4 ss | 70 × 170 |
| *Vesiculovirus* (vesicular stomatitis group) | Helical | | Yes | | 4 ss | |

**Table 31-2. Chemical and Physical Properties of Animal RNA Viruses (continued)**

| Families & Genera of RNA Viruses | Capsid Symmetry | Number of Capsomers | Envelope | Triangulation Number | Mol. Wt. (in millions of daltons) & Physical Properties of Virion Nucleic Acid | Approx. Dia. of Virion (nm) |
|---|---|---|---|---|---|---|
| ARENAVIRIDAE | | | | | | |
| Arenavirus (lymphocytic choriomeningitis) | ?[G] | | Yes | | [H] | 100–300 |
| BUNYAVIRIDAE | | | | | | |
| Bunyavirus (Bunyamwera supergroup) | Helical | | Yes | | | •90–100 |
| CORONAVIRIDAE | | | | | | |
| Coronavirus | Helical(?) | | Yes | | ? | 120 |
| RETROVIRIDAE (tumors) | ? | | | | 9–12[I] ss | 100 |
| REOVIRIDAE (ds RNA viruses) | | | | | | |
| Reovirus | Icosahedral | 120[J] | No | ? | 15[K] ds | 75–80 |
| Orbivirus[L] | Icosahedral | 32 | No | 3 | 15 ds | 65–80 |
| Rotavirus (possible genus) | Icosahedral | | No | ? | ? | ? |

[A] Details of symmetry unknown; probably 60 subunits clustered in groups of 5 about each of the 12 vertices.

[B] Includes approximately 20 viruses classified as Group A arboviruses, such as Western equine encephalitis (WEE), Eastern equine encephalitis (EEE), and Venezuelan equine encephalitis (VEE).

[C] Detailed structure unknown; values here are the result of "reasonable assumptions."

[D] Includes approximately 40 viruses serologically classified as Group B arboviruses, such as yellow fever, dengue fever, St. Louis encephalitis, and Japanese B encephalitis.

[E] Rubellavirus has been tentatively placed in the family Togaviridae on the basis of its physical and chemical similarities to the other togaviruses.

[F] RNA in 8 pieces, with a total mol. wt. of approximately 5 million daltons.

[G] Very pleomorphic virions.

[H] Characteristically host cell ribosomal RNA is contained also; viral RNA presumably in two pieces of ss RNA with molecular weights of 1.1 and 2.1 million daltons.

[I] Viral RNA presumably a single piece made up of 2 noncovalently linked subunits. Also, many retroviruses contain smaller pieces of RNA, believed to be host cell transfer RNA's and host cell ribosomal RNA's.

[J] Made up of an outer capsid surrounding an inner capsid; actual shape and number of capsomers not known for certain. Different interpretations of electron micrographs have yielded values of 92 to 180 capsomers.

[K] 10 separate pieces of ds RNA; total weight of all pieces is approximately 15 million daltons.

[L] A newly recognized virus structurally different from reoviruses, but containing 10 segmented pieces of ds RNA. Also, occasional enveloped virions have been described, but the envelope does not appear to be necessary for infectivity.

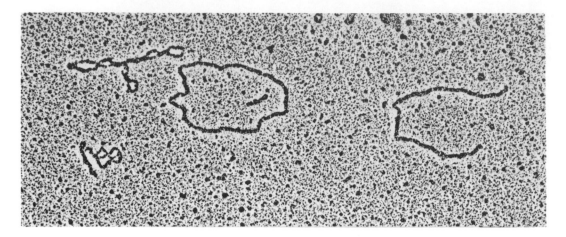

**Figure 31-5.** As shown in this electron micrograph of SV40 DNA, isolated viral DNA may be obtained as linear, circular, or coiled and supercoiled molecules. Supercoils are believed to be artifacts that arise during the isolation procedure as a result of protein removal and ionic strength. The supercoil results from an added twist within one strand of the double-stranded DNA, and if one strand is nicked, the strain is relieved and the molecule assumes a circular form.

DNA may exist within a virion as a linear structure or as a coiled or supercoiled nucleic acid (see Figure 31-5), but it always occurs as a single piece of DNA. Viral RNA may occur as a segmented genome in certain groups of viruses. For example, reovirus contains 10 fragments of ds RNA within each virion, and influenza virus contains eight pieces of ss RNA. Furthermore, the RNA in some viruses, such as the picornaviruses, acts as its own messenger RNA (positive or plus strand) and as a result, cells can be infected directly with the purified viral RNA. Other RNA viruses, such as influenza virus, contain RNA that must first be transcribed into messenger RNA by a viral RNA-dependent RNA polymerase before the virus can replicate. Such RNA is referred to as the negative or minus strand. Still other RNA viruses, such as the oncogenic cancer-producing viruses, must first have their RNA transcribed into DNA by a viral RNA-dependent DNA polymerase before they can replicate within the host cell. It is also interesting to note that many viruses add a long chain of polyadenylic acid (Poly A) to the 3′ end of their mRNA, analogous to that seen in host cell mRNA.

**Viral Envelopes**

We have thus far described a virion as consisting of a protein capsid enclosing the viral nucleic acid and, in some cases, one or more viral enzymes. This combination of capsid and nucleic acid is referred to as the nucleocapsid, and in the case of many animal virus groups, this comprises the completed virion. A large number of animal viruses, however, are surrounded by an additional envelope that they acquire during their final stage of replication as they bud through special areas of the host cell membrane. These special areas of host cell membrane are areas in which the host cell proteins have been replaced by viral-coded polypeptides and virus-specified glycoproteins—although it is likely that the carbohydrate moiety of the glycoproteins is specified by the host cell. Poxviruses provide an exception in that they acquire an outer membrane while still within the cytoplasm of the host cell. The glycoprotein usually occurs as projections or spikes on the outer surface of the envelope. These protrusions have been given the name peplomers.

In addition to protein and glycoprotein the viral envelope contains 20–30% lipid, totally derived from the host cell membrane. The presence of this lipid makes it simple to determine whether or not a virion possesses an envelope. The infectiousness of enveloped viruses is inactivated by lipid solvents such as ether, whereas most viruses existing as naked nucleocapsids are resistant to such treatment. Thus, the viral envelope is structurally similar to the host cell membrane, differing only in that it contains virus-coded proteins and virus-specified glycoproteins. A micrograph of an enveloped virus is shown in Figure 31-6a. Figure 31-6b shows a virus caught in the process of budding.

## CLASSIFICATION OF ANIMAL VIRUSES

As our knowledge of viruses has increased, the properties used to classify them into families, groups, or genera have shifted from the symptomology or pathology of infection to the physical characteristics of the virion. To prevent chaos in the naming of new viruses, an International Committee on Nomenclature of Viruses (ICNV) was set up at the Ninth International Congress for Microbiology in 1966. During the past decade, this committee has set forth the following criteria that it believes should be used for the classification of viruses: (1) the chemical nature of the nucleic acid, *i.e.*, DNA or RNA, single or double-stranded, single or segmented genome, approximate molecular weight of nucleic acid, and whether the virion contains a plus or minus strand of nucleic acid (plus strands of RNA may serve directly as mRNA whereas minus strands of RNA must be transcribed into complementary plus strands before protein synthesis can occur); (2) the symmetry of the nucleocapsid, *i.e.*, isometric or helical; (3) the presence or absence of an envelope; and (4) the number of capsomers for isometric virions, or the diameter of the nucleocapsids for helical viruses.

Based on these criteria, most of the viruses infecting mammalian hosts have been assigned to one of a number of virus families,

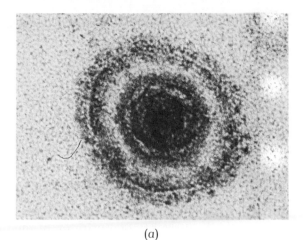

(a)

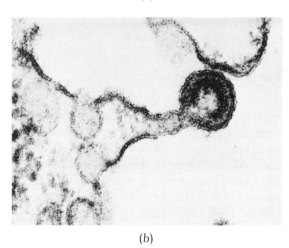

(b)

**Figure 31-6.** *a*. Section through a herpesvirus, showing envelope, capsid, and electron-dense internal DNA (about ×330,000). *b*. A C-type RNA virus budding from an infected cell (×168,000).

and these in turn have been subdivided into one or more genera. Table 31-1 lists the current classification for those DNA viruses that will be discussed in this text along with some of their chemical and physical properties, and Table 31-2 provides this information for the RNA-containing viruses with which we shall be concerned.

It should be emphasized to readers new to the field of medical virology that, although a generic-type classification of viruses is essential to provide a systematic handle for the animal viruses, some of the generic names are new and may be rarely used—especially by the medical virologist who is more likely to refer to many of the viruses by the name of the disease for which they are responsible. This text will briefly introduce the new generic terminology, but our discussions will for the most part utilize those virus names that are more commonly used by the medical virologist.

The following two sections will, therefore, list the recently formed families of animal viruses along with a brief description of the ones that will be discussed later in this text. Refer to Tables 31-1 and 31-2 for names of the newly established genera for each family.

### Families of DNA Viruses

ADENOVIRIDAE. Adenoviruses are large icosahedral viruses that cause various infections in humans. There are 33 known human serotypes, many of which will produce malignant tumors if injected into newborn hamsters. There is no evidence that they cause tumors in humans. They appear to persist in tissues for very long periods of time and in fact were originally isolated from seemingly normal human adenoids, as suggested by their name.

PARVOVIRIDAE. Parvoviruses are small icosahedral viruses that are sometimes referred to as picodnaviruses (pico—small, dna—DNA viruses). The parvoviruses are the only group of animal viruses that contain single-stranded DNA, and even more unusual, some virions will contain the plus strand of DNA, while other virions will contain the complementary minus strand of DNA. (The plus strand of DNA is the strand that is transcribed directly into mRNA). Subgenus A of the genus *Parvovirus* infects mice, rats, and swine, and recent evidence has now implicated a parvovirus-like agent as a cause of acute gastroenteritis in humans (Norwalk agent). Moreover, although it has not yet been cultivated, pre-

liminary evidence suggests that the etiologic agent of human infectious heptatis (hepatitis A) may be a parvovirus.

Subgenus B contains defective viruses called adeno-associated viruses; these viruses are unable to replicate even within susceptible cells and can grow only if they coinfect a cell with a helper adenovirus. Thus, they are found in association with adenoviruses, but are not known to cause disease in humans.

PAPOVAVIRIDAE. Papovaviruses are small double-stranded DNA viruses that have the ability to induce tumors. Human wart virus (*Papillomavirus*) and *Polyomavirus,* simian virus 40 (SV40), belong to this family. Polyomaviruses are known to produce a variety of cancers in susceptible animals, such as mice and hamsters. The papillomaviruses cause warts on the skin or mucous membranes in humans, rabbits, cows, pigs, dogs, and other animals.

HERPETOVIRIDAE. Herpesviruses are large, enveloped icosahedral viruses that cause a rather wide variety of infections in humans and other animals. The most common human diseases include fever blisters, chickenpox, and zoster (also known as shingles). Cytomegalovirus, a herpesvirus, causes serious congenital infections frequently manifested by mental retardation and defects of the central nervous system. Some herpesviruses are known to induce cancer in chickens, frogs, monkeys, and rabbits. Although there has been much speculation concerning the role of herpesvirus in human cancer, no indisputable proof is available at this time. There is, however, circumstantial evidence that a herpesvirus may be involved in a type of human cancer called Burkitt's lymphoma, and, curiously, this same herpesvirus appears to be the etiologic agent for infectious mononucleosis.

POXVIRIDAE. The poxviruses comprise a very large group of complex viruses that have been subdivided into six genera based primarily on the animal hosts that they infect. The human poxviruses (*Orthopoxvirus*) include the etiologic agent of smallpox as well as vaccinia and related viruses. Poxviruses are large oval-shaped or brick-shaped viruses that do not morphologically resemble either icosahedral or helical viruses; some of the genera share a common antigen, while others are included because of their morphologic similarities.

### Families of RNA Viruses

PICORNAVIRIDAE. The family Picornaviridae contains two genera that cause human disease. The members of the genus *Enterovirus* are transmitted to humans primarily via a fecal-oral route, and, although diarrhea may be the major result of most enteroviral infections, many can invade the blood stream and infect the central nervous system, causing aseptic meningitis and occasionally paralysis. Common human enteroviruses include the polioviruses, coxsackie viruses, and echoviruses (Enteric Cytopathic Human Orphan viruses).

The second genus of Picornaviridae, *Rhinovirus,* causes a great deal of misery in humans since it encompasses the major etiologic agents of the common cold. These viruses are morphologically identical to the enteroviruses but are much more labile to acid, being inactivated in one hour at pH 3–5 at 37°C. There are over 100 different serotypes of rhinoviruses, which undoubtedly accounts for the "commonness" of the common cold.

TOGAVIRIDAE. Togaviridae is the name given to a family of single-stranded RNA viruses possessing icosahedral symmetry. All are surrounded by a lipoprotein envelope—hence the prefix "toga" meaning coat or mantle. Included in this family are many of the arboviruses (arthropod-borne viruses). There are over 250 different arboviruses, all of which are transmitted from animal to animal (including humans) by a blood-sucking

arthropod vector. Mosquitoes and ticks are the usual vectors, and birds are the reservoir for many of these viruses. A few of the more common arboviral diseases are eastern equine encephalitis (EEE), western equine encephalitis (WEE), Venezuelan equine encephalitis (VEE), St. Louis encephalitis (SLE), and Japanese B encephalitis (JE). Yellow fever and dengue are also included in this group of viruses. On the basis of physicochemical similarities, rubella virus, the causative agent of German measles, is also classified with the togaviruses, although it is not carried by arthropods.

ORTHOMYXOVIRIDAE. Until recently, *Orthomyxovirus* has been the generic name for the viruses that cause influenza, but this genus has now been renamed as *Influenzavirus*. These agents are enveloped virions possessing helical symmetry. Projecting from their envelope are two different kinds of peplomers (spikes). One is called a hemagglutinin (HA) because it will react with a glycoprotein present on the surface of red blood cells, causing them to agglutinate. The second peplomer of the influenzaviruses is an enzyme called neuraminidase that can liberate neuraminic acid from the red blood cell glycoprotein, causing the spontaneous elution of the virus from the agglutinated red blood cells. Another characteristic of the influenzaviruses is that their single-stranded RNA exists within the virion in eight pieces. Furthermore, the RNA within the virion is the minus strand and thus cannot act as mRNA until it has been transcribed into the plus strand by a self-contained viral transcriptase (RNA-dependent RNA-polymerase).

PARAMYXOVIRIDAE. The paramyxoviruses include several animal pathogens such as Newcastle disease virus, simian virus 5, and five serotypes of parainfluenza virus that cause a mild respiratory disease in humans. These enveloped viruses possess a helical symmetry, but they can be rather pleomorphic (forming occasional filamentous virions); like the influenzaviruses, they carry a hemagglutinin and a neuraminidase on their surface. Paramyxovirus RNA exists as a single long minus strand that must be transcribed into messenger RNA by a viral transcriptase. The major human pathogens in this family are measles virus and respiratory syncytial virus.

RHABDOVIRIDAE. Rhabdoviruses are enveloped helical viruses that are characteristically bullet-shaped. The two best-studied members of this family are rabies virus and vesicular stomatitis virus (a pathogen for cattle). There are, however, many other rhabdoviruses, including a number of fish pathogens. The rhabdoviruses also carry the minus strand of RNA and, hence, their own RNA transcriptase.

BUNYAVIRIDAE. This family of viruses has been known for a number of years as the Bunyamwera supergroup. It comprises a large number of the arthropod-borne viruses, but unlike the togaviruses, the Bunyamwera supergroup is made up of helical viruses containing single-stranded RNA that probably exists in several segments. Presently they are all lumped into a single genus, *Bunyavirus,* but several other genera will probably be defined later.

ARENAVIRIDAE. Arenaviruses were originally grouped together because of their morphologic similarities, but little is known concerning their detailed structure. A common characteristic shared by the arenaviruses is that they all appear to contain a few host cell ribosomes within the viral capsid. The best studied arenavirus is lymphocytic choriomeningitis virus, which characteristically produces an asymptomatic infection in mice and occasionally causes meningitis in humans. Much more serious diseases produced by this group of viruses are the hemorrhagic fevers seen in South America.

CORONAVIRIDAE. Coronaviruses are enveloped RNA viruses that are so named because of the petal-like projections surrounding the envelope. They have been isolated from humans and other animals with upper respiratory disease.

RETROVIRIDAE. Retroviridae is the family name given to the RNA tumor viruses that were formerly called the leukoviruses or oncornaviruses. These viruses produce leukemias and sarcomas in birds and rodents. The symmetry of the capsid is not known, but the viral RNA appears to exist in several pieces that are noncovalently bound to each other—probably through complementary base pairing of short lengths of their RNA. One unusual property of these viruses is that they must first synthesize DNA complementary to the virion RNA before they can replicate. The virions accordingly contain an enzyme, called an RNA-dependent DNA-polymerase, that is often referred to as reverse transcriptase. It is because of this unusual method of replication that these viruses have been named retroviruses.

REOVIRIDAE. Reoviridae is a family of viruses that contains a genome of double-stranded RNA. The family comprises two recognized genera, *Reovirus* and *Orbivirus,* both of whose ds RNA is segmented into ten pieces within the virion. Reoviruses possess a double icosahedral capsid, but there is disagreement concerning the number of capsomers in the outer capsid. They are involved in mild respiratory infections in humans, but are also found in the human intestinal tract. In note of the fact that they are frequently not associated with disease, they are given the designation "Reo" (Respiratory Enteric Orphan).

Orbiviruses are arboviruses which possess an icosahedral capsid made up of 32 quite large, doughnut-shaped capsomers. They are primarily animal pathogens, causing diseases such as blue-tongue in cattle and a serious diarrhea in newborn calves, pigs, and mice.

A recently recognized virus that causes a severe human diarrhea, particularly in infants, also appears to belong to the family

Reoviridae. This virus has been given the tentative name of rotavirus by some virologists, while others refer to it as duovirus.

It should now be apparent that these "simple forms of life" are really not at all so simple and that in order to grow viruses in the laboratory it is necessary to provide a source of living susceptible host cells in which they can replicate. These procedures have become commonplace during the past several decades, and they will be discussed in some detail in the following chapter.

## REFERENCES

Dalton, A. J., and F. Hagoenau, eds. 1973. *Ultrastructure of Animal Viruses and Bacteriophages: An Altas.* Academic Press, New York.

Diener, T. O. 1974. Viroids: The smallest known agents of infectious disease. *Annu. Rev. Microbiol.* **28**:23–29.

Fenner, F. 1974. The classification of viruses: why, when and how. *Aust. J. Exp. Biol. Med. Sci.* **52**:223–250.

Fenner, F. 1976. The classification and nomenclature of viruses. *Intervirology* **6**:1–12.

Fraenkel-Conrat, H. 1974. Descriptive catalogue of viruses. In H. Fraenkel-Conrat and R. R. Wagner, eds. *Comprehensive Virology*, Vol. 1. Plenum Press, New York.

Gibbs, A. J., ed. 1973. *Viruses and Invertebrates.* North Holland Pub., Amsterdam.

Horne, R. W. 1974. *Virus Structure.* Academic Press, New York.

Melnick. J. L. 1975. Taxonomy of viruses. *Progr. Med. Virol.* **20**:208–211.

Rifkin, D. B., and J. P. Quigley. 1974. Virus-induced modification of cellular membranes related to viral structure. *Annu. Rev. Microbiol.* **28**:325–351.

# 32

## Growth, Purification, and Characteristics of Animal Viruses

**CELLS USED IN THE STUDY OF
ANIMAL VIRUSES**

Growth of viruses requires susceptible host cells capable of replicating the virus. The studies of early virologists were restricted to the use of whole animals from which they obtained virus from the blood or tissues. As scientists learned to grow animal cells in culture, however, the use of whole animals has been largely replaced by cell cultures consisting of animal cells.

Animal cell cultures can be classified either as primary cell cultures, diploid cell cultures, or permanent cell lines. Primary cell cultures used for the propagation of viruses may be obtained directly from an animal organ as follows: (1) the organ (e.g., monkey kidney) is minced and treated with trypsin to separate the cells; (2) the cells are dispersed into sterile tubes or dishes and covered with a serum containing a buffered growth medium; (3) after the cells have adhered to the surface of the container, they can be infected with the virus one wishes to propagate. Unlike a bacterial culture that can be transferred indefinitely, primary cell cultures can be subcultured at most five to ten times, after which they will die.

The second type of cell culture, diploid cell strains, can be derived from human embryonic tissue. They possess a normal chromosome karyotype (chromosome number and appearance) and will grow at a fairly constant rate. Diploid cell cultures can be grown for a number of generations; however, they will die after 40 to 50 generations.

During the growth of diploid cell strains, rare mutations may occur which give rise to a permanent cell line, capable of being cultivated for an unlimited number of generations. Stable cell lines of this type, however, possess an altered morphology from the parent cell culture and are more like cells derived from malignant tumors.

Cells derived from cancer tissue or which have been transformed into cancer cells by chemicals or oncogenic viruses can also be cultivated for an unlimited number of generations. Permanent cell lines of this type differ from diploid cells in that some will grow in suspension, and that they will frequently produce tumors if injected into susceptible animals. Table 32-1 lists some stable representative cell lines commercially available and the original source of the tissue from which they were isolated. Such cell lines (as well as diploid strains) may be kept frozen for

**Table 32-1. Selected Commercially Available Cell Lines**

| Cell Line | Source |
| --- | --- |
| Hela | Human carcinoma of the cervix |
| HEp-2 | Human carcinoma of the larynx |
| L-132 | Human embryonic lung |
| Raji | Human Burkitt lymphoma |
| RPMI 8226 | Human myeloma |
| WI-38 | Human normal diploid female |
| MDCK | Dog kidney |
| BHK-21 | Hamster kidney |
| BS-C-1 | African Green monkey kidney |
| LLC-MK$_2$ | Rhesus monkey kidney |
| MOPC-31-C | Mouse plasmacytoma |
| 3T3 | Mouse embryonic fibroblast |
| RTG-2 | Rainbow trout gonadal tissue |
| LLC-RK$_1$ | Rabbit kidney |
| P1-1-Ut | Racoon uterus |
| XC | Rat sarcoma |
| IgH-2 | Iguana heart |

Chick embryos and to a lesser extent duck embryos are also used for the propagation of certain viruses. Figure 32-1 shows a two-week-old chick embryo. The embryo is immersed in a fluid enclosed by the amniotic membrane, and this in turn is enclosed in a cavity that is bounded by the chorioallantoic membrane. Viruses can be inoculated directly into the allantoic or the amniotic cavity where they will grow in the corresponding membrane cells. After four to six days, the released viruses can be harvested from the respective fluid. Several viral vaccines, including influenza and mumps vaccines, are produced in this manner. Some viruses, such as herpesviruses and poxviruses, can be placed directly on the chorioallantoic membrane where they will produce pock-like lesions on the membrane.

very long periods of time, and after thawing, will begin to grow again.

The cell line most widely used during the past 25 years was derived from a cervical carcinoma of a black woman named Henrietta Lacks. This line, appropriately named Hela, has been extensively studied, and it can be cytologically differentiated from other cell lines because of the fusion of several normal chromosomes and because of the presence of an isoenzyme of glucose-6-phosphate dehydrogenase that does not occur in Caucasian cells but exists in the cells of approximately 30% of the Negro race. Interestingly, when these techniques were employed to study a wide variety of human cell lines currently in use, almost half of them appeared to be contaminated with the widely used Hela cell line. It is therefore obvious that, like bacterial cultures, one cell line can easily contaminate another culture, and scrupulous care must be used if more than one cell line is being used in a laboratory.

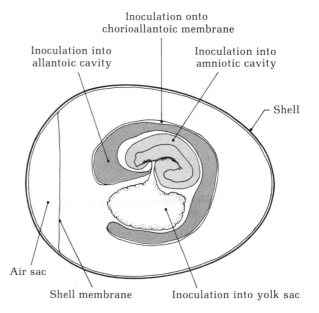

**Figure 32-1.** A chick embryo may be inoculated with virus suspension into the yolk sac, the amniotic cavity, the allantoic cavity, or directly onto the chorioallantoic membrane. In all cases the viruses grow in the membrane cells surrounding the cavity inoculated.

## REPLICATION OF VIRUSES

Viral multiplication in each infected cell occurs as a result of a series of independent events culminated by the assembly of the viral nucleic acid, viral protein, and any other viral components. The details of these reproductive steps vary for each type of virus, and will be discussed in some detail in subsequent chapters on the major viral families. However, we shall give here the general sequence of events.

1. Adsorption of the virion to specific receptor sites on the cell surface is probably the most specific reaction between virus and host cell. A cell lacking such receptor sites is resistant to infection by the virus.

2. Penetration of the virus occurs either by engulfment or phagocytosis of the intact virion (called viropexis) or by fusion of the viral envelope with the host cell membrane, allowing only the nucleocapsid to enter the cell. (Note the difference from the infection of a bacterium with bacteriophage, in which only the phage nucleic acid is injected into the infected cell.)

3. Uncoating occurs; the viral nucleic acid is released from the capsid and is accessible to enzymes necessary either to translate, transcribe, or replicate it. This process varies from one virus to another. In some cases the entire viral nucleic acid may be released; in others, parts are released at different times resulting in early and late transcription events; in still others the transcriptase appears able to function within a semi-intact nucleocapsid structure. The time from the uncoating until the assembly of mature virions is referred to as the eclipse period, because, if one were to rupture the host cell, no infectious virions would be found.

4. Transcription of the viral nucleic acid into messenger RNA (mRNA) is the next step for all viruses except those RNA viruses such as the picornaviruses whose viral RNA acts directly as mRNA. In the case of some complex viruses such as the poxviruses, one sees only part of the viral DNA transcribed at one time. The mRNA systhesized before the replication of viral DNA commences is called early mRNA, while late mRNA is made after the replication of DNA is underway. In general, early mRNA is used for the synthesis of early enzymes that are necessary for viral replication. Late mRNA, on the other hand, is most frequently translated into the structural proteins of the virion. The mRNA transcribed from most DNA viruses is usually very long and includes the message from several DNA genes on one molecule. However, before leaving the cell nucleus, this mRNA is cleaved into single gene products and a strand of 100 to 150 adenine molecules is added to the 3' end of each mRNA. This poly-A mRNA then enters the cytoplasm and is ready to be translated into protein. Those RNA viruses (orthomyxoviruses, paramyxoviruses, rhabdoviruses) that carry the minus strand of RNA must first transcribe their RNA to the plus strand before it can function as the viral mRNA. Poly-A is usually added to the 3' end before the message is translated.

5. Translation of mRNA into viral proteins occurs in the cytoplasm using ribosomes, transfer RNA's, and enzymes from the host cell. The translation of the mRNA yields one polypeptide which, in some cases, is subsequently cleaved into individual viral polypeptides.

6. Replication of viral nucleic acid begins as soon as the necessary viral polymerases have been translated from the viral mRNA. In the case of DNA viruses, this appears to occur by complementary base pairing in a manner identical to that occurring in host cells. The replication of the nucleic acid in RNA viruses is unique and will be discussed in greater detail in the chapters on the RNA viruses. In short, the single-stranded viral RNA must first form a complementary RNA (cRNA) which can then be simultaneously transcribed by a number of polymerase molecules to release viral RNA (vRNA). The

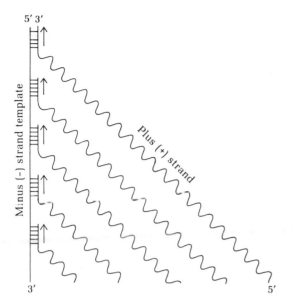

5' 3'

Minus (−) strand template

plus (+) strand

3'                    5'

**Figure 32-2.** Multiple plus strands of viral RNA simultaneously synthesized from one minus strand template. This structure is called a replicative intermediate.

synthesis of multiple vRNA molecules from a single cRNA template is depicted in Figure 32-2, and the entire structure is called a replicative intermediate (RI).

7. Assembly of the various viral components into nucleocapsids occurs shortly after the replication of the viral nucleic acid. This appears to be a self-assembly process not requiring energy, in which the virion is completed when the nucleic acid becomes enclosed within the capsid. In the case of the helical viruses, however, the capsid becomes assembled by incorporating the capsomers around the completed nucleic acid.

8. Release of the completed virions is the final step in virus multiplication. Those viruses that exist as naked nucleocapsids may be released by the lysis of the host cell, or they may be extruded by a process that could be called reverse phagocytosis. Enveloped viruses are released by budding through special areas of the host cell membrane where proteins and glycoproteins coded by

the virus have replaced those normally present in the host cell membrane. Bearing in mind the differences between groups, the above steps in viral replication are summarized in Figure 32-3.

## ASSAY OF VIRUSES

There are many methods for estimating the numbers of viruses, but essentially all of them depend upon diluting a virus suspension so that a measurable aliquot will contain a countable number of infectious virions. This aspect of the assay is identical to that done in the dilution method for enumerating bacteria. However, viruses must be grown in susceptible cells, and the infectious centers that develop are the entities that are actually counted. It is this latter technique that will vary depending upon the effect of the virus on its host cell. In general, various dilutions of virus are placed on the surface of a monolayer of susceptible cells. After allowing about an hour for the viruses to adsorb and penetrate, the entire surface is covered with medium containing agar to prevent free movement of released virions. In this manner, only the cells immediately adjacent to an infected cell are subsequently infected by newly synthesized viruses, and, at the end of several days, one will have a small plaque consisting of dead cells at each place that a virion infected a host cell. The assay can also be done by allowing a dilution of a virus to infect a suspension of cells; after adsorption and penetration of the virus the suspension is layered into a sterile petri dish or other appropriate container and covered with agar to prevent viral dissemination throughout the culture.

One need only count the number of infected areas of host cells and multiply that number by the viral dilution to calculate the number of infectious particles in the original material. Depending upon the ultimate fate of the infected cell, this may be rather simple, or it may require special techniques to locate infected areas. In those cases in which host

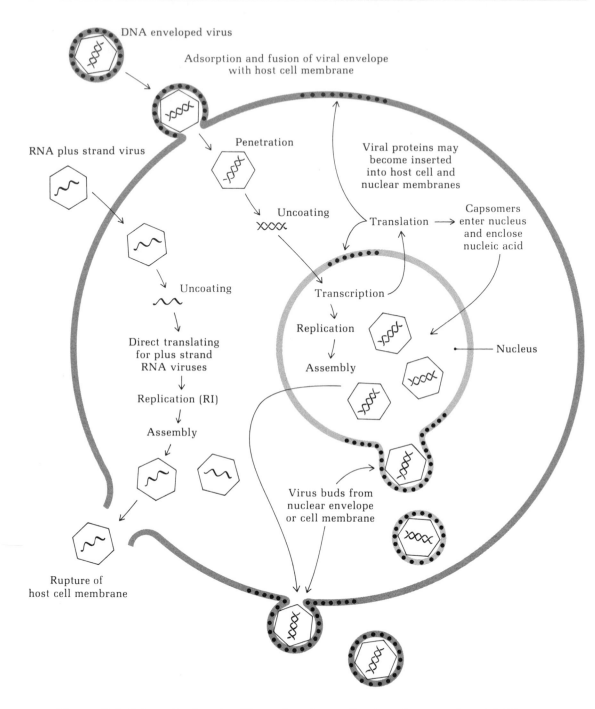

**Figure 32-3.** Schematic drawing illustrating the replication of an enveloped DNA virus and an RNA plus strand virus. Note, however, that with some DNA viruses, such as small-pox virus, the replication occurs solely in the cytoplasm of the host cell. In this and similar drawings of viral replication in the chapters to follow, the outer membrane of the nuclear envelope has been omitted for clarity.

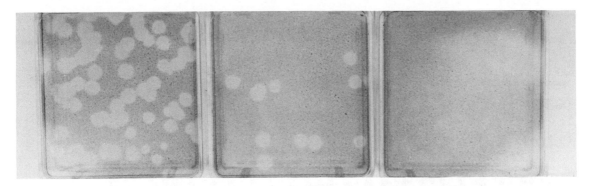

**Figure 32-4.** In the left and center flasks areas of duck embryo cells have been killed by viruses, as shown by the clear areas surrounded by living cells stained with neutral red. On the right is an uninfected culture of stained duck embryo cells.

cells are killed by the infection, the layer of cells can be stained with a vital dye such as neutral red. Living cells take up the dye, while dead cells remain colorless. Thus, each infected area appears as a colorless plaque, as shown in Figure 32-4. The histological changes that occur as a result of damage and death of the host cell are known as cytopathic effect (CPE) and the infecting virus is said to be cytopathic. Plaques caused by viruses which do not kill their host cells must be located by different means. For those viruses with receptors for red blood cells, one can flood the culture plate with red blood cells and after an appropriate time count the plaques where hemadsorption has occurred, in other words, where red blood cells adhere to the infected cells. Fluorescent antibody to the virus may be used in a similar manner, with the sites of fluorescence counted. Oncogenic viruses (those viruses that transform host cells into cancer cells) may be enumerated by counting the plaques of morphologically transformed cells. In any case, the final number of infectious virions is expressed as plaque-forming units (pfu).

A relative quantitation of viruses which possess hemagglutinins (for example, orthomyxoviruses and paramyxoviruses) can be obtained using techniques similar to those used for antibody titration. The viral suspension is serially diluted 10 or 12 times, and red blood cells are added to each dilution. The reciprocal of the highest dilution of virus which will still cause hemagglutination is referred to as the hemagglutination titer. As shown in Figure 32-5, hemagglutinated red blood cells show a diffuse area of agglutination, whereas nonagglutinated cells settle as a small compact button on the bottom of the well.

One can visualize the number of virus particles with an electron microscope, but this would be of value only with a highly purified suspension of virus particles. Moreover, electron microscopy gives a total number of physical particles, but not all particles may be infective. Hence, it usually gives a much higher value than the plaque method, which measures only infective virions.

Finally, for those viruses that do not form plaques, one can inoculate serial dilutions of virus into embryonated eggs or animals and observe for the death of the host. This type of measurement, called a quantal assay, does not actually measure the number of infectious particles in a suspension but rather determines the extent to which a virus suspension can be diluted and still contain infectious viruses.

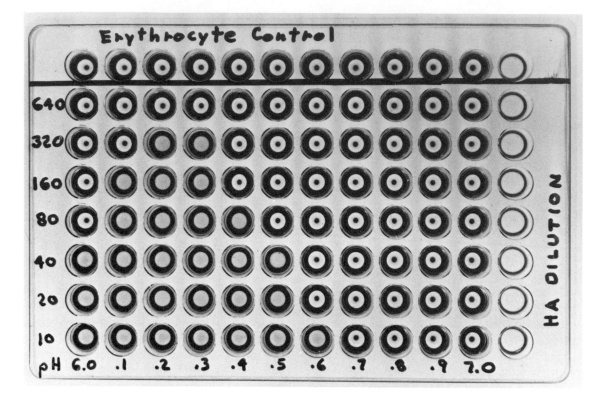

**Figure 32-5.** Microtiter plate showing hemagglutination. Numbers to the left are the reciprocal of the antigen dilution. (The antigen here is western equine encephalitis virus.) Across the bottom on this plate are the pH values of the diluent in which the erythrocytes are suspended. A button of cells in the center of a well indicates no agglutination; therefore the erythrocyte controls across the top—containing cells but no antigen—are satisfactory. Western encephalitis virus is seen to have a titer of 1:40 at pH 6.0, 1:160 at pH 6.1, 1:320 at pH 6.2 and 6.3, 1:80 at pH 6.4, 1:40 at pH 6.5, 1:10 at pH 6.6, and less than 1:10 at higher pH values.

## REACTION OF HOST CELL
## TO VIRAL INFECTION

In the introduction to Unit Four we enumerated some reactions of the host cell to viral infection, which are summarized in Table 32-2. It can be seen that some viruses may produce different effects depending on the type of host cell infected.

In addition, some viruses produce intracellular inclusions in the infected host cell. These "inclusion bodies" are frequently but not always areas of viral assembly, and their intracellular location and appearance is constant for a particular virus. As a result, many inclusion bodies have been given specific names, and their appearance within a cell is a diagnostic criterion for infection. Figure 32-6 shows one such body.

A more subtle effect of viral infection is the subsequent interference of a later infection by other viruses. This interference may be quite specific, being manifested only by the prevention of a subsequent infection by a closely related virus, or it may be of a type in which the host cell is induced to

**Table 32-2. Reaction of Host Cell
to Viral Infection**

| Reaction | Representative Viruses Causing These Effects |
|---|---|
| Death of host cell | Most viruses |
| Proliferation of host cells | Poxvirus, Papovaviruses Papillomavirus |
| Fusion of membranes of adjacent cells to form multinucleate hybrid cells | Respiratory syncytial virus Measles virus Sendai virus Herpesvirus |
| Transformation of normal cells into malignant cancer cells | Polyomaviruses Herpesvirus Adenovirus RNA oncogenic viruses |
| No histologic change in host cell appearance for several weeks | Rubella virus Some adenoviruses |

produce and secrete a substance which protects uninfected cells from a wide spectrum of viruses.

## VIRAL INTERFERENCE

The infection of a cell by a virus frequently results in that cell becoming resistant to infections by other viruses. This resistance is due to interference by the primary infecting virus, and it can be manifested in several different ways. One obvious type occurs when the virus causing the initial infection destroys or alters the receptor sites of the host cell. Such an effect renders the cell resistant to infection by closely related viruses which require similar receptor sites. Examples are seen following the infection of chicken cells with leukemia viruses which destroy the receptors for Rous sarcoma virus, or the treatment of cells with ultra-violet-light-irradiated Newcastle disease viruses, which remove host cell neuraminic acid and render the host cell resistant to infection by other paramyxoviruses. How-

ever, because this is effective only against closely related viruses that require the same receptor site, one would not expect this type of interference to be a major mechanism of controlling virus infections.

A more important type of viral interference was first described in 1951 by von Magnus, who reported that the infection of chick embryos with an undiluted influenza virus suspension resulted in a markedly decreased yield of infectious virus. Furthermore, if a harvested suspension of low infectivity was mixed with a high titer virus preparation, it interfered with the growth of the highly infective influenza virus preparation. An explanation for these observations (known as the von Magnus phenomenon) emerged when it was discovered that the low infectivity influenza suspension contained a large number of virus particles that possessed less nucleoprotein per virion than did the high infectivity influenza particles and that these incomplete defective particles interfered with the growth of the standard virus.

It is now known that essentially all virus–cell systems produce varying amounts of incomplete viruses which contain only part of the virus genome (see Figure 32-7). These particles interfere with the replication of complete virions, and are called defective-interfering particles (DI). Infection of cells with high concentrations of virus (as was done originally by von Magnus) is not essential for the production of DI, but since DI can replicate only when a host cell is coinfected with a complete virion, the use of high concentrations of virus insures that most cells become infected with both a DI and a complete virion. Little is known concerning the mechanism whereby DI is preferentially replicated over that of standard virus. It may be that DI from different viruses have different mechanisms of interference. This is suggested by reports that the DI from vesicular stomatitis virus inhibits the replication of standard viral RNA and that from poliovirus inhibits the

456

GROWTH, PURIFICATION, AND CHARACTERISTICS OF ANIMAL VIRUSESGROWTH, PURIFICATION, AND CHARACTERISTICS OF ANIMAL VIRUSES

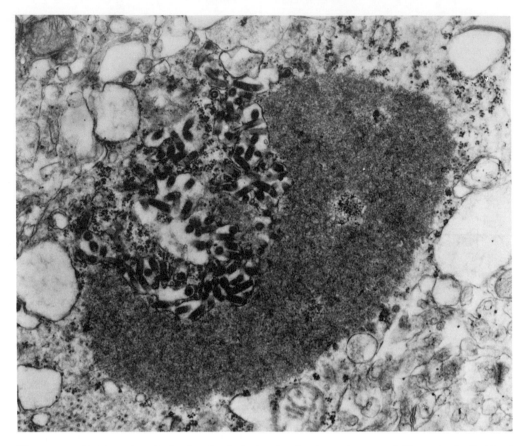

**Figure 32-6.** Rabies virus inclusion body in fox brain tissue ($\times$50,000). Note the individual virions in close proximity to the inclusion.

production of capsids by the host cell. As more is learned, however, it seems possible that a common step in viral replication may prove to be involved and that it is only the final manifestation of this interference which varies from one viral system to another.

The importance of DI in the usual viral infection (as proposed by Alice Huang) is illustrated in Figure 32-8. This model shows that when the number of viral particles becomes high, DI are produced and the number of infective virions is drastically decreased. In the case of viral diseases, specific host defenses would usually prevent a resurgence of viral growth; however, in the absence of such a response, virus growth again increases until the production of DI interferes with the production of standard virions. Passages 16 to 34 in the figure repre-

sent subacute or persistent infections in which host defenses are unable to completely eliminate the infection. Thus, DI may act as a normal regulator for the control of virus replication.

## INTERFERON–TYPE INTERFERENCE

Interferon-mediated resistance is the result of the production of a protein coded in the genome of the infected animal cell. This type of interference was originally described when it was discovered that allantoic fluid obtained from a chick embryo infected with influenza virus would prevent the subsequent infection of uninfected chick embryos. In other words, something was produced during the initial infection that, when injected into other chick embryos, made

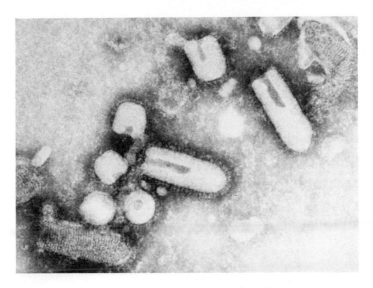

**Figure 32-7.** Electron micrograph of defective-interfering (DI) particles and normal virions of vesicular stomatitis virus (VSV). The much shorter DI particles can be readily differentiated from the elongated, bullet-shaped virions. Note also the helical nucleoprotein visible in one virion. (×144,300.)

them resistant to viral infection. Interferon was later shown to be a soluble protein produced by cells infected with almost any animal virus and, furthermore, produced both in tissue culture and in an intact animal.

An interesting property of interferon is that it is not virus-specific; rather, it is host-species specific. This means that the interferon produced by chick embryo cells infected with influenza virus is effective in preventing the infection of other chick embryo cells with almost any virus. On the other hand, interferon produced in a mouse as a result of virus infection is effective in protecting other mice from a virus infection but of little value when used with chicken or human cells. In fact, interferons from different host cells vary in their molecular weight as well as other physical properties. Thus, one can generalize by stating that interferon inhibits viral replication most effectively in the species in which it was produced and that it is nonspecific with respect to the types of viruses it can inhibit.

Interferon is secreted in exceedingly small amounts by the virus-infected cell.

**Figure 32-8.** A model for the oscillating interactions between standard virus and DI particles during continuous passage. Note that when the concentration of DI becomes high, standard virus falls, followed by DI. Once the number of DI particles falls to a certain level, standard virus can again increase to begin another cycle. It is proposed that passages 16–34 may represent subacute or persistent infections in which host responses do not completely eliminate the infectious agent.

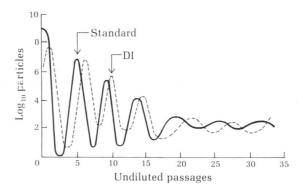

**Figure 32-9.** *a.* Translation inhibition model of interferon action. One or a few molecules of interferon (1) act to derepress a host cell cistron, initiating transcription of the mRNA, TIP-mRNA (2), which encodes for the translation inhibitory protein (TIP). TIP in turn is synthesized and accumulates in the cytoplasm (3), where it binds to ribosomes and contributes TIP units to the ribosome pool (4). Polysomes composed of TIP-ribosomes and host cell mRNA are translated normally (5), whereas polysomes formed from TIP-ribosomes and viral mRNA are not translated (6), producing a state of interferon-mediated interference. *b.* Transcription inhibition model of interferon action. Interferon (1) acts to derepress a cell cistron, initiating transcription of the mRNA, AVP-mRNA (2), which encodes for the antiviral protein (AVP) (3). AVP then binds to the viral RNA polymerase (4), preventing transcription of viral RNA and thus producing a state of interferon-mediated interference.

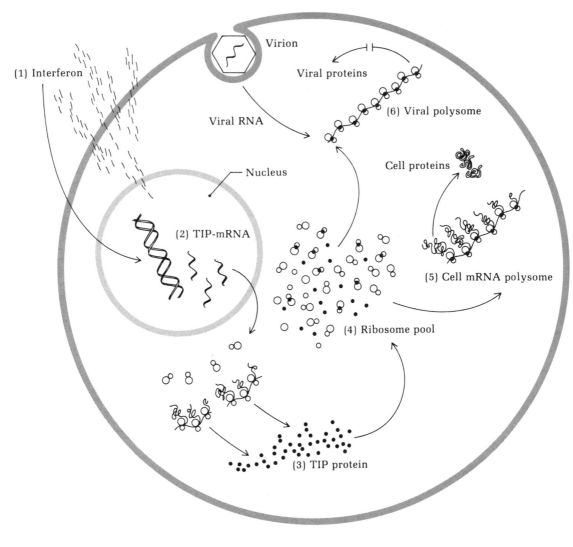

(a)

It is inactive against viruses in cell free extracts, and only after it enters or reacts with an animal cell can it exert its antiviral activity. There is disagreement concerning its mode of action, and some investigators have good evidence that the ultimate effect of interferon is to inhibit the translation of viral mRNA, while other researchers have convincing data that interferon blocks the transcription of viral RNA. In either case, it is generally assumed that interferon reacts with a repressor in the cell in a manner similar to the mechanism explained for inducible enzymes (Chapter 7). This allows the cell to synthesize a new antiviral protein which acts directly to inhibit translation or transcription.

Experiments suggesting that translation is the ultimate target for the inhibiting effect of interferon have shown that ribosomes isolated from interferon-treated cells could combine with viral mRNA but could not translate it. These same ribosomes, however, were able to translate host cell mRNA. These investigators concluded that the antiviral protein (also called "translation inhibitory protein") combined with the ribosome in a manner that specifically

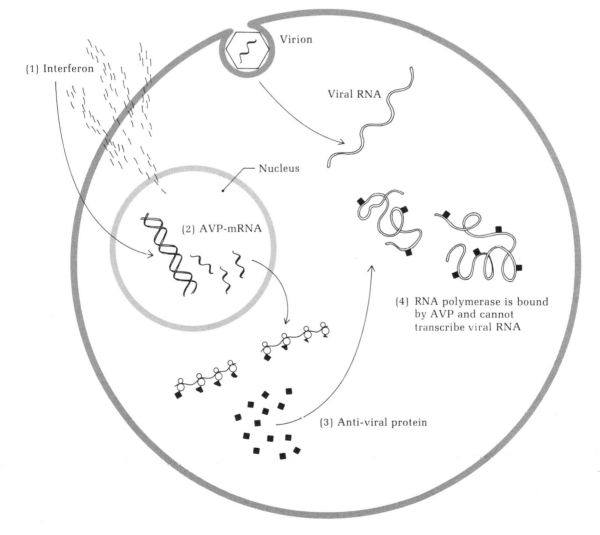

(b)

prevented the ribosome from translating viral mRNA.

Data supporting the conclusion that transcription of viral RNA is the step inhibited by interferon are also convincing. A model for this concept proposes that the antiviral protein (synthesized by the interferon-treated cell) reacts with the viral RNA polymerase. Thus, viruses possessing their own RNA polymerase are blocked immediately, while those such as the togaviruses and picornaviruses are blocked after synthesis of their RNA polymerase. Figure 32-9 has schematic diagrams summarizing the two explanations proposed for the inhibition of viral replication by interferon.

Regardless of the specific step that is blocked by interferon, its possible therapeutic value is being investigated in many laboratories throughout the world. The production of interferon for use in the treatment or prevention of viral diseases seems almost impossible because, in the first place, the interferon must be produced in humans or in human cells to be effective in humans, and, in the second place, the amounts produced are exceedingly small. A far more promising approach is to use some nontoxic material which, when injected into an individual, would cause that person to synthesize interferon. It has been found that double-stranded RNA will act as an inducer for interferon. Moreover, the best inducer yet found is a synthetic polynucleotide called poly-IC. This is a small double-stranded RNA molecule consisting of paired homopolymer (all the same base) strands of polyriboinosinic acid (poly-I), and its complementary base, polyribocytidylic acid (poly-C).

In tests with mice, a small quantity of poly IC was instilled into their nostrils; all survived a lethal dose of pneumonia virus of mice (PVM). In tests with humans, interferon could be detected in the blood as early as two hours after the injection of poly-IC, and persisted in some patients as long as 72 hours. Although there did not seem to be serious clinical symptoms following the injection of poly-IC into humans, there was a marked rise in temperature.

Other nonviral inducers of interferon have been described, of which bacterial endotoxins have been the most intensively studied. Endotoxin-induced interferon appears earlier and is more heat and acid-labile than virus or poly-IC-induced interferon. There is also evidence that endotoxin-induced interferon is specifically synthesized and released by macrophages. Preliminary data suggest that different inducers stimulate different cell types to produce interferon, resulting in a heterogenous mixture of interferons.

An unusual application of interferon has been reported from Scandinavia, in which interferon isolated from human leukocytes was successfully used to treat patients with osteogenic sarcoma. At this time, the number of persons so treated is too small to draw final conclusions concerning the efficacy of interferon therapy for this malignancy, but early results appear promising. In addition, interferon treatment is being tried for a number of serious diseases, some known to be caused by viruses, and others only potential virus infections. These include cytomegalovirus infections in neonates (Chapter 33), herpesvirus infections of the eye (Chapter 33), hepatitis (Chapter 36), and breast cancer.

## PURIFICATION OF VIRUSES

The ability to grow viruses in tissue culture has made it possible to obtain large amounts of very pure virions. The methods by which viruses are purified from the culture medium will vary from one virus to another, but in general the following basic techniques are used: (1) precipitation of the virus using either salts or organic solvents, (2) column chromatography of the partially concentrated virus, and (3) ultracentrifugation.

Purification using centrifugation may be done with either rate zonal centrifugation or isopycnic (equilibrium density) centrifugation. Rate zonal centrifugation is achieved by carefully filling a centrifuge tube with a solution of sucrose or glycerol that is added in a linear decreasing concentration to the tube. When filled, the contents of the centrifuge tube will have a continuous increase in density from the top to the bottom of the tube. A virus suspension is then carefully layered over the top of the gradient, and the tube is subjected to high-speed centrifugation. The rate at which the virus sediments through the gradient is a function of its size and weight. The centrifuge is stopped when the band of virus has moved part way through the gradient, and a hole is punched in the bottom or side of the centrifuge tube to collect the contents in a series of fractions. Isopycnic, or equilibrium density, centrifugation is done by suspending the virus preparation in a solution of an alkali metal chloride, such as cesium chloride. When such a solution is subjected to high-speed centrifugation, a gradient is automatically established during the time of centrifugation, and the virus will form a narrow band in the centrifuge tube at that depth where its buoyant density exactly equals the density of the solution in which it is being centrifuged. The band of virus, free of host cell proteins and nucleic acids, can then be collected as described above and further purified by dialysis or gel filtration.

A simpler technique may be used for the partial purification of viruses that hemagglutinate and subsequently spontaneously elute from red blood cells. Orthomyxoviruses or paramyxoviruses can be mixed with red blood cells, and after hemagglutination the red cells can be centrifuged down and gently washed. Following elution of the virus, the red cells can be pelleted and discarded, leaving a partially purified viral suspension in the supernatant solution.

## EFFECT OF PHYSICAL AND CHEMICAL AGENTS ON VIRUSES

Because of considerable variation in the sensitivity of different viruses to either physical or chemical agents, one can only generalize when speaking of the viruses as a whole. For the most part, however, icosahedral viruses are more stable to both heat and cold than are the helical-enveloped viruses. Most viruses lose their infectivity if heated to 60°C for 30 minutes; however, as with bacteria, the suspending medium will influence their stability. Many viruses can be preserved for long periods of time if kept at −70°C; again, in general, the enveloped helical viruses lose infectivity more rapidly than the isometric viruses.

There are a few antibiotics that can affect viral replication, but these are substances that interfere with nucleic acid metabolism and hence are also toxic to the host cell. A few other chemicals that have been used with limited success to treat or prevent viral infections will be discussed in the appropriate chapters on virus groups.

## VIRAL GENETICS

It is beyond the scope of this text to more than summarize a few genetic properties of viruses; however, the application of viral genetics in the research laboratory is providing new knowledge concerning the functions of the viral nucleic acid. Obviously, spontaneous or induced changes in the viral nucleic acid result either in the death of the virus or the production of a mutant with altered properties. Some of the most useful mutants used today are referred to as "conditionally lethal mutants." These mutants can be considered in two general categories: (1) host-range mutants (HR) are viruses that have lost the ability to infect cells from one animal but are still able to infect cells from other animals, or that require a helper virus for growth to complement a mutant defect; and (2) temperature-sensitive mutants (ts) that are able to replicate normally at a low temperature (e.g., 35°C), but are unable to replicate at a nonpermissive temperature (e.g., 42°C). Temperature-sensitive mutants usually produce a protein that is defective at the nonpermissive temperature, and studies of these mutants have provided some answers to the sequence of events that occur during viral replication and the functions of various viral proteins.

Studies have also shown that if two different but related viruses simultaneously infect a cell, their nucleic acids may break and recombine to yield recombinant progeny with some properties of both parental viruses. A similar type of event occurs during a process called multiplicity reactivation, in which the simultaneous infection of a cell with two or more inactive viruses yields progeny virus as a result of the recombinations of their nucleic acids. And, as we shall see, several viruses are able to exist within the host cell without the production of protein capsids. In such cases, the viral nucleic acid appears to be incorporated into the host cell genome, as was described for the specialized transducing phages. This may result in either a latent infection that can be activated later or the morphological change of the host cell into a malignant cell.

## VIRAL VACCINES

Since viral capsids are made of protein and viral envelopes contain both proteins and glycoproteins, it is not surprising that many viral infections will induce immunological responses. Specific responses will be discussed in more detail for the major groups, but suffice it to say at this point that viral vaccines are widely used to induce active immunity to many viral diseases. These vaccines contain either killed virulent viruses which are injected into the individual or living attenuated (mutant) viruses still possessing the same antigenic properties as the virulent virus but having lost the ability to produce disease. Attenuated vaccines may be administered by injection, or, in some cases, orally.

## REFERENCES

Bablanian, R. 1975. Structural and functional alterations in cultured cells infected with cytocidal viruses. *Progr. Med. Virol.* **19**:41–84.

Bialy, H. S., and C. Colby. 1972. Inhibition of early vaccinia virus ribonucleic acid synthesis in interferon-treated chick embryo fibroblasts. *J. Virol.* **9**:286–289.

Casjens, S., and J. King. 1975. Virus assembly. *Annu. Rev. Biochem.* **44**:555–611.

Cole, C. N. 1975. Defective interfering (DI) particles of poliovirus. *Progr. Med. Virol.* **20**:180–207.

Dales, S. 1973. Early events in cell-animal virus interactions. *Bacteriol. Rev.* **37**:103–135.

Geralds, A., ed. 1975. *Effects of Interferon on Cells, Viruses and the Immune System.* Proceedings of a meeting in Oeiras, Portugal in Sept. 1973. Academic Press, New York.

Ho, M., J. A. Armstrong, and M. C. Breinig. 1975. Interferon. *Annu. Rev. Microbiol.* **29**:131–161.

Huang, A. 1973. Defective interfering viruses. *Annu. Rev. Microbiol.* **27**:101–117.

Kleinschmidt, W. J. 1972. Biochemistry of interferon and its inducers. *Annu. Rev. Biochem.* **41**:517–542.

Levy, H. B., G. Baer, S. Baron, C. E. Buckler, C. J. Gibbs, M. J. Iadarola, W. T. London, and J. Rice. 1975. A modified polyriboinosinic-polyribocytidilic acid complex that induces interferon in primates. *J. Infect. Dis.* **132**:434–439.

Maehara, N., and M. Ho. 1977. Cellular origin of interferon induced by bacterial lipopolysaccharide. *Infect. Immun.* **15**:78–83.

Marcus, P. I., and J. M. Salb. 1966. Molecular basis of interferon action: Inhibition of viral RNA translation. *Virology* **30**:502–516.

Metz, D. H. 1975a. Interferon and interferon inducers. *Adv. in Drug Research* **10**:101–156.

Metz, D. H. 1975b. The mechanism of action of interferon. *Cell* **6**:429–439.

Mozes, L. W., and J. Vilček. 1975. Distinguishing characteristics of interferon induction with poly(I)-poly(C) and Newcastle disease virus in human cells. *Virology* **65**:100–111.

Oxman, M. N., and M. J. Levine. 1971. Interferon and transcription of early virus-specific RNA in cells infected with simian virus 40. *Proc. Nat. Acad. Sci. U.S.A.* **68**:299–302.

Pollack, R. 1973. Compiler. *Readings in Mammalian Cell Culture.* Cold Spring Harbor, New York.

Raghow, R., and D. W. Kingsbury. 1976. Endogenous viral enzymes involved in messenger RNA. *Annu. Rev. Microbiol.* **30:**21–39.

Russell, W. C. 1975. Assembly of viruses. *Progr. Med. Virol.* **19:**1–40.

Samuel, C. E., and W. K. Joklik. 1974. A protein synthesizing system from interferon-treated cells that discriminates between cellular and viral messenger RNAs. *Virology* **58:**476–491.

Siminovitch, L. 1976. On the nature of hereditable variation in cultured somatic cells. *Cell* **7:**1–11.

Smith, H. 1972. Mechanisms of virus pathogenicity. *Bacteriol. Rev.* **36:**291–310.

# 33

# Herpetoviridae

The Herpetoviridae are a large group of viruses extremely widespread throughout the animal kingdom. The property most, if not all, herpesviruses share is their ability to produce latent infections which, after months or years, may be activated to produce identical symptoms for each sporadic reoccurrence or may produce a disease totally unlike the original infection. In humans, herpesvirus infections occur in many forms. The more common manifestations are fever blisters (which may involve the eye), varicella (chickenpox), and zoster (shingles). Herpesviruses may also cause congenital defects in newborns and severe encephalitis in adults, and there is strong evidence that a herpesvirus is the etiologic agent for infectious mononucleosis. In addition, there is good evidence that a herpesvirus is involved in a human cancer (Burkitt's lymphoma), and there is circumstantial evidence that herpes simplex type 2 may be involved in human cervical carcinoma.

## STRUCTURE AND REPLICATION OF HERPESVIRUSES

Herpesviruses have double-stranded DNA and are icosahedral viruses surrounded by an envelope which is acquired as the virion buds from the host cell's nucleus (see Figure 33-1). The diameter of the enveloped virion is 180 to 200 nm and that of the naked capsid is approximately 100 nm. The capsids of all herpesviruses are composed of 162 capsomers, and the molecular weight of the DNA from different herpesviruses may vary from 64 to 100 million daltons.

Attachment of the virus to a host cell will occur at 4°C; however, the subsequent penetration requires energy and appears to result from pinocytosis into a cell vesicle or from fusion of the viral envelope with the cell membrane to release the naked capsid into the cytoplasm.

Very little is known about the uncoating or initial processing of the herpesvirus capsid, but transcription of viral DNA and the final assembly of the nucleocapsid occur in the nucleus of the host cell, so intranuclear inclusion bodies can be seen. During infection certain sequences of viral DNA are transcribed as early mRNA, before the initiation of viral DNA replication, and other sequences are transcribed as late mRNA, occurring after viral DNA synthesis has begun. In either case, host-cell RNA synthesis is inhibited, and viral mRNA is synthesized as large polycistronic strands, containing several cistrons in sequence. These strands are subsequently cleaved into monocistronic mRNA's that are polyadenylated (having a long strand of poly-A added to the 3' end) before entering the cytoplasm to be translated.

Translation of viral mRNA results in the formation of both structural proteins and nonstructural proteins that are necessary for the replication of the viral DNA (namely DNA polymerase, thymidine kinase, and DNase). The structural proteins are transported into the nucleus where they are assembled into nucleocapsids. The remaining structural proteins are integrated into both the nuclear and the cell membranes, resulting in a complete replacement of the membrane proteins of the host cell. The completion of the glycoprotein that will be incorporated into the envelope occurs when carbohydrate moieties are added to regions of viral membrane protein.

Curiously, even though the cell membrane contains viral glycoprotein, the nucleocapsid appears to obtain its envelope as it buds through the nuclear membranes. Various mechanisms have been proposed for the release of the virus from the host cell: a reverse-type phagocytosis in which the virion becomes enclosed in a vacuole that fuses with the cell membrane; release from some types of host cells through channels in the plasma membrane; or in some cases a disruption of the cell membrane may release the completed virions. Whatever the case, the production of infective viruses results in the eventual death of the host cell. Herpesvirus replication is schematically shown in Figure 33-2.

## HERPESVIRUS CLASSIFICATION

The nomenclature of the herpesviruses has evolved rather haphazardly: one virus is named after the disease it causes (varicella-zoster virus), another named for its codiscoverers (Epstein-Barr virus), and still another named to describe the pathology of the infection (cytomegalovirus). Two other herpesviruses are each referred to by two separate names, i.e., herpes simplex type 1 or *Herpesvirus hominus* type 1 and herpes

**Figure 33-1.** Virions of herpesvirus acquire an envelope as they bud through a nuclear envelope ($\times$100,000). To the left in the nucleus are icosahedral capsids containing DNA; viruses in the cytoplasm to the right are enveloped following budding. In this section one bud has not yet pinched off from the nuclear envelope.

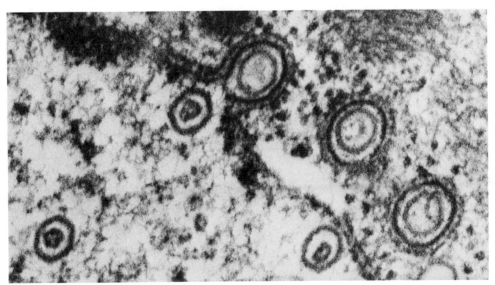

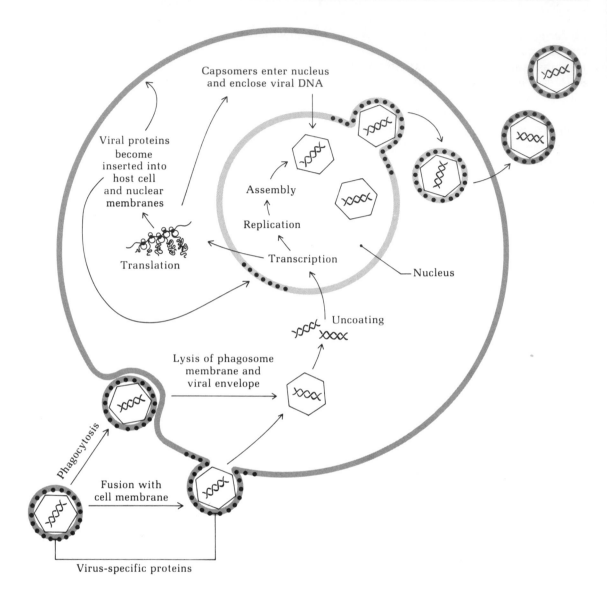

**Figure 33-2.** Replication of herpesvirus. It is thought that the infecting virus enters the host
cell by both phagocytosis and fusion with the cell membrane. After uncoating, viral DNA
enters the nucleus where it is transcribed and replicated. The mRNA is translated in the
cytoplasm, forming viral glycoproteins and structural proteins. The glycoproteins replace
host cell glycoproteins in both the cell membrane and the nuclear envelope, and the structural proteins enter the nucleus to take part in the assembly of the herpesvirion. The viral
envelope is thought to be acquired as the herpes capsid buds through the inner nuclear
membrane; but the pathway of the virion from this perinuclear space to the extracellular
space is unknown.

simplex type 2 or *Herpesvirus hominus* type 2.

In an attempt to put some uniformity into herpesvirus nomenclature, the International Committee on Viral Nomenclature decided in 1973 to use the designations shown in Table 33-1. However, neither virologists nor scientific journals have adhered to the newly proposed names, and so this text will continue to use the more common designation for the herpesviruses.

## HERPESVIRUS INFECTIONS IN HUMANS

Until recently, it was believed that a single type of herpesvirus was responsible for recurrent fever blisters in humans (see Figure 33-3). However, it is now possible to divide these agents into two types, on the basis of antigenic and biological differences. Herpes simplex type 1 is characteristically responsible for oral infections, whereas herpes simplex type 2 is normally found in the genital tract.

### Herpes Simplex Type 1

A primary infection with herpes simplex type 1 may be asymptomatic and is usually undiagnosed; however approximately 15% of primary infections are manifested by an acute gingivostomatitis in which the gums become red and swollen and multiple ulcerated lesions occur on the membranes of the mouth. The lesions may also involve the tonsils, pharynx, or nose. Normally, the disease is self-limiting, and lesions disappear in two to three weeks. More serious primary infections occur if the virus infects multiple sites on the skin of an individual with eczema, causing the loss of large areas of epithelium and resulting in the subsequent loss of body fluids and frequent secondary bacterial infections. Traumatic (wound) herpes may follow the infection of an open injury. Such infections occur most frequently on the fingers and are an occupational hazard to dentists, physicians, and nurses.

Infection of the eye by herpes simplex type 1 causes an extremely painful ulceration of the cornea. These infections are usually resolved in 2 or 3 weeks, with blindness a not infrequent result.

Herpetic encephalitis in adults is probably the most devastating disease produced by herpes simplex type 1. The virus produces necrotic lesions (areas of dead cells) in localized areas of the brain, frequently causing death or residual neurological abnormalities such as partial paralysis, mental retardation, or abnormal behavior patterns.

### Latent Infections

Recovery from a primary infection by herpes simplex type 1 may be followed by an asymptomatic latent infection. During latency, the virus appears to be harbored in the nervous system within the sensory ganglion cells. The physical state of the virus during latency is not known; however, it has been reported that the virus could not be found in ganglia at the time of autopsy in animal experiments, but herpesvirus could subsequently be detected when the ganglia were maintained in cell culture. Such results seem to support the concept that the herpesvirus exists as naked DNA within the host cell nucleus.

During the latent period, it is likely that small amounts of infective virions are sporadically produced, since the virus can occasionally be isolated from oral secretions, and humoral antibody levels remain high.

**Table 33-1. Nomenclature Proposed for Human Herpesviruses by the International Committee for the Nomenclature of Viruses**

| New Designation | Older Designation |
| --- | --- |
| Human herpesvirus 1 | Herpes simplex type 1 |
| Human herpesvirus 2 | Herpes simplex type 2 |
| Human herpesvirus 3 | Varicella-zoster virus |
| Human herpesvirus 4 | Epstein-Barr virus (EB virus) |
| Human herpesvirus 5 | Cytomegalovirus |

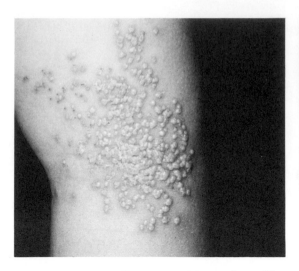 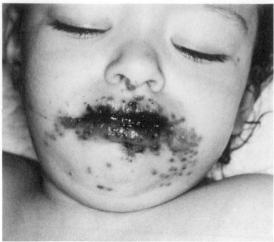

**Figure 33-3.** Herpes fever blisters on leg and on lips and face.

The molecular events that trigger secondary recurrent disease are not known, although it is well established that reactivation frequently follows fever, menstruation, emotional stress, or exposure to sunlight, resulting in clusters of vesicles at the muco-cutaneous junction of the lips. Recurrent herpes may also occur in the nose, eyes, or areas of the skin which have experienced a primary infection as in eczema or traumatic infections. It appears that recovery from the overt infection is due more to a cellular-type immunity than a result of humoral anti-bodies. Patients with defects in cellular immune functions or those who have had their cellular immune system suppressed following organ transplants are much more likely to suffer chronic herpetic ulcers or a severe disseminated herpetic infection, par-ticularly of the skin or respiratory tract.

### Herpes Simplex Type 2

Herpes simplex type 2 appears to be trans-mitted during sexual intercourse. Primary infections may be asymptomatic, or in the female, lesions may occur on the vulva, vagina, cervix, or the perineum. In the male, lesions may occur on the glans, pre-puce, or shaft of the penis, producing symptoms of burning, itching, and painful urination. The primary lesions disappear after two to three weeks, but like the oral infections of type 1, the virus becomes latent and may cause sporadic reoccurrences of overt disease.

### Neonatal Herpesvirus Infections

Childbirth during an episode of herpes sim-plex type 2 infection may result in an un-usually severe infection in the newborn during the first month of life. Such infections are frequently fatal, and survivors may have residual damage of the central nervous system or the eyes, although current evi-dence also indicates type 2 infections of the newborn may in some instances be asymp-tomatic. In addition, type 2 infections during pregnancy may result in abortions or congen-ital defects in the child.

### Oncogenic Potential

There is currently a growing volume of cir-cumstantial information linking herpes simplex type 2 infections to cervical cancer. This postulation is based, in part, on the fact that in several large, worldwide studies antibodies to the type 2 virus were found in a much higher percentage of women with cervical carcinoma than in appropriate control groups. The virus has also been isolated from degenerating cervical tumor cells, and hybridization studies have suggested such tumor cells do contain herpes simplex type 2 DNA. Furthermore, if one infects hamster embryo fibroblasts with type 2 virus which has been partially inactivated with U.V. light to prevent it from completing its lytic cycle, such fibroblasts are transformed into cancer cells that produce highly malignant tumors after inoculation into hamsters. Thus, at least in this *in vitro* situation, the potential oncogenicity of the virus has been demonstrated.

### Treatment

Several drugs, such as 5-iodo-2'-deoxyuridine (IUDR) and cytosine arabinoside (AraC), have been used topically to treat herpetic keratitis (eye infections). However, drug-resistant mutants may occur. There have also been reports of the successful treatment of herpes encephalitis with IUDR, but there has not been a sufficient number of cases to establish the efficacy of the therapy.

## VARICELLA–ZOSTER VIRUS

Varicella (chickenpox) is prinicpally a disease of childhood, characterized by pock-type lesions (raised skin lesions containing pus) occurring over essentially the entire body surface. Zoster (shingles) is a disease of adults characterized by similar pock-type lesions. These are restricted, however, to an area of the skin supplied by the sensory nerves of a single or small group of dorsal root ganglia. It is known that both diseases are caused by the same virus and that zoster represents a reactivation of a latent chickenpox infection in a partially-immune individual.

### Viral Properties

The varicella-zoster virus is morphologically identical to the herpes simplex viruses. It can be propagated in human diploid fibroblast cells, but attempts to grow the virus in experimental animals have been unsuccessful. Inasmuch as assembly of the varicella-zoster virus occurs in the host cell nucleus, it is not surprising that, like all herpesvirus-infected cells, intranuclear inclusion bodies are seen (see Figure 33-4).

### Varicella (Chickenpox)

Varicella occurs worldwide, usually in children, and frequently in epidemics during the winter and spring. The virus is probably acquired via the respiratory route, and during an incubation period of 14 to 16 days it multiplies in the respiratory tract and in the regional lymph nodes. It is released into the blood stream and disseminated throughout the body. Fever, headache, and malaise are the usual symptoms that precede a maculopapular rash, a rash containing macules (flat discoloration) and papules (spots elevated above the level of the skin in the same area). The rash develops into vesicles that eventually form scabs and in the absence of secondary bacterial infection heal without leaving a scar. A prominent characteristic of the lesions of chickenpox is that they occur in crops—that is, new lesions begin to develop in the same areas where older lesions are crusting-over and healing. Neutralizing antibodies can be detected about one week after the rash, and recovery is usually complete two weeks after the initial symptoms.

Although varicella is considered to be a mild disease of childhood, it can be quite severe in adults or in individuals whose immune response is defective or suppressed. Meningoencephalitis is a rare complication with a high fatality rate occurring in all age groups. Varicella pneumonia is seen more frequently as an adult complication.

### Zoster (Shingles)

Zoster is the result of the reactivation of a latent varicella virus infection. It appears

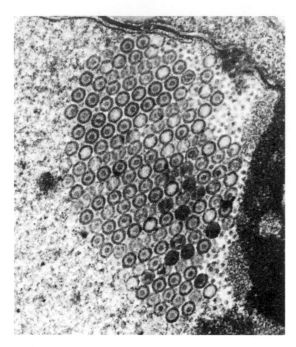

**Figure 33-4.** Electron micrograph of an intranuclear inclusion body of herpesvirus; note the presence of both "empty" and DNA-containing particles. (×32,400.)

a clinical picture similar to chickenpox, and the differentiation between these two diseases can be made by the histological observation of cells occurring in the vesicles. Varicella lesions characteristically contain giant cells and cells with typical intranuclear inclusion bodies. Also, the virus can be grown in cell culture, permitting a positive identification using serologic techniques with known antiserum.

### Control of Varicella-Zoster Virus

Preventive measures against chickenpox are not particularly effective because an infected individual spreads the virus before clinical symptoms are apparent; also, since the source of infective virus for zoster appears to be internal, there is no known way to prevent this secondary disease. Children with leukemia or immunodeficiency syndromes or persons who are taking immunosuppressive drugs may be given zoster-immune globulin to prevent or modify the disease.

### CYTOMEGALOVIRUS

Cytomegaloviruses (CMV) are typical herpesviruses both in their structure and in the manner in which they replicate. Infected cells become distinctly enlarged (i.e., cytomegaly) and possess both intranuclear and cytoplasmic inclusion bodies (see Figure 33-5). This unusual appearance of salivary gland cells of children who died from congenital infections prompted the name salivary gland virus disease, although it is more frequently called cytomegalic inclusion disease. These viruses can be grown in a number of human embryonic fibroblast cell lines, but human CMV appears to be species-specific, and no experimental animal model is available to study the human strains. Cytomegaloviruses do exist for other animals, but the congenital defects seen in humans have not been observed in infected animals.

probable that all persons who have recovered from chickenpox continue to carry the latent varicella virus in their ganglionic nerve cells. Activation of the latent virus may occur following physical trauma, tuberculosis, cancer, and undoubtedly other unknown factors. Following activation, the virus travels along a nerve (or nerves) to the skin, where it produces lesions over that area of the skin supplied by the affected nerves. Paralysis can result from infection of the spinal cord, but the more usual result is recovery in two to four weeks. Children who are exposed to an adult with zoster may develop a typical case of chickenpox.

### Diagnosis of Chickenpox and Shingles

The diagnosis of either disease entity caused by varicella-zoster virus is almost always made on the basis of the clinical picture. Smallpox is the only major disease that has

## Pathogenicity of Cytomegalovirus Infections

There are at least three antigenic types of CMV which infect humans, and although geographical areas differ, worldwide surveys show that approximately 80% of adults over 35 years of age have circulating antibody to these viruses. For the most part, however, adult infections appear to be asymptomatic, and the importance of these viruses lies primarily in their ability to infect the fetus before birth.

Current evidence indicates that following a primary infection, CMV is excreted in the urine and saliva for very long periods of time. If this primary infection occurs during pregnancy, the virus is thought to be capable of crossing the placenta and infecting the fetus. This may cause the death of the fetus; it may cause a wide variety of congenital defects; or it may produce no immediately obvious effects in the newborn.

**Figure 33-5.** A number of dark CMV inclusion bodies are evident in these Giemsa-stained human fibroblast cells three days after infection (×3000).

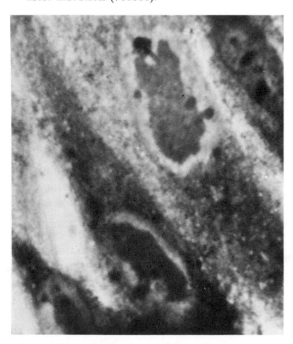

The congenital effects caused by CMV are extremely varied, but it is postulated that CMV is the most common viral cause of mental retardation, surpassing even rubella virus in this regard. Current estimates indicate that approximately one percent of all infants are infected with CMV when born. Many such infants do not show obvious abnormalities, but about ten percent of those infected in utero have many congenital abnormalities, such as microcephaly (an abnormally small head), central nervous system damage resulting in seizures and deafness, mental retardation, psychomotor retardation, ocular abnormalities, chronic gastroenteritis, jaundice, pneumonia or thrombocytopenia (lack of thrombocytes). It is also known that the newborn may show no signs of CMV infection and yet have extensive abnormalities that are seen only later in life. One study of such infants born at Strong Memorial Hospital in Rochester, New York, has revealed that the average IQ score of infants born with a CMV infection is significantly lower than that of a control group. Although this finding has yet to be confirmed, it is generally agreed that such children may have other subtle defects not normally associated with a congenital CMV infection. Several studies, for example, have shown a significant hearing defect in many congenitally infected children, and it is now thought that fetal infection by CMV may be a major cause of congenital deafness.

Since the disease in the mother is asymptomatic, it is not generally possible to determine the age of the fetus when it becomes infected. Like other herpesviruses, CMV is believed to produce infections which may persist in a latent state and periodically flare up, resulting in the excretion of infectious virus. It is not certain whether fetal infection can result from such a flare-up of CMV during pregnancy or whether the mother must experience a primary infection during pregnancy for the fetus to become infected. The latter possibility seems likely, since subsequent children are usually not infected *in utero* even though the mother may be excreting CMV during the pregnancy.

Another syndrome caused by CMV, similar to infectious mononucleosis, occurs in young adults. This disease has been named cytomegalovirus mononucleosis. It resembles the more common infectious mononucleosis (also caused by a herpesvirus) but apparently does not cause the severe sore throat or the rise in heterophile antibodies (that agglutinate sheep's red blood cells) usually seen in infectious mononucleosis.

### CMV in Immunodepressed Individuals

Organ transplant recipients receiving immunosuppressive drugs to prevent rejection of their transplant appear to be unusually susceptible to cytomegalovirus infections. A large number of studies have reported the isolation of CMV from the lungs of such patients. Such infections may be asymptomatic, or they may cause pneumonia or a disseminated infection in these patients. It seems that the maintenance of the latent state requires a functioning immune system and that any deficiency in this system might result in an activation of the latent infection.

### Diagnosis of CMV

Urine or saliva can be cultured on human fibroblasts which are then observed for the the cytopathic characteristics of swollen, rounded cells possessing large intranuclear inclusion bodies.

Antibodies formed in response to a CMV infection may be measured either by the determination of neutralizing antibodies that destroy the infectivity of a known strain of cytomegalovirus or by an assay for the presence of complement-fixing antibodies formed in response to the virus. Since all human strains of CMV possess the same complement-fixing antigen, the determination of antibodies to this antigen is routinely used as a diagnostic aid for suspected infec-

tions by CMV. In addition, infected infants produce IgM antibodies against the virus, and one can use an indirect fluorescent-antibody test for IgM directed against CMV.

### Control of CMV

Since adult infections are usually asymptomatic, controlling the spread of this virus is difficult. The virus is excreted primarily in the urine, and it is thought that CMV may be frequently transmitted as a venereal disease; however, blood transfusions containing infected lymphocytes are also a source of infection.

Considerable efforts are being expended to produce an attenuated vaccine to immunize women before they become pregnant. The efficacy of such a vaccine is based on the unproven premise that fetal invasion occurs only during a primary infection with CMV during pregnancy.

A major problem in the isolation of an attenuated mutant of CMV for a vaccine is that even the nonattenuated virus usually produces an asymptomatic infection in adults. Thus, how can one be certain that the vaccine is truly attenuated? Moreover, the propensity of herpesviruses to induce the transformation of normal cells into malignant cells is also a major concern for any herpesvirus vaccine.

## EB VIRUS

EB virus, named for its codiscoverers, Epstein and Barr, was originally isolated during a search for an etiologic agent for Burkitt's lymphoma (BL), a malignancy originating in the cells of the lymph nodes. In this disease, the malignant cells are not found circulating in the blood, and the lower jaw is the most common site of the tumor, although tumors may occur in the kidneys, liver, ovaries, thyroids, adrenals, or upper jaw.

Burkitt's lymphoma first received worldwide attention in 1958 when Burkitt reported a large number of African children in Uganda suffering from this malignancy. The rarity of the disease elsewhere prompted a search for an infectious agent as the cause of BL. Although no virus could be seen in (BL) tumor cells, continued cultivation of the tumor cells revealed that some cells contained herpes-like virus particles which upon subsequent isolation were shown to be a previously undescribed herpesvirus.

The infectious nature of BL is also suggested by a report in 1976 that three children in Winchester, Virginia, died of the disease within a very short time span. Two were boys who lived two houses apart and the third case of BL occurred in a boy who lived about half a mile away. Because BL occurs so rarely outside of Africa, an explanation for the almost simultaneous occurrence of three cases in a small Virginia town is not available.

## Properties of EB Virus

EB virus appears to be morphologically identical to other human herpesviruses. The virus can infect only human lymphoid cells, and when these lymphocytes are infected with EB virus, the normal sequence of events is a cytopathic effect in which the virus multiplies and the lymphocyte degenerates and dies. An occasional host cell is "transformed" into a permanent EB-virus-carrying lymphoblastoid cell. Unlike normal lymphocytes which are unable to divide in cell culture, cells transformed by EB virus can proliferate continuously and have an unlimited life span. Electron microscopic studies of these transformed cell lines show that only a small percentage of the cells are actually producing EB virus. The isolation and cultivation of a single nonproducer clone, however, also gives rise to a population of cells in which only a few cells actually produce EB virus, indicating that nonproducers, as well as producers, are infected with EB virus. The fact that all "transformed" cells actually carry the EB virus genome was confirmed when it was shown that purified EB virus DNA would hybridize with

the nucleic acid of the so-called "nonproducer" cells. Furthermore, some transformed cell lines in which no virus could be detected could be induced (with bromodeoxyuridine) to produce EB virus. Thus, there appears little doubt that EB virus DNA can exist in the transformed cell in the absence of any virus replication.

The physical state of the EB virus DNA within the transformed cell is not known. One report claimed that by treating the cells with alkali, followed by high speed centrifugation, the viral DNA (which was detected by hybridization with known radioactive viral DNA) could be separated from the host cell DNA. It was postulated that the viral DNA existed in close association with the cellular DNA but was not covalently linked to it. Other workers claim that the viral DNA is linearly integrated with the host cell DNA but is released on treatment with the alkali.

## Infectious Mononucleosis

Before discussing the possible role of EB virus in human malignancies, let us turn to its well established role as the etiologic agent of infectious mononucleosis (IM).

Infectious mononucleosis is primarily a disease of young adults in which the usual clinical symptoms are high fever, headache, chills and sweats ("shake and bake"), fatigue, and a severe sore throat. The duration of the illness may vary from several days to several weeks and may occasionally be accompanied by mild hepatitis or signs of meningitis (see Table 33-2).

Clinically the disease is diagnosed by the above symptoms and by the presence of abnormal, large lymphocytes in the blood. In addition, most patients develop high titers of heterophile antibodies which are characterized by their ability to agglutinate red blood cells from sheep.

The first indication that EB virus might be the causal agent of IM occurred when a laboratory technician developed IM while working with EB virus. After recovery, it was found that she had developed antibodies to

**Table 33-2. Some Differential Diagnostic Problems in Infectious Mononucleosis**

| Signs and Symptoms | Anatomic Lesions | Analogous Disorders |
|---|---|---|
| SORE THROAT | Ulcerative or membranous pharyngitis | Diphtheria |
| PAINFUL AND STIFF NECK; occasionally convulsions and coma | Rapidly enlarged retrocervical lymph nodes. Acute hyperplastic lymphadenitis. Pleocytosis in cerebrospinal fluid may be present | Meningitis (serous meningitis may be present) |
| GENERALIZED LYMPHADENOPATHY | Acute hyperplastic lymphadenitis | Leukemia |
| ABDOMINAL PAIN AND TENDERNESS | Rapidly enlarged abdominal lymph nodes | |
| right lower quadrant | | Acute appendicitis |
| left upper quadrant | Acute splenomegaly Acute diffuse hyperplasia | Acute pleuritis; perinephritic abscess |
| acute tenderness and pain in right upper quadrant | Acute diffuse hepatitis; periportal infiltrations; enlarged lymph nodes around common bile duct | Acute hepatitis, especially if jaundice present |
| acute general abdominal pain, followed by shock | Ruptured spleen | Acute abdominal emergency |
| COUGH (resembling whooping cough) | Enlarged mediastinal lymph nodes | Pertussis; Hodgkin's disease; tuberculosis |
| CUTANEOUS RASHES | | Exanthematous disease (measles); scarlet fever especially if angina is present; secondary syphilis, especially if enlarged inguinal lymph nodes and positive test for syphilis are present |
| PUFFINESS AROUND EYES | Swelling of retrobulbar tissues | Trichinosis |
| TOOTHACHE | Acutely swollen submandibular lymph nodes | Pulpitis |
| HEMATURIA | Specific infiltration of renal parenchyma or purpuric renal hemorrhage | Acute glomerulonephritis |

EB virus, and, furthermore, her lymphocytes could be cultivated in a continuous cell line which, after growing several months, yielded infectious EB virus. Four months after recovery, it was no longer possible to cultivate her lymphocytes as a continuous cell line. Subsequent studies with other patients recovering from IM have provided similar results. Table 33-3 summarizes the relation of EB virus and antibody to IM.

It seems, therefore, that IM is an excellent example of a self-limiting malignancy, since infected lymphocytes are transformed into established cell lines characteristic of malignant cells. The disappearance of these transformed lymphocytes following recovery from IM may result from the host's immune response to new membrane antigens occurring in the transformed lymphocytes and to neutralizing antibodies that appear during the course of the disease.

### Control of Infectious Mononucleosis

IM has frequently been referred to as the "kissing disease," a term arising from the belief that the disease is transmitted through close oral contact. The observation that throat washings from individuals with IM could transform EB-negative lymphocytes into EB-positive lymphocytes certainly supports this assertion.

### EB Virus and Human Cancer

There are several human malignancies with which EB virus is at least associated. A nasopharyngeal carcinoma (NPC) consisting of proliferating epithelial cells has been grown in cultures, and from these cultures a virus which appears to be EB virus has been isolated. Interestingly, NPC occurs much more frequently among the Chinese than in individuals in the Western Hemisphere. In addition, patients with Hodgkin's disease (a malignancy of the lymphatic system) usually have high titers of antibodies to EB virus. The same is true of patients with acute lympho-

cytic leukemia. But, in neither of these latter diseases has EB virus been directly implicated.

We still have not come to grips with the question of whether or not EB virus is the etiologic agent of the human cancer Burkitt's lymphoma (BL), and, if so, why does this widespread virus produce so few actual malignancies? There is at present no answer, but several hypotheses have been proposed: (1) Perhaps a cofactor of some type must also be present with the EB virus to produce a malignancy. Areas where BL is most prevalent also have high incidences of malaria. Malaria is known to suppress the immune system and to stimulate lymphocyte proliferation, so simultaneous infection with EB virus and malaria may be required to produce BL; (2) perhaps there are subtypes of EB virus which differ in their oncogenic potential, and the subtype causing infectious mononucleosis possesses little or no oncogenic potential, but that causing BL possesses a higher oncogenic potential; (3) because many herpesviruses seem to be species-specific, perhaps there are genetic variations within the human population which allow the oncogenic expression of EB virus; (4) finally, a "passenger hypothesis" has been proposed stating that EB virus is a very widespread but usually inocuous inhabitant of the lymphoid tissue, even though it may cause infectious mononucleosis, and it is only carried along by the malignant cells and is unrelated to the malignancy. At this time, any one or none of the above possibilities may be correct in explaining the paradoxical association of EB virus with Burkitt's lymphoma.

### HERPES B VIRUS

B virus, also named *Herpesvirus simiae*, occurs as a latent virus infection in monkeys. A person becomes infected with B virus as a result of a bite by an infected monkey or by contact with infected monkeys or monkey tissue cultures; hence B virus is an occupational hazard to laboratory personnel who handle monkeys.

**Table 33-3. Relation of EB Virus and EB Virus Antibodies to Infectious Mononucleosis**

| EB Virus | EBV Antibody |
| --- | --- |
| Regularly present in cultured lymphocytes from infectious mononucleosis | Absent before illness |
| | Appears during illness |
| Persists in lymphocytes for years after infectious mononucleosis | Persists for years after illness |
| May be necessary for lymphocyte proliferation *in vitro* | Shows no such relation to any other illness |
| Produces infectious mononucleosis in susceptible recipients via blood transfusion | When present indicates immunity to infectious mononucleosis |
| Has produced infectious mononucleosis in one transmission experiment | When absent indicates susceptibility to infectious mononucleosis |

In humans, the B virus invades the central nervous system causing an acute ascending paralysis. The disease has a mortality rate greater than 75%, and death usually results from a paralysis of the respiratory system.

## HERPESVIRUS TUMORS IN ANIMALS

Because of the intense interest in the role of herpesvirus in human cancer, it may be appropriate to mention briefly examples in which a herpesvirus has been proven to be the etiologic agent of animal tumors.

Marek's disease of chickens is a disease of the lymphatic system in which malignant cells invade the nerve cells of the bird. When injected into healthy chickens, a herpesvirus isolated from these tumors causes a lymphatic tumor characteristic of Marek's disease. An encouraging aspect of the disease is that it has been almost eliminated by immunization with either a live, attenuated Marek's disease virus or a related live turkey herpesvirus.

Lucké kidney tumor of frogs is an example in which Koch's postulates have at least partially been fulfilled. There seems little doubt that a herpesvirus is the etiologic agent of this tumor. The tumor can be transmitted using cell-free tumor extracts; however, no single isolated herpesvirus is able to induce the tumor. It has been postulated that the production of a tumor may require the presence of more than one form of virus, perhaps a defective virus and a helper virus.

*Herpesvirus saimiri* was initially isolated from kidney cell cultures derived from apparently healthy squirrel monkeys, and subsequent isolations of this virus have been made from their circulating lymphocytes. The high incidence of antibodies to this virus in squirrel monkeys indicates that infection must be frequent and probably mild. However, inoculation of this virus into a large number of other nonhuman primates results in the production of a variety of highly malignant lymphomas and leukemias.

A herpesvirus has been isolated from primary kidney-cell cultures obtained from healthy cottontail rabbits, and inoculation of other cottontail rabbits with this virus induces a malignant lymphoma in the inoculated rabbits. Table 33-4 lists those herpesviruses with known or suspected oncogenic potential.

Undoubtedly, there will be additional reports of malignancies in animals attributed to herpesviruses, and perhaps the role of herpesviruses in human cancer can soon be known as facts and not circumstantial evidence. Since immunization is effective in preventing animal tumors caused by herpesviruses, we can hope for the possibility of preventing some human cancers.

**Table 33-4. Transforming Herpesviruses with Known or Suspected Oncogenic Potential**

| Virus | Cell transformation | Host cell DNA stimulation | Oncogenicity |
|---|---|---|---|
| Marek's Disease Virus (chicken) | Leukocytes | Yes | Lymphoma (chicken) |
| Herpesvirus saimiri and H. ateles (monkey) | Leukocytes | Unknown | Lymphoma (monkey) |
| Lucké frog virus | Unknown (has not been replicated in vitro) | Unknown | Adenocarcinoma (frog) |
| Herpesvirus sylvilagus (rabbit) | Leukocytes | Unknown | Lymphoma (rabbit) |
| Guinea pig herpesvirus | Leukocytes | Unknown | Suspected leukemia (guinea pig) |
| Epstein-Barr virus (humans) | Leukocytes | Yes | Suspected lymphoma (humans) |
| Herpes simplex virus (humans) | Hamster, mouse, and human fibroblasts | Unknown | Adenocarcinoma and fibrosarcoma (hamster) |
| Cytomegalovirus (humans) | Hamster embryo fibroblasts | Yes | Fibrosarcoma (hamster) |

## REFERENCES

Anderson, M., G. Klein, J. L. Ziegler, and W. Henle. 1976. Association of Epstein-Barr viral genomes with American Burkitt lymphoma. *Nature* **260**:357–358.

Aurelian, L. 1973. Virions and antigens of herpesvirus type 2 in cervical carcinoma. *Cancer. Res.* **33**:1539–1547.

Breidenbach, G. P., N. S. Skinner, J. H. Wallace, and M. Mizell. 1971. In vitro induction of a herpes-type virus in "summer phase" Lucké tumor explants. *J. Virol.* **7**:679–682.

Bryson, Y. J., and J. D. Connor. 1976. In vitro susceptibility of varicella-zoster virus to adenine arabinoside and hypoxanthine arabinoside. *Antimicrob. Agents Chemother.* **9**:540–543.

Burkitt's lymphoma—Winchester, Virginia. 1976. *Morbidity Mortality Weekly Reports* **25**:173.

Docherty, J. J., and M. Chopan. 1974. The latent herpes simplex virus. *Bacteriol. Rev.* **38**:337–355.

Dowling, J. N., A. R. Saslow, J. A. Armstrong, and M. Ho. 1976. Cytomegalovirus infection in patients receiving immunosuppressive therapy for rheumatologic disorders. *J. Infect. Dis.* **133**:399–408.

Epstein, M. A., and B. G. Achong. 1973. The EB virus. *Annu. Rev. Microbiol.* **27**:413–436.

Epstein, M. A., B. G. Achong, and Y. M. Barr. 1964. Virus particles in cultured lymphoblasts from Burkitt's lymphoma. *Lancet* **1**:702–703.

Geder, L., R. Lausch, F. O'Neill, and F. Rapp. 1976. Oncogenic transformation of human embryo lung cells by human cytomegalovirus. *Science* **192**:1134–1137.

Gentry, G. A., and J. F. Aswell, 1975. Inhibition of herpes simplex virus replication by ara T. *Virology* **65**:294–296.

Hampar, B., A. Tanaka, M. Nonoyama, and J. G. Derge. 1974. Replication of the resident repressed Epstein-Barr virus genome during the early S phase (S-1 period) of nonproducer Raji cells. *Proc. Natl. Acad. Sci. U.S.A.* **71**:631–633.

zur Hausen, H., and H. Schulte-Holthausen. 1970. Presence of EB virus nucleic acid homology in a "virus-free" line of Burkitt tumour cells. *Nature* **227**:245–248.

Kaplan, A. S. 1973. A brief review of biochemistry of herpesvirus-host cell interaction. *Cancer Res.* **33**:1393–1398.

Kaplan, A. S., ed. 1973. *The Herpesviruses.* Academic Press, New York.

Levine, P. H., R. R. Connelly, C. W. Berard, G. T. O'Conor, R. F. Dorfman, J. M. Easton, and V. T. DeVita. 1975. The American Burkitt lymphoma registry: A progress report. *Ann. Internal Med.* **83**:31–41.

Marx, J. L. 1975. Cytomegalovirus: A major cause of birth defects. *Science* **190**:1184–1186.

Miller, G. 1975. Epstein-Barr herpesvirus and infectious mononucleosis. *Progr. Med. Virol.* **20**:84–112.

Nonoyama, M., and J. S. Pagano. 1973. Homology between Epstein-Barr virus DNA and viral DNA from Burkitt's lymphoma and nasopharyngeal carcinoma determined by DNA-DNA reassociation kinetics. *Nature* **242**:44–47.

Pagano, J. S. 1975. Diseases and mechanisms of persistent DNA virus infection: Latency and cellular transformation. *J. Infect. Dis.* **132**:209–223.

Rafferty, K. A., Jr. 1973. Herpesviruses and cancer. *Sci. American* **229**:26–33.

Rapp, F., and W. R. Koment. 1974. Herpesvirus etiology of abnormal growth. Chapter 8 in E. Kurstak and K. Maramorosch, eds. *Virus, Evolution and Cancer.* Academic Press, New York.

Rawls, W. E., E. Adam, and J. L. Melnick. 1973. An analysis of seroepidemiological studies of herpesvirus type 2 and carcinoma of the cervix. *Cancer Res.* **33**:1477–1482.

Roizman, B., and N. Frenkel. 1973. The transcription and state of herpes simplex virus DNA in productive infection and in human cervical cancer tissue. *Cancer Res.* **33**:1402–1416.

Roizman, B., and D. Furlong. 1974. The replication of herpesviruses. In H. Fraenkel-Conrat and R. R. Wagner, eds. *Comprehensive Virology,* Vol. 3. Plenum Press, New York.

Stevens, J. G. 1975. Latent herpes simplex virus and the nervous system. *Current Topics in Microbiol. and Immunol.* **70**:31–50.

Wagner, E. K. 1974. The replication of herpesviruses. *Amer. Scientist* **62**:584–593.

# 34

## Adenoviridae, Papovaviridae,
## and Parvoviridae

### Adenoviridae

In 1953 the first of the viruses that comprise the large group of adenoviruses was isolated from cultures of normal adenoids. Subsequently 33 serological types of adenoviruses have been found that produce a variety of respiratory and conjunctival infections in humans. Interestingly, these viruses have been frequently isolated from normal (or at least apparently normal) adenoids and tonsils, as well as from respiratory secretions and secretions of the eye. In fact, adenoviruses are found in the majority of adenoids removed by surgery, even though they appear normal at the time of removal. The mechanism of this apparent "latency" is still obscure, but some investigations suggest that the viruses are not truly latent, for viral DNA is not integrated into host DNA in a manner analogous to latent herpesvirus. Instead, the viruses seem to be replicating at a very slow or uneven rate. Using surgically removed tissue, these investigations showed that less than one out of ten million cells were actually infected with adenovirus, even though the minced adenoids eventually grew out virus.

On the other hand, there is no doubt that under special circumstances (discussed later in this chapter) adenoviruses can induce tumors in animals, and in this situation DNA from the virus seems to be integrated into the host cell genome. Infectious adenovirus, however, has never been obtained from tumor cells, and one might presume that such cells may not possess the complete genome of the virus in a state that could ever be reactivated to produce infectious virus. The current hypothesis, then, is that adenoviruses replicate in a very asynchronous manner, and when adenoids become infected with very small numbers of virions, there may be a long or even indefinite lag before the appearance of newly replicated virus particles. As a result, even though adenoviruses are frequently observed following the prolonged culture of apparently normal adenoids and tonsils, they do not seem to arise from the activation of a latent infec-

479

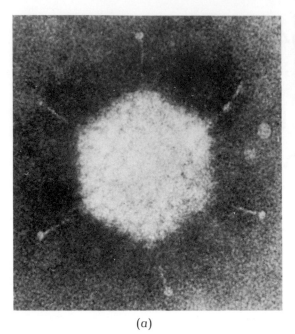

(a)

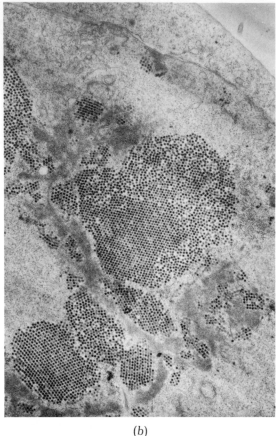

**Figure 34-1.** *a.* Negatively-stained virion of adenovirus (about ×500,000); note fibers extending from vertices. *b.* Crystalline aggregates of adenovirus in the nucleus of a Hela cell 24 hours after infection (×8,870).

(b)

tion. Moreover, individuals harboring adenoviruses do not experience recurrent overt disease from them, possibly due to the presence of a specific cellular and humoral immune response.

## STRUCTURE AND REPLICATION OF ADENOVIRUSES

Adenoviruses are icosahedral virions containing double-stranded DNA. They are 60–90 nm in diameter and are not enclosed in an envelope. Each capsid is composed of 252 capsomers, and from the vertex at each of the 12 penton capsomers extends a long fiber which attaches to specific receptor sites on the host cell (see Figure 34-1a).

Following adsorption, the virus is rapidly taken into the cell, either by phagocytosis or

direct penetration of the membrane (see Figure 34-2). It then penetrates the nuclear envelope and the viral DNA is released into the nucleus. Once in the nucleus, part of the DNA is immediately transcribed into early mRNA (made prior to DNA replication) which is then translated into a number of nonstructural proteins. Two of the best-studied ones are designated T and P antigens. The T antigen is so named because of its association with adenovirus-induced tumors or transformed cells; however, its function in the replication of adenovirus in human host cells is not known. The P antigen is an arginine-rich protein which becomes associated with the replicated viral DNA to form the final core nucleoprotein. The major observed effect of the early gene products is to stop host cell DNA synthesis and to redirect host cell enzymes to the synthesis of viral DNA and viral structural proteins. The mechanism by which the virus causes this switch-over is not known; however, it has been proposed that one of the early gene products may preferentially stimulate the initiation of translation of viral mRNA.

Approximately 12 to 14 hours after infection of the host cell, the structural proteins that make up the complete virion can be detected. These late gene products consist of the hexons, fibers, and penton subunits. Like all proteins, they are synthesized in the cytoplasm of the cell, but they are then transported into the nucleus. These proteins, particularly the fibers and pentons, are frequently made in such excess that they form crystalline inclusion bodies within the nucleus (see Figure 34-1b).

Final assembly of the virion occurs in the nucleus. The core nucleoprotein plus one or two other proteins becomes enclosed in the hexon structure, the penton subunit assembles with the fiber to form the penton capsomers, and the penton capsomers are then incorporated with the hexons to form the infective virion.

**Figure 34-2.** Electron micrograph of a replica of a freeze-etched KB cell infected with adenovirus type 2 for 10 minutes prior to cleaving and 30 minutes of deep etching. Adenovirions are shown embedded in the plasma membrane. (×114,000).

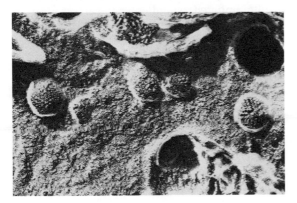

## FATE OF THE HOST CELL

Adenoviruses can be grown in continuous human cell lines such as KB or Hela cells, or they can be grown in primary cell cultures, particularly human embryo kidney cells. They are cytopathic for such permissive cells, and plaque assays can be carried out in cell monolayers. Death is manifested by a "rounding-up" of the infected cell; however, since lysis is not a normal event, only a small amount of virus is released into the culture medium. To obtain large yields of adenovirus, infected cells must be disrupted (by sonication or mechanical grinding) to release the virions from the cell nucleus. The cytopathic effect appears to result from the toxicity of the penton subunit, since the addition of purified pentons to a growing cell culture will cause the cells to round-up and detach from the glass on which the cells are growing.

## CLASSIFICATION OF ADENOVIRUSES

All adenoviruses except chicken adenoviruses contain a common group-specific antigen in the hexon capsomers and a second group-specific determinant in the penton subunit. In addition, hexons also possess an additional antigenic determinant that is used to subdivide these viruses into specific serotypes. The fiber contains a hemagglutinin, which exists as a knob at its outer end, that can bind to receptors on the surface of a red blood cell. The antigenic determinants on the hemagglutinin are moderately distinct for each serotype. As a result one can determine type specificity using a hemagglutination-inhibition test (the ability of the specific antihemagglutinin to prevent hemagglutination). However, because there are some crossreactions with this antigen, hemagglutination-inhibition does not provide as reliable a test for type specificity as do antibody reactions (e.g., neutralizing infectivity) directed toward the type-specific hexon antigen.

Adenoviruses have also been separated into groups based on whether they will hemagglutinate only rhesus monkey cells (group A), only rat cells (group B), or have no effect on rhesus and little effect on rat red blood cells (group C).

## ONCOGENIC ADENOVIRUSES

The discovery that at least 12 of the 33 types of human adenoviruses produce malignant carcinomas if injected into newborn hamsters, mice, or rats has provided a great deal of information concerning the properties of virally-induced malignancy in cells (see Figure 34-3). All attempts to obtain the infectious virus from the resulting tumor cells have failed. However, special hybridization techniques with viral nucleic acids show that tumor cells possess both viral DNA and viral mRNA (see Figure 34-4). Furthermore, it is possible to transform normal newborn hamster or rat kidney cells into malignant cells *in vitro,* and these transformed cells will then produce tumors when inoculated into hamsters or rats. Cells transformed *in vitro* fail to produce any infectious virus (and hence are called nonpermissive cells) but do contain viral DNA and mRNA.

Virally-induced tumor cells have been shown to contain significant amounts of a virus-coded antigen designated the T antigen (for tumor antigen). This antigen is apparently made by all adenoviruses but persists only in the transformed tumor cells. One can make antibody to the various types of adenovirus T antigens and the antibody can be made fluorescent by attaching fluorescein isothiocyanate to it. This fluorescently labeled anti-T antibody has been used in numerous attempts to show adenovirus T antigens in human malignancies. All have failed, and the consensus is that adenoviruses do not induce human tumors. Tumor cells also acquire a new tumor-specific transplantation antigen (TSTA), also specified by the virion, since all tumors produced by a specific virus will possess the same TSTA.

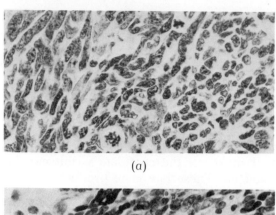

(a)

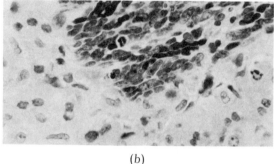

(b)

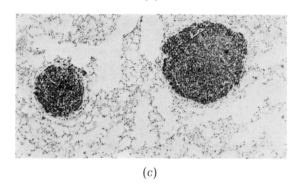

(c)

**Figure 34-3.** Histology of adenovirus type 2 tumor in rats (all H and E stained). *a.* Undifferentiated spindle cell sarcoma. *b.* Tumor infiltrating normal liver. *c.* Secondary tumor foci in lung.

Why some adenoviruses produce tumors and others do not is not known. It has been reported that those groups of human adenovirus possessing a low guanine plus cytosine (G + C) content in their DNA are more highly oncogenic than those having a high G + C content. As shown in Table 34-1, this correlation does exist; however, the fact

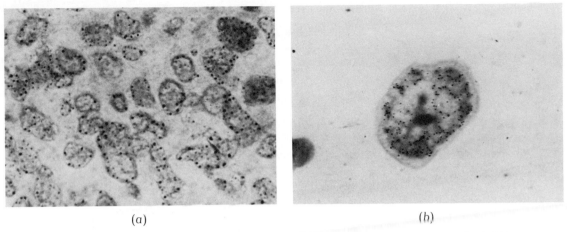

(a)                                                              (b)

**Figure 34-4.** a. Frozen section of an adenovirus-12-induced rat tumor after *in situ* hybridization with a complementary ³H-RNA viral probe. The autoradiographic grains are over areas of viral DNA synthesis and are over tumor cell nuclei only. b. Adenovirus-12-infected human embryo kidney cell nucleus treated in same manner as in a; note localization of autoradiographic grains indicating viral DNA synthesis over the nucleus.

that other highly oncogenic viruses, such as simian virus 40 (SV40), possess a high G + C content has cast doubt on the validity of this concept. Further, in the group of simian (monkey) adenoviruses, those with a high G + C content are more oncogenic than those containing a lower amount of G + C.

## ADENOVIRUS HYBRIDS

It has been found that adenoviruses form hybrids with a papovavirus called simian virus 40 (SV40) in which the resulting virions contain covalently linked nucleic acid from both viruses. In some such hybrids the adenovirus genome is defective, and the hybrid can replicate only if a cell is coinfected with a normal adenovirus. Other hybrids have been isolated in which the adenovirus genome is essentially complete but is still linked to part of the SV40 genome. Because this latter hybrid is able to replicate in the absence of a helper, it provides a valuable tool for genetic studies on the SV40 genome.

**Table 34-1. Oncogenicity of Human Adenoviruses for Newborn Hamsters Related to the Percentage of G + C in Their DNA**

| Group | Members | Oncogenicity | % DNA | DNA % G + C |
|-------|---------|--------------|-------|-------------|
| A | Ad 12, 18, 31 | Highly oncogenic[a] | 11.6–12.5 | 48–49 |
| B | Ad 3, 7, 11, 14, 16, 21 | Weakly oncogenic[a] (except Ad 11) | 12.5–13.7 | 49–52 |
| C | Ad 1, 2, 5, 6 | Nononcogenic, but transform rat embryo cells | 12.5–13.7 | 57–59 |

[a]Highly oncogenic adenoviruses induce tumors in a large proportion of newborn hamsters within two months after injection with a purified virus; weakly oncogenic adenoviruses induce tumors in a small proportion of animals after 4–18 months.

**Table 34-2. Adenovirus Types Related to Various Diseases**

| Types | Disease |
|---|---|
| 3, 4, 7, and 14 | Acute respiratory disease, primarily in military recruits |
| 1, 3, and 7A | Pneumonia (mostly in infants) |
| 3, 4, 7, and 14 | Acute respiratory disease in adults |
| 1, 2, 3, 4, 5, 6, 7A, and 14 | Pharyngitis and pharyngoconjunctival fever |
| 2, 3, 4, 6, 7A, 9, 10, and 15 | Conjunctivitis |
| 3, 8, and 7A | Epidemic keratoconjunctivitis |

## ADENOVIRUS INFECTIONS IN HUMANS

The incidence of overt respiratory infection caused by adenoviruses appears to be quite low. However, the observation that adenoviruses can be grown from 50–80% of tonsils and adenoids surgically removed certainly suggests that the vast majority of adenovirus infections occur as undiagnosed infections. As shown in Table 34-2, different serological types may cause various manifestations of respiratory and conjunctival infections. Major epidemics seem to occur primarily in new army recruits in the form of an acute respiratory disease caused by types 3, 4, and 7. For unknown reasons, these types occur much less frequently in civilian populations. Adenovirus causes epidemic keratoconjunctivitis (pink-eye), primarily in an environment in which the eyes are subjected to mild trauma by the presence of dust.

### Control of Adenovirus Infections

Since human beings seem to be the only reservoir for the human adenoviruses, the spread from person to person appears to occur directly via respiratory or conjunctival discharges; transmission of these discharges via swimming pools has also been suggested.

Recovery from adenovirus infections results in a long-lasting, type-specific immunity, and it seems possible that the long duration of immunity might be the result of a subclinical infection. One would expect vaccines to be effective for the prevention of adenovirus infections, and the Army has shown that to be the case using inactivated viral vaccines. In addition, live vaccines incorporated into a capsule which dissolves in the intestine have recently been shown to produce solid immunity (probably by stimulating the synthesis of specific IgA antibodies) without causing overt disease. The general absence of epidemics of acute respiratory disease in the civilian population, however, and the multiplicity of serological types of adenoviruses rules out the widespread use of adenovirus vaccines.

### Diagnosis of Adenovirus Infections

The diagnosis of adenovirus infections can be accomplished either by the isolation and identification of the virus or by the demonstration of a rise in specific antibody titer during a patient's convalescent period. Isolation is accomplished by placing respiratory or conjunctival secretions on monolayers of tissue culture cells and observing the cultures for cytopathic effect. General identification of an adenovirus is accomplished using known complement-fixing antibody which will react with all adenoviruses. Neutralizing or hemagglutination-inhibition antibodies are required to determine type specificity.

## Papovaviridae

The family Papovaviridae comprises a group of DNA viruses that essentially all produce either benign or malignant tumors. The name, papovavirus, was coined by using the first two letters of the original three viral types included in this family: (1) human and animal papillomaviruses, (2) mouse polyomavirus, and (3) simian vacuolating virus (SV40). All three types are naked icosahedral virions with 72 capsomers (see Figure 34-5) containing double-stranded circular DNA that apparently can exist as either a twisted supercoil or a simple circular structure. Although papillomavirus has not been successfully grown in vitro, all papovaviruses appear capable of causing an infection in which virus is synthesized in permissive cells and released by the death and lysis of the host cell. Papovaviruses also are capable of inducing a nonproductive infection in nonpermissive cells, resulting in cell transformation and the disappearance of infectious virions.

### POLYOMAVIRUS AND SV40

Polyomavirus can be routinely isolated from secretions of wild and laboratory mice; under natural conditions the infected mouse appears asymptomatic, even though it may excrete the virus for long periods of time. Inoculation of polyomavirus into mouse embryo or kidney cells results in a productive infection—virions are produced and infected host cells are destroyed. If, however, the virus is injected into newborn mice, hamsters, or rats, the animals develop multiple malignant tumors in essentially every organ of the body. Furthermore, the in vitro infection of nonpermissive hamster or rat cells results in their transformation into malignant cells. Thus, this virus appears to

**Figure 34-5.** Negatively-stained virions of SV40 ($\times$198,450).

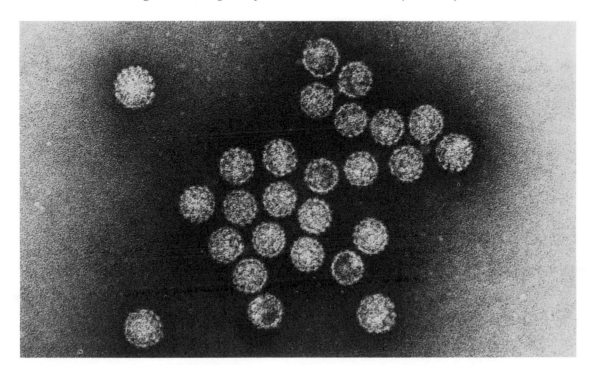

be essentially harmless when acquired naturally by the adult mouse but causes highly
fatal malignancies if injected into a newborn
animal that is not immunologically competent.

Simian vacuolating virus (SV40) is frequently isolated from cultured rhesus and
cynomolgus monkey kidney cells. It does
not produce a cytopathic effect in such cells,
and its presence in tissue cultures was undetected for many years. However, African
green monkey kidney cells infected with
SV40 virus show a cytopathic effect and are
killed. Furthermore, injection of SV40 virus
into newborn hamsters results in the production of a malignant sarcoma or lymphoma,
and the *in vitro* infection of nonpermissive
cells from a number of animals (including
humans) results in their transformation and
the loss of all infectious virus.

This latter fact was particularly disquieting when it became known that both the
Salk and the Sabin poliovirus vaccines were
grown in rhesus monkey kidney cells which
were unknowingly contaminated with SV40
virus, and as a result millions of individuals
were given live SV40 virus. Such persons
excreted the virus for weeks, but insofar as
is known, no human tumors resulted from
these infections. (See Progressive Multifocal
Leukoencephalopathy, described as a slow
SV40 virus infection in Chapter 40).

## Reproduction of Polyoma and
## SV40 Viruses

After penetration of the host cell, these
viruses are uncoated in cytoplasmic vacuoles and the DNA enters the nucleus where
they are transcribed into mRNA. Viral capsids are synthesized in the cytoplasm and
then enter the nucleus where assembly with
viral DNA occurs. Release follows rupture
of the nuclear envelope and lysis of the
host cell.

Transformation requires that at least a
part of the viral DNA become covalently
integrated into specific areas of the host cell

DNA. Even in nonpermissive cells this is an
infrequent event, and thus infection of most
nonpermissive cells results in an abortive
infection in which the cell undergoes transient transformation but later returns to
normal. However, if eventually transformed,
neither infectious particles nor free viral
DNA can be isolated from the malignant
cell, although the presence of viral DNA in
the host genome can be detected by hybridization with viral DNA. Furthermore, in some
cases if the transformed cell is fused with a
permissive cell (using an irradiated paramyxovirus to induce the fusion), infective
virus is sometimes produced, indicating that
viral replication is controlled at least in
part by the host cell.

## Characteristics of Transformed Cells

After transformation, cells are found to possess all or most of the following new properties: (1) they may form colonies in soft
agar; (2) they may have a reduced requirement for serum factors; (3) loss of contact
inhibition allows transformed cells to grow
to much higher densities than normal cells;
(4) the rate of sugar transport across the
cell membrane is accelerated; (5) frequent
chromosomal abnormalities are seen; (6)
changes in surface glycolipid concentration
or orientation allow increased agglutination
by plant lectins such as conconavalin A;
(7) they may produce malignancies when
injected into susceptible animals; (8) new
antigens are synthesized by the transformed
cells; (9) the concentration of 3'5'-adenosine
monophosphate (cAMP) within the transformed cell decreases.

## Evidence that the Virus Encodes
## for Transformation

Both polyoma and SV40 virus have a genome
believed to contain five genes with a molecular weight of 3 million daltons. By using
temperature-sensitive (ts) mutants, it has
been shown that two of these genes are

required to initiate transformation, but once transformation has occurred, only one gene is required to maintain this state. Experimental evidence for these conclusions is as follows: two different ts mutants, ts-a and ts-3, are capable of transforming cells at the permissive temperature (35°C), but not at the nonpermissive temperature (39°C). When cells transformed at 35° with the ts-3 mutant were raised to 39°C, they reverted to normal cells, indicating that the ts-3 gene must function continually in order to maintain the transformed state. On the contrary, cells transformed at 35°C by the ts-a mutant did not revert when raised to 39°C. Thus, this gene product must be necessary only for the initial transformation event and not for its maintenance.

### Antigenic Changes in Transformed Cells

T antigen appears in the nucleus of all cells infected with polyoma or SV40 virus. Antibodies to this new antigen do not react with the viral capsid, and in a productive infection T antigen is released from the nucleus during lysis of the host cell. However, virally transformed cells continue to express this antigen in their nuclei, and, as a result it has been named the T (for "tumor") antigen. It is virus-specific; any cell type transformed by polyomavirus will possess the same T antigen. Similarly, any cells transformed by SV40 will possess the same T antigen, but it differs from the polyomavirus T antigen. Thus, it is possible to screen cancer cells for the presence of specific T antigens by immunofluorescence or complement fixation tests to determine whether they are the result of a specific virus transformation.

Tumor-specific transplantation antigen (TSTA) is an antigen which is found on the surface of virally transformed cells. Like T antigen, it is probably coded by the viral genome, since it is specific for the transforming virus. Animals that are immunized with this antigen will destroy similar in-

fected malignant cells—presumably as a result of a cell-mediated immune response.

As previously stated, neither polyoma nor SV40 virus appears to cause tumors in humans. They have, however, provided the first model system for the induction of animal tumors and in vitro cell transformation by a DNA virus, and investigations of these two viruses will undoubtedly continue to elucidate the molecular mechanisms through which viruses induce malignant tumors in animals.

## PAPILLOMAVIRUS

Papillomaviruses, though slightly larger than polyoma and SV40 viruses, also possess a circular double-stranded DNA with a molecular weight of 5 million daltons enclosed in a naked icosahedral capsid.

Various papillomaviruses infect dogs, cattle, rabbits, and humans, producing benign growths on the skin called papillomas or warts. Virus can be demonstrated in these benign growths by transmission to a susceptible animal, by electron microscopy, or by immunofluorescence with specifically-labeled antibody. Studies of these viruses, however, have been hampered because it has not been possible until recently to get productive infection in tissue cultures, and assay of this virus has been therefore based on wart formation on the skin of a susceptible animal.

Rabbit papillomas were the first to be described and have been the most extensively studied of this group. In the usual course of events, proliferation of skin cells at the point of infection results in the formation of the papilloma or wart. Such growths may remain static for months or years and then spontaneously regress—presumably as a result of immunological destruction by the host.

Rabbit papillomas may occasionally convert into malignant tumors, after which, as described for polyoma and SV40 virus transformation, the papillomavirus can no longer be found. This transformation is particularly frequent when extracts of the papillomas from wild rabbits are injected into the skin of domestic rabbits, indicating that a host factor present in the domestic rabbits may be involved in this transformation. Once converted, malignant cells do not convert back to virus-producing cells and will routinely produce cancer if injected into a susceptible animal.

## Parvoviridae

Parvoviruses are the smallest icosahedral viruses found in vertebrates. They contain single-stranded linear DNA with a molecular weight of 1.6 million daltons and have been divided into two subgenera on the basis of whether they are defective or nondefective.

Subgenus A contains nondefective viruses that infect rats, mice, hamsters, cats, dogs, pigs, and possibly humans. In some of these animals, such as rats, they produce a variety of congenital defects in the fetus. Because of this ability to produce congenital defects in rats and inasmuch as some parvoviruses can be grown in human cells, the possible role of viruses in subgenus A in human infections cannot be ignored, and, in fact, recent observations suggest that parvoviruses do cause human disease. The first of these reports was concerned with an outbreak of nonbacterial gastroenteritis that occurred in an elementary school in Norwalk, Ohio. The infectious nature of the etiologic agent was demonstrated by infecting human volunteers. The disease is characterized by mild diarrhea and vomiting that occurs about 48 hours after exposure. The agent appears to be highly infectious, since over 50% of the student population was striken. Electron micrographs of concentrated fecal extracts have supported the conclusion that the Norwalk agent is a parvovirus (see Figure 34-6). However, the virus is extremely difficult to cultivate, and proof of a relationship between the Norwalk agent and other parvoviruses is still lacking. Infectious hepatitis (also called hepatitis A, see Chapter 36) is also believed to be a parvovirus, but this agent has not yet been cultivated and this possibility is still equivocable.

Subgenus B contains four serologic types of defective viruses named adeno-associated viruses or sometimes adenosatellite viruses (see Figure 34-7). These viruses are unable to grow in any cell unless the host cell is coinfected with an adenovirus. The nature of the helper function provided by the adenovirus is unknown, but since temperature-sensitive mutants unable to replicate their DNA at a nonpermissive temperature in a host cell are still capable of providing the helper function, the help must come from the early protein synthesis of the adenovirus.

All adeno-associated viruses contain single-stranded DNA, but they are additionally unusual in that some virions contain a plus

**Figure 34-6.** Norwalk agent virions (diameter = 27 nm; bar = 100 nm).

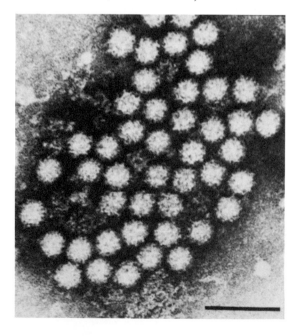

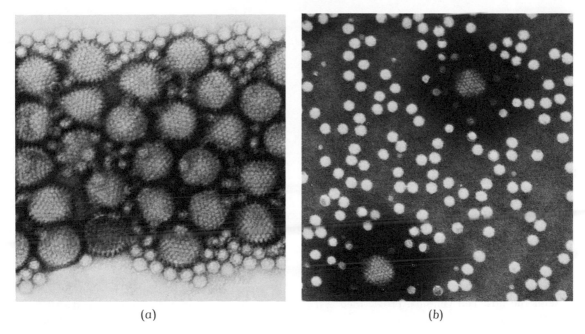

(a)                                             (b)

**Figure 34-7.** *a.* Adenovirus type 18 (diameter = 80 nm) contaminated with adeno-associated virus type 2 (diameter = 20 nm). This preparation is from a CsCl density gradient and is negatively-stained with PTA (×159,000). *b.* Human adenovirus type 31 (diameter = 70 nm) with adeno-associated virus type 1 (diameter = 20 nm). (×120,000.)

strand of DNA, while others contain the complementary minus strand. Types designated 1, 2, and 3 are human viruses, and type 4 is a monkey virus. They appear to be very widespread, based on the observation that most children acquire antibodies to the human types prior to reaching their teens. As far as is known, however, none of these viruses produce disease in humans.

Parvoviruses are very resistant to physical destruction; they can survive heating at 56°C for hours, are resistant to treatment with either ether or chloroform, and remain viable after years of storage. This resistance to physical destruction may well be important for their transmission as fecal-oral agents—Norwalk agent and hepatitis A.

## REFERENCES

Acheson, N. H. 1976. Transcription during productive infection with polyoma virus and simian virus 40. *Cell* **8:**1–12.

Bellett, A. J. D. 1975. Covalent integration of viral DNA into cell DNA in hamster cells transformed by avian adenovirus. *Virology* **65:**427–435.

Berns, K. I. 1974. Molecular biology of the adeno-associated viruses. *Current Topics in Microbiol. and Immunol.* **65:**1–20.

Brown, D. T., and B. T. Burlingham. 1973. Penetration of host cell membranes by adenovirus 2. *J. Virol.* **12:**386–396.

Butel, J. S. 1975. The role of SV40 viral genes in cellular transformation. *Progr. Med. Virol.* **21:**88–102.

Doerfler, W. 1970. Integration of the deoxyribonucleic acid of adenovirus type 12 into the deoxyribonucleic acid of baby hamster kidney cells. *J. Virol.* **6:**652–666.

Dolin, R., N. R. Blacklow, H. DuPont, R. F. Buscho, R. G. Wyatt, J. A. Kasel, R. Hornick, and R. M. Chanock. 1972. Biological properties of the Norwalk agent of acute infectious nonbacterial gastroenteritis. *Proc. Soc. Exp. Biol. Med.* **140:**578–583.

Fujinaga, K., and M. Green. 1970. Mechanism of viral carcinogenesis by DNA mammalian viruses. VII. Viral genes transcribed in adenovirus type 2 infected and transformed cells. *Proc. Nat. Acad. Sci. U.S.A.* **65**:375–382.

Khoury, G., and N. P. Salzman. 1975. Replication and transformation by papovaviruses. In F. F. Becker, ed. *Cancer 2.* Plenum Press, New York.

Levine, A. J., P. C. van der Vliet, and J. S. Sussenbach. 1976. The replication of papovavirus and adenovirus DNA. *Current Topics in Microbiol. and Immunol.* **73**:67–124.

Mayor, H. D., and E. Kurstak. 1974. Viruses with separately encapsulated complementary DNA strands. Chapter 3 in E. Kurstak and K. Maramorosch, eds. *Viruses, Evolution and Cancer.* Academic Press, New York.

McDougall, J. K. 1975. Adenoviruses—interaction with the host cell genome. *Progr. Med. Virol.* **21**:118–132.

Nernut, M. V. 1975. Fine structure of adenovirus type 5. I. Virus capsid. *Virology* **65**:480–495.

Philipson, L., and V. Lindberg. 1974. Reproduction of adenoviruses. In H. Fraenkel-Conrat and R. R. Wagner, eds. *Comprehensive Virology,* Vol. 3. Plenum Press, New York.

Rose, J. A. 1974. Parvovirus reproduction. In H. Fraenkel-Conrat and R. R. Wagner, eds. *Comprehensive Virology,* Vol. 3. Plenum Press, New York.

Salzman, N. P., and G. Khoury. 1974. Reproduction of papovaviruses. In H. Fraenkel-Conrat and R. R. Wagner, eds. *Comprehensive Virology,* Vol. 3. Plenum Press, New York.

Sundquist, B., E. Everitt, L. Philipson, and S. Hoglund. 1973. Assembly of adenoviruses. *J. Virol.* **11**:449–459.

Westphal, H., and R. Dulbecco. 1968. Viral DNA in polyoma and SV40 transformed cell lines. *Proc. Nat. Acad. Sci. U. S. A.* **59**:1158–1165.

# 35

## Poxviridae

Poxviruses are large, complex, oval viruses which are classified into genera on the basis of their natural hosts and the possession of specific group antigens. All poxviruses are morphologically similar, and all induce cell proliferation to some degree in a susceptible host. The most common manifestation of this proliferation is the pox lesion—the external signs of such diseases as smallpox, cowpox, rabbitpox, sheeppox, and fowlpox. In these cases, the lesion disappears in one to two weeks as a result of the death of the infected cells.

Other poxviruses induce the formation of nodules or benign tumors which may persist for several months before disappearing. Still others have become so well adapted to their normal host that they are able to induce host cell proliferation without causing the death of the infected cell. This results in large superficial masses of cells called fibromas, benign and seldom fatal. One poxvirus causes a benign fibroma in South American rabbits and a highly fatal myxomatosis in European rabbits, demonstrating that the final manifestation of an infection can be a function of both the virus and the host.

## STRUCTURE AND REPLICATION OF POXVIRUSES

Poxviruses are structurally the most complex of any of the animal viruses. Their double-stranded DNA, capable of coding for several hundred proteins, is enclosed in a dense, dumbbell-shaped core, along with a number of enzymes necessary for viral replication. The core is surrounded by a lipoprotein membrane, and fitting into the concave portions of the dumbbell-shaped core are dense structures which have been named lateral bodies. Very little is known concerning either the composition or function of these bodies. This entire structure is enclosed in a second lipoprotein envelope which may possess thread-like or globular subunits on its external surface (see Figure 35-1). A better concept of poxvirus structure may be gained by examining the events which occur during the replication of vaccinia virus, the avirulent virus used to vaccinate against smallpox.

## REPLICATION OF VACCINIA VIRUS

The replication of vaccinia virus is in all likelihood identical to that occurring in hu-

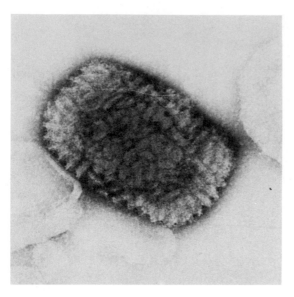

**Figure 35-1.** Smallpox (variola) virus (×147,000). Note "brick" shape and globular subunits on surface.

membrane, and a second uncoating must occur to release the naked DNA. This step puzzled virologists for years, because inhibitors of RNA or of protein synthesis prevented the second uncoating, indicating that either the cell or the virus must synthesize an uncoating enzyme before viral replication could continue. It was then discovered that the virus core contains a DNA-dependent RNA polymerase which can function within the virus core. Thus, the polymerase synthesizes early mRNA's corresponding to about 14% of the viral DNA genome. These early mRNA's are extruded from the viral core and are translated on host cell ribosomes, producing several proteins. One of these early proteins is an uncoating enzyme which degrades the viral core membrane, releasing the naked DNA.

Following release of the DNA, additional early transcription occurs (before DNA replication begins), producing several structural proteins and several enzymes, including a DNA polymerase. The appearance of the DNA polymerase is followed by the replication of the viral DNA. At the same time, the synthesis and translation of late mRNA's begins, resulting in the formation of more viral enzymes and most of the structural proteins of the virus. During this time, host cell protein synthesis is inhibited and transport of host cell mRNA from the nucleus is blocked. The molecular mechanism by which the virus prevents these cellular events is not known.

Two aspects of poxvirus replication should be noted as different from DNA viruses such as adenoviruses and herpesviruses. First, the entire replication occurs in the cytoplasm

man smallpox infection and is probably quite similar to that of most other poxviruses (see Figure 35-2).

Following the inoculation of a cell culture, the virus is rapidly adsorbed to receptors on the host cell. The nature or specificity of these cellular receptor sites is not known. Penetration occurs as a result of phagocytosis of the intact virion into a host cell phagocytic vesicle. At this stage the first uncoating step occurs, the degradation of the outer viral membrane by host cell enzymes. The viral core, without the lateral bodies, then leaves the phagocytic vesicle and enters the cytoplasm of the host cell.

At this point in the replicative cycle the viral DNA is still enclosed within its own

**Figure 35-2.** *a.* Replication of vaccinia. Note that replication takes place entirely within the cytoplasm of the host cell. *b.* Insertion of nucleoprotein into viral membranes to form immature vaccinia "proviruses." The first frame shows deoxyribonucleoprotein at midstage of condensation and insertion, the second shows insertion nearly completed with some material still extending into the host cell's cytoplasm, and the third frame shows a fully developed nucleoid, or provirus, with a small orifice remaining to close. (Each frame ×102,900.)

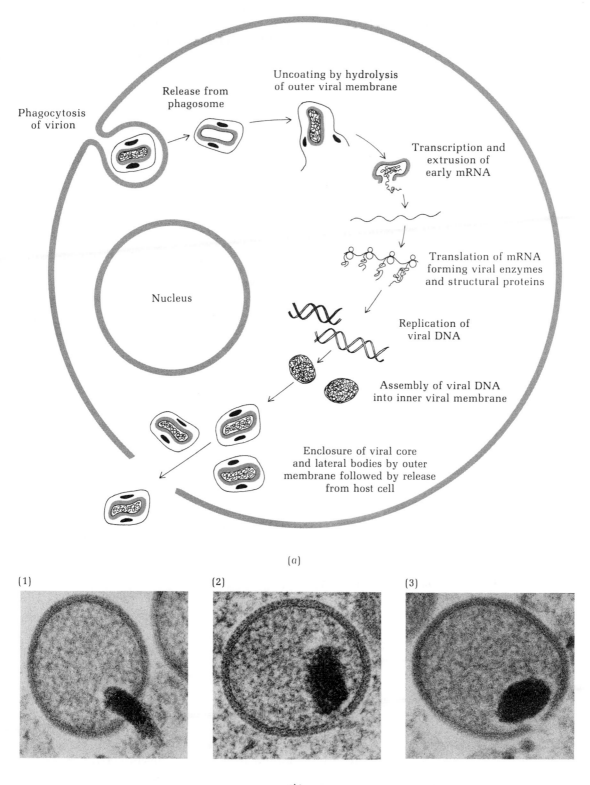

Phagocytosis
of virion

Release from
phagosome

Uncoating by hydrolysis
of outer viral membrane

Transcription and
extrusion of
early mRNA

Translation of mRNA
forming viral enzymes
and structural proteins

Replication of
viral DNA

Nucleus

Assembly of viral DNA
into inner viral membrane

Enclosure of viral core
and lateral bodies by outer
membrane followed by release
from host cell

(a)

(1)        (2)        (3)

(b)

of the host cell; and second, viral assembly does not begin until viral DNA replication is essentially complete. The assembly of the viral DNA and viral enzymes into this very complex virion is not fully understood, but events appear to occur in reverse order to those in its degradation. Thus, the DNA is enclosed in a viral membrane, which is then surrounded by a second membrane enclosing the lateral bodies to form the completed virion. The release of completed virions from the host cell is a very inefficient process, and at least 90% of the virions remain in the cell. Those virions which leave the cell may exit through the microvilli, or perhaps they fuse with portions of the plasma membrane of the host cell. Preliminary evidence suggests that those virions exiting from the host cell may acquire new antigens from the host membrane.

## POXVIRUS INFECTIONS IN HUMANS

### Smallpox

Smallpox is an ancient disease, causing the death of untold millions of people during its 3000-year recorded history. As recently as 50 years ago there were thousands of cases of smallpox occurring annually in the United States.

Two variants of the smallpox virus are pathogenic for humans. The first, variola major, causes a severe illness which may have a mortality rate of 25–50%. It is undoubtedly this variant of the virus which has claimed so many lives. The second variant, variola minor (frequently called alastrim), produces a much milder disease, with a mortality of less than 1%. Although there is no doubt that these two variants actually exist as separate entities, they are morphologically and antigenically identical. It is claimed, however, that they have different growth characteristics when grown at 38°C on the chorioallantoic membrane of chick embryos or mouse brain: variola minor will not produce pox lesions at this elevated temperature although variola major does. For both viruses the pathogenesis of infection is nearly identical, although the skin lesions of variola minor are more superficial.

PATHOGENICITY OF SMALLPOX. The usual site of entry for the smallpox virus is the respiratory tract. An incubation period of 12 to 16 days follows, during which the virus multiplies, probably in the regional lymph nodes. Symptoms (characterized by chills, fever, headache, back pains, and prostration) begin when the virus enters the blood stream. Viremia (virus in the blood stream) results in the spread of the virus throughout the body, infecting internal organs, mucous membranes, and skin. Several days later pox lesions appear on the face and then spread to the forearms, hands, and lower extremities. Lesions occur over the entire body, but they are usually more abundant on the shoulders and chest than on the abdomen (see Figure 35-3). Unlike those of chickenpox, the lesions of smallpox are usually in the same stage of development in any given body area, that is, they occur as a single crop which progresses from a macule (unraised discoloration) to a papule (raised lesion) to a vesicle (containing fluid) and finally rupture, followed by crusting over and healing.

Spread of the virus is probably most often from direct or indirect contact with the pox lesions of an infected individual. However, since mucous membranes may also be infected, any contact with secretions or discharges of an infected patient can serve to spread the disease.

DIAGNOSIS OF SMALLPOX. The diagnosis may be made on the basis of appearance and clinical symptoms, but a positive confirmation requires one or more laboratory procedures. The best technique is to inoculate the chorioallantoic membrane of a 12 to 14-day-old chick embryo with scrapings obtained from the pox lesions. Growth of the virus is manifested after two to three days by the appearance of lesions on the membrane.

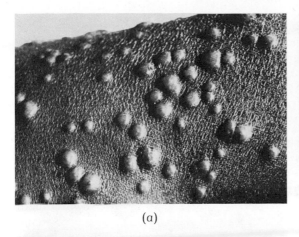

(a)

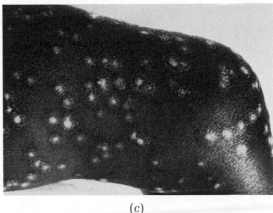

(c)

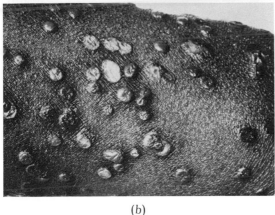

(b)

**Figure 35-3.** Smallpox lesions on leg of 3-year-old girl. *a*. Day 5 of eruption. *b*. Day 9. *c*. Day 14; healing is well along.

The identity of the virus can be confirmed by treating virus isolated from the chick embryo with known neutralizing antiserum and inoculating additional embryos with the treated specimen.

The direct microscopic examination of stained cells from pox lesions (or the lesions occurring on the chick embryo) will show characteristic cytoplasmic inclusion bodies called Guarnieri bodies (see Figure 35-4). These bodies are the virus assembly areas, and their appearance provides a presumptive diagnosis of smallpox.

One may also use serologic tests, employing antigen from the human lesions and immune rabbit serum for the complement fixation test. A retrospective diagnosis can be made by showing a rise in antibody titer against smallpox virus; however, this method would not be of value until about one week after the occurrence of symptoms.

CONTROL OF SMALLPOX. Although smallpox is no longer common in the Western Hemisphere, epidemics still occur in some parts of the world. For example, during the first five months of 1973, 66,185 cases of smallpox were reported to the World Health Organization. Most of these cases were from epidemics in northern India and Bangladesh. Because smallpox can be controlled by vaccination, it should be possible to eliminate the disease, and the World Health Organization (WHO) has predicted that for the first time in thousands of years smallpox may be eradicated from the earth by the end of 1976. (Unfortunately, several African outbreaks delayed fulfillment of this goal.)

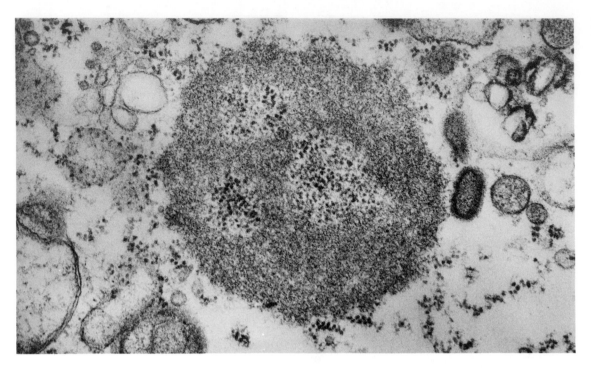

**Figure 35-4.** Electron micrograph of inclusion body in an L cell 3 hours after infection with vaccinia virus (×49,200). The appearance of inclusions resulting from smallpox virus infections is identical, and under the light microscope with appropriate staining such bodies are termed Guarnieri bodies.

The potential for this significant event began when Edward Jenner pointed out in 1798 (long before anyone had any concept of a virus) that in a population where essentially everyone contracted smallpox, many of the milkmaids in England were immune to the disease. He postulated that their immunity stemmed from an earlier infection with cowpox acquired from milking infected cows. In spite of a great deal of ridicule and opposition for proposing such an unorthodox concept, a vaccination program using ground scabs obtained from the lesions of infected cows was instigated in both Europe and the United States. The efficacy of this program is now readily apparent.

A number of viral strains called vaccinia virus are currently used for vaccination against smallpox; although their origin is somewhat hazy, they probably represent mutants of cowpox virus which occurred during the production of the vaccine.

In modern vaccination practice the vaccinia virus is introduced into the skin of a susceptible person. About a week later a local lesion develops, healing about two weeks later and leaving a scar. This series of events is called a primary take. Sometimes one does not get a primary take, even in individuals who are known not to have been vaccinated previously. In such cases, the person is vaccinated repeatedly until a primary take occurs. In a previously vaccinated individual the severity of the vaccination reaction varies according to the degree of residual immunity. In comparison with a primary take, the lesion progresses through its stages more rapidly and heals considerably sooner in a partially immune individual. This is called a vaccinoid reaction. The completely immune person gets only a small red papule, which appears two or three days after vaccination and heals in a few more days, leaving no scar. It is important to remember that inactive virus may give a response identical with that of an immune reaction. Therefore, one must not interpret such a result as an immune reaction in a previously unvaccinated person.

The normal smallpox vaccination does not usually provide lifelong immunity, and there is no general agreement as to the length of its protection. However, it is believed to be effective for at least three to seven years.

Several complications may follow vaccination with vaccinia virus. Progressive vaccinia, or vaccinia necrosum, occurs when the primary lesion fails to heal and continues to enlarge and spread. This is extremely rare and seems to occur in those persons unable to make a cellular immune response. Although it has in the past been invariably fatal, treatment with vaccinia immune globulin might be effective.

A condition known as generalized vaccinia is seen in persons with eczema. It is characterized by the presence of vaccinia lesions all over the eczematous area, resulting from a transplantation of the virus (usually by fingers) from the original vaccination site. It is an extremely severe and sometimes fatal complication. Thus, an individual with eczema or one who lives with an unvaccinated person who has eczema should not be vaccinated.

Postvaccinal encephalitis is another rare complication that may follow smallpox vaccination. The incidence seems to vary from year to year, but it probably occurs in about one out of every 50,000 persons vaccinated. The symptoms of encephalitis usually begin about 10 to 12 days after vaccination, and the mortality may run as high as 50%.

Fetal vaccinia has also been reported to occur in women who receive their primary vaccination during pregnancy. This, also, is quite rare. It is thought that vaccinia virus cannot normally pass through the placental membrane; however, since reported cases have resulted in the death of the fetus, primary vaccination during pregnancy should be avoided.

There has been no case of smallpox in the United States for over 25 years, and many public health officials maintain that in most Western countries the risks of complications from smallpox vaccination far outweigh the risks of contracting smallpox. The official policy of the U.S. Public Health Service is now to vaccinate only those persons returning from endemic areas in the Far East and Africa.

It should be emphasized that vaccination is a very effective control for smallpox, and it is only as a result of intensive vaccination programs that smallpox has been essentially eliminated from the Western World. Current efforts by the World Health Organization (WHO) to eradicate this disease from endemic areas by vaccination programs are proving successful. Complete eradication of smallpox is possible because there are no nonhuman hosts for the virus.

TREATMENT OF SMALLPOX. Immunity to smallpox is probably due to both humoral antibody production and to a cellular immune response. Vaccinia immune globulin is available in the United States, and, although it may provide protection prior to infection, it appears to be of little value if given during the overt disease.

Much effort has been directed toward finding chemotherapeutic agents that are effective for the treatment of smallpox. Although some antibiotics, such as rifampicin, will prevent the replication of vaccinia virus in tissue culture, the concentrations required are too high to be of value for therapeutic use. One compound which does inhibit the replication of poxviruses in humans is N-methyl isatin-$\beta$-thiosemicarbazone. This chemical appears to block the translation of viral mRNA. It is ineffective for the treatment of smallpox symptoms, but it seems to be of prophylactic value in reducing the attack rate during smallpox epidemics.

Since poxvirus replication is inhibited by the presence of interferon, a mechanism for the stimulation of interferon production might also be of value, particularly as a prophylactic measure during epidemics.

## Cowpox

This disease occurs in cows as a mild infection which is transmitted to humans by direct contact. Thus, human infections usually occur on the hands and fingers, causing lesions not unlike a primary take from vaccinia virus. The disease is self-limiting, and following healing of the lesions, infected humans possess immunity to the much more virulent smallpox virus. Although early vaccinations used cowpox, the vaccinia virus used today is not identical to cowpox virus, as we mentioned earlier.

## Molluscum Contagiosum

This disease involves a lesion which proliferates on the skin, most frequently on the face, arms, buttocks, genitals, and legs. The lesions appear as small, white nodules, about 2 mm in diameter, and result from the proliferation of epithelial cells. Infected cells contain very large cytoplasmic inclusion bodies containing poxvirus, which have been given the name molluscum bodies.

The nodules usually disappear after several months, probably following the development of a cellular immune response. The virus has not been extensively studied and the mechanism by which it stimulates cell proliferation is unknown.

## Yaba Monkey Poxvirus

This poxvirus causes a benign tumor in Asian and African monkeys, and it regresses after

five or six weeks. People can be infected accidentally or experimentally by laboratory strains, but no spontaneous human infections have been reported.

## Miscellaneous Animal Poxviruses That May Infect Humans

Orf, a poxvirus that causes a contagious pustular dermatitis in sheep, may occasionally infect a person by direct contact with an infected sheep. Milker's nodules is a disease of cattle which is immunologically distinct from cowpox. Milkers may become infected, usually on their hands, as a result of milking infected cows. Human infection with either of these two viruses is an occupational hazard. Both infections result in local lesions at the point of infection, which spontaneously regress after four to eight weeks.

## REFERENCES

Baxby, D. 1975. Identification and inter-relationships of the variola/vaccinia subgroup of poxviruses. *Progr. Med. Virol.* **19**:215–246.

DeHarven, E., and D. S. Yohn. 1966. The fine structure of the Yaba monkey tumor virus. *Cancer Res.* **26**:995–1008.

Gaylord, W. H., and J. L. Melnick. 1953. The intracellular forms of poxviruses as shown by the electron microscope (vaccinia, ectromelia, molluscum contagiosum). *J. Exp. Med.* **98**:157–172.

Ito, Y. 1975. Papilloma-Myxoma Viruses. In F. F. Becker, ed. *Cancer 2.* Plenum Press, New York.

Katz, E., and E. Margalith. 1973. Location of vaccinia virus structural polypeptides on the surface of the virus particle. *J. Gen. Virol.* **18**:381–384.

Kaverin, N. V., N. L. Varich, V. V. Surgay, and V. I. Chernos. 1975. A quantitative estimation of poxvirus genome fraction transcribed as "early" and "late" mRNA. *Virology* **65**:112–119.

Langer, W. L. 1976. The prevention of smallpox before Jenner. *Sci. American* **234**:112–117.

Moss, B. 1974. Reproduction of poxviruses. In H. Fraenkel-Conrat and R. R. Wagner, eds. *Comprehensive Virology,* Vol. 3. Plenum Press, New York.

Sarov, I., and W. K. Joklik. 1973. Isolation and characterization of intermediates in vaccinia virus morphogenesis. *Virology* **52:**223–233.

# 36

# Hepatitis

Although over 50,000 cases of viral hepatitis (inflammation of the liver) are reported annually in the United States (Table 36-1), the causative agents for this disease have not yet been grown in cell cultures. Essentially everything known about the epidemiology and pathogenesis of viral hepatitis has been learned by infecting human volunteers with extracts such as blood, feces, urine, and duodenal contents obtained from patients suffering from hepatitis.

Such studies have shown that human hepatitis is caused by at least two distinctly different viruses which can be clinically differentiated from one another by the length of their incubation periods and by the epidemiology of the infection. In one case, the incubation period averages about 35 days, and the virus is usually transmitted from person to person via a fecal-oral route, the origin of the original name, infectious hepatitis. In the second case, the incubation period is considerably longer, varying from 50 to 180 days, and the mode of transmission was thought to be restricted to the injection of blood or serum from an infected individual, giving rise to the name serum hepatitis. Several decades of research have confirmed the concept of two distinct agents of viral hepatitis, although it is now known that the mechanism of transmission of serum hepatitis is not restricted to the mechanical injection of infectious blood products. In 1974, a Committee on Viral Hepatitis of the National Research Council of the National Academy of Sciences proposed a standard terminology for the nomenclature of the various particles and antigens found associated with serum hepatitis. This terminology refers to infec-

**Table 36-1. Cases of Viral Hepatitis Reported in the U.S. 1966–1973**

| Calendar Year | Acute Hepatitis A and Unspecified | Hepatitis B |
|---|---|---|
| 1966 | 32,859 | 1,497 |
| 1967 | 38,909 | 2,458 |
| 1968 | 45,893 | 4,829 |
| 1969 | 48,416 | 5,909 |
| 1970 | 56,797 | 8,310 |
| 1971 | 59,606 | 9,556 |
| 1972 | 54,074 | 9,402 |
| 1973 | 50,749 | 8,451 |

tious hepatitis as hepatitis A and serum hepatitis as hepatitis B.

## NATURE OF THE HEPATITIS VIRIONS

Since neither hepatitis A nor hepatitis B virus has been grown in cell cultures, much of our current information about these agents has resulted from observations of blood and feces of infected individuals and the use of human volunteers to determine the infectiousness of treated material.

Hepatitis A virus appears to be one of the most stable viruses infecting humans. Its resistance to treatment with ether suggests that it does not possess an envelope. It can withstand heating at 56°C for 30 minutes and is remarkably resistant to many disinfectants. Electron microscopy of fecal extracts, which have been mixed with antibody to hepatitis A virus, has revealed clumps of virus-like particles approximately 27 nm in diameter which appear to possess an icosahedral sym-

**Figure 36-1.** Immune electron microscopy of hepatitis A virus purified from a chimpanzee stool (×256,300). The coating of IgM antibody produces the "halo" around individual particles.

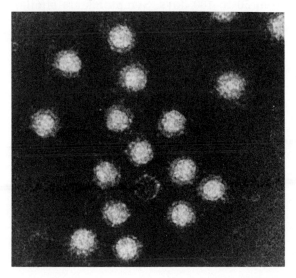

metry (Figure 36-1), and it has been postulated that this agent may be a parvovirus (see Chapter 34).

Hepatitis B virus is also an unusually stable virus; however, as a result of tremendous numbers of virus-like particles which occur in the blood of both infected individuals and asymptomatic carriers, a great deal more is known about this virus. These virus-like particles, originally discovered in the serum of an Australian aborigine, have until recently been referred to as Australian antigen, or hepatitis-associated antigen. The particles are uniformly 22 nm in diameter, existing as both spherical particles and filaments (see Figure 36-2). Treatment with ether removes a 2 nm coat, but the nature or significance of the material removed is unknown. These particles do not, however, contain nucleic acid and are assumed to represent excess viral-coat particles. Standard terminology now refers to these coat particles as $HB_sAg$ to designate that they are the surface antigen of hepatitis B. In addition, it has been established that $HB_sAg$ contains a group-specific determinant, $a$, and subtype determinants, $d$ or $y$, plus $w$ or $r$. Thus, there is a total of four subtypes of hepatitis B virus, which are designated as $adw$, $adr$, $ayw$, and $ayr$.

In 1970 another particle 42 nm in diameter was found in the serum of hepatitis B patients. These larger particles (named Dane particles, after their discoverer) occurred in much lower concentration than did the $HB_sAg$ particles. Treatment of the Dane particles with a nonionic detergent caused them to dissociate into $HB_sAg$ particles and an inner core 27 nm in diameter. This inner core, now called $HB_cAg$, has been shown to contain circular double-stranded DNA (see Figure 36-3). Furthermore, the core contains a DNA polymerase which can synthesize DNA using the circular DNA as a template for replication.

It appears that the 42 nm Dane particle represents the intact hepatitis B virus composed of an inner, double-stranded, DNA-

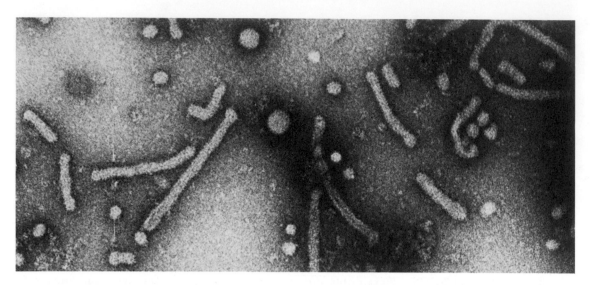

**Figure 36-2.** Fraction of the blood serum from a severe case of human hepatitis; the patient's immune system failed to counteract the infection. The larger spherical particles, or Dane particles, are 42 nm in diameter and are thought to be the complete hepatitis B virus. The smaller, more numerous spherical particles may be the cores (HB$_c$Ag) of the larger ones. Also seen are filaments of capsid protein (HB$_s$Ag).

protein core (HB$_c$Ag) and an outer surface coat (HB$_s$Ag).

## PATHOGENESIS OF HEPATITIS

Both hepatitis A and hepatitis B viruses appear to be widely disseminated throughout the body, but the major area of cell necrosis (death) occurs in the liver. The resulting necrosis and enlargement of the liver frequently cause blockage of the biliary excretion, resulting in jaundice.

Hepatitis A infections have an asymptomatic incubation period of 15 to 40 days. Symptoms usually begin abruptly, with fever, nausea, and vomiting, as shown in Table 36-2. After several days, jaundice may become apparent, and at that time the acute symptoms usually subside. Complete recovery may require eight to twelve weeks, and during the convalescent period the patient frequently remains weak and occasionally depressed. Virus is present in the blood and feces for about two weeks before symptoms

begin and for one to two weeks after the disappearance of jaundice. The severity of the disease varies considerably with age; most cases occurring in young children are mild and undiagnosed.

Hepatitis B infections are characterized by a considerably longer incubation period, from 50 to 180 days. Symptoms are similar to those described for hepatitis A infections, but their onset is usually more insidious. Virus is only rarely present in feces or urine but does occur in the blood during the latter half of the incubation period. In most cases virus disappears from the blood by the time liver-function tests return to normal. However, in 10–30% of hepatitis B infections, both virus (Dane particles) and tremendous amounts of HB$_s$Ag may be found in the blood for months or years after recovery from the overt disease. It has been estimated that there are over 100 million carriers of hepatitis B in the world. The over-all higher fatality rates of hepatitis B over hepatitis A infections (about 2%) may be a reflection of

**Table 36-2. Reported Signs and Symptoms in an Outbreak of Hepatitis A from Fecally Contaminated Water**

| Signs and Symptoms | Percent |
| --- | --- |
| Nausea | 91 |
| Lethargy | 85 |
| Abdominal pain | 83 |
| Anorexia | 71 |
| Vomiting | 71 |
| Fever | 70 |
| Dark urine | 63 |
| Jaundice | 55 |
| Sore throat | 36 |
| Diarrhea | 21 |

the size of the infecting dose, the health of the patient receiving a transfusion (a major source of infection), or the result of a more destructive virus.

## EPIDEMIOLOGY OF HEPATITIS

### Hepatitis A

It is well established that hepatitis A is most often spread from person to person via a fecal-oral route and that the majority of infections occur during the fall and winter. The 34,570 cases reported in the United States during 1975 probably represent only a small percentage of actual infections, since the vast majority of hepatitis A infections are undiagnosed. This is particularly true for children, in whom jaundice is not a common manifestation of the disease.

Epidemics have resulted from drinking fecally-contaminated water or by eating food which has been prepared by a subclinically infected individual. The ingestion of raw oysters or clams from fecally-contaminated water has also caused a large number of hepatitis A infections.

Because hepatitis A virus is present in the blood for about two weeks before symptoms, the disease during this period can be passed from person to person by transfusions or by the use of improperly sterilized needles or syringes. It has been estimated that about one-fourth of all cases of post-transfusion hepatitis are caused by hepatitis A virus; however, because of the relatively short incubation period in which the virus is present in the blood, other investigators believe this figure is too high.

### Hepatitis B

Early volunteer studies with this disease failed to show a normal portal of exit for hepatitis B virus, and for years it was believed that an individual could become infected

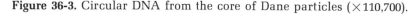

**Figure 36-3.** Circular DNA from the core of Dane particles (×110,700).

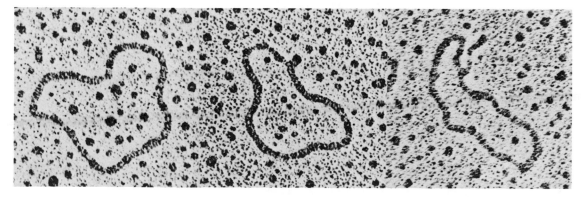

only by the injection of blood or serum from an infected person or through the use of contaminated needles or syringes. It has now been shown that this supposition is not true. Using serologic techniques, $HB_sAg$ has been found in the feces, urine, and other body secretions of infected persons. Also, the disease has been transmitted by feeding infected serum to human volunteers. But, even though a fecal-oral transmission does occur, the vast majority of hepatitis B infections appear to result from an injection of the virus.

The frequency of this disease is primarily caused by the large number of undiagnosed hepatitis B infections; even more important, an individual may be asymptomatic and continue to carry extremely large amounts of virus in his blood for months or even years. Thus, not only the injection of blood or serum but the use of improperly sterilized syringes, needles, or dental instruments has been shown to be the source of infection. Drug addicts are, of course, particularly susceptible. One series of infections was traced to a jewelry store using soiled instruments to pierce ears, and other cases have been traced to instruments used in tattooing. Table 36-3 summarizes the major characteristics of hepatitis A and B.

## DIAGNOSIS OF HEPATITIS

The diagnosis of individual cases of viral hepatitis is not usually possible in the absence of supporting laboratory findings. Abnormal liver function is indicated by increased levels of serum glutamic-oxaloacetic transaminase (SGOT) and serum glutamic-pyruvic transaminase (SGPT). The presence of $HB_sAg$ confirms a diagnosis of hepatitis B. Since a number of other viral and bacterial infections may cause liver damage, the diagnosis of hepatitis A is more difficult and may depend upon a history of an injection 15 to 40 days prior to symptoms or the simultaneous occurrence of a number of cases in which the epidemiology and incubation period is con-

**Table 36-3. Differential Characteristics of Hepatitis A and Hepatitis B**

| Characteristic | Hepatitis A | Hepatitis B |
|---|---|---|
| Length of incubation period | 15–40 days | 50–180 days |
| Source of infection | Mostly fecal-oral | Mostly from parenteral injections |
| Host range | Humans and possibly nonhuman primates | Humans and some non-human primates |
| Seasonal occurrence | Higher in fall and winter | Year round |
| Age incidence | Much higher in children | All ages |
| Occurrence of jaundice | Much higher in adults | Higher in adults |
| Virus in blood | 2–3 weeks before illness to 1–2 weeks after recovery | Several weeks before illness to months or years after recovery |
| Virus in feces | 2–3 weeks before illness to 1–2 weeks after recovery | Rarely present, or present in very small amounts |
| Probable size of virus | 27 nm ? | 42 nm |
| Diagnosis based on | Liver function tests, clinical symptoms, & history | Liver function tests, clinical symptoms, history, & presence of $HB_sAg$ in blood |
| Value of gamma globulin for prophylaxis | Good | Ineffective |

sistent for that disease. Such a situation has been known to arise in summer camps or military installations.

The serologic detection of $HB_sAg$ is now routinely carried out in diagnostic laboratories and blood banks. This can be accomplished by reacting the patient's serum with serum known to contain antibody to $HB_sAg$, using any of the following techniques: (1) complement fixation, (2) immunodiffusion in which the patient's serum and the anti $HB_sAg$ diffuse toward each other to form a precipitin band, (3) counter-immunoelectrophoresis in which the serum and the antiserum are electrophoresed toward each other to hasten the precipitin reaction, (4) red cell agglutination in which red cells are coated with anti-$HB_sAg$ prior to the addition of unknown serum, and (5) radioimmune assay in which antigen in the patient's serum competes with known radioactively-labeled antigen for reaction with the specific antibody. Of these, counter-immunoelectrophoresis is the most rapid, but red cell agglutination and the radioimmune assay are many times more sensitive and, as a result, are being increasingly used to detect $HB_sAg$. Table 36-4 compares the sensitivity of these procedures in several classes of patients.

## CONTROL OF HEPATITIS

Proper sanitation to prevent fecal contamination of water and food is certainly the most effective way to interrupt the fecal-oral transmission of hepatitis A and to a lesser extent of hepatitis B. In addition, scrupulous attention to the adequate sterilization of syringes and needles would eliminate a number of needless infections with hepatitis virus. One must bear in mind, though, that viral hepatitis is caused by at least two different agents, and thus different specific control measures may be directed toward these infectious agents.

### Control of Hepatitis B

The examination of all donor blood for the presence of $HB_sAg$ is now routine, and this practice has done much to control the occurrence of post-transfusional hepatitis B infections.

Passive immunization of human volunteers with hyperimmune hepatitis B antiserum prevents active disease when challenged with infectious material. But the use of immune serum is not effective for the treatment of the disease and, since exposure to hepatitis B is usually not known until the appearance of symptoms, passive immunization appears to be of no practical value. Pooled gamma globulin has little, if any, value for the prevention of hepatitis B—probably because the level of antibodies to this agent in the general population is not high enough to provide an adequate level of immunity.

The possibility of an effective vaccine has been reported by investigators who have

**Table 36-4. Comparison of Techniques for the Detection of Antibodies Against $HB_sAg$**

| Technique | Relative Sensitivity | PREVALENCE OF ANTI-$HB_s$ IN THE U.S.A. | | |
|---|---|---|---|---|
| | | Blood Donors | Hemophiliacs | Patients Convalescing from Hepatitis Type B |
| Immunodiffusion | 1 | <1% | 20–30% | 1% |
| Counter-Immunoelectrophoresis | 1–4 | <1% | 40–50% | 1% |
| Complement fixation | 2–10 | <1% | 15–20% | 1% |
| Passive hemagglutination | 1000–10,000 | 3–5% | 75–80% | 70–80% |
| Solid-phase radioimmunoassay | 1000–10,000 | 5–7% | 75–80% | 70–80% |
| Radioimmunoprecipitation | 10,000–100,000 | 10–15% | 80–85% | 75–85% |

purified the $HB_sAg$ from human carriers, eliminating infectious virus, blood proteins, and blood group substances in the process. The use of this purified antigen as a vaccine in chimpanzees was found to be 100 percent effective in preventing infections when challenged with an infectious dose of the same subtype of infectious virus. When animals immunized with $HB_sAg$ subtype *ayw* were challenged with subtype *adr,* they became infected but did not develop any overt signs of the disease, suggesting that at least partial immunity occurs across subtypes.

Should this vaccine be proved safe and be approved for use by the Food and Drug Administration, it would be given to high-risk individuals such as blood bank workers, doctors, dentists, nurses, and persons who might be expected to require multiple blood transfusions.

An additional antigenic complex, called the e-antigen, has been reported to occur in the Dane particles but not in $HB_sAg$. Little is known about this component, but initial investigations indicate that individuals with high levels of anti-e also possess high levels of the supposedly infectious Dane particles and also show signs of active disease as manifested by liver damage. On the contrary, persons lacking antibodies to the e-antigen appear to possess very few Dane particles. Although they may be carriers of $HB_sAg$, they are asymptomatic and do not appear to represent an important source for transmitting the hepatitis B virus. For the present, however, the exact location or significance of the e-antigen complex is unknown.

### Control of Hepatitis A

Until recently, there were no procedures for the detection of hepatitis A virus and therefore no effective scheme to prevent its transmission via blood obtained from an individual during the asymptomatic period. Recently, though, there have been several reports from different laboratories that human hepatitis A virus has been transmitted to marmoset monkeys. The conclusion that this virus is actually the human hepatitis type A virus and not a contaminating marmoset virus is questioned by some investigators, but the evidence that this is the human virus seems convincing. For example, antiserum obtained from humans who have recently recovered from a hepatitis A infection will specifically neutralize the infectivity of the hepatitis virus growing in marmosets. Data from such experiments, moreover, have led to the conclusion that there are at least two different serological types of human hepatitis A virus. Hepatitis B virus will not infect marmosets, nor is there any cross-immunity between the hepatitis A and B viruses.

Several laboratories have successfully demonstrated virus-like particles in the feces of hepatitis A patients by the use of immune electron microscopy. This procedure is carried out by mixing immune serum with fecal extracts to cause an agglutination of virus particles. Electron micrographs of the resulting clumps reveal virus particles, as was shown in Figure 36-1.

The current status of the hepatitis A virus and control of hepatitis A are still in a state of flux. At a 1976 symposium in Milan and Washington, D.C., it was reported that patients with hepatitis A developed complement-fixing antibodies and positive immune adherence tests (see Chapter 13). Using these serologic techniques, it was reported that most individuals of a low socioeconomic level possessed antibodies to hepatitis A virus, and these antibodies were detectable for at least seven years after infection. On the other hand, most persons from a high socioeconomic status appeared to reach adulthood without experiencing a hepatitis A infection. When one considers the fecal-oral route of transmission and the importance of effective sewage disposal for the prevention of this disease, such results are not surprising.

A new era of hepatitis research is under way, and methods may soon be routinely available for the assay of hepatitis A virus in human blood, the development of an effective vaccine, and, hopefully, the propagation of the virus in cell culture.

## REFERENCES

Bradley, D. W., R. M. Fields, and J. E. Maynard. 1976. Distinct deoxyribonucleic acid polymerase activities associated with Dane particles and naked Dane cores. *Infect. Immun.* **13**:1001–1004.

Committee on Viral Hepatitis of the Division of Medical Sciences of the National Academy of Sciences. 1974. Current trends: The public health implications of hepatitis B antigen in human blood—a revised statement. *Morbidity Mortality Weekly Reports* **23**:125–126.

Deinhardt, E., A. W. Holmes, R. B. Capps, and H. Popper. 1967. Studies on the transmission of human viral hepatitis to marmoset monkeys. *J. Exp. Med.* **125**:673–688.

Feinstone, S. M., A. Z. Kapikian, and R. H. Purcell. 1973. Hepatitis A: Detection by immune electron microscopy of a virus-like antigen associated with acute illness. *Science* **182**:1026–1028.

Feinstone, S. M., A. Z. Kapikian, R. H. Purcell, H. J. Alter, and P. V. Holland. 1975. Transfusion-associated hepatitis not due to hepatitis type A or B. *New Eng. J. Med.* **292**:767–770.

Gerin, J. L. 1976. Hepatitis: The search for viral and subviral antigens. *Fractions* **1**:1–9.

Holmes, A. W., F. Deinhardt, L. Wolfe, G. Froesner, D. Peterson, and B. Casto. 1973. Specific neutralization of human hepatitis type A in marmoset monkeys. *Nature* **243**:419–420.

Mascoli, C. C., O. L. Ittensohn, W. M. Villarejos, J. A. Arguedas G., P. J. Provost, and M. R. Hilleman. 1973. Recovery of hepatitis agents in the marmoset from human cases occurring in Costa Rica. *Proc. Soc. Exp. Biol. Med.* **142**:276–282.

Maugh, T. II., II. 1975. Hepatitis B: A new vaccine ready for human testing. *Science* **188**:137–138.

Maugh, T. H., II. 1976. Chemotherapy: Antiviral agents come of age. *Science* **192**:128–132.

Melnick, J. L., G. R. Dreesman, and F. B. Hollinger. 1977. Viral hepatitis. *Sci. American* **237**:44–52.

Nordenfelt, E., and L. Kjellen. 1975. Dane particles, DNA polymerase, and e-antigen in two different categories of hepatitis B antigen carriers. *Intervirology* **5**:225–232.

Provost, P. J., O. L. Ittensohn, V. M. Villarejos, J. A. Arguedas G., and M. R. Hilleman. 1973. Etiological relationships of marmoset-propagated CR326 hepatitis A virus to hepatitis in man. *Proc. Soc. Exp. Biol. Med.* **142**:1257–1267.

Robinson, W. S., D. A. Clayton, and R. L. Greenman. 1974. DNA of a human hepatitis B virus candidate. *J. Virol.* **14**:384–391.

Robinson, W. S., and R. L. Greenman. 1974. DNA polymerase in the core of the human hepatitis B virus candidate. *J. Virol.* **13**:1231–1236.

Stevens, D. P., K. S. Warren, and A. A. F. Mahmoud. 1977. Acute viral hepatitis. *J. Infect. Dis.* **135**:126–130.

Waterson, A. P. 1976. Infectious particles in hepatitis. *Annu. Rev. Med.* **27**:23–35.

Zuckerman, A. J. 1974. Viral hepatitis, the B antigen, and liver cancer. *Cell* **1**:65–67.

Zuckerman, A. J. 1974. The antigen complexity of hepatitis B virus. *Cell* **1**:157–159.

Zuckerman, A. J. 1975. *Human Viral Hepatitis.* American Elsevier Pub., New York.

# 37

## Togaviridae and Bunyaviridae

The viruses comprising the families Togaviridae and Bunyaviridae are often collectively called arboviruses, for arthropod-borne viruses. They acquired this name because they possess the ability to multiply in both an arthropod vector (most frequently mosquitoes and ticks) and in a wide variety of vertebrates—including humans. As a result, the infections they produce share a common epidemiology, that is, the virus is ingested by a blood-sucking arthropod from an infected animal, and, after multiplication within the arthropod, is injected into an uninfected animal during a subsequent blood meal.

## Togaviridae

Togaviruses appear to be icosahedral in shape, contain single-stranded RNA (molecular weight = 4.2 million daltons), and are surrounded by a membrane envelope (toga = mantle). Based on antigenic similarities in their envelope hemagglutinin (as measured by cross-reactions in the hemagglutination-inhibition test), they are divided into two distinct groups. Group A (genus *Alphavirus*) contains about 20 types, and Group B (genus *Flavivirus*) about 40 types. Antigenic cross-reactions within each group can be detected by neutralization and complement fixation tests, indicating that each of these large groups possibly evolved from a common ancestor.

### REPLICATION OF TOGAVIRUSES

Reproduction appears to occur entirely within the cytoplasm of the infected cell. Following adsorption, penetration, and uncoating, the virion RNA acts as its own mRNA to code for the production of an RNA polymerase and the structural proteins which will be incorporated into both the nucleocapsid and the envelope of the completed virion.

Replication of the viral RNA has not been extensively studied, but experimental data support the concept that its synthesis proceeds through a multistranded replicative intermediate similar to that described for poliovirus (Chapter 38).

Completed Group A virions (25–70 nm) contain three proteins. A single polypeptide is found in the capsid, while the envelope contains two different glycosylated (carbohydrate-containing) polypeptides. Both neutralizing antibody and hemagglutination-inhibition antibody are directed against one or both of these glycosylated envelope proteins.

Group B virions (20–50 nm) also possess three proteins, a single capsid polypeptide and two envelope polypeptides; however, only one of the envelope polypeptides is glycosylated.

Togaviruses obtain their envelopes as they bud through areas of the host cell membrane which have been modified by the incorporation of viral proteins (see Figure 37-1). Thus, release of the virions does not result in lysis of the host cell but does, generally, cause the eventual death of vertebrate cells. Infection of cultures of arthropod cells frequently results in a chronic situation in which small amounts of virus continue to be produced over a long period of time without causing destruction of the infected cell. This corresponds to the *in vivo* situation in which the virus multiplies without apparent damage to its arthropod vector.

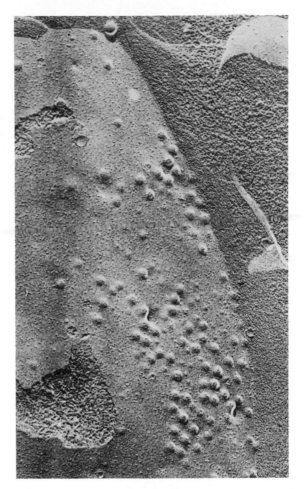

**Figure 37-1.** Numerous viral buds are seen here on the outer surface of the inner leaflet of the plasma membrane surrounding a cell infected with Sindbis virus (×69,000).

## EPIDEMIOLOGY OF TOGAVIRUS INFECTIONS

As can be seen in Table 37-1, many togavirus names correspond to the region where the virus was first isolated or to that area of the world where the virus is endemic. A person acquires the virus from the bite of an infected mosquito, or in the case of some Group B viruses from the bite of an infected tick.

Those togaviral diseases in which humans are the primary or secondary vertebrate hosts include yellow fever, dengue fever, chikungunya, and o'nyong-nyong. Lower mammals are a reservoir for the tick-borne encephalitides, but wild birds constitute the major vertebrate reservoir for most other togaviruses. Thus, it appears that many human infections occur when people enter an area where a natural virus cycle involving wild vertebrates and blood-sucking arthropods exists, and humans are accidental hosts who play no role in maintaining these natural virus cycles. Figure 37-2 summarizes the general epidemiology of the togaviruses.

It is likely that the arthropod-vertebrate cycle is a continuous one in the tropical areas of the world; however, where colder climates

**Table 37-1. Classification and Description of Togaviruses and Other Arthropod-Borne Viruses**

| Family | Group (genus) | Sub-group | Viral species | Vector | Clinical diseases in humans | Geographic distribution |
|---|---|---|---|---|---|---|
| Togaviridae | A | I | Eastern equine encephalitis (EEE) | Mosquito | Encephalitis | Eastern U.S.A., Canada, Brazil, Cuba, Panama, Philippines, Dominican Republic, Trinidad |
| | | | Venezuelan equine encephalitis (VEE) | Mosquito | Encephalitis | Brazil, Columbia, Ecuador, Trinidad, Venezuela, Mexico, U.S.A. (Florida and Texas) |
| | | | Western equine encephalitis (WEE) | Mosquito | Encephalitis | Western U.S.A., Canada, Mexico, Argentina, Brazil, British Guiana |
| | | | Sindbis | Mosquito | Subclinical | Egypt, India, South Africa, Australia |
| | | II | Chikungunya | Mosquito | Headache, fever, rash, joint and muscle pains | East Africa, South Africa, Southeast Asia |
| | | | Semliki Forest | Mosquito | Fever or none | East Africa, West Africa |
| | | | Mayora | Mosquito | Headache, fever, joint and muscle pains | Bolivia, Brazil, Colombia, Trinidad |
| | | | (13 others named) | Mosquito | Subclinical or none known | |

Table 37-1. Classification and Description of Togaviruses and Other Arthropod-Borne Viruses (continued)

| Family | Group (genus) | Sub-group | Viral species | Vector | Clinical diseases in humans | Geographic distribution |
|---|---|---|---|---|---|---|
| Togaviridae | B | I | St. Louis encephalitis | Mosquito | Encephalitis | U.S.A., Trinidad, Panama |
| | | | Japanese B encephalitis | Mosquito | Encephalitis | Japan, Guam, Eastern Asian mainland, Malaya, India |
| | | | Murray Valley encephalitis | Mosquito | Encephalitis | Australia, New Guinea |
| | | | Ilheus | Mosquito | Encephalitis | Brazil, Guatemala, Trinidad, Honduras |
| | | | West Nile | Mosquito | Headache, fever, myalgia, rash, lymphadenopathy | Egypt, Israel, India, Uganda, South Africa |
| | | II | Dengue (4 types) | Mosquito | Headache, fever, myalgia, prostration, rash (sometimes hemorrhagic) | Pacific Islands, South and Southeast Asia, northern Australia, New Guinea, Greece, Caribbean islands, Nigeria, Central and South America |
| | | III | Yellow fever | Mosquito | Fever, prostration, hepatitis, nephritis | Central and South America, Africa, Trinidad |
| | | IV | Tick-borne group (Russian spring-summer encephalitis group) 9 viruses | Tick | Encephalitis; meningo-encephalitis, hemorrhagic fever | Russian spring-summer encephalitis: U.S.S.R.; Powassan: Canada, U.S.A. Others: Japan, Siberia, Central Europe U.S.S.R., India, Malaya, Great Britain (Louping Ill) |
| | | | Bat salivary gland (12 others) | Unrecognized | Encephalitis | California, Texas |

**Table 37-1. Classification and Description of Togaviruses and Other Arthropod-Borne Viruses (continued)**

| Family | Group (genus) | Sub-group | Viral species | Vector | Clinical diseases in humans | Geographic distribution |
|---|---|---|---|---|---|---|
| Bunyaviridae | C | | Marituba and 12 others | Mosquito | Headache, fever | Brazil (Belém), Panama, Trinidad, Florida |
| | Bunyamwera | | Bunyamwera and 13 others | Mosquito | Headache, fever, myalgia; just fever; or none | Uganda, South Africa, India, Malaya, Colombia, Brazil, Trinidad, West Africa, Finland, U.S.A. |
| | California group | | California encephalitis and 8 others | Mosquito | Encephalitis, or none | U.S.A., Trinidad, Brazil, Canada, Czecho-slovakia, Mozambique |
| Phlebotomus fever group | | | 3 species | Phlebotomus | Headache, fever, myalgia | Italy, Egypt |

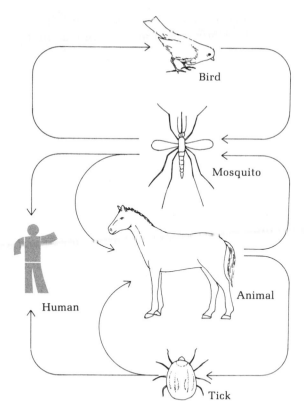

**Figure 37-2.** Epidemiology of togavirus infections. Although the bird-mosquito cycle is probably most important for the maintenance of these viruses, lower animals and ticks also participate in the epidemiology of the togaviruses. Humans become infected by either mosquitos or ticks (varying, of course, among the different togaviruses) when they come into contact with one of these cycles.

result in the temporary disappearance of the vector, the diseases are seasonal. It is not known for certain where the viruses are harbored during the winter months, but several possibilities have been proposed: (1) it has been shown experimentally that the viruses may exist in a latent state in cold-blooded animals such as snakes or frogs and in hibernating bats; (2) they may be reintroduced into an area by migratory birds; (3) they may remain viable in the inactive mosquitoes; or (4) they may remain in secondary vertebrate hosts such as rodents. It is plausible that all of these possibilities provide for the seasonal reintroduction of the infectious viruses.

## GROUP A TOGAVIRUS INFECTIONS IN HUMANS

Human infections by Group A togaviruses may be divided roughly into two categories, infections of the central nervous system causing encephalitis and infections without central nervous system involvement.

The major Group A encephalitides occurring in the western world include western equine encephalitis (WEE), eastern equine encephalitis (EEE), and Venezuelan equine encephalitis (VEE). Each is confined to a specific geographical area, i.e., WEE in the western United States and Canada, EEE in the eastern and southern United States, and VEE in South America, Central America, and southern United States. All are transmitted to humans, horses, and birds (including domestic game birds such as pheasants and partridges) by mosquito species of the genus *Culex*. All infect horses, but it does not seem that the horse is an important reservoir for the spread of the virus to humans.

Human infections may give rise to a biphasic fever curve. The first bout of fever results from a systemic infection, while the second phase of fever occurs when the virus enters the central nervous system and multiplies in the brain.

By far the most serious of the Group A encephalitides is EEE, producing lesions througout the brain and causing a high mortality rate with frequent severe neurological damage in survivors. WEE is less severe, and it is believed that many cases may consist only of a systemic infection without progression to an involvement of the central nervous system. VEE causes huge epidemics in horses, but the disease is usually mild in humans.

Group A viruses such as chikungunya and o'nyong-nyong are found primarily in Africa, although isolation of the virus has occurred in Thailand and South America. They are also carried by mosquitoes and cause a systemic infection in which the major symptoms are fever, headache, and joint pain. It is likely that humans and subhuman primates are the reservoir for these viruses. Control of all of the Group A encephalitides is directed primarily at the elimination of the mosquito vector. A live attenuated vaccine for VEE has been very successful in preventing the disease in horses, but it has not yet been used in humans. Inactivated viral vaccines have been prepared for the other encephalitides but have not been very effective.

## GROUP B TOGAVIRUS
## INFECTIONS IN HUMANS

The diseases produced by the Group B togaviruses can be grouped into three categories: (1) encephalitis, (2) yellow fever, and (3) dengue and dengue-like infections.

### Group B Encephalitides

St. Louis encephalitis (SLE) is the most common Group B infection in the United States. Epidemics occur sporadically throughout the southern and southeastern United States. It appears that the epidemiology is similar to the Group A encephalitides in that birds constitute the major reservoir and mosquitoes are the vectors. In humans the disease is usually mild, but epidemics reported during the past several decades have had approximately a 10% mortality rate.

Japanese B encephalitis (JBE) is a more serious disease, and a high percentage of survivors have neurological and mental disturbances. The disease occurs throughout the Far East, and epidemics in Japan and Korea have occasionally resulted in mortality rates above 50%. Apparently, the reservoir is birds, and spread occurs via mosquitoes.

Russian spring summer encephalitis (RSSE) is one of the Group B togaviruses in which the vector is the wood tick. Undoubtedly, wild animals can serve as the reservoir, but since the virus can be passed transovarily

(from mother to egg) in the tick, an additional reservoir is not necessary for the maintenance of this disease. RSSE can also be transmitted to humans via the milk of infected goats. In humans the disease is characterized by headache, fever, nausea, and, occasionally, coma. The virus is found in both the blood and the spinal fluid and may cause paralysis early in the infection. Mortality can reach as high as 30%, although the use of a vaccine grown in mouse brains has been beneficial in reducing the incidence and the severity of the disease. Table 37-2 lists the overall arboviral infections and deaths occurring in the United States during 1975.

At least nine other tick-borne Group B togaviruses infect animals, including occasional infections of humans causing mild to severe symptoms. Several of the best-studied ones include louping ill (primarily a disease of sheep), Omsk hemorrhagic fever (from USSR), and Kyasanur Forest disease (from India). The latter two may cause severe hemorrhagic diseases in humans.

### YELLOW FEVER

The yellow fever virus is a small icosahedral particle, approximately 38 nm in diameter, that antigenically belongs to the Group B togaviruses. It can be grown in chick embryos, tissue cultures, and certain animals, particularly monkeys. There is only one antigenic strain of yellow fever virus, so a single vaccine is effective.

### Pathogenesis and Epidemiology
### of Yellow Fever

Yellow fever is an acute infectious disease characterized by severe liver damage. Symptoms include headache, backache, fever, prostration, nausea, and vomiting. As a result of liver damage, jaundice may be evident as early as the fourth or fifth day of the illness. The incubation period is three to six days, and recovery from the disease results in lifelong immunity.

Table 37-2. Confirmed and Presumed Infections and Deaths in the U.S. during 1975 Caused by St. Louis Encephalitis (SLE), California Encephalitis (CE), and Western Equine Encephalitis (WEE).

| State | SLE | | | CE | | | WEE | | |
|---|---|---|---|---|---|---|---|---|---|
| | $C^A$ | $P^A$ | $D^B$ | C | P | D | C | P | D |
| Alabama | 38 | 19 | 3 | — | — | — | — | — | — |
| Arizona | 4 | — | — | — | — | — | — | — | — |
| Arkansas | 10 | 7 | 2 | 1 | — | — | — | — | — |
| Colorado | 3 | — | — | — | — | — | 17 | — | — |
| Georgia | 2 | — | — | — | — | — | — | — | — |
| Illinois | 381 | 188 | 20 | 25 | 2 | — | 3 | — | — |
| Indiana | 251 | 54 | 4 | 8 | — | — | — | — | — |
| Iowa | 15 | — | 2 | 11 | — | — | 5 | — | — |
| Kansas | 31 | 20 | 1 | — | — | — | 8 | — | 1 |
| Kentucky | 54 | 19 | 3 | — | — | — | — | — | — |
| Louisiana | 7 | 6 | 1 | — | — | — | — | — | — |
| Maryland | 8 | 1 | — | — | — | — | 1 | — | — |
| Michigan | 59 | 25 | 1 | 6 | 2 | — | — | — | — |
| Minnesota | — | — | — | 23 | — | — | 15 | — | — |
| Mississippi | 109 | 80 | 23 | — | — | — | — | — | — |
| Missouri | 21 | 18 | 2 | — | — | — | 1 | — | — |
| Montana | — | — | — | — | — | — | 3 | 1 | — |
| Nebraska | 3 | — | — | — | — | — | 5 | — | — |
| New Jersey | 29 | — | 1 | 2 | — | — | — | — | — |
| New Mexico | 1 | — | — | — | — | — | 3 | — | — |
| New York | 6 | — | — | 1 | — | — | — | — | — |
| North Carolina | 1 | — | — | — | — | — | — | — | — |
| North Dakota | 13 | — | 1 | — | — | — | 40 | — | 3 |
| Ohio | 195 | 90 | 11 | 15 | 10 | 1 | — | — | — |
| Oklahoma | 3 | — | — | — | — | — | 1 | — | — |
| Pennsylvania | 9 | 4 | 5 | — | — | — | — | — | — |
| South Dakota | 11 | 4 | — | — | — | — | 17 | 7 | — |
| Tennessee | 56 | 29 | 13 | 1 | — | — | — | — | — |
| Texas | 37 | — | 2 | — | — | — | — | — | — |
| West Virginia | — | 9 | — | 2 | — | — | — | — | — |
| Wisconsin | 4 | — | — | 25 | — | — | — | — | — |
| Washington, D.C. | 6 | 1 | — | — | — | — | — | — | — |
| Total | 1,367 | 574 | 95 | 120 | 14 | 1 | 119 | 8 | 4 |

[A]Reported confirmed (C) and presumptive (P) cases.

[B]Reported deaths related to C and P categories combined.

A great advance in medicine occurred when Dr. Walter Reed and his associates worked out the epidemiology of yellow fever. Their research resulted in the elimination of this dread disease from many urban areas of the world, including Panama (which, at least indirectly, made the completion of the canal construction possible). It is now known that the disease is transmitted from person to person, monkey to human, or monkey to monkey by one or another species of mosquito. Humans are the reservoir of infection in urban areas, and the mosquito *Aedes aegypti* is the vector for urban yellow fever. Monkeys, marmosets, and perhaps marsupials serve as reservoirs in the jungle. Jungle yellow fever differs from urban yellow fever only in the fact that different genera of mosquitoes are the vectors for its transmission.

### Diagnosis and Control of Yellow Fever

Clinical observations are usually sufficient for diagnosis during epidemics, but mild cases may be difficult to diagnose. Diagnosis may be accomplished by the microscopic examination of liver biopsies for necrotic lesions and for intranuclear inclusion bodies characteristic for yellow fever, by isolation of the virus from mice after intracerebral inoculation with a patient's serum, or by demonstration of a rise in neutralizing antibodies during convalescense.

The eradication of *Aedes aegypti* mosquitoes in urban areas is an effective control measure. This sort of attack on the vector has virtually eliminated the disease from the urban populations of Central and South America, as well as the southern cities of the United States in which the disease had occurred. Inasmuch as monkeys are a major reservoir of the disease, elimination of mosquitoes is not possible for control in forest and jungle areas.

A living attenuated vaccine for yellow fever—the 17D strain of the virus—is grown in chick embryos and has proved to be very effective in stimulating active immunity to the disease. There is no specific treatment.

## DENGUE

Dengue fever virus is also a very small Group B togavirus which is transmitted from person to person by several species of mosquitoes of the genus *Aedes* (see Figure 37-3).

The disease dengue is an acute infection which is usually manifested by headache, backache, fatigue, stiffness, loss of appetite, chilliness, and occasionally a rash. Probably the most characteristic symptom is emphasized by the other name for this disease—break-bone fever. Many of the symptoms may precede the first rise in temperature. In some cases the onset may be sudden with a sharp temperature rise, severe headache, backache, pain behind the eyes, and muscle and joint pains.

The virus of dengue fever is found in the blood of the infected person shortly before the onset of fever. There are four serologic types of dengue fever virus. They possess considerable antigenic cross-reactivity, but recovery from an infection by one type does not provide cross-immunity against infection by other types.

### Dengue Shock Syndrome

Dengue shock syndrome (DSS) appears to be a new manifestation of this disease and has become more and more prevalent since the

**Figure 37-3.** Dengue virus particles (about ×150,000).

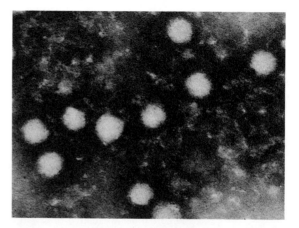

early 1950's. Prior to that time, the disease had a low fatality rate and was particularly mild in children. However, in the Philippines and in Southeast Asia the disease appears to have become much more severe, with symptoms of shock and hemorrhage and a mortality rate that approaches 10%. The cause of this severe manifestation is not attributed to a new strain of dengue virus but, at least indirectly, to better transportation facilities, resulting in an increased movement of persons between the various endemic areas of dengue fever. Thus, the severe hemorrhagic aspect of this disease is believed to be the result of a second infection with a different serologic type of dengue virus. Because of the cross-reacting antigens, the individual responds with an anamnestic antibody response, producing large amounts of antibody directed against the common antigens present in different strains of dengue virus. It is believed that the resulting production of immune complexes and the activation of complement causes a hypersensitivity reaction that is responsible for the severe fever and hemorrhaging (see Chapter 16).

The normal incubation period is 5–8 days, but this seems to be influenced by the amount of infecting virus and may vary from three to fifteen days. Humans and the *Aedes* mosquito are the recognized reservoir and vector respectively; however, as in yellow fever, monkeys may also serve as a major reservoir.

### Diagnosis and Control of Dengue

Serologic tests that are useful as diagnostic aids include tests for complement-fixing, neutralizing, and hemagglutination-inhibition antibodies. The major types of the virus are adapted for growth in mice, and mice are used for the preparation of specific antigen for the diagnostic serologic tests.

Control measures are directed toward the elimination of *Aedes* mosquitoes. A vaccine has been effective in experimental work, but it is not available for general use. Also, the possibility of provoking or enhancing the dengue shock syndrome in vaccinated individuals may be a serious objection to the use of dengue vaccines. There is no specific treatment that is effective against the virus.

# Bunyaviridae

Until the late 1960's the viruses that comprise the Bunyamwera (a locality in Africa) supergroup were lumped together with other groups in the large taxonomic group known as the arboviruses. Enough has now been learned about this group to give it the status of a family, called the Bunyaviridae. At present the group contains over 100 viruses and is divided into subgroups based on complement-fixing cross-reactions. Subgroups are further divided by the use of hemagglutination-inhibition and neutralizing antibodies.

## STRUCTURE AND REPLICATION

Although the Bunyamwera supergroup comprises the largest number of arboviruses, very little is known concerning the structure and multiplication of many of these viruses.

Structurally they are unlike the togaviruses in that they possess a helical nucleocapsid (see Figure 37-4). Those that have been investigated appear to possess a single protein in their nucleocapsid and a glycosylated protein in an envelope which surrounds the nucleocapsid. The viruses contain single-stranded RNA, but it is not known for certain whether it exists in one or two pieces within the virion.

## DISEASES IN HUMANS

All members of the Bunyaviridae have been isolated from mosquitoes, but only a few subgroups have been shown to infect

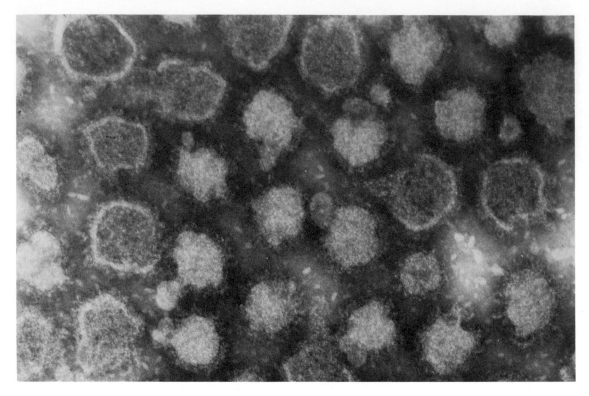

**Figure 37-4.** Nucleocapsids of California encephalitis virus, a representative bunyavirus (×212,500).

humans. Group C contains 11 serotypes isolated from South and Central America and the southeastern United States. Human infections are mild and usually undiagnosed.

The California encephalitis group contains 10 serotypes found in California and many other geographical areas of the world. They have been isolated from rabbits and rodents as well as mosquitoes of the genera *Aedes* and *Culex*. Human infections have been reported throughout the Midwest and Far West of the United States. Symptoms may be moderately severe, including central nervous system involvement; death is rare and recovery is usually complete.

### Sandfly Fever and Colorado Tick Fever

The viruses causing sandfly fever are helical viruses with single-stranded RNA, spread to humans via the bite of the female sandfly, *Phlebotomus papatasii*. The disease, found primarily around the Mediterranean Sea, causes headache, nausea, fever, photophobia, and abdominal pain. Complete recovery is usual.

Colorado tick fever is a mild disease which occurs throughout much of the western United States. Major symptoms in humans include fever, headache, joint pain, nausea, and vomiting. Mortality is very low. Little is known concerning the etiologic agent, but the virus appears to contain double-stranded RNA and may well be related to the orbivirus group (see Chapter 38). The wood tick constitutes both the vector and a major reservoir for the disease, since the virus is passed transovarily from generation to generation.

### REFERENCES

Bardos, V., ed. 1969. Arboviruses of the California complex and the Bunyamwera group. *Proceedings of the Symposium held at Smolenice in*

*1966.* Publishing House of the Slovak Academy of Sciences, Bratislava.

Brown, D. T., M. R. F. Waite, and E. R. Pfefferkorn. 1972. Morphology and morphogenesis of Sindbis virus as seen with freeze-etching techniques. *J. Virol.* **10:**524–536.

Burge, B. W., and J. H. Strauss. 1970. Glycopeptides of the membrane glycoprotein of Sindbis virus. *J. Mol. Biol.* **47:**449–466.

Casals, J. 1971. Arboviruses: Incorporation in a general system of viral classification. In K. Maramorosch and E. Kurstak, eds., *Comparative Virology*. Academic Press, New York.

Casals, J., and L. Whitman 1960 A new antigenic group of arthropod-borne viruses. The Bunyamwera group. *Amer. J. Trop. Med. Hyg.* **9:**73–77.

Inoue, Y. K. 1975. An attenuated Japanese encephalitis vaccine. *Progr. Med. Virol.* **19:**247–257.

Matsumara, T., V. Stollar, and W. Schlesinger. 1971. Studies on the nature of dengue virus. V. Structure and development of dengue virus in Vero cells. *Virology* **46:**344–355.

Mussgay, M., P. J. Enzmann, E. Weiland, and M. C. Horzinek. 1975. Growth cycle of arboviruses in vertebrate and arthropod cells. *Progr. Med. Virol.* **19:**258–323.

Pfefferkorn, E. R., and D. Shapiro. 1974. Reproduction of togaviruses. In H. Fraenkel-Conrat and R. R. Wagner, eds. *Comprehensive Virology,* Vol. 2. Plenum Press, New York.

Porterfield, J. S., J. Casals, M. P. Chumakov, S. Ya Gaidamovich, C. Hannoun, I. H. Holmes, M. C. Horzinek, M. Mussgay, N. Oker-Blom, and P. K. Russell. 1976. Bunyaviruses and Bunyaviridae. *Intervirology* **6:**13–24.

# 38

## Picornaviridae, Reoviridae, and Coronaviridae

The viruses included in this chapter cause diseases which include central nervous system disorders resulting in paralysis and death, aseptic meningitis and myocarditis (inflammation of the muscular walls of the heart), and mild or asymptomatic upper respiratory diseases. All are RNA viruses which infect humans via an oral or respiratory route.

## Picornaviridae

Human pathogens in the family Picornaviridae (pico = small) have been sub-divided into two large genera, *Enterovirus* and *Rhinovirus,* and each of these genera has been further divided into serotypes. The enteroviruses include three major subgroups: (1) poliovirus—three serotypes; (2) echoviruses—thirty-four serotypes; and (3) coxsackievirus—twenty-three serotypes of type A and six serotypes of type B. The rhinoviruses include approximately one hundred different serotypes.

There are also several groups of nonhuman pathogens that probably also belong to the picornavirus group, such as the cardioviruses and foot-and-mouth viruses. But we shall restrict our discussion to the human pathogens.

### STRUCTURE AND REPLICATION OF PICORNAVIRUSES

In spite of the diversity of human diseases caused by these viruses, there do not appear to be major differences in their modes of replication or general structures. Minor differences in structure do exist and can be deduced from the observation that the enteroviruses can maintain their structural stability and infectivity at pH 3, whereas the rhinoviruses are inactivated at this level of acidity. However, since the subtle differences in structure which account for this acid stability, or lability, are not known, we shall discuss the physical characteristics and reproduction of the entire family, Picornaviridae, as a unit.

Picornaviruses contain a single molecule of linear single-stranded RNA (molecular weight of 2.6 million daltons) enclosed in a naked isometric capsid. Because of the very small size of the virion, there is still doubt as to the total number of capsomers included in the completed capsid; however, interpretations of electron micrographs suggest that they contain 60 capsomers (see Figure 38-1).

## Adsorption, Penetration, and Uncoating of Picornaviruses

The adsorption of picornaviruses requires the presence of specific viral receptors on the surface of the host cell. Little is known about the nature of these receptors, and they may differ for the various subgroups of picornaviruses. It does appear that only a small percentage of the specifically adsorbed virions actually penetrate the host cell membrane and that the remaining are eluted from the membrane. Eluted picornaviruses lose one capsid protein (VP4, see below), which is necessary for cellular adsorption, and cannot be readsorbed to other host cells.

There is also some doubt concerning the mechanism of penetration and uncoating, since evidence both for engulfment into a vacuole and for the direct penetration of the virion has been proposed. The removal of VP4 is actually the first uncoating step, even though it occurs extracellularly, and it seems possible that the loss of VP4 may weaken the capsid sufficiently to cause its dissolution upon penetration. After uncoating, however, the translation of the viral RNA causes an inhibition of cellular protein synthesis by preventing the attachment of cellular mRNA to the ribosomes. Inhibition of cellular RNA synthesis also may be due to the presence of a virally coded protein, since infection with irradiated virus or the use of antibiotics preventing protein synthesis will allow host-cell RNA synthesis to continue.

## Synthesis of Viral Protein

Since picornaviruses contain the plus strand of RNA, protein synthesis uses the infecting viral RNA directly as mRNA. The virion

**Figure 38-1.** *a.* Crystalline array of poliovirus particles in a Hela cell (×59,400). *b.* Highly-purified, negatively-stained, type 1 Mahoney poliovirions (×290,000).

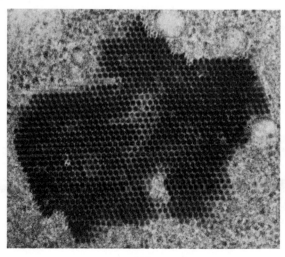

(a)

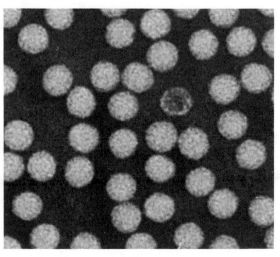

(b)

RNA is translated as one message into a single polypeptide with a molecular weight of over 200,000 daltons, which is subsequently cleaved by cellular enzymes into four structural proteins and a number of nonstructural proteins. (Presumably one of the nonstructural proteins is the RNA-dependent RNA-polymerase necessary for viral RNA replication.) According to the nomenclature of polioviruses, which are picornaviruses, the four structural proteins of picornaviruses have been designated VP1, VP2, VP3, and VP4. It appears that during the initial assembly of the capsid, VP4 and VP2

**Figure 38-2.** Replication of poliovirus. As shown, all steps occur in the cytoplasm of the host cell. Since the virion contains the plus strand of RNA, translation occurs immediately after uncoating, forming one long protein molecule that is subsequently cleaved into individual enzymes and structural proteins. The viral RNA is then replicated by the formation of a replicative intermediate, particles are assembled, and the intact virions are released from the host cell.

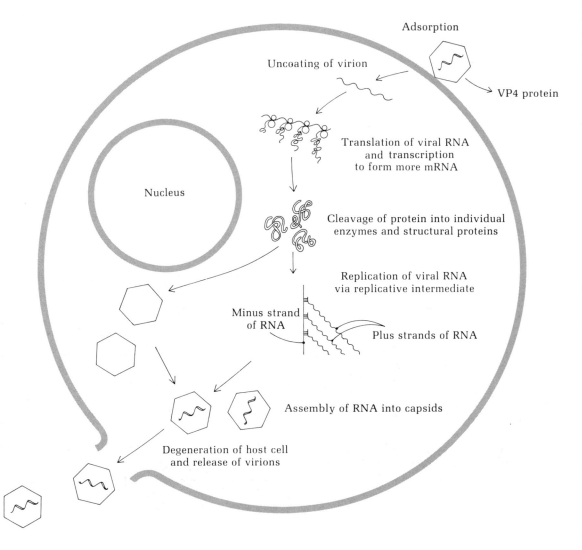

remain bonded as a single polypeptide (called VPO), and it is only after the incorporation of the viral RNA into the capsid that VPO is cleaved into VP4 and VP2 peptides.

## Synthesis of Viral RNA

The general events occurring during infection of a host cell by poliovirus have been quite well established, even though the molecular controls determining the time sequence of the various phases of viral replication are not known. Based on experimental results and in small part on a few educated guesses, the following events occur after the uncoating of the infecting virion: (1) protein synthesis results in the formation of a single protein which is subsequently cleaved into structural proteins, RNA replicase, and other products which inhibit cellular macromolecule synthesis; (2) during the early part of infection, mRNA is produced exponentially and is translated into viral proteins; and (3) approximately three hours after infection, mRNA begins to be incorporated into the preformed capsids, forming infectious virus. If one adds radioactively-labeled poliovirus RNA to infected cells during this latter phase of replication, it is incorporated into infectious virions within 5 minutes, in spite of the presence of a large pool of poliovirus mRNA. This suggests that in some way the cell differentiates between the plus strands of RNA which were destined for protein synthesis and the supposedly identical molecules which become enclosed in viral capsids.

It has also been established that the plus strands of RNA are replicated in a semiconservative manner using minus strands of viral RNA as templates. This results in the formation of a replicative intermediate (RI) that consists of a single minus strand of RNA simultaneously copied by several molecules of RNA replicase. Thus, an RI is an RNA molecule made up of one minus strand and multiple plus strands, with each new plus strand displacing the one being synthesized immediately ahead of it. Thermal denaturation of an RI results in the liberation of a single complete minus strand, a complete plus strand, and a series of plus strands of various lengths.

One other species of RNA found in cells infected with poliovirus is a double-stranded RNA consisting of one complete minus strand and its complete complementary plus strand. These molecules are named replicative forms (RF), and it could be that they are formed when two complementary RNA's pair up to form a double-stranded RNA. However, this form of double-stranded RNA is probably not available for the replication of new plus strands of RNA.

## Assembly of Picornaviruses

Empty pro-capsids are formed from the structural proteins designated VP0, VP1, and VP3. By an as-yet-unknown mechanism, viral RNA enters the pro-capsid, after which the VP0 protein is cleaved into two polypeptides designated VP2 and VP4. The completed virions (about 150,000 per infected cell) are then released by lysis of the host cell. Figure 38-2 summarizes the replication of polioviruses.

## PICORNAVIRUS INFECTIONS IN HUMANS

### Epidemiology and Pathogenesis of Poliovirus Infections

As far as is known, poliovirus occurs naturally only in humans, probably disseminated primarily via a fecal-oral route. However, since early multiplication occurs in both the oropharynx and the intestinal mucosa, spread of the virus through pharyngeal secretions during the first week of illness appears possible. Following initial multiplication, primarily in the tonsils and the Peyer's patches of the ileum, the virus is found in both the cervical and mesenteric lymph nodes; at this stage blood stream invasion and dissemination of the virus throughout the body occurs. It appears that at this point the clinical illness in humans may take one of three forms.

1. Abortive poliomyelitis is undoubtedly the most common form of this disease for all persons; but it is most characteristic in infants who still possess a small amount of maternal antibody to the virus. It may be essentially asymptomatic or may be characterized by fever, headache, malaise, drowsiness, sore throat, nausea, and vomiting. Recovery is usually rapid, and because the illness is mild, it is rarely diagnosed.

2. Aseptic meningitis is a generalized term given to meningeal infections in which a bacterium cannot be cultured from the spinal fluid. Moreover, unlike bacterial meningitis, glucose and protein levels in the spinal fluid are about normal. Poliovirus may enter the central nervous system causing an aseptic meningitis, which, in addition to the symptoms of the abortive cases, is characterized by stiffness of the neck and back. Recovery is usually complete in about a week.

3. Paralytic poliomyelitis is an extension of the aseptic meningitis syndrome, and is characterized by destruction of the large motor neurons in the anterior horn of the spinal cord. Since these cells give rise to motor fibers of peripheral nerves, their destruction is accompanied by paralysis. In bulbar poliomyelitis there is involvement of neurons in the medulla, and the respiratory or vasomotor center may be affected.

The incubation period of poliomyelitis may vary from three to 35 days but most often is a period ranging from seven to 14 days.

### Diagnosis of Poliovirus Infections

By far, the majority of poliovirus infections result in a mild illness without involvement of the central nervous system; therefore, most cases are not diagnosed clinically or by laboratory techniques.

Laboratory diagnosis is based on the isolation of the virus from throat swabs, feces, or rarely spinal fluid, or by demonstrating an increase in neutralizing antibody to one of the three serotypes of poliovirus during convalescence.

Feces or rectal swabs can be treated with antibiotics to destroy bacteria present and the material inoculated on cell lines derived from human or monkey cells. After growth, identification of the virus is confirmed by demonstrating a loss of infectivity following treatment with known neutralizing antiserum for poliovirus.

### Control of Poliovirus Infections

Because of the devastating crippling effects of paralytic poliomyelitis, it became one of the most feared diseases of the twentieth century. As recently as 1958, almost 6000 cases of paralytic polio were reported in the United States; however, during 1974 only five such cases were reported. Figure 38-3 summarizes the incidence of poliomyelitis occurring in the United States between 1958 and 1972. Interestingly, the increase in paralytic polio in some geographical areas during the early part of the century can be attributed in part to better sanitation; that is to say, since polio is primarily transmitted by a fecal-oral route, the better sanitation became, the older an average individual would be before becoming infected with the virus. The incidence of paralysis increases markedly with age, and infection in an infant —particularly one still partially protected by maternally acquired antibodies—is much less likely to lead to paralysis.

Prior to the development of vaccines, pooled gamma globulin provided effective protection if administered before the time of infection. The effectiveness of pooled gamma globulin could be attributed to the fact that the majority of adults had already recovered from undiagnosed abortive polio

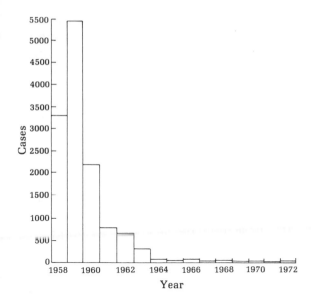

**Figure 38-3.** Best available paralytic poliomyelitis case count by year in the United States between 1958 and 1972. Note the dramatic decrease in paralytic poliomyelitis with the advent of the Salk and Sabin vaccines during the early 1960's.

infections, probably by all three serotypes, and therefore possessed neutralizing antibodies to the virus. The obvious disadvantage of gamma globulin prophylaxis was that it had to be administered prior to infection, and, like all passively acquired immunity, was effective in adults for only about six weeks.

Effective vaccines are now available. The original vaccine, developed by Jonas Salk, contained formalin-killed viruses of each of the three serotypes. The injection of this vaccine stimulated the production of antibodies in the serum. Following infection, a virulent virus was neutralized as it entered the viremic stage (blood stream), thus preventing involvement of the central nervous system.

A live vaccine, the Sabin vaccine, has now replaced the Salk vaccine. The Sabin vaccine

is composed of attenuated polioviruses of each of the three types. The vaccine is administered orally, usually on a sugar cube. Initially, only one type was given at a time, but current practice is to administer all three types together in three successive doses. The live vaccine multiplies in the cells of the gastrointestinal tract and oropharynx, stimulating the same solid immunity that the natural infection would provide. Supposedly, however, it is unable to multiply in the cells of the central nervous system.

The efficacy of the Salk and Sabin vaccines in preventing paralytic polio is now well established, but the safety of the live Sabin vaccine is still a matter of dispute. This was emphasized in 1976 when several eminent virologists, including Jonas Salk, testified before a United States Senate hearing that, in their opinion, a large percentage of the 140 cases of paralytic polio that have occurred in the United States since 1961 were due to the use of the live vaccine. This supposition was based in part on the observation that there have been no incidences of paralytic polio in countries such as Finland, where only the killed Salk vaccine is used, as contrasted with Norway, where the live vaccine is used and where at least eight cases have been recorded. It therefore appears possible that there may be a return to use of the killed vaccine in the United States in spite of the fact that many experts question whether the killed virus vaccine equals the oral version in effectiveness.

It should be kept in mind that while the polio vaccine has essentially eliminated the paralytic aspects of this disease, the virus is still widespread. Thus, public complacency could easily result in a large population lacking immunity, and the return of paralytic poliomyelitis is possible.

## COXSACKIEVIRUSES

Coxsackieviruses were named for Coxsackie, New York, where they were isolated from stools in 1948 and were originally believed to be a new type of poliovirus. Though their structure and replication appears to be that of a typical poliovirus (see Figure 38-4), their high virulence for newborn mice resulted in their assignment into a new group of picornaviruses.

### Classification of Coxsackieviruses

These viruses are placed into one of two groups based on the pathology observed following the infection of newborn mice. Group A viruses, serologically divided into 23 types by the possession of type-specific neutralizing and complement-fixing antigens, produce a fulminating, lethal infection resulting in total flaccid paralysis and death of the mouse. Pathologically, Group A virus

**Figure 38-4.** An array of coxsackievirus, Group B-3, in a thin section of mouse muscle (×70,000). Compare with the poliovirus array in Figure 38-1a.

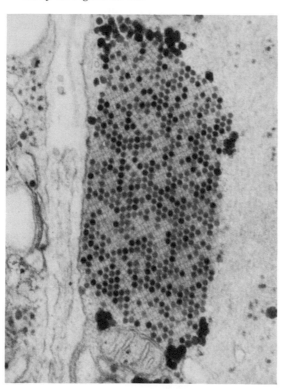

lesions are restricted to the necrosis and degeneration of skeletal muscle. Group B viruses, divided into six serotypes, produce a less severe infection in mice; however, these viruses may produce localized lesions in the liver, pancreas, myocardium, brain, and brown fat pads as well as in the skeletal muscle. There have been recent reports that some types of Coxsackie Group B virus may produce a diabetes-like syndrome in mice, and this has renewed speculation concerning the possible viral etiology of human juvenile diabetes. In addition, all Group B coxsackieviruses share a common group antigen while no common antigen has been observed with Group A coxsackieviruses.

### Epidemiology and Pathogenesis of Coxsackievirus Infections

Coxsackieviruses occur worldwide, and, like polioviruses, humans appear to be their only natural host. They also seem to be easily transmitted, and the majority of infections are asymptomatic or mild (and hence, undiagnosed). This is supported by the fact that pooled gamma globulin will neutralize all of the coxsackieviruses and is confirmed by the observation that most close contacts of infected persons become infected.

The virus grows in the pharynx and intestines, and spread can probably occur via oral secretions or a fecal-oral route. Since most cases occur in the summer and fall during swimming season, it seems probable that the fecal-oral spread is the more prevalent.

The diseases produced in humans vary considerably from one virus type to another. Table 38-1 lists the more common clinical syndromes, along with the virus usually involved.

Aseptic meningitis may be caused by any of the Group B viruses and also several of the Group A types. The usual symptoms for this syndrome include fever, headache, nausea, and stiffness in the neck. Recovery is usually complete, although rare cases with residual paralysis do occur.

**Table 38-1. Clinical Syndromes Associated with Coxsackieviruses**

| Syndrome | Coxsackievirus Group |
|----------|---------------------|
| Aseptic meningitis | A and B |
| Herpangina | A |
| Pleurodynia | B |
| Summer grippe | A and B |
| Myocarditis | B |
| Pericarditis | B |

The disease herpangina may be caused by several of the Group A viruses. This disease is an acute illness characterized by fever and lesions on the tonsils, soft palate, and pharynx. Difficulty in swallowing (dysphagia), loss of appetite (anorexia), vomiting, and abdominal pain may also occur. The duration is usually one to four days.

Pleurodynia (also called Bornholm disease or devil's grip) is primarily a Group B disease that is characterized by fever, headache, severe pleuritic pain, and malaise. Symptoms may last several days to several weeks.

Summer grippe is an illness of short duration in which the patient has fever, sore throat, headache, malaise, and vague pains. Many cases may be considered to be common colds.

Myocarditis, particularly that caused by Group B coxsackieviruses, may occur in both adults and children, causing permanent cardiac abnormalities. This type of infection is frequently fatal when contracted by the newborn. Furthermore, if the mother becomes infected during pregnancy, it appears that the virus can pass the placental wall and cause congenital heart defects.

### Diagnosis and Control of Coxsackievirus Infections

The virus can be isolated from throat washings, spinal fluid, or feces. Injection into newborn mice or the use of tissue cultures which show cytopathic effects will allow recovery of the virus. Identification requires the use of specific neutralizing antiserum.

A retrospective diagnosis can also be made by showing a rise in neutralizing antibodies between the acute and convalescent phases of the disease.

There are no effective control measures. Although vaccines would likely be effective, the multiplicity of virus types would make their development and production highly impractical.

## ECHOVIRUSES

The echoviruses illustrate the dilemma virologists faced as they discovered many new viruses in the feces of persons who had no clinical illness. At one time these viruses were facetiously referred to as "viruses in search of disease." Later, they were given the rather long name of enteric cytopathogenic human orphan viruses, indicating that they were isolated from human feces, caused a cytopathic effect in tissue cultures, and could not be associated with any disease. From this name came the acronym "echovirus."

### Classification of the Echoviruses

Echoviruses appear to be typical picornaviruses whose structure and replication are similar to poliovirus (see Figure 38-5).

**Figure 38-5.** Virions of echovirus type 19 ($\times$120,000).

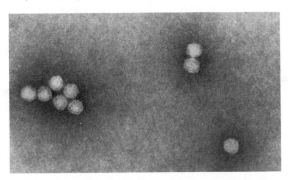

They have been subdivided into 31 types based on the presence of a type-specific neutralizing antigen in their capsid. However, they do not possess a group antigen, and the designation of a virus as an echovirus is sometimes slightly arbitrary. Echoviruses were originally differentiated from the coxsackieviruses by their lack of pathogenicity for suckling mice; however, a few variant types have now been shown to produce lesions in newborn mice.

### Epidemiology and Pathogenicity of Echoviruses

Most echoviruses are no longer "orphans," inasmuch as they are now known to produce a number of clinical manifestations in humans. It is interesting to note that although humans are the only hosts for echoviruses, other animals harbor similar enteroviruses. Monkeys have their ecmoviruses, swine their ecsoviruses, and cattle their ecboviruses.

Echoviruses occur worldwide, and a person becomes infected via either a fecal-oral route or respiratory contact. Multiplication of most echoviruses appears to occur in either the intestinal or respiratory tract, although some echoviruses cause a more widely disseminated infection.

The illnesses caused by the echoviruses are similar to coxsackievirus infections, and like other enterovirus infections, they are frequently unapparent or undiagnosed in infants and somewhat more severe in adults. The specific illness depends on the type of echovirus involved. Some of the echoviruses are still "orphans" in that they have not yet been associated with any disease entity.

In general, echovirus illnesses can be subdivided into four categories: (1) aseptic meningitis from which recovery is usually complete; (2) respiratory infections which are clinically similar to the common cold; (3) gastroenteritis resulting in a diarrhea which can be particularly severe in the newborn; and (4) disseminated infections which are characterized by skin rashes, fever, and malaise.

### Diagnosis and Control of Echovirus Infections

Echoviruses can be grown in tissue cultures of both monkey and human kidney cells. They produce a cytopathic effect and can be isolated and identified serologically using known antiserum.

However, since echoviruses occur frequently in the complete absence of any clinical disease, the mere isolation of an echovirus during an illness cannot be used as evidence that the echovirus is the etiologic agent for the disease in question. Furthermore, it is not possible to diagnose an isolated infection on clinical grounds alone. Thus, to establish that an echovirus is the etiologic agent for a disease, it is necessary to show a rise in antibody to the virus during convalescence or to isolate the virus consistently during an epidemic of some specific disease.

Because of the multiplicity of serological types and the fact that many infections are mild to asymptomatic, control through vaccination would be impractical.

### RHINOVIRUSES

The very "commonness" of the common cold was a stumbling block for many years in understanding the etiology of this disease. Although initially a single viral agent was sought, it is now known that a large variety of viruses may cause the mild respiratory infections we refer to as the common cold. The largest number of these common cold viruses have been classified into a group known as rhinoviruses.

#### Classification of the Rhinoviruses

Only a few of the viruses in this group have been extensively studied, but current information indicates they are small RNA viruses which morphologically and biochemically belong to the picornavirus family (see Figure 38-6). They can be differentiated from the enteroviruses on the basis of their acid lability, buoyant density, and temperature

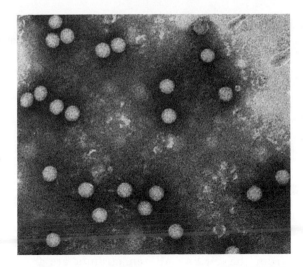

**Figure 38-6.** Virions of human rhinovirus type 14 (×120,000).

sensitivity. If rhinoviruses are maintained at a pH of 3 at 37°C for one hour, the virions will be disrupted and infectivity is lost. This same treatment has little or no effect on the enteroviruses. Immunologically, the rhinoviruses have been subdivided into over 100 serotypes based on a type-specific antigen in their capsid.

## Epidemiology and Pathogenesis of Rhinovirus Infections

Infections in humans appear to be restricted to the cells of the upper respiratory tract, and during the first five or six days of an illness the virus can be isolated from nasopharyngeal secretions. It therefore follows that a person acquires the virus by coming into contact with infected secretions, either by the inhalation of infected droplets or by direct contact with infected objects.

Humans and chimpanzees are the only animals known to be susceptible to rhinovirus infections; much of the early work on these agents was carried out (in England, by Sir Christopher Andrewes) using human volunteers. Since this type of research required complete isolation of the volunteers, many of the subjects were newlywed couples who were offered free accommodations in

isolated honeymoon cottages in return for serving as guinea pigs for the common cold. One interesting product of this research showed that exposure to inclement weather does not result in "catching a cold." It appears that the major effect of cold weather is to place people closer together in poorly ventilated locations, enhancing the opportunity for transmission of the virus.

These studies also demonstrated that immunity to rhinovirus infections is type-specific and that it is probably effective for at least two years. As one might expect, immunity can be better correlated with the amount of IgA present in the nasal mucous secretions than with the serum IgG.

## Diagnosis and Control of Rhinovirus Infections

The clinical symptoms of the common cold hardly need description to anyone old enough to read this text.

The virus can be grown in Hela cells, human embryo kidney cells, human embryonic nasal or tracheal epithelium, and in human diploid cell lines. Some strains grow in both monkey and human cell lines. These are designated as M strains to differentiate them from H strains that grow only in human cells. Identification of isolated viruses is accomplished using standard known neutralizing antiserum.

An unusual and unexpected property of rhinoviruses is that on initial isolation their growth and cytopathic effect occur maximally at 33°C (a condition similar to that of the nasal mucosa) and hardly at all at normal tissue-culture temperatures of 36 or 37°C. This unexpected property undoubtedly delayed the isolation of rhinoviruses for a number of years, since cells are routinely grown at 37°C.

The impracticality of a vaccine can be easily understood, given the following reasons: (1) immunity is type-specific for over 100 serotypes; (2) immunity appears to result from IgA antibody, and experimental vaccines must be administered intranasally;

and (3) two years is probably the longest period of immunity one could expect from even the best vaccine. Therefore, the control of rhinovirus infections continues to rely on avoiding infected individuals.

# Reoviridae

The family Reoviridae was recently established to include those icosahedral viruses (60–80 nm in diameter) whose genome consists of 10 to 12 segments of double-stranded RNA. Many virologists have objected to the name "reovirus" because it has no real meaning to the uninitiated. The name was coined because original isolates obtained from the respiratory and intestinal tracts did not appear to cause disease. As a result, the current generic name of *Reovirus* arose from the first letter of each word in the designation respiratory enteric orphan. The five morphologically similar but entirely unrelated groups of viruses included in this family are: (1) reoviruses which have been isolated from both humans and animals; (2) orbiviruses which are arthropod-borne diseases of animals; (3) rotaviruses that cause acute diarrhea in humans; (4) cytoplasmic polyhedrosis viruses that infect insects; and (5) plant viruses that are spread from plant to plant via leafhoppers.

## REOVIRUSES

### Structure and Replication of Reoviruses

Reoviruses are unusual, not only because they contain ten separate segments of double-stranded RNA but also because this complex genome is enclosed in a double-walled icosahedral capsid (see Figure 38-7).

After adsorption, the virion enters the cell by phagocytosis and the phagocytic vacuole fuses with a lysosome. Hydrolytic enzymes from the lysosome remove the outer capsid wall, and this action activates the RNA transcriptase present in the inner capsid wall.

Transcription occurs within the intact inner capsid, and mRNA molecules are extruded from holes at the 12 pentomer vertices (see Figure 38-8). Transcription occurs semiconservatively, since only one strand of the double-stranded RNA is copied and only plus strands of RNA (i.e., mRNA) are released from the virion. All ten strands are transcribed and then translated simultaneously.

The mRNA for each segment of RNA must also serve as a template for the production of a minus strand of RNA to form the final double-stranded RNA for the completed virion. This occurs later in the infection cycle after the mRNA's have been translated into polypeptides and enzymes, including an RNA replicase required for the synthesis of the minus strand. Once the minus strand is completed on the mRNA template, the two strands remain together, and free minus strands of RNA are not found within the host cell.

Assembly of these complex virions, so that each capsid receives its total complement of ten double-stranded RNA molecules, is not well understood. It appears that replication of the mRNA to form double-stranded RNA occurs within a polypeptide structure which eventually becomes the virion core. These "cytoplasmic factories" form crystalline aggregates of virions and empty capsids. The completed virions are released from the cell without budding.

### Epidemiology and Pathogenesis of Reovirus Infections

Reoviruses are extremely widespread in nature, and essentially all mammals possess antibodies to these agents. There are only

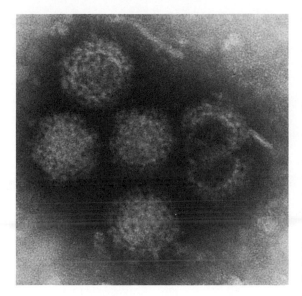

**Figure 38-7.** Reovirus capsids (×272,000).

by both a respiratory and a fecal-oral route. Attempts at control seem unwarranted in view of the mildness of the diseases for which they may be responsible.

## ROTAVIRUSES

Acute infectious diarrhea is a major cause of death in the very young, and until recently no infectious agent could be ascribed to this very serious disease. However, a previously unknown virus has now been found in the feces of about half of the children with acute diarrhea. These agents have not yet been given an official generic name, and the term rotavirus stems from the morphological similarity of their double-walled capsid to a wheel (see Figure 38-9). Because these

three serologic types that infect humans, and since the antigenic differences reside in their surface hemagglutinin, they can be typed either by hemagglutination-inhibition or by neutralization tests.

Reoviruses have been isolated from individuals with mild respiratory disease, diarrhea, and from many completely healthy persons. Experimental infections have frequently been unsuccessful in the production of symptoms, and when illness is occasionally produced, it is a mild respiratory disease. Hence, the acronym "reovirus" appears to be appropriate.

### Diagnosis and Control of Reovirus Infections

The virus can be isolated from throat washings or feces and grown on a number of human or monkey tissue cultures. All human strains possess a common complement-fixing antibody, which allows a single screening test for human reoviruses.

It would seem very probable that reoviruses are spread from person to person

**Figure 38-8.** Reovirus reaction cores with RNA extruded from the vertices. Note the loops in some strands of RNA. Bar = 0.2 μm.

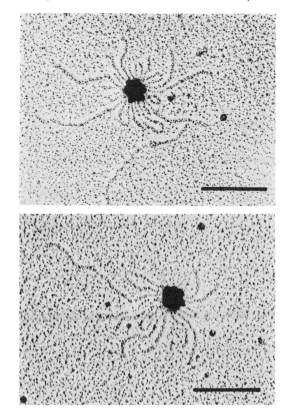

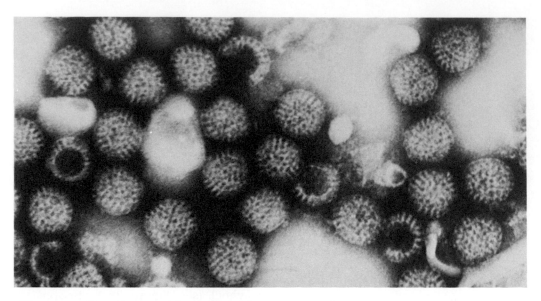

**Figure 38-9.** Rotavirus particles; each is about 70 nm in diameter. Note the resemblance of some capsids to a wheel with spokes.

viruses also contain double-stranded RNA within their double-walled capsid, the name duovirus has also been suggested for a generic name.

The ubiquity of rotaviruses throughout the animal kingdom is supported by the observation that piglets and calves that are deprived of colostrum (the first milk, containing high concentrations of the mother's antibodies) will invariably die from a severe diarrhea caused by a virus related to human rotavirus. Approximately 75% of newborn humans possess maternally acquired antibodies to rotavirus. The antibody titer declines during the first six months of life, but by five or six years of age approximately three-fourths of all children will have acquired an active immunity to rotavirus infections.

The incubation period of the gastroenteritis is one to three days; in the newborn it may result in death due to dehydration and loss of electrolytes from the diarrhea and vomiting. Early hospitalization with fluid and electrolyte replacement essentially eliminates the mortality, but newborns in under-developed countries undoubtedly continue to suffer

many infant deaths from these ubiquitous viruses. For reasons that remain to be explained, the incidence of this disease is higher in the winter months than during the summer. This is curious since infections with enteroviruses such as poliovirus have a higher incidence during the summer season.

As far as is known, there is only one serological type of human rotavirus, and the potential to produce an avirulent vaccine is good. A vaccine, however, would be of no value to the newborn, but it could be used to immunize expectant mothers. Breast feeding seems to be the best means of preventing rotavirus infections, since the mother's milk is very high in immunoglobulins, especially IgA. Even long after a child is able to absorb these antibodies, the milk will continue to contain secretory IgA that will provide local intestinal immunity to rotaviruses as well as many other infectious agents.

## ORBIVIRUSES

*Orbivirus* is a genus comprised of animal pathogens that are transmitted to animals via a mosquito vector. They contain a segmented genome of ten double-stranded RNA molecules, and their icosahedral capsid is morphologically similar to that of *Reovirus*.

As far as is known, orbiviruses do not cause disease in humans, but they do produce serious diseases in domestic animals. Of these, African horsesickness and blue tongue of sheep have been the most extensively studied.

# Coronaviridae

Coronaviruses cause gastroenteritis in swine and calves, and hepatitis in mice; however, it seems that human strains of these viruses are associated only with an upper respiratory tract infection indistinguishable from the common cold caused by the rhinoviruses.

## STRUCTURE AND REPLICATION OF CORONAVIRUSES

Coronaviruses were so named because of a series of petal-like projections that cover the surface of their envelope, resembling a solar corona (see Figure 38-10). Although they have not been extensively studied, they appear to be RNA-containing virions that multiply in the cytoplasm of infected cells.

The coronaviruses are difficult to grow in tissue culture. Some will grow only in human ciliated embryonic tracheal or nasal tissues, whereas others grow only in human kidney cells. A few strains have been adapted to grow in the brains of newborn mice, but, in general, research has been difficult because of the lack of experimental host cells.

## EPIDEMIOLOGY AND PATHOGENESIS OF CORONAVIRUS INFECTIONS

Coronavirus infections occur mainly in the winter and spring and are undoubtedly spread via respiratory secretions. Surprisingly, they seem to infect adults more frequently than children, but this observation may be an erroneous conclusion, since complement-fixing antibodies may not reach measurable or lasting titers until after multiple infections. If this is the case, a survey for complement-fixing antibodies in children will show a low level of infectivity.

Because of the very limited range of cells in which coronaviruses can be propagated, it seems probable that during a human infection the virus grows only in the cells of the respiratory tract. Volunteer studies have shown an average incubation period of three days and an illness lasting about a week. Symptoms include a sore throat plus other effects normally associated with an acute upper respiratory infection.

## DIAGNOSIS AND CONTROL OF CORONAVIRUS INFECTIONS

Virus isolation is difficult and is not routinely done. The most common laboratory diag-

**Figure 38-10.** Human coronavirus. Surface projections create a corona effect around each virion. ($\times$230,000.)

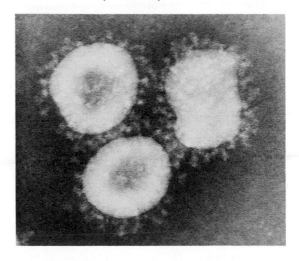

nostic procedure is the demonstration of complement-fixing antibodies against the human prototype strain 229E. One can also coat red cells with the coronavirus antigen and then test the serum for hemagglutination.

It is not known whether control with vaccines is feasible. Thus, at the present time control must rely on avoidance of individuals with upper respiratory illnesses.

## REFERENCES

Bartlett, N. M., S. C. Gillies, S. Bullivant, and A. R. Bellamy. 1974. Electron microscopy study of reovirus reaction cores. *J. Virol.* **14:**315–326.

Joklik, W. K. 1974. Reproduction of Reoviridae. In H. Fraenkel-Conrat and R. R. Wagner, eds. *Comprehensive Virology*, Vol. 2. Plenum Press, New York.

Levintow, L. 1974. Reproduction of picornaviruses. In H. Fraenkel-Conrat and R. R. Wagner, eds. *Comprehensive Virology*, Vol. 2. Plenum Press, New York.

McIntosh, K. 1974. Coronaviruses: A comparative review. *Current Topics in Microbiol. and Immunol.* **63:**86–129.

Petric, M., M. T. Szymanski, and P. J. Middleton. 1975. Purification and preliminary characterization of infantile gastroenteritis virus. *Intervirology* **5:**233–238.

Phillips. B. A. 1972. The morphogenesis of poliovirus. *Current Topics in Microbiol. and Immunol.* **58:**157–174.

Rodger, S. M., R. D. Schnagl, and I. H. Holmes. 1975. Biochemical and biophysical characteristics of diarrhea viruses of human and calf origin. *J. Virol.* **16:**1229–1235.

Rueckert, R. R. 1976. On the structure and morphogenesis of picornaviruses. In H. Fraenkel-Conrat and R. R. Wagner, eds. *Comprehensive Virology*, Vol. 6. Plenum Press, New York.

Salk, J., and D. Salk. 1977. Control of influenza and poliomyelitis with killed virus vaccines. *Science* **195:**834–847.

Shatkin, A. J., and G. W. Both. 1976. Reovirus mRNA: Transcription and translation. *Cell* **7:**305–313.

Silverstein, S. C., J. K. Christman, and G. Acs. 1976. The reovirus replicative cycle. *Annu. Rev. Biochem.* **45:**375–408.

Spector, D. H., and D. Baltimore. 1975. The molecular biology of poliovirus. *Sci. American* **232:**24–31.

Tyrrell, D. A. J., J. D. Almeida, C. H. Cunningham, W. R. Dowdle, M. S. Hofstad, K. McIntosh, M. Tajima, L. Ya Zakstelskaya, B. C. Easterday, A. Kapikian, and R. W. Bingham. 1975. Coronaviridae. *Intervirology* **5:**76–82.

White, D. O. 1974. Influenza viral proteins: Identification and synthesis. *Current Topics in Microbiol. and Immunol.* **63:**1–48.

# 39

# Orthomyxoviridae, Paramyxoviridae, and Rubella

The original designation of "myxovirus" included a large group of enveloped viruses capable of adsorbing to glycoprotein receptors on the surface of erythrocytes and host cells. As more was learned about the structure and replication of these viruses, it became obvious that this designation included two distinct viral groups. Consequently, the International Committee on Viral Nomenclature has proposed the family Orthomyxoviridae to include the influenza viruses and Paramyxoviridae for the remainder of this group. Table 39-1 lists some major characteristics of these viruses.

## Orthomyxoviridae

### STRUCTURE, REPLICATION, AND CLASSIFICATION OF THE ORTHOMYXOVIRUSES

Since all orthomyxoviruses are influenza viruses, virologists tend to use the name orthomyxovirus and the newly created genus, *Influenzavirus,* interchangeably. *Influenzavirus* is a somewhat spherical particle (although filamentous forms are produced by some strains), whose ribonucleoprotein core possesses helical symmetry. The internal ribonucleoprotein (total molecular weight of single-stranded RNA = 4 million daltons) is surrounded by a protein membrane which, in turn, is enclosed in a lipid bilayer envelope.

The viral envelope is covered with closely packed spikes about 10 to 14 nm in length. Electron microscopy of isolated spikes shows that they exist as two different morphological entities, of which one is a hemagglutinin and the other the enzyme neuraminidase (see Figure 39-1).

The hemagglutinin spike allows the virus to attach to a glycoprotein on the surface of erythrocytes, causing them to agglutinate. After about an hour at 37°C, the neuraminidase spike cleaves the terminal neuraminic acid from the hemagglutinin receptor on the red blood cell, causing the release of the virus. Such eluted virions can again agglutinate fresh erythrocytes. After elution the red blood cells originally agglutinated no

### Table 39-1. Comparison of Orthomyxoviruses and Paramyxoviruses

| Characteristics | Orthomyxoviruses | Paramyxoviruses |
|---|---|---|
| Major viruses | Influenza A, B, & C | Parainfluenza 1 thru 5 |
| | | Mumps |
| | | Measles |
| | | Respiratory syncytial virus |
| | | Newcastle disease virus |
| Particle size | 80–100 nm | 120–250 nm |
| Ribonucleoprotein core size | 9 nm | 18 nm |
| Nature of virion RNA | 8 segmented molecules of ss RNA | 1 molecule of ss RNA |
| Replication of virion RNA | Host cell nucleus | Host cell cytoplasm |
| Inclusion bodies | None | Cytoplasmic |
| Presence of virion neuraminidase | All | Some |

longer possess the hemagglutinin receptor.

Influenza viruses can be grown in chick embryos as well as in a number of mammalian tissue culture cell types. However, newly isolated strains grow poorly in tissue culture, and it usually requires several passages before a mutant can be selected that grows to high yields.

Adsorption is a specific reaction between the hemagglutinin spike and a glycoprotein on the host cell surface. Antibodies directed specifically against the viral hemagglutinin will neutralize infection by preventing adsorption of the virus. Also, treatment of potential host cells with neuraminidase to remove terminal neuraminic acid residues from the specific glycoprotein receptor will prevent adsorption of the virus. Crude enzyme preparations which carry out this reaction have been isolated from *Vibrio cholerae* and are called receptor-destroying enzyme (RDE).

There is still no general concurrence on the actual mechanism of penetration and uncoating of the infecting virion. Engulfment into a cytoplasmic vacuole as well as fusion of the viral envelope with the host cell membrane have been proposed. In either event, the ribonucleoprotein (RNP), which contains eight fragmented minus strands of single-stranded RNA and a viral transcriptase, is released into the cytoplasm of the cell.

The RNP enters the cell nucleus where the viral transcriptase transcribes each distinct fragment of viral RNA (vRNA) into a complementary strand (cRNA) which then enters the cytoplasm to act as mRNA. Thus, the vRNA consists of minus strands which must first be transcribed into functional mRNA before viral protein synthesis can begin. For reasons that are not readily apparent, RNA transcription is inhibited by the presence of actinomycin D.

At least eight different viral polypeptides are synthesized, and although not proven, it is tempting to believe that each segment of vRNA contains the information for one polypeptide. There appears to be some control regulating the synthesis of viral proteins, and it now appears that not all proteins are synthesized simultaneously, as previously believed. Neither the control mechanism nor the function of early and late proteins is understood.

About three hours after infection, vRNA synthesis begins. The molecular mechanism which controls the change from the preferential formation of cRNA to vRNA is not known, nor is it known whether the responsible replicase carries out this synthesis of

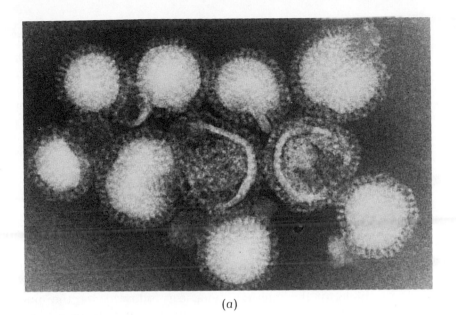

(a)

**Figure 39-1.** *a*. Negatively-stained influenza virus type A/Hong Kong (strain A $H_3N_2$). Note the surface spikes on the viral envelopes ($\times 214,200$). *b*. Diagram of a partial section through an influenza virion, illustrating the components making up a virus particle. Neuraminidase and hemagglutinin exist on separate, morphologically distinct spikes.

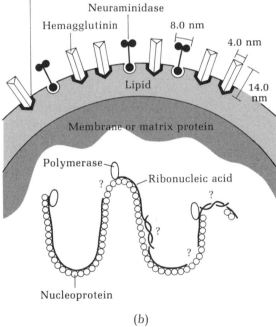

(b)

vRNA in the cytoplasm or in the nucleus of the host cell.

Meanwhile, out in the cytoplasm, spikes of hemagglutinin and neuraminidase develop on areas of the plasma membrane, and a new protein layer (named M protein) is laid down inside the host cell lipid bilayer. RNP associates with these morphologically-altered areas of host cell membrane, and the viruses, surrounded by the protein and lipid bilayer envelope, are released by budding from the infected cell (see Figure 39-2).

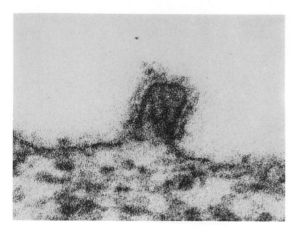

**Figure 39-2.** A budding influenza virus ($\times 200,000$).

Based on the antigenicity of the internal nucleoprotein, there are three completely unrelated serological types of influenza virus. Type A has been isolated from humans, animals, and birds; types B and C appear to infect only humans. In addition, type A and to a lesser extent type B can be subdivided into strains based on antigenic differences in their hemagglutinin and neuraminidase spikes. Neutralizing, and thus protective, antibodies are directed against the hemagglutinin. There is apparently only one strain of type C influenza virus.

### INFLUENZA IN HUMANS

Infections in humans are normally characterized by fever, chills, headache, generalized muscular aching, and loss of appetite. The virus is generally restricted to the upper respiratory tract, where spread is facilitated by the ability of the viral neuraminidase to hydrolyze the mucoproteins lining the respiratory tract. The death and sloughing off of ciliated epithelial cells may be responsible for many of the respiratory symptoms.

Although a patient may be very ill during the acute infection, an uneventful recovery after three to seven days is the usual prognosis. Deaths from influenza are most frequently due to an invasion of the lower respiratory tract by virus or bacteria resulting in severe pneumonia (see Figure 39-3). Although cases occur in which the influenza virus is the sole etiologic agent of the pneumonia, secondary bacterial pneumonias are far more frequent causes of death. As a result, it is difficult to obtain accurate statistics of the number of deaths directly attributable to an influenza epidemic. However, it is estimated that the influenza pandemic (worldwide outbreak) of 1918–1919 caused over 20 million deaths. The most recent pandemics in 1957 (Asian influenza) and in 1968 (Hong Kong influenza) also resulted in many fatalities but did not approach the 20 million of the 1918 pandemic. The most common bacterial invaders are the staphylococci followed by the pneumococcus, *Haemophilus influenzae,* and somewhat less frequently a beta-hemolytic *Streptococcus.*

### DIAGNOSIS AND TREATMENT OF INFLUENZA

Although a presumptive diagnosis can be made on the basis of clinical evidence, a positive diagnosis requires either the isolation of the virus or the demonstration of a rise in antibody following the acute illness.

Virus can be recovered from throat garglings during the acute illness and grown in the amniotic membranes of 11–12-day-old fertile chicken eggs. After several days, amniotic and allantoic fluids can be harvested from the eggs and assayed for the presence of influenza virus. Virus can be detected by mixing serial dilutions of the harvested fluid with a 1% suspension of human or guinea pig erythrocytes. Agglutination of the erythrocytes provides presumptive evidence for the presence of influenza virus, but confirmation requires the demonstration that type-specific influenza antisera will inhibit hemagglutination (hemagglutination-inhibition).

Throat washings (after treatment with antibiotics to destroy bacteria) can also be plated on primate cell cultures, and infected cells can then be located by hemadsorption or reaction with type-specific fluorescently-labeled antibody.

Hemagglutination-inhibition assays using dilutions of the patient's acute and convalescent phase sera with a known influenza virus are the easiest method to detect an antibody increase. However, sera must first be treated with trypsin or neuraminidase to destroy any mucoproteins which may nonspecifically inhibit hemagglutination. Complement-fixing antibodies also increase following an influenza infection. Those di-

rected against the nucleocapsid have broad specificity, while those directed against the hemagglutinin spike are type-specific.

## EPIDEMIOLOGY OF INFLUENZA INFECTIONS

Epidemics of influenza A occur every two or three years, while those caused by influenza B virus are usually seen at four to six-year intervals. Also, influenza A epidemics are more widespread and the illnesses more severe than those caused by influenza B

**Figure 39-3.** Pneumonia-influenza death rates by month and excess mortality during epidemic periods in the United States from 1934–1972. Note that type A epidemics result in a higher mortality and that they occur about twice as often as type B epidemics.

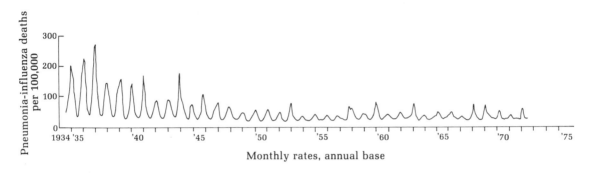

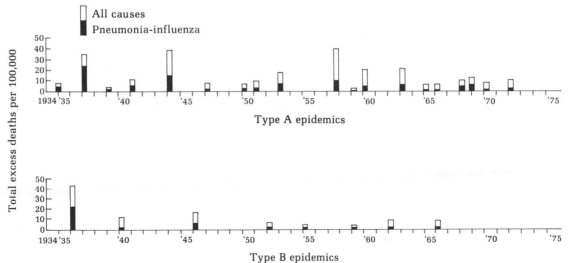

virus. Influenza C produces a very mild illness and has not been associated with epidemics.

To comprehend the epidemiology of influenza infections it is necessary to review the antigenic components of the virus and their role in the immune response of an infected individual. These facts can be summarized as follows:

1. Antibodies to the nucleoprotein are used to differentiate the three serologic types (i.e., A, B, and C) of influenza virus. These antibodies are not protective and will not prevent infection.

2. Antibodies induced by the M protein surrounding the nucleocapsid are also unable to neutralize infectivity.

3. Antibodies directed against the neuraminidase spike will not prevent infection, but it is believed that they may inhibit at least partially the release of mature virions from an infected cell. It thus seems possible that such antibodies play some role in the course of influenza infections.

4. Antibodies to the hemagglutinin spike will neutralize viral infectivity and hence are protective.

Since recovery from influenza results in immunity to the infecting virus, it appears obvious that the frequent major epidemics of influenza could not occur unless each succeeding epidemic was caused by a virus possessing a hemagglutinin antigenically different from that which was present in earlier epidemics. This is now verified, and, interestingly, two entirely different mechanisms occur to account for this variability.

The first, termed antigenic drift, is caused by minor antigenic changes in the hemagglutinin, the neuraminidase, or both. Such changes occur as mutations which enable the virus to survive in a population immune to the parent strain. Furthermore, there seems to be a finite possible number of such changes, so that with each succeeding influenza epidemic the adult population acquires a greater immunity. This results in either mild disease, unapparent infection, or complete resistance to the virus. Epidemics resulting from antigenic drift of the virus are, therefore, more likely to cause disease in children and young adults. Antigenic drift occurs in both influenza types A and B but not in type C.

The second, termed antigenic shift, occurs as a major change in the antigenic nature of either the hemagglutinin or the neuraminidase or both. This type of major alteration occurs only in influenza A, and it is the viruses of this origin that cause devastating pandemics in an essentially nonimmune population.

The most recent examples of antigenic shift occurred in 1957 and 1968, when Asian influenza and the Hong Kong strain, respectively, appeared. In both cases the viral hemagglutinin had undergone an extensive antigenic change. Two theories have been proposed to explain the source of major changes in type A virus: (1) direct mutation, and (2) recombination between an avian, animal, or human strain.

The mutational theory seems unlikely because peptide maps of the hemagglutinin are so unrelated to earlier strains that they could arise only from multiple simultaneous mutations (see Figure 39-4). Furthermore, such mutations have never occurred in laboratory strains.

The recombination theory appears plausible for several reasons: influenza A virus is found in birds, animals, and humans; and influenza virus is known to have a high recombination frequency—possibly because of its highly segmented genome. One can produce antigenic hybrids between avian and animal influenza viruses by the multiple infection of host cells with different viruses. Since many major pandemics begin in China and since birds migrating from Australia to China as well as swine in China carry type A virus, it has been proposed that these two reservoirs are the progenitors for the major antigenic shifts responsible for worldwide influenza epidemics.

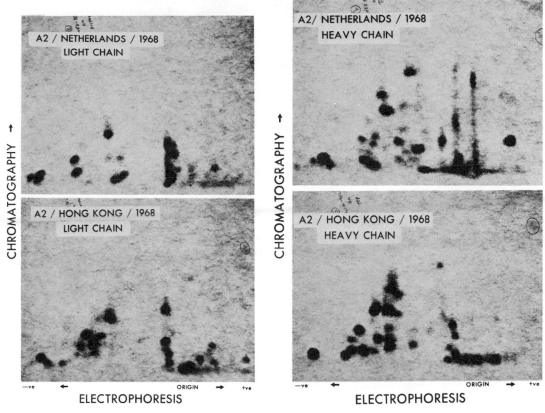

**Figure 39-4.** Maps of tryptic peptides from the light and heavy polypeptide chains of the hemagglutinin subunits of $A_2$ Netherlands/68 ($H_2N_2$) and the $A_2$ Hong Kong/68 ($H_3N_2$) influenza viruses. Since the Hong Kong strain represents a sudden antigenic shift, the differences in the tryptic digests between the two hemagglutinins are not unexpected.

## CONTROL OF INFLUENZA VIRUS

The parenteral injection of formalin-inactivated, chick embryo-grown influenza virus remains our major control mechanism. The efficacy of such vaccines has been the subject of much debate, and a general consensus is that even though such immunization does not always provide absolute protection, it will at least modify the disease. Maximum protection would require annual immunization with concentrated vaccines; in the event of an antigenic shift of the virus, even these would be ineffective. The development of protection against new influenza strains requires that the virus be isolated, adapted to give high yields in chick embryos, and then grown in tremendous quantities that can be concentrated and dispensed for use in vaccines.

Forewarning of the appearance of new variants is essential, and surveillance teams are continually isolating and identifying current strains. Since antibodies to the hemagglutinin (H) and to a lesser extent the neuraminidase (N) are protective, current strain terminology identifies these antigens as well as the type-specific antigen. For example, the epidemic in 1934 was caused by strain A ($H_0N_1$); the outbreak in 1947 by A ($H_1N_1$); the Asian epidemic in 1957 by A ($H_2N_2$); and the Hong Kong epidemic by

A ($H_3N_2$) (see Table 39-2). Thus, the isolation of any strain, particularly with a new antigenic hemagglutinin, sets the wheels in motion to produce a vaccine to the new strain.

This very situation arose during the spring of 1976 when a swine-like strain of influenza type A virus was isolated from a case of human influenza. Such a finding might not normally evoke much excitement among medical personnel, but all available data indicate that it was a swine strain that caused the devastating influenza pandemic of 1918. The virus from this pandemic was never isolated, but essentially all persons who lived through this period possessed antibodies to swine influenza virus. The magnitude of this pandemic can be appreciated by some mortality statistics from 1918. The United States death toll over a period of a few weeks is listed as 548,452 persons, over ten times the number killed during World War I (53,513). India put its toll at 12.5 million, and the Dutch East Indies at 800,000. Many villages throughout the world were entirely wiped out by this virus, whose worldwide mortality was finally placed at 20 million persons. Proof that swine and human influenza viruses will recombine to form hybrid agents is shown by the experiment illustrated in Figure 39-5.

It is, therefore, no wonder that the isolation of a swine-like influenza virus from human disease evoked great worldwide concern. In April 1976, the United States government appropriated 135 million dollars to produce sufficient vaccine to immunize all Americans to this agent. Since the swine-like virus does not grow well in fertile eggs, a clever trick was used to obtain an agent that would grow rapidly and still stimulate an effective immunity to the virus. This was accomplished by simultaneously infecting

**Table 39-2. Hemagglutination and Neuraminidase Composition of Human Influenza A Viruses**

| Year Isolated | Composition |
|---|---|
| 1934 | $H_0N_1$ |
| 1947 | $H_1N_1$ |
| 1957 | $H_2N_2$ |
| 1968 | $H_3N_2$ |

fertile eggs with the swine-like virus and a fast growing strain of type A influenza virus. Recombinants were subsequently isolated that possessed the hemagglutinin and neuraminidase antigens of the swine-like virus but, in addition, had acquired the rapid growing potential of the human type A strain.

Immunization of the American population was begun by late September, 1976, and by mid-December over 35 million individuals had received the swine influenza vaccine. At this time, however, a disturbing problem came to light; namely, a number of individuals experienced an ascending paralysis (known as Guillain-Barré syndrome) that began a few days after receiving the swine influenza vaccine. The cause of Guillain-Barré syndrome is unknown, and the statistical data connecting the syndrome with swine influenza vaccine were far from absolute. Until more is learned concerning the etiology of Guillain-Barré syndrome, the possibility must be considered that something related to the swine influenza vaccine may have precipitated this disease.

Chemical prophylaxis by 1-adamantanamine hydrochloride (amantadine) appears to be effective. However, most individuals are reluctant to obtain a prescription, purchase the drug, and take it daily during the duration of an epidemic. This, coupled with reports of

**Figure 39-5.** Recombination between Hong Kong (HK) and swine (SW) influenza viruses under conditions of natural transmission. One pig was infected with HK influenza virus, and a second pig was infected with SW influenza virus. Six hours later the infected animals were put into a room with four contact pigs. Beginning on the fifth day after introduction of the infected animals, one pig was sacrificed each day and lung suspensions were

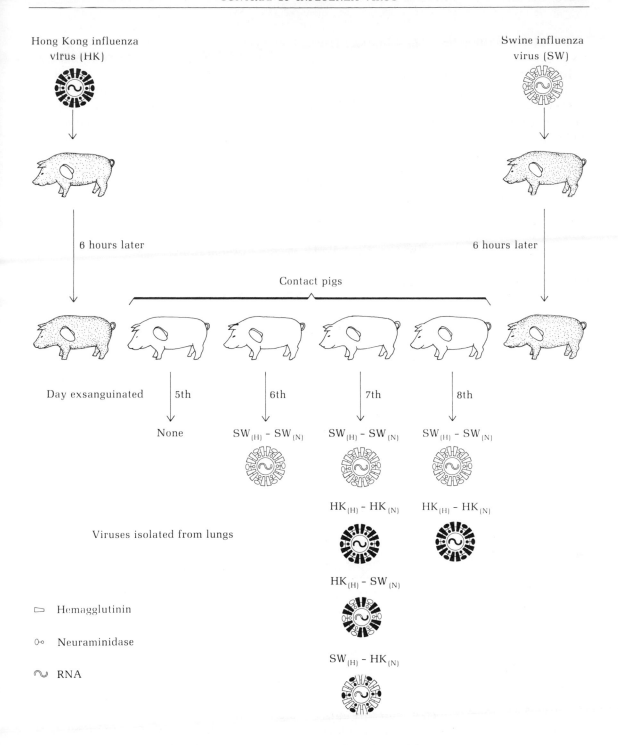

Hong Kong influenza virus (HK)

Swine influenza virus (SW)

6 hours later

6 hours later

Contact pigs

Day exsanguinated    5th    6th    7th    8th

None    SW$_{(H)}$ - SW$_{(N)}$    SW$_{(H)}$ - SW$_{(N)}$    SW$_{(H)}$ - SW$_{(N)}$

HK$_{(H)}$ - HK$_{(N)}$    HK$_{(H)}$ - HK$_{(N)}$

Viruses isolated from lungs

HK$_{(H)}$ - SW$_{(N)}$

▱  Hemagglutinin

SW$_{(H)}$ - HK$_{(N)}$

o⚬  Neuraminidase

∿  RNA

examined for recombinant viruses. As can be seen, both HK and SW influenza virus were isolated from pigs sacrificed on the 7th and 8th days, and recombinant viruses containing HK hemagglutinin–SW neuraminidase and SW hemagglutinin–HK neuraminidase were isolated from the contact pig sacrificed on the 7th day.

the toxicity of the drug, has hindered its extensive use.

Research on the future control of influenza is following two approaches. One is concerned with the isolation of attenuated strains which retain their antigenicity but no longer cause overt disease. Such vaccines are now used experimentally, wherein they are administered intranasally, resulting in the production of high IgA and IgG antibodies. However, mutants for new strains might be extremely difficult to produce in time to be effective.

A second approach is based on the belief that even antigenic shifts are limited to a reasonable finite number of variations. This is supported, in part, by the observation that the pandemic in 1897 was caused by a virus thought to have the same hemagglutinin antigen as the Asian influenza epidemic of 1957; only persons 65 or 70 years old possessed neutralizing antibody to the new virus. Consequently, some laboratories are attempting to make new mutants by recombination experiments so that when a new variant appears in nature, a high-yield laboratory strain would be immediately available for vaccine preparation.

# Paramyxoviridae

Most of the paramyxoviruses possess properties which outwardly resemble the more obvious characteristics of the orthomyxoviruses, the most notable of which are the ability to adsorb to neuraminic-acid-containing glycoproteins (causing hemagglutination) and the possession of neuraminidase activity in the spikes extending from their envelopes. However, their structure, mode of replication, and even the types of infections differ markedly from those of the influenza viruses; obviously they constitute a different group of viruses.

## STRUCTURE AND REPLICATION OF THE PARAMYXOVIRUSES

Paramyxoviruses contain a single piece of single-stranded RNA (molecular weight = 6.5–7.5 million daltons), and they exhibit helical symmetry within the ribonucleoprotein core. The ribonucleoprotein (RNP) is enclosed in a protein coat, and this entire structure is surrounded by a lipid bilayer membrane containing numerous spikes (see Figure 39-6). Thus, the over-all structure is similar to that of the influenza viruses, but it differs in the following properties:

(1) the nucleic acid exists as a single long piece of RNA; (2) the diameter of the enveloped virions is about twice that of the orthomyxoviruses, and there tends to be greater pleomorphism (more distinct forms) with the frequent formation of filamentous forms; and (3) hemagglutinin and neuraminidase activities both reside on the same glycoprotein spike, and a second morphologically similar spike on the virion possesses the ability to cause fusion of infected host cells. Measles virus, respiratory syncytial virus, and the animal pathogens of distemper and rinderpest viruses do not possess a neuraminidase.

Adsorption, penetration, and uncoating of paramyxoviruses are not completely understood; however, those possessing a hemagglutinin and a neuraminidase appear to bind to neuraminic-acid-containing glycoprotein receptor sites on the cell surface in a manner similar to that described for the influenza virus. Penetration may require the action of the virion spike involved in cell fusion, but there is no specific evidence for this speculation.

Transcription of the viral genome into mRNA occurs in the cytoplasm and is cata-

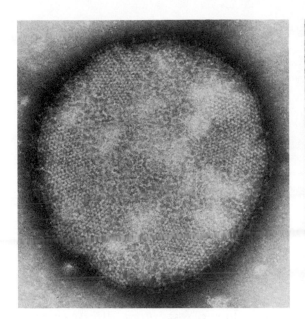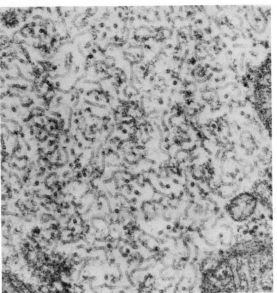

**Figure 39-6.** *a.* Electron micrograph of parainfluenza virus type 4A (×116,800). *b.* Portions of a paramyxovirus inclusion body consisting of nucleocapsids (×58,400).

lyzed by a viral transcriptase. Thus, like the influenza viruses, the paramyxoviruses carry their genetic information on minus strands of single-stranded RNA, which must be transcribed before viral protein synthesis begins. Although viral RNA exists as a single molecule, mRNA is found in seven or eight pieces within the infected cell. Available evidence suggests that there are multiple initiation sites for the viral transcriptase, and apparently each mRNA is synthesized independently.

Replication of viral RNA is not catalyzed by the viral transcriptase, and a replicase must be synthesized after cell infection. Very little is known about this enzyme, since its instability has prevented *in vitro* studies. It is also not clear whether one or two enzymes are involved, i.e., one to transcribe the infecting virion RNA into a single molecule of mRNA and a second to replicate that mRNA into viral RNA.

Capsid proteins are synthesized in large excess, and the majority remain as capsomers, forming cytoplasmic inclusion bodies (Figure 39-6*b*). The capsid binds to the newly-synthesized viral RNA, after which the RNP migrates to areas of the host cell membrane where viral proteins have replaced cell proteins. The arrival of the nucleoprotein at the cell membrane is quickly followed by the appearance of the glycoprotein spikes in the lipid bilayer of the host cell. The nucleocapsid is then enclosed by a lipid bilayer membrane containing the glycoprotein spikes, and the virion is released by budding from the host cell. The observation that the completed virions also contain varying amounts of mRNA which will anneal to viral RNA has been interpreted as an "accidental" incorporation of some mRNA during the assembly process.

The fate of the host cell varies considerably, depending both on the particular virus involved and on the type of cell infected. However, two general properties of paramyxovirus infections deserve emphasis. First, many paramyxoviruses will cause adjacent host cells to fuse into multinucleate giant cells. This eventually results in the death of the cell; perhaps even more important, it has become a very useful laboratory technique to cause the fusion of cells for genetic studies. Cell fusion is caused by one of the glycoprotein spikes on the surface of the envelope, possibly in conjunction with lysolecithin in the cell membrane. The same viral protein responsible for cell fusion will also cause hemolysis of red blood cells. Second, essentially all of the paramyxoviruses have been shown to establish persistent infections in cultured cells. These infections may result in the production of small amounts of virus, or they may be manifested only by the intracellular presence of viral antigens. Still, the fact that such persistently infected cells may continue to survive indefinitely has broad implications in animal infections. Measles virus is the only proven instance where a persistent infection in humans can reoccur as a neurological disease, called subacute sclerosing panencephalitis (SSPE), but indirect evidence has suggested the possible role of paramyxoviruses in other chronic diseases such as multiple sclerosis, lupus erythematosus, and polymyositis.

## PARAMYXOVIRUS INFECTIONS IN HUMANS

### Parainfluenza Virus

There are five serological types of these viruses; but since type 5 was isolated from monkey kidney cells, it is usually referred to as simian virus 5 (SV5).

All parainfluenza viruses produce upper respiratory infections in adults, although illnesses from type 4 are usually asymptomatic. Types 1 and 2 and to a lesser extent type 3 cause infections in adults that would be diagnosed clinically as a common cold. In infants and children these viruses may invade the lower respiratory tract, causing pneumonia. Types 1 and 2 seem to be particularly frequent invaders of the larynx in infants, causing a syndrome called laryngotracheobronchitis, or croup.

All types can be grown in human or monkey tissue cultures, but usually they produce few cytopathic changes. Infected areas can be recognized by hemadsorption or the use of specific immunofluorescent antibody. Antibody can be determined by hemagglutination-inhibition or by complement fixation, but because of its widespread occurrence, the mere presence of antibody is not diagnostic.

Inactivated vaccines have been used against parainfluenza viruses, but the stimulated IgG response is not protective. Living attenuated vaccines to be administered intranasally are being developed and if successful may be of value in preventing the serious lower respiratory disease caused by these viruses in infants and young children. Because immunity to reinfection is not solid, attenuated vaccines would hardly seem practical for adult use.

### Mumps

The usual, familiar clinical picture of mumps hardly needs description. Infection of the parotid glands produces inflammation, with marked swelling behind the ears and difficulty in swallowing.

PATHOGENESIS OF MUMPS. The paramyxovirus causing mumps is transmitted via respiratory secretions; it multiplies in the upper respiratory tract and in the local lymph nodes. It then enters the blood stream, and viremia results in the spread of the virus throughout the body. Most commonly, the major symptom is the painful swelling of one or both parotid glands, occurring 18 to 21 days after exposure. Also, infection may develop in the meninges, the pancreas, the ovaries, the testes, or the heart. Of these, the most feared complication is the infection of the testes (orchitis) which occurs in 20–30% of infected males who have reached puberty. This complication is extremely painful, primarily because the lining surrounding the testes will not allow the inflamed testes to swell and, as a result, may lead to sterility. Infection of the ovaries may also occur, but since swelling is not prevented it is not as painful nor is it likely to result in sterility. Aseptic meningitis is also a frequent but usually not severe complication.

DIAGNOSIS AND CONTROL OF MUMPS. A diagnosis is most frequently made by observing the clinical picture. In cases of atypical mumps, the diagnosis can be confirmed by injecting saliva or spinal fluid into either eight-day-old chick embryos or monkey kidney cell cultures. Virus can be detected in embryo amniotic fluid by its hemagglutination and in tissue culture cells by either immunofluorescent antibody or hemadsorption of chicken or guinea pig erythrocytes. In either case, positive identification can be completed by demonstrating hemagglutination-inhibition with known antiserum.

Mumps is not nearly as contagious as many of the other childhood diseases, and it is therefore quite common for persons to reach adulthood and still be completely susceptible to infection by mumps virus.

Following recovery, an individual develops antibodies to both the nucleocapsid protein and the hemagglutinin surface antigen. Antibodies induced by the hemagglutinin are protective; but even though immunity is life-long, detection of these antibodies several years after recovery may not be possible.

Since there is only one antigenic type of mumps virus, a live attenuated vaccine grown in chick embryos has been widely used since 1967. It appears that at least 95% of susceptible individuals develop adequate antibody titers as a result of vaccine administration. Although the duration of the vaccine-induced immunity is not known, it appears to be permanent. The vaccine is of particular value for males who have no history of the natural disease. Because inapparent (or at least undiagnosed) infections account for approximately 30% of all infections by mumps virus, many persons who are in fact immune may give no history of having had the disease. In such cases a skin test may be used in which inactivated mumps virus is injected into the skin. Usually those who are immune develop a delayed skin reaction that reaches maximum inflammation in about 24 to 48 hours. However, the U.S. Public Health Service claims the test is not a reliable indicator of immunity.

## Measles

Measles virus is also classified as a paramyxovirus, although its position in this group is somewhat less solid than that of the other paramyxoviruses. It is an RNA virus morphologically similar to other paramyxoviruses. Furthermore, it possesses a hemagglutinin which will weakly hemagglutinate monkey erythrocytes, but it does not contain a neuraminidase nor are its erythrocyte receptor sites destroyed by neuraminidase.

PATHOGENESIS AND EPIDEMIOLOGY OF MEASLES. Measles (rubeola, or morbilli) is a severe, acute, highly-contagious disease which is spread via respiratory secretions and may occur in epidemics every two to three years. Humans are the only normal reservoir of the virus, although, if exposed, monkeys will readily develop the disease.

The virus multiplies in the upper respiratory tract and conjunctiva during the early phase of the incubation period. Late in the incubation period, the virus enters the blood stream (viremia) and is transported to all parts of the body. The severity of the clinical infection is frequently not fully appreciated. High fever (often leading to convulsions), delirium, cough, and eye pain from light (photophobia) are accompanied by severe conjunctivitis and a rash over the entire body.

As a result of the spread of the virus throughout the body, complications are not uncommon. As in influenza, secondary infections causing pneumonia and ear infections may frequently be the result of bacterial invaders. By far the most feared complication is encephalitis, which can cause permanent neurologic injury and even death. Although encephalitis is relatively rare, it does follow approximately one out of 10,000 cases of measles. When this does occur, symptoms of encephalitis appear about five to seven days after the appearance of the rash.

The incubation period is quite uniform, with the first symptoms of fever, cough, headache, · sore throat, and conjunctivitis beginning 11 days after exposure; the rash appears three days later. Infected individuals secrete virus from their respiratory tract, conjunctiva, and in their urine from approximately three days before to about five days after the appearance of the rash. Measles is one of the most contagious of all infectious diseases.

DIAGNOSIS AND CONTROL OF MEASLES. A diagnosis is almost always made on clinical grounds. Early diagnosis, before the rash appears, frequently can be made by observing Koplik spots—small bluish-yellow spots—that occur in the mouth on the buccal mucosa two to three days before the rash appears. In addition, the virus from specimens taken from respiratory secretions may be grown in tissue cultures of a large number of primary or continuous cell lines. Virus can be detected by the hemadsorption of infected cells with chicken erythrocytes.

The presence of giant cells in nasal secretions, resulting from the property of measles virus to cause cell fusion of infected cells, is also a characteristic of measles infections (see Figure 39-7). Serologic tests may be carried out for neutralizing and complement-fixing antibodies. Fortunately (for us), there is only one antigenic type of measles virus, and recovery from the disease imparts lifelong immunity.

Isolation of persons who have measles has not been an effective control measure

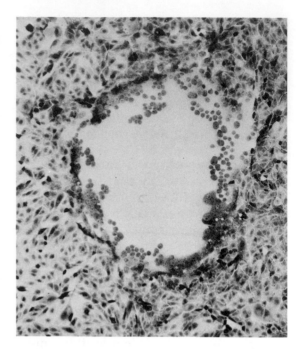

**Figure 39-7.** Giant cell formed of fused Vero cells in culture 48 hours after infection with measles virus ($\times 70$).

because individuals are infective several days prior to the appearance of the rash and are usually undiagnosed during that period. Antibodies to this virus pass through the placenta and protect infants for about the first six months of life.

VACCINES FOR MEASLES. Because measles is a severe disease with frequent grave complications, much effort has been expended in developing an effective vaccine. The first vaccine used was a formalin-killed virus prepared from virus grown in cell cultures. The use of this vaccine did stimulate the formation of neutralizing antibodies, but since killed vaccines do not provide lifelong immunity, efforts persisted to obtain a live attenuated strain of measles virus that could be used as a vaccine. The first such attenuated strain was isolated by John Enders after passage of the virus through human kidney cells, human amnion cells, and finally, chick embryo tissue culture. This strain, called the Edmonston vaccine, caused rather severe symptoms in about a third of the recipients, but pooled gamma globulin, given at the same time in the early days of this vaccine, minimized these symptoms.

Newer attenuated vaccines produce symptoms far milder than the original Edmonston strain. These are usually given at 12 to 18 months of age without gamma globulin, and a single injection results in antibody production in over 95% of the recipients. Mass immunization has reduced the incidence of measles in the United States by about 90% (see Figure 39-8) and has the potential for essentially eliminating the disease.

Before vaccines the prophylactic use of pooled gamma globulin was the only method of modifying the disease. The administration of large amounts to an individual within five or six days after exposure completely prevents the disease. However, because such passive immunity to measles was only temporary, it left the individual susceptible to a later measles infection. Therefore, it became a routine procedure to administer only

enough gamma globulin to lessen the severity of the disease but still allow the individual sufficient clinical expression of measles to acquire a permanent immunity. This procedure is not used for persons who have received the measles vaccine, but gamma globulin treatment would still be very important to a person who has been exposed to measles but has never received the vaccine. Unfortunately, the modification of the disease by the limited use of gamma globulin has not succeeded in preventing the rare complications of encephalitis. It is thus better to give adequate gamma globulin to exposed nonimmune individuals to prevent the disease completely, and then follow with the normal vaccination three to six months later.

### Respiratory Syncytial Virus

This paramyxovirus appears to be morphologically related to measles virus, but it does not possess a hemagglutinin, a neuraminidase, or any hemolytic activity on erythrocytes. The fact that it causes respiratory infections and the fusion of infected cells into giant multinucleated cells (syncytia—Figure 39-9) prompted its designation as respiratory syncytial virus (RSV).

There are three antigenic strains of RSV that can be differentiated on the basis of neutralizing antibodies. The virus is very fragile, difficult to grow, and apparently very widespread. Adult infections resulting in upper respiratory disease can be grouped in that great category called the "common cold syndrome." Serious RSV infections occur in infants under six months of age, and in such cases the lower respiratory tract becomes infected. The fact that 95% of children possess antibodies to RSV by age five attests to the ubiquity of this agent.

The relationship between the severity of RSV infections and the age of the patient seems paradoxical, since the most severe disease is seen in infants who possess circulating maternal antibodies to respiratory

Figure 39-8. Reported cases of measles by four-week periods occurring in the United States from 1969 through 1973. Incidence rates are related to the intensity of the immunization efforts.

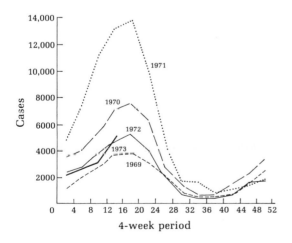

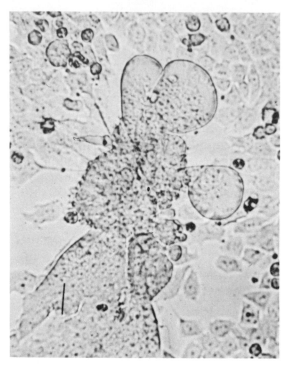

**Figure 39-9.** Cell culture infected with RSV. A number of giant cells and a large syncytium are seen in the late cytopathic effect shown here.

syncytial virus. Furthermore, in a clinical trial where inactivated virus was injected into infants in an attempt to immunize them to RSV, those infants receiving the vaccine suffered from more serious infections during a subsequent RSV epidemic than did the nonimmunized controls. These observations have led to the postulation that the severity of the disease is a function of a hypersensitivity reaction between circulating IgG and the infecting virus. Protective antibodies are, no doubt, of the IgA type, but since IgA does not pass through the placenta, the newborn receives only antiviral IgG. It therefore appears that any vaccine will have to specifically stimulate an IgA response if it is to be effective.

Laboratory diagnosis requires the isolation of the virus from respiratory secretions. In cell cultures, giant syncytia develop after one to two weeks which can be detected and identified using specific immunofluorescent antibody.

Immunity following recovery is only temporary, and inactivated vaccines have proved ineffective.

# Rubella

The agent causing rubella is definitely not an orthomyxovirus or a paramyxovirus. Actually, it is closely related to and classified with the togaviruses, but since it is not arthropod-borne, it seems appropriate to discuss it here with the viruses that are spread from person to person via respiratory secretions.

## STRUCTURE AND REPLICATION OF RUBELLA

Rubella virus contains a single linear molecule of single-stranded RNA (molecular weight = 3 million daltons) which itself is infectious. Thus, unlike the orthomyxoviruses and the paramyxoviruses, rubella virion RNA acts directly as mRNA.

The virus can be grown in a variety of human and primate cell cultures; in some no noticeable cytopathic effect occurs, but in others an effect is readily detectable. Rubella virus grows in the cytoplasm of infected cells, and based on the formation of double-stranded RNA during replication, it appears to form replicative intermediates (RI), as described for the picornaviruses (See Chapter 38).

Assembly of the virions occurs at the cell membrane, where the rubella virus acquires an envelope as it buds through the virally-altered host membrane.

## PATHOGENESIS AND EPIDEMIOLOGY OF RUBELLA

Rubella is a rather mild disease spread via respiratory secretions. After replication in the cervical lymph nodes, the virus is disseminated via the blood stream throughout the body, with the first overt signs of disease being moderate catarrhal symptoms, mild fever, and a rash that tends to be variable. The incubation period varies from two to three weeks, but virus can be isolated from nasopharyngeal secretions for as much as a week before recognizable illness. The illness is of short duration and recovery is usually complete within three or four days after the appearance of the rash. Transient arthritis is a fairly frequent symptom in adult women, but other complications are rare.

A tragic aspect of rubella may come to the fore if infection occurs during pregnancy. The virus can cross the placental wall and infect the fetus, where it disseminates and grows in every fetal organ. Infection may result in the death of the fetus or in a large variety of congenital defects, which have been collectively referred to as the rubella syndrome. Defects may include mental retardation, cerebral palsy, cataracts, microcephaly, and heart abnormalities, as well as other congenital anomalies. Infected fetuses who survive may continue to shed rubella virus for one to two years after birth in spite of the presence of circulating antibody to the virus, and it is estimated that 10–20% of such babies die during the first year following birth.

The prognosis of an infected fetus born with the rubella syndrome is in large part dependent upon its stage of development at the time the mother becomes infected. Thus, congenital defects may occur in as many as 80% of the fetuses of mothers infected during the first month of pregnancy, but this will drop to about 15% by the third month, and by the end of the first trimester the percentage of fetuses with congenital defects is small. It appears obvious that the most serious congenital abnormalities occur when the fetus is infected during the period of maximum cell differentiation. The observations that most rubella-infected tissue cultures do not show cytopathic effects and that infected cells grow much slower and eventually cease to divide may shed light on the reasons for the congenital defects. Thus, infection of the fetus before cell differentiation is complete could easily interfere with development, causing a variety of defects.

## DIAGNOSIS AND CONTROL OF RUBELLA

Laboratory diagnosis of rubella requires the isolation of the virus—usually from nasopharyngeal secretions. The lack of cytopathic effect in some types of cell cultures can be overcome by utilization of the fact that rubella-infected cells, though outwardly normal, are resistant to infection by a number of picornaviruses which ordinarily cause cytopathic effects. Also, since rubella virus possesses a hemagglutinin, infected areas can be located by hemadsorption. Other methods of diagnosis measure a rise in antibody titer using hemagglutination-inhibition, complement-fixation, or neutralization tests.

There is only one antigenic strain of rubella virus, and immunity appears to be life-long, although second infections may occur occasionally as unapparent disease. Rash does not occur in some cases of rubella, even though such individuals are excreting virus. Thus, there are three major unapparent sources for virus spread: (1) unapparent infections, (2) the asymptomatic period of about one week before apparent symptoms, and (3) congenitally infected babies who may appear normal even though they are excreting virus. Control through isolation of individuals diagnosed as having the disease is, therefore, impossible.

There are several live attenuated rubella vaccines now available that appear to induce

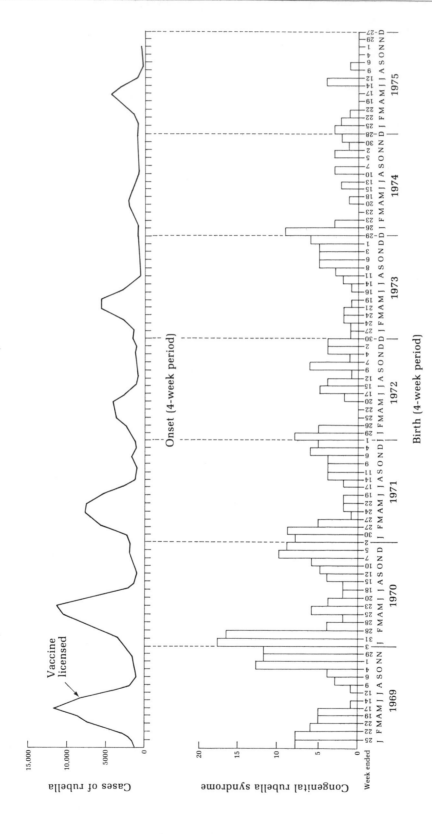

**Figure 39-10.** Cases of rubella and congenital rubella syndrome occurring in the United States from 1969 through 1975.

some immunity (see Figure 39-10). The vaccines may cause fever, mild rash, and, in adult women, transient arthritis. In addition, the level of antibody response to the vaccine is considerably lower than that seen in individuals recovering from the overt disease, and it appears that vaccinated persons can subsequently experience mild to unapparent rubella virus infections. The frequency of fetal infections in partially immune vaccinated women is unknown.

A major disadvantage of the available vaccines is that they can infect the fetus, although as yet the vaccines have not been associated with congenital abnormalities. However, the risk of this possibility makes it imperative for women who may become pregnant within three months to avoid being vaccinated. The recommended time for vaccination of women is either at 11 or 12 years of age or immediately after delivery of a baby, when the risk of pregnancy is minimal.

## REFERENCES

Beare, A. S. 1975. Live viruses for immunization against influenza. *Progr. Med. Virol.* **20:**49–83.

Choppin, P. W., and R. W. Compans. 1975. Reproduction of paramyxoviruses. In H. Fraenkel-Conrat and R. R. Wagner, eds. *Comprehensive Virology,* Vol. 4. Plenum Press, New York.

Choppin, P. W., E. D. Kilbourne, W. Dowdle, G. K. Hirst, W. K. Joklik, R. W. Simpson, and D. O. White. 1975. Genetics, replication and inhibition of replication of influenza virus—summary of influenza workshop VII. *J. Infect. Dis.* **132:**713–723.

Compans, R. W., and Choppin, P. W. 1975. Reproduction of myxoviruses. In H. Fraenkel-Conrat and R. R. Wagner, eds. *Comprehensive Virology,* Vol. 4. Plenum Press, New York.

Compans, R. W., H. Klenk, L. A. Caliguiri, and P. W. Choppin. 1970. Influenza virus proteins. I. Analysis of polypeptides of the virion and identification of spike glycoproteins. *Virology* **42:**880–889.

Dowdle, W. R., M. T. Coleman, and M. B. Gregg. 1974. Natural history of influenza type A in the United States, 1957–1972. *Progr. Med. Virol.* **17:**91–135.

Glass, S. E., D. McGeoch, and R. D. Barry. 1975. Characterization of the mRNA of influenza virus. *J. Virol.* **16:**1435–1443.

Hirst, G. K. 1973. Mechanism of influenza virus recombinations. *Virology* **55:**81–93.

Hovi, T., and A. Vaheri. 1970. Infectivity and some physiochemical characteristics of rubella virus ribonucleic acid. *Virology* **42:**1–8.

Joseph, B. S., P. W. Lampert, and M. B. A. Oldstone. 1975. Replication and persistence of measles virus in defined subpopulations of human leukocytes. *J. Virol.* **16:**1638–1649.

MacKenzie, J. S., and M. Houghton. 1974. Influenza infections during pregnancy: Association with congenital malformations and with subsequent neoplasms in children, and potential hazards of live virus vaccines. *Bacteriol. Rev.* **38:** 356–370.

Maugh, T. H., II. 1976. Amantadine: An alternative for prevention of influenza. *Science* **192:** 130–131.

Parkes, D. 1974. Amantadine. *Adv. in Drug Res.* **8:**11–81.

Salk, J., and D. Salk. 1977. Control of influenza and poliomyelitis with killed virus vaccines. *Science* **195:**834–847.

Shope, R. E. 1931. Swine influenza. III. Filtration experiments and etiology. *J. Exp. Med.* **54:** 373–385.

Shvartsman, Y. S., and M. P. Zykov. 1976. Secretory anti-influenza immunity. *Adv. in Immunology* **22:**291–330.

Spenser, M. J., J. D. Cherry, K. R. Powell, C. V. Sumaya, and A. J. Garakian. 1975. Clinical trials with Alice strain, live, attenuated, serum-inhibitor resistant intranasal influenza A vaccine. *J. Infect. Dis.* **132:**415–420.

Stephenson, J. R., and N. J. Dimmock. 1975. Early events in influenza virus multiplication. I. Location and fate of the input RNA. *Virology* **65:**77–86.

Vaheri, A., and T. Hovi. 1972. Structural proteins and subunits of rubella virus. *J. Virol.* **9:**10–16.

Webster, R. G. 1972. On the origin of pandemic influenza viruses. *Current Topics in Microbiol. and Immunol.* **59**:75–105.

Webster, R. G., C. H. Campbell, and A. Granoff. 1971. The *in vivo* production of new influenza A viruses: I. Genetic recombination between avian and mammalian influenza viruses. *Virology* **44**:317–328.

Webster, R. G., C. H. Campbell, and A. Granoff. 1973. The *in vivo* production of new influenza viruses: III. Isolation of recombinant influenza viruses under simulated conditions of natural transmission. *Virology* **51**:149–162.

# 40

## Rhabdoviridae, Arenaviridae, and Slow Viruses

### Rhabdoviridae

Rhabdoviruses form a large family of agents which infect both animals and plants. The assignment of a virus to this family has in the past been based primarily on the structure of the virion; to be more specific, all rhabdoviruses are rod-shaped or bullet-shaped (see Figure 40-1). Current biochemical studies support this classification by demonstrating extensive similarities in spite of the diversity of the hosts they infect. Rabies virus is the only agent of this group which normally infects humans, although laboratory infections with vesicular stomatitis virus (a pathogen of cattle) have occasionally occurred. We are concerned here only with rabies virus infections, but as far as is known the general structure and mode of replication for all rhabdoviruses is similar.

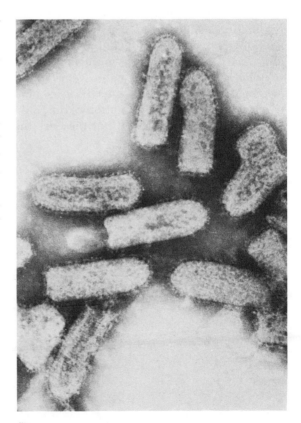

**Figure 40-1.** Virions of vesicular stomatitis virus, a typical rhabdovirus that infects animals. Note the external spikes protruding from virion membranes and striations within the core resulting from spirally-wound RNA within the nucleoprotein.

## STRUCTURE AND REPLICATION OF RHABDOVIRUSES

The rhabdoviruses differ in shape from the paramyxoviruses, but they are similar in the helical symmetry of their virion RNA and their mode of replication. The glycoprotein spikes of the enveloped rod-shaped virion appear to attach to specific host cell receptor sites. Removal of the spikes with trypsin causes a marked decrease in infectivity, presumably because the virus can no longer attach to the host cell.

Fusion of the viral envelope with the host cell membrane allows the liberation of the nucleocapsid into the host cell cytoplasm. The nucleocapsid contains one molecule of single-stranded RNA, and, because this is a minus strand, it must first be transcribed into mRNA before protein synthesis can occur. This is accomplished in the host cell cytoplasm by a viral transcriptase without further uncoating of the nucleocapsid. Rabies virus replication differs from that of most other rhabdoviruses in that infected cells develop characteristic cytoplasmic inclusion bodies which have been given the name Negri bodies (see Figure 40-2). There is some disagreement concerning the origin or function of the Negri bodies, but it seems likely that they are the site of virus replication.

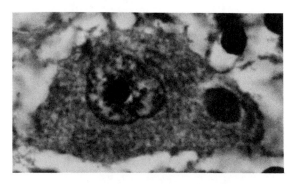

**Figure 40-2.** An oval Negri body is seen to the right of the nucleus in this brain cell from a human rabies case. Lendrum's stain was used in this instance, although most manuals call for Seller's stain.

The details of RNA replication to form molecules for inclusion in progeny virions are not well understood, but the process may well be similar to that which occurs in the paramyxoviruses, where the infective RNA is transcribed into a single plus strand of RNA—a strand that can then serve as a template for the production of minus strands of viral RNA.

Assembly of virions occurs at specific locations in the host cell where viral spikes have been inserted into the membrane and a viral protein has replaced host cell membrane proteins. Liberation occurs as the completed virion buds from the cell membrane.

## RABIES

Few diseases can induce the psychological terror caused by the bite of a "mad" dog. The scope of this fear is indicated by the thousands of persons who receive treatment for potential rabies following dog bites each year, even though the development of the disease may be unlikely in any single case because rabies in domestic dogs is rare in the United States.

### Pathogenesis and Epidemiology of Rabies

Rabies infections are almost always acquired from the bite of a rabid animal, although animals placed in caves inhabited by rabid bats have contracted rabies via a respiratory route. Once infected, the most unusual feature of rabies is the long and variable incubation period before the appearance of overt symptoms. Reports vary from 13 days to 9 months, but the average is about 30 days. Controversy surrounds explanations of the variable incubation period, the route by which the virus reaches the brain, and the mechanism by which the virus infects the salivary glands of the rabid animal. Although absolute answers must wait future research, experimental observations support the conclusion that the length of the incubation period is determined by the severity of the lacerations due to the bite, the amount of virus introduced, and the distance the virus must travel in the body to reach the brain. Thus, head and face wounds usually show a short incubation period because wounds are usually extensive and the brain is nearby.

Once introduced into a wound, the virus may remain at the site of injection for one to four days, after which it appears to progress along nerve paths to the central nervous system. Once in the central nervous system it produces an encephalitis, which is usually fatal. Experimental evidence supports the possibility of dissemination via the blood stream, and it may be possible that spread occurs through both nerves and blood vessels. The exact mechanism whereby the salivary glands become infected is also unknown, but such infection could occur from the centrifugal spread of the virus via nerve paths or as a result of viremia.

Initial symptoms of headache, nausea, sore throat, and sensitivity around the original wound site are followed by a period of excitation and nervousness. During this stage, the individual has great difficulty in swallowing, and even the sight of liquid may induce painful contractions of the throat muscles, inspiring the older, common name of "hydrophobia" for this disease. This is followed by convulsions, coma, and death.

Rabies virus seems capable of infecting all warm-blooded animals, and wild mammals are a major reservoir for the virus. The type of animal most frequently involved will vary from one part of the world to another, but skunks, foxes, coyotes, and raccoons appear to be common sources in North America. Dogs and cats, particularly in rural areas, may become infected by a wild animal, and these animals constitute a dangerous source of infection for humans. In addition, both vampire and insectivorous bats make up an exceedingly dangerous reservoir for rabies virus, inasmuch as it appears that these animals may be asymptomatic carriers of the latent virus.

## Diagnosis and Control of Rabies

The major criterion for a laboratory diagnosis of rabies is based on the presence of the characteristic Negri bodies in the cytoplasm of infected brain cells (see Figure 40-2). In addition, a suspension of brain or salivary gland cells can be injected intracerebrally into mice, and following paralysis of the mice, their brains can be examined for the presence of Negri bodies.

Antibody to rabies virus is also available with a fluorescent label, and tissue slices treated with such antibody will show areas of fluorescence in infected cells. This technique is much more sensitive than the older method of staining for Negri bodies and is now preferred in most laboratories.

Rabies control in the United States is primarily directed toward the prevention of rabies in domestic dogs. This is accomplished by mandatory vaccination of all dogs, using a living attenuated virus (Flury LEP) which has been adapted to grow in chick embryos. Vaccinated animals may become mildly ill, but the resulting immunity is effective for about three years. Control in wild animals is more difficult, but wide-spread trapping during a rabies epidemic is effective in breaking the epidemiologic chain of the animal disease.

## Treatment of Rabies

Although there is now one documented case of recovery from overt rabies in humans, the disease can still be considered essentially 100% fatal once symptoms have appeared. Thus, treatment is designed to induce an effective immune response in a potentially infected individual during the long incubation period of the disease. This was first done by Pasteur in 1885; he used ground-up spinal cords of rabies-infected rabbits which had been dried for various lengths of time to partially inactivate the virus. This somewhat altered rabies virus was called "fixed" virus to differentiate it from the wild type strain which Pasteur referred to as "street" virus. Although the viral vaccine used today is somewhat different from that used in 1885, the principle is the same, and the daily injections of rabies vaccine into an individual bitten by a rabid animal is still spoken of as the Pasteur treatment. The vaccines used today consist of either a phenol-inactivated virus grown in rabbit brain or a β-propiolactone-inactivated virus grown in duck embryos. The vaccine grown in rabbit brains induces a better immunologic response, but because of the presence of brain tissue in the vaccine, a small percentage of treated individuals develop a very severe and often fatal allergic encephalitis. This allergic encephalitis is an autoimmune disease in which the patient receiving the rabies vaccine may form antibodies against the rabbit brain tissue used for growing the viral vaccine. These antibodies possess reactive sites that will also react with and destroy the patient's own brain cells. Because there is no nervous tissue in the duck vaccine, it is the more widely used of the two. With either modern vaccine, immunization requires daily injections for as many as 21 days.

The newest and most promising rabies vaccine is currently being tested experimentally in several countries. It consists of killed rabies virus that has been grown in human diploid cell strains. It is postulated that this new vaccine will provide complete protection after only six injections, and since the vaccine contains essentially no extraneous foreign proteins, allergic reactions do not occur. Another promising experimental rabies vaccine contains only the glycoprotein spikes isolated from rabies virus grown in human diploid cells.

However, these new vaccines are not yet

**Figure 40-3.** In the United States during 1973, rabies was reported in 2930 wild animals, 767 domestic animals, and one human. The map below shows the number of cases of reported rabies from each state.

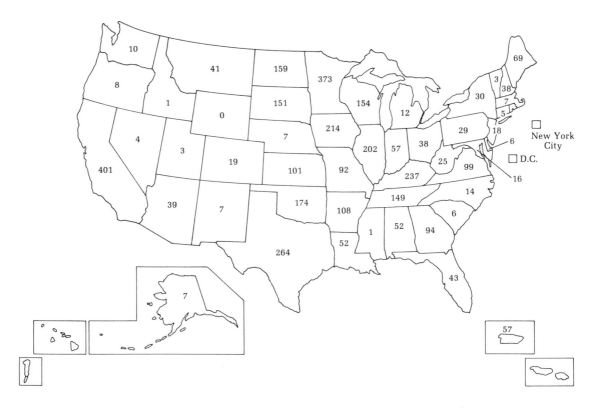

available, and one must still rely on the rabbit brain or duck embryo. Because such immunization is painful and not without some danger, the decision to use these vaccines can be a difficult one. An unprovoked bite by a wild animal, bat, or dog must be considered a potential exposure to rabies. If the animal can be apprehended, it should be confined for observation. If no symptoms develop in the animal during the subsequent ten days, there is no danger of rabies from the bite. However, if the animal is destroyed immediately after

the bite, the brain should be examined for Negri bodies, and brain suspensions should be injected intracerebrally into mice. The extent to which rabies is present in the animal population is shown in Figure 40-3, and this undoubtedly represents only a small fraction of actual infections.

Hyper-immune rabies antiserum is also available. It should be used to wash the wound and should be injected parenterally to provide instant passive immunity to the virus.

# Arenaviridae

The establishment of this taxonomic group was based primarily on the morphology and grainy appearance of the virions when viewed in thin section with the electron microscope (arenosus = Latin for sandy; see Figure 40-4). Subsequent investigations have shown serologic similarities to exist within this diverse group of viruses.

## STRUCTURE AND REPLICATION

The arenaviruses are very pleomorphic and various types exhibit a range of diameters from 60 to 350 nm. Virtually nothing is known about the series of events involved in replication except that arenaviruses are enclosed in envelopes which they acquire as they bud through the host cell plasma membrane.

The virions contain single-stranded RNA which can be shown to exist as four major discernable components. Two of these RNA strands (18S and 28S) arise from host cell ribosomes which are incorporated into the nucleocapsid of the virion, providing the characteristic sandy appearance. The other two segments of RNA (31S and 22S) appear to be the viral RNA.

Based on shared complement-fixing antigens, the arenaviruses can be subdivided as follows: (1) lymphocytic choriomeningitis virus, (2) the Tacaribe complex of viruses, and (3) Lassa fever virus.

## LYMPHOCYTIC CHORIOMENINGITIS VIRUS (LCM)

LCM virus possesses the unique ability to cause a congenital infection in mice that leads to an essentially asymptomatic condition in which the adult animal continues to excrete the virus. The ability of most congenitally infected mice to become permanent virus carriers results from the development of an immunological tolerance to the virus and from the fact that replication of the virus

**Figure 40-4.** Lassa fever virus in a Vero cell culture (×173,000). Ribosomes incorporated from the host cell may be seen within the virus particles.

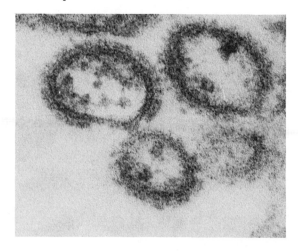

does not result in the cytopathic destruction of the infected host cell. Tolerance is not always complete, and virus may be present in the bloodstream as a virus-IgG complex. The IgG does not, however, neutralize the virus, and such complexes are infectious.

Injection of LCM virus into adult mice may, in contrast, cause acute disease and death. Since LCM virus did not appear to cause a cytopathic effect in mouse cells, a simple explanation for this observation was not immediately available. This phenomenon can now be explained as follows: the virus grows in the adult mouse, and although no major cytopathic changes take place, new virally coded antigens are inserted into the infected host cell membranes; the adult mouse reacts with both a humoral and a cell-mediated immune response directed against the LCM-infected cells; the cell-mediated immunity results in the destruction of the host cells in a manner analogous to a graft-versus-host reaction (see Chapter 17). The important lesson to be learned concerning LCM infections is not that they cause a mild respiratory infection in humans but rather that the disease in mice may be a model for certain autoimmune diseases that occur in humans. Thus, any virus that reproduces without causing apparent injury to the host cell but modifies the host cell membrane by inserting virally coded foreign proteins certainly sets up conditions that could induce an autoimmune disease.

**Pathogenesis and Epidemiology of LCM Infections in Humans**

Although it was at one time believed that LCM was a major cause of aseptic meningitis in humans, careful studies have shown that meningitis is a fairly rare manifestation of human disease caused by LCM virus. Most human infections are influenza-like, with symptoms of fever, headache, malaise, and nausea. When central nervous invasion does occur, the symptoms are ordinarily mild, and recovery is usually complete within one to three weeks.

It is fairly well established that the house mouse is the major reservoir for this virus. Infected mice excrete the virus in their feces, urine, nasal secretions, milk, and sperm. In geographical areas where mouse infection is prevalent, more than 10% of the human population may have neutralizing antibody to LCM, even though the vast majority of such sero-positive individuals have no history of meningitis.

Pet Syrian hamsters have been shown to be the source of human infections, but the virus does not persist in the hamster as it does in the mouse, and the hamster thus appears to be only an intermediate host between the mouse and humans.

**Figure 40-5.** Partial map of the Western Hemisphere showing the geographic localities in which viruses of the Tacaribe complex have been recognized.

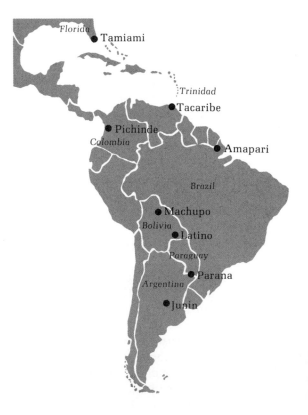

## TACARIBE VIRUS COMPLEX

As shown in Figure 40-5, eight serotypes of this complex have been isolated from Florida and South America. They appear to be rodent-associated, and, like LCM, some (if not all) cause a silent chronic infection in their rodent host. This infection is characterized by a persistent viremia in the absence of detectable circulating antibodies.

Only two of the Tacaribe viruses have been shown to infect humans—Junin and Machupo viruses, which cause Argentine and Bolivian hemorrhagic fever respectively. Both of these diseases are characterized by bleeding from the mouth, stomach, intestines, nose, and occasionally the vagina. Although blood loss is not great, patients may go into shock and die. Overall mortality varies from 10–50%. These diseases were once believed to be arthropod-borne; however, there is no evidence to support this concept, and human infection probably results from contact with infected rodent secretions.

## LASSA FEVER VIRUS

This disease was first described in Nigeria in 1969, and several epidemics have since been described in other areas of Africa.

The virus, which is morphologically and biochemically an arenavirus, has been isolated in nature only from humans; however, inapparent infections can be established in newborn mice. In humans subcutaneous hemorrhages on the arms and legs occur; other clinical features include most of the influenza-like symptoms. The disease has a very high mortality rate, and death is usually attributed to cardiac failure.

# Slow Virus Diseases in Humans

The final section of this chapter is designed for contemplative reading. We shall be concerned with relatively rare syndromes that are characterized as chronic central nervous system diseases. Because of incubation periods that may last for years, the diseases in question are spoken of as slow virus diseases. Etiologic agents for these diseases shall be divided into two categories: (1) conventional viruses that have been isolated and grown; and (2) unconventional agents that, although apparently infectious agents, have never been grown or visualized.

## DISEASES ASSOCIATED WITH CONVENTIONAL SLOW VIRUSES

Subacute sclerosing panencephalitis (SSPE) is a chronic central nervous system infection which is characterized by behavioral changes, mental deterioration, loss of vision, and coma. It is fairly well established that it is caused by measles virus. The series of events that culminate in this disorder is not understood, but it appears to follow a reactivation of a latent measles virus in an individual with an immune deficiency.

Progressive multifocal leukoencephalopathy (PML) is a rare degenerative central nervous system infection which usually occurs in persons with severe immunodeficiency disorders. The disease is characterized by memory loss, difficulty in speaking, and uncoordination. The causative agent is one of several viruses—classified as papovaviruses (see Chapter 34)—named JC virus, BK virus, and SV40 virus. In one case, the isolated SV40 from PML appeared to be identical to the virus routinely found in rhesus monkey kidney cells that contaminated much of the early poliovaccines. Other SV40 isolates from PML are slightly different and are referred to as "SV40-like." The fact that about 70% of normal adults possess neutralizing antibody to one or more of these agents supports the concept that central nervous system involvement is a rare event.

## DISEASES ASSOCIATED WITH
## SLOW UNCONVENTIONAL AGENTS

Kuru is a degenerative disease of the central nervous system that is characterized by tremors, progressive ataxia (uncoordinated movements), mental deterioration, and death about one year after the onset of symptoms. The disease has been described only in a tribe in New Guinea, and its transmission appears to have resulted from the tribal custom of eating the uncooked brains of deceased persons by the tribal women and children. Injection of human brain suspensions from Kuru victims into chimpanzees results in a similar disease in the chimpanzee after an incubation period of one to five years. However, no infectious agent of any kind has been found, and since cannibalism is now forbidden, the disease has essentially disappeared from the Melanesian tribe.

Creutzfeldt-Jakob disease (CJD) is a rare presenile (resembling senility but occurring earlier in life) dementia which closely resembles Kuru, and which has also been successfully transmitted to nonhuman primates. However, like Kuru no agent of any kind has been associated with this syndrome.

Scrapie, a disease of sheep, and transmissible mink encephalopathy (TME), a disease of minks, also appear to be analogous to Kuru and Creutzfeldt-Jakob disease in humans. It has been proposed that all of these chronic, progressive, and ultimately fatal neurological syndromes might be caused by a class of agents called "viroids." This term is used to describe "subviral" pathogens of plants that appear to exist solely as short strands of low-molecular-weight, naked RNA. There seems little doubt that such agents do exist and cause plant diseases; however, their occurrence in the animal kingdom has not as yet been demonstrated. Since naked RNA would induce neither an immunological nor an inflammatory response, it is tempting to think of animal "viroids" as potential agents for the unconventional neurological diseases in humans.

## OTHER NEUROLOGICAL DISEASES
## IN HUMANS

There are yet other neurological diseases occurring in humans which are not known to be even infectious, much less of viral etiology. However, circumstantial evidence is accumulating which indicates a latent virus may be reactivated and become the etiologic agent of these disorders. It must, however, be stressed that *all* of the following postulations are based on circumstantial data, analogies, and conjecture.

Multiple sclerosis (MS) is a chronic demyelinating (the myelin sheath surrounding the nerves is destroyed) disease in which IgG antibody to measles virus has been found in the spinal fluid, and laboratory research has suggested that the reticuloendothelial cells of MS patients may not be able to recognize measles virus or other lipid-containing viruses. Data are, however, still much too inconclusive to assign measles virus as the etiologic agent of multiple sclerosis.

Guillain-Barré syndrome (GBS) has been associated with a number of viral entities, including the swine influenza vaccine (see Chapter 39). Echo viruses and *Mycoplasma pneumoniae* have been isolated from the spinal fluid of such patients, and a recent study has shown that GBS patients possess a higher level of antibody to the herpes EB virus than do age-marked controls.

Amyotrophic lateral sclerosis (ALS) is a fatal, chronic, degenerative disease which appears to be infectious. On the basis of conjecture and pathologic analogies, it has been proposed that ALS could be the result of the activation of latent poliovirus.

Parkinson's disease is also of unknown etiology, but influenza virus antigen has been reported to occur in the brains of post-encephalitic Parkinson patients.

It will be interesting to re-read this section in one or two decades to see how many of these postulations prove to be correct and to check whether or not the etiology of these chronic degenerative central nervous system diseases is still in the category of conjecture.

# REFERENCES

Albrecht, P., T. Burnstein, M. J. Klutch, J. T. Hicks, and F. A. Ennis. 1977. Subacute sclerosing panencephalitis: Experimental infection in primates. *Science* **195**:64–66.

Black, F. L. 1975. The association between measles and multiple sclerosis. *Progr. Med. Virol.* **21**:158–164.

Constantine, O. G., R. W. Emmons, and J. D. Woodie. 1972. Rabies virus in nasal mucosa of naturally infected bats. *Science* **175**:1255–1256.

Craighead, J. E. 1975. The role of viruses in the pathogenesis of pancreatic disease and diabetes mellitus. *Progr. Med. Virol.* **10**:163–214.

Diener, T. O. 1973. Viroids as prototypes or degeneration products of viruses. In E. Kurstak and K. Maramorosh, eds. *Viruses, Evolution and Cancer.* Academic Press, New York.

Emerson, S. U. 1976. Vesicular stomatitis virus: Structure and function of virion components. *Current Topics in Microbiol. and Immunol.* **73**:1–34.

Fuccillo, D. A., J. E. Kurent, and J. L. Sever. 1974. Slow virus diseases. *Annu. Rev. Microbiol.* **28**:231–264.

Haase, A. T. 1975. The slow infection caused by visna virus. *Current Topics in Microbiol. and Immunol.* **72**:101–156.

Holland, J. J. 1974. Slow, inapparent and recurrent viruses. *Sci. American* **230**:32–40.

Hotchin, J. E., ed. 1974. Slow virus diseases. *Progr. Med. Virol.* **18**:1–371.

Johnson, K. M., P. A. Webb, and G. Justines. 1973. Biology of the Tacaribe-complex viruses. In F. Lehmann-Grub, ed. *Lymphocytic Choriomeningitis Virus and Other Arenaviruses.* Springer-Verlag, New York.

Lehmann-Grub, F. ed. 1973. *Lymphocytic Choriomeningitis Virus and Other Arenaviruses.* Springer-Verlag, New York.

Minimoto, N., K. Kurata, I. Kaizuka, and H. Sazawa. 1976. Use of the hemadsorption phenomenon for determining virus and neutralizing antibody titers of rabies. *Infect. Immun.* **13**:1454–1458.

Murphy, F. A., S. G. Whitfield, P. A. Webb, and K. M. Johnson. 1973. Ultrastructural studies of arenaviruses. In F. Lehmann-Grub, ed. *Lymphocytic Choriomeningitis Virus and Other Arenaviruses.* Springer-Verlag, New York.

Notkins, A. L., and H. Koprowski. 1973. How the immune response to a virus can cause disease. *Sci. American* **228**:22–31.

Parker, J. C., H. J. Igel, R. K. Reynolds, A. M. Lewis, Jr., and W. P. Rowe. 1976. Lymphocytic choriomeningitis virus infections in fetal, newborn and young adult Syrian hamsters. *Infect. Immun.* **13**:967–981.

Pasteur, L. 1885. Méthode pour prévenir la rage apres morsure. *Compt. Rend. Acad. Sc.* **101**:765–772.

Weissenbacher, M. C., C. E. Coto, and M. A. Calello. 1976. Cross-protection between Tacaribe-complex viruses. Presence of neutralizing antibody against Junin virus (Argentine hemorrhagic fever) in guinea pigs infected with Tacaribe virus. *Intervirology* **6**:42–49.

Yoon, J., and A. L. Notkins. 1976. Virus-induced diabetes mellitus. VI. Genetically determined host differences in the replication of encephalomyocarditis virus in pancreatic beta cells. *J. Exp. Med.* **143**:1170–1185.

# 41

# Retroviridae

The concept that both DNA and RNA viruses can induce benign and malignant tumors is now a well-established fact. Many of the DNA tumor-producing viruses, however, are also etiologic agents for a variety of other diseases, and this text has chosen to correlate their oncogenicity with a general discussion of the viral family. Therefore, for a review of the oncogenic DNA viruses the reader is referred to Chapter 33 (herpesviruses), Chapter 34 (adenoviruses and papovaviruses), and Chapter 35 (poxviruses). This chapter will be limited to a discussion of the RNA tumor viruses.

## RETROVIRIDAE

The first of this large group of tumor-producing RNA viruses was described in the early 1900's when it was shown that leukemias and sarcomas of chickens could be transmitted to newborn healthy chickens using cell-free extracts of the tumors. At that time the phenomenon was an intellectual curiosity, and few scientists visualized the importance that this discovery would have on the role of viruses in cancer.

It is now known that the RNA tumor viruses are widespread in nature, having been isolated from tumors of birds (especially chickens), mice, cats, hamsters, and nonhuman primates. Since most of these RNA-containing viruses cause either leukemia (a malignancy of primitive blood cells such as lymphoblasts, myeloblasts, or erythroblasts) or sarcoma (a solid tumor that can metastasize to any organ of the body), they have also been called oncornaviruses (onco-RNA), leukoviruses, or simply the leukemia sarcoma viruses.

## STRUCTURE AND REPLICATION OF RETROVIRUSES

Retroviruses are generally spherical with an overall diameter varying from 65 to 150 nm. The mature virion is composed of three morphologic components: (1) an outer envelope made up of a lipid membrane and containing strain-specific viral glycoprotein spikes; (2) an internal core shell containing protein and RNA; and (3) within the core, an electron-dense nucleoid containing the RNA and several enzymes necessary for viral replication. The one linear piece of 60–70S single-stranded RNA (molecular weight = 9–12 million daltons) appears to consist of two identical segments joined together through complementary base pairing of a part of each segment. Thus, heat denaturation of viral RNA results in the formation of identical molecules of RNA. In addition, several different tRNA's are hydrogen-bonded to each segment of the viral genome. The role of these complementary tRNA's is not well understood except that the tryptophanyl tRNA has been shown to be a primer for the RNA-dependent DNA-poly-merase (reverse transcriptase) in the avian retroviruses, and proline tRNA is believed to provide a similar function for the mouse RNA tumor viruses.

Electron micrographs of the RNA tumor viruses reveals several morphological types of particles. The most common is a spherical, enveloped virus with a centrally located dense nucleoid. This structure has been designated by Bernhard as a C-type particle (see

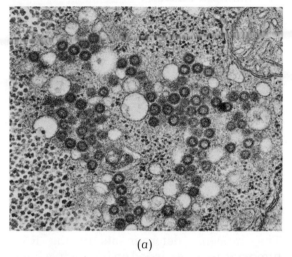

(a)

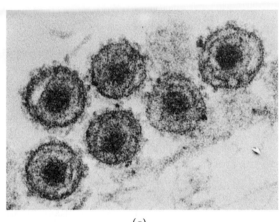

(c)

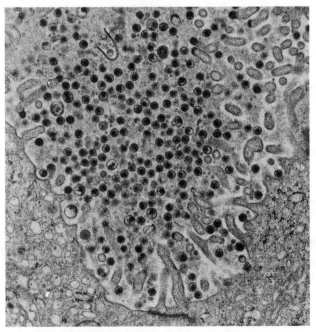

(b)

**Figure 41-1.** *a.* A developing cytoplasmic inclusion body of A-type particles (mouse mammary tumor virus; ×36,750). *b.* B-type particles of mouse mammary tumor virus in an intercellular lumen (×20,800). Note the eccentric nucleoids within the particles. *c.* Typical C-type particles of Rous sarcoma virus (×147,000). The central, dense nucleoids are characteristic of all C-type particles.

Figure 41-1) to differentiate it from B-type particles (morphologically similar but whose spherical dense nucleoid is eccentrically located within the particle) and A-type particles (that are seen only within the cytoplasm of a host cell and thus do not possess an envelope). A-type particles are believed to be precursors of B-type viruses. All of the leukemia and sarcoma RNA viruses are C-type particles. The only known B-type virus is the mouse mammary tumor agent (to be discussed later in this chapter).

## Replication of Retroviruses

The replication of the RNA tumor viruses begins with the interaction of the viral envelope glycoprotein spikes on specific areas of the host cell membrane. Removal of the spike proteins with proteolytic enzymes will prevent infection of the host cell. Following fusion of the viral envelope with the host cell membrane, the viral core is released into the cell. At this point the replication of the RNA tumor viruses differs from all other viruses because the first step is the transcription of their viral RNA into complementary DNA. This reaction is catalyzed by a viral enzyme which is correctly named an RNA-dependent DNA-polymerase; however, since this transcription is the opposite to the normal transcription—DNA to RNA—the enzyme is frequently called a reverse transcriptase (the basis for the name "retroviruses"). Based on the observation that retrovirus RNA can be transcribed into DNA even though protein synthesis is completely blocked and on the fact that reverse transcriptase activity can be demonstrated in purified virions, one can also conclude that the transcriptase must enter the cell as a preformed viral enzyme.

The location of DNA synthesis within the host cell is not known, nor are some of the details of viral replication completely understood, but a model consistent with experimental data would be as follows:

1. Newly-synthesized DNA is replicated to form double-stranded DNA which is subse-quently cyclized to form a molecule of circular double-stranded DNA.

2. One or two such DNA molecules integrate into specific sites in the host cell genome, and the continued production of viral progeny is transcribed from the integrated viral DNA.

3. Viral proteins, including viral enzymes and structural core proteins, migrate to specific areas of the host cell membrane where viral glycoproteins have been incorporated into the lipid bilayer.

4. The assembly of RNA, viral enzymes, and structural proteins occurs at the cell membrane, and the virus is released by budding from the membrane. It is important to note that, unlike most other viral infections, the RNA tumor viruses do not ordinarily kill the host cell, and both cell division and virus production can continue indefinitely. Figure 41-2 summarizes the probable steps in RNA tumor virus replication.

## Retrovirus Antigens

The antigenic determinants of the RNA tumor viruses are carried on four or five internal structural proteins (P-antigens), two glycoproteins (GP-antigens), and the reverse transcriptase. These antigens can be divided into the following three categories: (1) type-specific antigens which distinguish different viruses derived from the same species of animal; (2) group-specific antigens which are common to different viruses infecting the same animal species; and (3) interspecies antigens which are found in all mammalian C-type tumor viruses.

The two glycoproteins in the viral envelope contain type-specific, group-specific, and interspecies determinants; strain designations, however, are based on the effect of neutralizing antibody to the glycoprotein type-specific determinants. Similarly, multiple antigenic determinants, which can be assayed by complement fixation or radioimmune precipitation reactions, are found on individual internal protein antigens

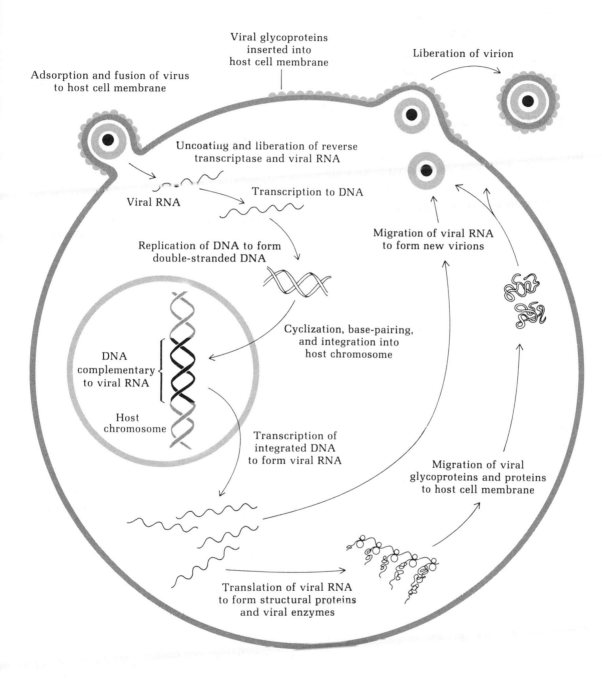

**Figure 41-2.** Replication of an RNA tumor virus. Note that the viral RNA must be transcribed to a complementary DNA which becomes integrated into the host genome before viral replication can occur.

such as the reverse transcriptase (which also carries both group and interspecies determinants).

## AVIAN LEUKEMIA VIRUSES

The avian leukemia viruses are divided into five subgroups, A, B, C, D, and E, on the basis of their envelope antigens, host specificity, and the ability of one subgroup to interfere with infection by an exogenous virus (see Tables 41-1 and 41-2). Susceptibility to infection is manifested by the presence of specific cell receptors for the virus, and resistance results from the genetic absence of virus receptors on the cells.

### Avian Leukemia

Normally, immature blood cells undergo differentiation in the bone marrow and emerge into the blood stream as mature circulating cells such as lymphocytes, granulocytes (polymorphonuclear leukocytes), erythrocytes, and so forth. However, animals with leukemia are characterized by having pathologically excessive numbers of immature cells in their circulating blood stream. Thus, the pathological manifestations of leukemia seem to involve progenitors to lym-

**Table 41-2. Interference Patterns among Avian Tumor Viruses in C/O Cells**

| Preinfecting ALV Subgroup | SUBGROUP OF CHALLENGE RSV | | | | |
|---|---|---|---|---|---|
| | A | B | C | D | E |
| A | I | + | + | + | + |
| B | + | I | + | I | I |
| C | + | + | I | + | + |
| D | + | I | + | I | I |
| E | + | + | + | + | I |

I, Interference; (+) susceptible, no interference.

phocytes (a condition known as lymphoblastosis), granulocytes (myeloblastosis), or erythrocytes (erythroblastosis). Leukemia may occur as a malignancy of only one cell type or may involve more than one cell type, as in erythromyeloblastosis; it is not known, however, whether more than one virus is involved in the etiology of multiple cell type leukemias.

The observation that avian leukemia could be transferred to baby chicks was reported almost 70 years ago, and research during the past few decades has demonstrated that avian leukemias may be caused by any one of a number of avian leukemia viruses (ALV). However, since ALV's are capable of transforming only progenitors to leukocytes, they cannot transform mature cells *in vitro,* and the inability to culture leukocyte progenitors has hindered research concerning the mechanism whereby ALV transforms normal cells into malignant cells.

### Natural Transmission of Avian Leukemia Virus

Avian leukemia virus can be passed from chicken to chicken both horizontally through secretions and vertically through eggs and possibly sperm. The virus is widespread throughout a large number of flocks of chickens and constitutes a considerable economic loss to chicken raisers throughout the

**Table 41-1. Host Range of Avian Tumor Viruses in Several Avian Species**

| | VIRUS SUBGROUP | | | | |
|---|---|---|---|---|---|
| | A | B | C | D | E |
| Red jungle fowl | + | + | + | + | +, − |
| Japanese quail | + | − | ± | − | + |
| Ring-necked pheasant | + | − | ± | − | + |
| Bobwhite quail | − | − | − | ± | − |
| Turkey | + | − | + | − | + |
| Duck | − | − | + | ± | Not tested |
| Goose | − | − | ± | ± | − |

world. In general, horizontal transmission to adult chickens does not routinely result in overt leukemia. The virus apparently multiplies in a number of mature cells (which it does not transform) and, for the most part, the chicken seems to carry these viruses without developing disease. On the other hand, vertical transmission is much more likely to cause clinical leukemia. In this situation the chicken is infected with multiplying ALV at the time of hatching but is immunologically tolerant to the foreign virus and does not therefore make antibodies to the infecting ALV. After two to four months, however, many of the chickens will develop leukemia and die.

### Assay of Avian Leukemia Viruses

Since these viruses do not cause a morphological transformation of mature cells, assays of ALV are a little less quantitative and more subtle than for those viruses that produce an observable cytopathic effect. However, the following general procedures are used to quantitate ALV: (1) assay for reverse transcriptase activity, (2) assay for the ability to act as a helper virus for defective Rous sarcoma virus, (3) use of fluorescently-labeled antibody to locate infected foci, (4) use of complement fixation tests in infected culture, and (5) ability to interfere with a subsequent infection by Rous sarcoma virus.

### AVIAN SARCOMAS

Sarcomas differ from leukemias in that they are solid tumors which characteristically originate from a malignancy of the connective tissue. In 1911 Peyton Rous demonstrated that chicken sarcomas could be passed from one chicken to another using cell-free filtrates of the tumors, thus establishing the viral etiology of this malignancy. Since that time, the many strains of avian sarcoma virus that have been isolated have, in general, been called Rous sarcoma viruses (RSV), although the broader term of avian sarcoma virus (ASV) is also used.

### Morphology and Replication of Avian Sarcoma Viruses

Morphologically, RSV is a C-type retrovirus that is essentially identical to that of the ALV, and, like ALV, it can continue to replicate in host cells without causing their death. Unlike ALV, however, RSV causes morphological transformation of many different types of cells, and, as a result, can be easily assayed by counting the foci of transformed cells occurring in a monolayer of chicken fibroblasts (see Figure 41-3).

As far as is known, RSV is acquired in nature only via a vertical route through eggs or sperm, not as a result of contact with infected animals, but the susceptibility to infection and tumor production varies considerably from one flock of chickens to another. This is due to genetic differences (since susceptibility of chickens is controlled by at least four dominant alleles of loci on the autosomal chromosomes) and to the fact that some flocks are asymptomatically infected with an ALV

**Figure 41-3.** A single focus of cells transformed by Rous sarcoma virus in a culture of chick embryo cells.

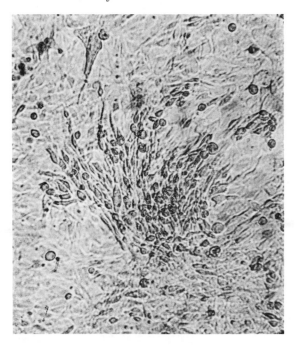

(previously called resistance-inducing factor or RIF) which blocks the cellular receptor sites for RSV.

### Defective Sarcoma Strains

Strains of RSV isolated by Bryan have yielded a great deal of information concerning the RNA sarcoma viruses. It was found that tumors produced by very low doses of Bryan strain RSV (BS.RSV) do not produce infectious virus, even though they do cause sarcomas. Briefly, this observation can be explained as follows:

1. BS.RSV is a defective virus which can infect and transform cells alone, but it lacks the genetic information to make its own envelope and thus cannot produce infectious virus.

2. The original strains of BS.RSV were contaminated with a second virus, called Rous associated virus (RAV), which when simultaneously infecting a cell with BS.RSV provided the necessary genetic information to produce the envelope for both the RAV and the BS.RSV.

3. A large series of RAV's, or as they are frequently called, helper viruses, have now been isolated, so that a particular Bryan strain of Rous sarcoma virus must be designated with its helper virus, for example, BS.RSV (RAV 1), BS.RSV (RAV 6), and so forth.

4. All of the RAV helper viruses are actually avian leukemia viruses, and essentially any avian leukemia virus can act as a helper virus for the defective avian sarcoma viruses. Figure 41-4 schematically illustrates the replication of a defective RSV.

All strains of avian sarcoma virus are not defective, and nondefective viruses can both transform infected host cells and replicate without the aid of a helper virus. (Inasmuch as all known mammalian sarcoma viruses are defective, the nondefective avian sarcoma strains would appear to be the exception, rather than the rule).

### ENDOGENOUS VIRAL GENES IN CHICKENS

It is now an accepted fact that even completely normal chicken cells carry RNA tumor virus DNA as an apparently normal component of their host genome. Evidence supporting the presence of endogenous viral genes in normal, nontransformed cells is as follows:

1. Many normal chicken cell lines can be shown to produce a group-specific antigen (gs+) that is found in avian leukemia viruses even though these cells are from chickens selected from virus-free flocks.

2. Infection of gs+ cells with a defective Bryan RSV results in the production of intact RSV, indicating that an endogenous factor, named chicken helper factor (chf), provides the genetic information for the production of the RSV envelope.

3. Treatment of gs+ cells with X-rays (which are known to activate the lytic cycle in lysogenic bacteria) releases small quantities of an avian leukemia virus.

4. Tumor virus RNA will specifically hybridize with the host cell DNA from both gs+ and gs− cells, suggesting that all chicken cells possess the endogenous viral genome but that the expression of the gs antigen in gs− cells is somehow repressed. As shown in Figure 41-5, it seems that chicken leukemia viruses can be transmitted horizontally as infectious virions, vertically as infectious virions, and genetically as integrated cellular DNA.

### MURINE LEUKEMIA VIRUSES

A number of C-type murine (mouse) leukemia viruses have been isolated and named for their discoverers. The most studied strains of murine leukemia virus (MLV) are the Gross, Friend, Moloney, and Rauscher MLV's. The last three form a single group (FMR) which can be differentiated from the Gross strain (G) on the basis of the antigenic deter-

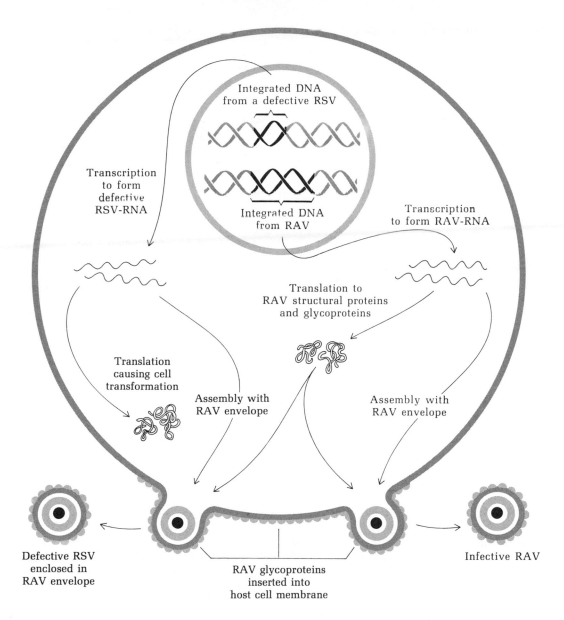

**Figure 41-4.** Replication of defective Rous sarcoma virus. Defective RSV becomes integrated as DNA into the host genome; transcription and subsequent translation form proteins that transform the host cell into a malignant cell. However, the defective RSV is unable to code for its own viral envelope and is thus released as a free virion only when a host cell is coinfected with a helper virus (Rous associated virus, RAV) which provides a viral envelope for the defective RSV genome.

minants that are deposited in the membranes of leukemic cells. Murine leukemia viruses can additionally be divided into three groups based on their ability to grow on mouse cells derived from two different inbred strains of mice. Thus, those MLV that grow on NIH Swiss (N) cells are designated N-tropic, while those viruses that readily grow on Balb/C

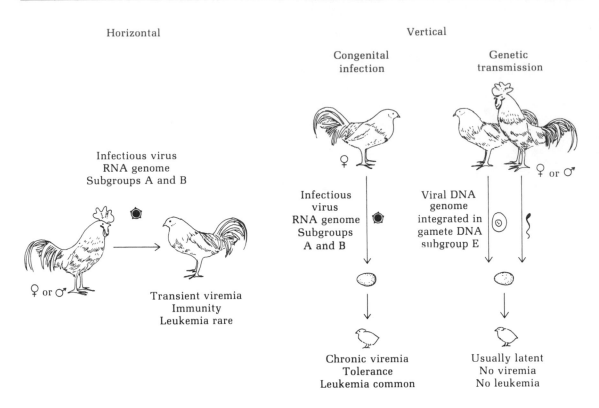

Horizontal

Vertical

Congenital
infection

Genetic
transmission

Infectious virus
RNA genome
Subgroups A and B

♀ or ♂

Transient viremia
Immunity
Leukemia rare

Infectious
virus
RNA genome
Subgroups
A and B

Viral DNA
genome
integrated in
gamete DNA
subgroup E

♀ or ♂

Chronic viremia
Tolerance
Leukemia common

Usually latent
No viremia
No leukemia

**Figure 41-5.** Modes of transmission of avian leukosis (leukemia) virus.

(B) cells are termed B-tropic. A third category (NB-tropic) contains the viruses that grow equally well on N and B cells. As is suggested from this classification, various strains of mice differ in the frequency of spontaneous leukemia and in the ease with which MLV will induce leukemia following infection of the virus. This resistance (or susceptibility) appears to be a result of both the host's genetic control of susceptibility and viral genome components. It is interesting that different MLV will usually give rise to specific tumors. Gross-MLV characteristically causes a thymic lymphosarcoma, but if injected into thymectomized mice will generally produce a myeloblastoma (granulocytic leukemia) after a latent period of several months. On the other hand, Friend and Rauscher MLV will more frequently cause an erythroblastoma after an incubation period of 1 to 3 weeks.

## MURINE SARCOMA VIRUSES

Murine sarcoma viruses (MSV) have generally been isolated from stocks of MLV, and like MLV, the various strains have been named for their discoverers. All MSV are defective, but unlike avian sarcoma viruses, whose defect lies only in their ability to produce a viral envelope, the types of defects in MSV vary from one strain to another and may include deficiencies other than the inability to synthesize envelope glycoproteins. Thus, all MSV's require that a host cell also be infected with a helper leukemic virus in order to produce progeny, even though all can transform cells and produce sarcomas in the absence of helper virus. Actually, leukemia viruses obtained from other mammals, such as hamsters, rats, and cats, can also serve as a helper virus for MSV. Assays for MSV are usually done by counting the foci of transformed cells in monolayers of cell cultures.

## ENDOGENOUS MURINE VIRUSES

Murine leukemia viruses can be transmitted horizontally from one animal to another as well as vertically through milk, semen, or the uterus. However, a genetic transmission, in which the virus is transmitted as DNA—which is integrated in the mouse chromosome—is by far the most common method of transmission. In some strains, such as AKR mice, the genetically-transmitted virus is activated soon after birth and these mice are characterized as high incidence strains. In other mice, known as low incidence strains, the virus may fail to induce sarcoma until late in life, if at all. A large number of mating experiments between low incidence and high incidence strains have revealed that AKR mice possessed two dominant loci ($V_1$ and $V_2$) and that the presence of either locus results in the expression of the MLV genome. Final proof that MLV exists as endo-

genous integrated DNA came when it was shown that the addition of 5-bromodeoxyuridine (BrdU) or 5-iododeoxyuridine (IdU) would readily induce nonproducing cultures of mouse fibroblasts to produce MLV.

## FELINE LEUKEMIA AND SARCOMA VIRUSES

Feline leukemia viruses can be isolated from about 60% of cats with leukemia, and feline sarcoma viruses from a number of feline sarcomas. These viruses are all morphologically typical C-type retroviruses, and like the murine leukemia viruses, feline leukemia viruses can infect and replicate in cell culture but cannot transform cells, whereas feline sarcoma viruses can infect and transform cells but cannot replicate in the absence of a helper virus.

Epidemiologically, feline tumor viruses appear to be transmitted horizontally, and animals infected as adults are infectious for other adults. Whether vertical transmission via egg or sperm occurs is not known.

**Figure 41-6.** B-type particles of mouse mammary tumor virus at high magnification, clearly showing the off-center nucleoids ($\times 136,000$).

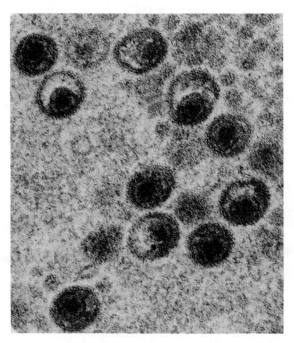

## MURINE MAMMARY TUMOR VIRUS

In 1936 Bittner discovered the first of these agents in the milk of a strain of mice showing high incidences of mammary carcinomas. All are generally similar to the other RNA tumor viruses, but their dense RNA nucleoid is slightly off-center in the spherical virion, and hence they are called B-type particles (see Figure 41-6). In addition, these viruses do not contain the same interspecies antigens that are common to the mammalian RNA C-type particle viruses, but the five different strains of mouse mammary tumor viruses (MMTV) do share group-specific antigens among themselves.

None of the MMTV can be grown in cell culture, and their classification is currently based on their route of transmission and pathology *in vivo*.

Bittner's original virus, now called MMTV-S, is highly oncogenic and is passed from parent to offspring only through milk. Therefore, strains of mice can be freed from the virus if they are removed from their mothers before nursing. Those newborns who are infected via the mother's milk will usually develop mammary carcinomas after a latent period of six to twelve months.

A virus discovered by Muhlbock, now designated MMTV-P, is also highly oncogenic, but it is passed via the eggs and sperm as well as the milk of infected mice. Other strains, MMTV-L, MMTV-O, and MMTV-X, are apparently of very low oncogenicity and are transmitted only via the eggs and sperm of infected parents.

The production of mammary carcinomas by MMTV is, in part, both a genetic and a hormonal function. Some strains of mice are much more resistant to infection than others, and tumors do not develop in infected male mice unless they are treated with female hormones. Table 41-3 summarizes the properties of a number of MMTV's.

### Other RNA Tumor Viruses

RNA-containing C-type particles have been isolated from leukemias, lymphomas, and sarcomas of rats, guinea pigs, cows, vipers, monkeys, and gibbons. Like the leukemia viruses, many of these are nontransforming, but some can serve as a helper for defective strains of sarcoma virus.

### VIRUSES IN HUMAN CANCER

The etiology of viral malignancies in many animals is unequivocal, and it would seem naive to suppose that humans are not subject to such infections. Indeed, the evidence is exceedingly convincing that some human malignancies do result from oncogenic viruses. For example, the presence of antigens of herpes simplex type 2 in human cervical carcinomas and the actual recovery of the virion from tumor cells grown in culture provide strong circumstantial evidence for the association of this virus with human cervical carcinoma. The causal relationship of herpes EB virus with both lymphoma and nasopharyngeal carcinomas, though unproven, is equally strong.

The search for human leukemia viruses has been frustrating. Virus-like particles have been observed from human leukemias, and several early isolations were subsequently shown to be contaminants that were nonhuman in origin. However, there has been a report that a human C-type virus associated with acute myelocytic leukemia has been isolated. The virus was obtained after culture of human malignant cells, and preliminary characterizations indicate that the major proteins of this virus are immunologically identical to proteins previously isolated from other patients with acute myelocytic leukemia. However, the proteins of this "human"

### Table 41-3. Properties of Strains of Mouse Mammary Tumor Viruses

| Strain | Common Name | Natural Host | Characteristic | Transmission |
|--------|-------------|--------------|----------------|--------------|
| MMTV-S | Bittner Virus | C3H | Virulent | Milk |
| MMTV-P | Mühlbock Virus | GR | Virulent; induces hormone-dependent plaques | Milk, egg, sperm |
| MMTV-L | Nandi Virus | C3HF | Low oncogenicity | Egg, sperm |
| MMTV-O | Van Leeuwenhoek Virus | Balb/c | Very low oncogenicity | Egg, sperm |
| MMTV-X | Timmermans Virus | 020 | Induced by X-irradiation | Egg, sperm |
| MMTV-Y | | C57BL | Only antigens detected | |

virus are also very closely related to proteins from viruses that cause leukemia in subhuman primates, i.e., wooly monkeys, and there is considerable disagreement as to whether this virus represents a human leukemia virus that happens to be closely related to wooly monkey leukemia virus or whether it is a contaminant and totally unrelated to human leukemia.

The postulation that human breast cancer is virally induced has also been both tantalizing and frustrating. Virus-like B-type particles have been frequently observed in the milk of women from families having a history of breast cancer and rarely in women with no such familial history. Furthermore, a reverse transcriptase has been found in these milk samples, and further characterization suggests that they may well be a human counterpart of the mouse mammary tumor viruses. However, absolute proof is lacking, even though a recently isolated RNA virus from human breast cancer has some nucleic acid homology with the RNA in human tumors and the DNA in human placental tissue. If, however, a human breast cancer virus exists, epidemiological studies of breast-fed and non-breast-fed babies indicates that the virus is not transmitted via milk as is the case for Bittner's MMTV.

The widespread occurrence of RNA-tumor viruses and virus-like particles associated with tumors (see Table 41-4) certainly suggests that humans would be very unusual animals if they were not subject to virally-induced malignancies known to occur in other animals.

## EPIDEMIOLOGY OF THE RNA TUMOR VIRUSES

It has been well established that RNA tumor viruses may exist in a latent endogenous condition that is somewhat analogous to that of a prophage, and the induction of such "proviruses" in many animals has been accomplished using X-rays and physical or

**Table 41-4. RNA Tumor Viruses as Defined by Morphological, Biochemical, and Other Biological Properties**

1. Avian RNA tumor viruses
   (a) Avian leukosis-sarcoma (subgroups A, B, C, D, E, F, G)
   (b) Avian reticuloendotheliosis viruses
2. Mammalian C-type RNA tumor viruses
   (a) Murine leukemia-sarcoma viruses, strains Gross, Friend, Moloney, Rauscher, Kirsten, Harvey
   (b) Endogenous viruses of mice (AKR: N- and S-tropic; Balb/c: N- and S-tropic; xenotropic viruses of other mouse strains, etc.)
   (c) Feline leukemia-sarcoma viruses, strains Gardner, Rickard, Theilen
   (d) Endogenous viruses of cats (RD-114, CCC, etc.)
   (e) Hamster leukemia-sarcoma viruses
   (f) Rat leukemia viruses
   (g) Simian leukemia-sarcoma viruses, strains simian sarcoma (= wooly monkey), gibbon ape leukemia
   (h) Endogenous viruses of primates (M7, M28, other baboon viruses)
   (i) Virus-like particles in human leukemias, lymphomas, and sarcomas; SSV-related C-type viruses
3. Reptilian RNA tumor viruses
   (a) Viper C-type virus
4. B-type viruses
   (a) Mouse mammary tumor virus
   (b) Virus-like particles in human milk
5. Mason-Pfizer monkey viruses (MPMV, X381, Hela particles, AO-virus, etc.)
6. "Slow" (visna, maedi) viruses
7. Syncytium-forming "foamy" viruses

chemical carcinogens. This observation has led to the concept that, in general, RNA tumor viruses may be acquired by one of three mechanisms:

1. Horizontal infection in which the adult animal is infected exogenously and usually recovers as a result of an immune response to the virus or to the transformed cells.

2. Congenital infection in which the newborn becomes infected by the virus, either *in utero* or via infected milk, resulting in an immunological tolerance to the newly acquired antigens and a malignancy as an adult.

3. Genetic transmission whereby the viral genome is vertically transmitted from one generation to another as a DNA provirus linked to the genome of the gamete.

There are now many data supporting the concept of genetic transmission in birds and rodents, and many scientists believe that all mammals and birds contain genetic elements capable of specifying RNA tumor viruses. Based on this hypothesis, two somewhat similar concepts for the origin of RNA tumor viruses have arisen.

### Oncogene-Virogene Theory

The oncogene-virogene theory, as proposed by Huebner and Todaro, postulates that stable genes—which evolved in the distant past—possess the capability of specifying virus particles (virogene) or of transforming normal cells into malignant cells (oncogene). According to this theory, these genes are transmitted vertically like other genetic information, and under normal conditions they are repressed and remain unexpressed. However, any interference with this repressor system, such as irradiation, chemical carcinogens, the normal aging process, or perhaps an infection by an exogenous virus, would permit the expression of the oncogene, resulting in cell transformation. The validity of this theory is supported by a number of observations. For example: (1) many apparently normal cell lines can be induced by irradiation or chemicals (BrdU, IdU) to produce C-type particles—which may or may not be oncogenic; (2) normal cells may produce proteins or glycoproteins that are antigenically indistinguishable from RNA tumor virus antigens; and (3) endogenous viruses of mice and chickens are known to

be vertically transmitted, and in some animals, the expression of these endogenous viral genes remains repressed unless activated by irradiation or chemical carcinogens. It is apparent that many of our current concepts of virally-induced tumors are compatible with the concepts proposed by the oncogene-virogene theory.

### Provirus–Protovirus Theory

The provirus theory was proposed in 1960 by Howard Temin, and, although it is not mutually exclusive of the oncogene theory, it suggests that provirus genes arise from an infection with an exogenous RNA tumor virus. Such an infection would lead to the transcription of the viral RNA into DNA and the subsequent integration of the DNA into the host cell genome. This hypothesis is certainly supported by the observation that many animal tumors can be horizontally transmitted with infectious RNA tumor viruses.

The protovirus theory, also proposed by Temin, provides an explanation for the origin of RNA tumor viruses that does not require either a vertical or horizontal transfer of genetic information. This theoretical hypothesis proposes that RNA tumor viruses (called ribodeoxyviruses by Temin) evolved from genetic accidents occurring during the normal transcription or reverse transcription of cellular DNA which could result in the formation of stable nucleic acid capable of independent replication. If such "protoviruses" contained information involving cellular multiplication or differentiation, they could give rise to a neoplastic transformation. Temin also proposes that small DNA viruses, such as the parvoviruses and perhaps papovaviruses, could originate in a similar manner. In this case, unintegrated DNA—arising from the reverse transcription of a ribodeoxyvirus—could continue to replicate as DNA and, if enclosed in a capsid, would be transmitted as a new virus.

In light of our current knowledge con cerning the vertical and horizontal transmission of viruses and viral genes, as well as the theoretical plausibility that replicating viruses could arise from a series of transcription mistakes followed by information exchange between cells, one might consider that the events proposed by all of these theories could occur and that perhaps at least part of each proposal is correct.

## REFERENCES

Axel, R., C. Gulati, and S. Spiegelman. 1972. Particles containing RNA-instructed DNA polymerase and virus-related RNA in human breast cancers. *Nature* **226**:1209–1211.

Baldwin, D. S. 1976. Tumor antigens and tumor-host relationships. *Annu. Rev. Med.* **27**:151–163.

Baltimore, D. 1976. Viruses, polymerases, and cancer. *Science* **192**:632–636.

Bernhard, W. 1960. The detection and study of tumor viruses with the electron microscope. *Cancer Res.* **20**:712–727.

Bishop, J. M., and H. E. Varmus. 1975. The molecular biology of RNA tumor viruses. In F. F. Becker, ed. *Cancer 2*. Plenum Press, New York.

Bittner, J. J. 1936. Some possible effects of nursing on the mammary gland tumor incidence in mice. *Science* **84**:162.

Callahan, R., M. M. Lieber, G. J. Todaro, D. C. Graves, and J. F. Ferier. 1976. Bovine leukemia virus genes in the DNA of leukemic cattle. *Science* **192**:1005–1007.

Dulbecco, R. 1976. From the molecular biology of oncogenic DNA viruses to cancer. *Science* **192**:437–440.

Hehlmann, R. 1976. RNA tumor viruses and human cancer. *Current Topics in Microbiol. and Immunol.* **73**:141–215.

Huebner, R. J., and G. J. Todaro. 1969. Oncogenes of RNA tumor viruses as determinants of cancer. *Proc. Nat. Acad. Sci. U. S. A.* **64**:1087–1094.

Kaplan, A. S., ed. 1974. *Viral Transformation and Endogenous Viruses*. Academic Press, New York.

Lieber, M. M., and G. J. Todaro. 1975. Mammalian type C RNA viruses. In F. F. Becker, ed. *Cancer 2*. Plenum Press, New York.

Martin, M. A., and G. Khoury. 1976. Integration of DNA tumor virus genomes. *Current Topics in Microbiol. and Immunol.* **73**:35–65.

Moore, D. H. 1975. Mammary tumor viruses. In F. F. Becker, ed. *Cancer 2*. Plenum Press, New York.

Nooter, K., A. M. Aarssen, P. Bentvelzen, F. G. DeGroot, and F. G. van Pelt. 1975. Isolation of infectious C-type oncornavirus from human leukemic bone marrow cells. *Nature* **256**: 595–597.

Rawls, W. E., and W. A. F. Tompkins. 1975. Consideration of the role of viruses in human cancer. *Progr. Med. Virol.* **21**:72–87.

Rous, P. 1911. A sarcoma of the fowl transmissible by an agent separable from the tumor cells. *J. Exp. Med.* **13**:397–411.

Shoyab, M., and M. A. Baluda. 1975. Homology between avian oncornavirus RNAs and DNA from several avian species. *J. Virol.* **16**:1492–1502.

Teich, N. M., R. A. Weiss, S. Z. Salahuddin, R. E. Gallagher, D. H. Gillespie, and R. C. Gallo. 1975. Infective transmission and characterization of a C-type virus released by cultured human myeloid leukaemia cells. *Nature* **256**:551–555.

Temin, H. M. 1972. RNA-directed DNA synthesis. *Sci. American* **226**:24–33.

Temin, H. M. 1976. The DNA provirus hypothesis. *Science* **192**:1075–1080.

Todaro, G. J., C. J. Sherr, R. E. Benveniste, and M. M. Lieber. 1974. Type C viruses of baboons: Isolation from normal cell cultures. *Cell* **2**:55–61.

Tooze, J., ed. 1973. *The Molecular Biology of Tumor Viruses*. Cold Spring Harbor, New York.

Tooze, J., and J. Sambrook, eds. 1974. *Selected Papers in Tumor Virology*. Cold Spring Harbor, New York.

# 42

## Diagnosis of Viral Infections

The majority of viruses causing human disease can be isolated from clinical material and grown in the laboratory. It is therefore not surprising that laboratories for the identification of viruses are becoming standard facilities in many large hospitals. However, it should be emphasized that virus isolation requires many specialized items such as readily available sources of cell lines, chick embryos, and a variety of susceptible animals and highly trained personnel; thus the cost is prohibitive for using these facilities for routine illnesses or those diseases that can be readily diagnosed by their clinical appearance. Moreover, many of these procedures may require several weeks, and in many cases such a delayed answer would be of little value to the physician.

Then, when would one want to actually isolate and identify the etiologic virus from a patient? There is no complete answer, but there are certainly instances in which isolation would be exceedingly important. Important instances would include potential epidemics which could be prevented by specific immunization of community members, for example, polio, smallpox, or influenza. Also, early knowledge of arthropod-borne encephalidites such as EEE and WEE could initiate mosquito control measures to halt the epidemic. Another example results from the fact that certain echovirus infections can mimic rubella, and diagnosis by viral isolation during pregnancy is an indispensable measure against a suspected rubella infection.

Finally, virus isolation from diseases of unknown etiology are important, since once the agent has been grown, there is always a possibility of future prevention through the use of effective vaccines.

### DIRECT OBSERVATION

Direct observation of cells from an infected lesion will sometimes provide an immediate diagnosis, particularly if the infected cells contain characteristic inclusion bodies that can be definitively recognized. One can also treat infected cells, whether from lesions or cell cultures, with specific viral antibodies that have been conjugated to a fluorescent dye. In such cases infected cells will appear fluorescent when viewed under a special fluorescence microscope. An indirect "sandwich" technique also may be employed in which nonlabeled human viral antibodies are reacted with infected cells—followed by treatment with a goat-antihuman fluorescently-labeled globulin to ascertain whether the cells had bound the specific viral antibodies. Table 42-1 lists some of the viral diseases for which these immunofluorescent techniques would be of value.

Electron microscopy would not routinely be of value, but a modification known as immunoelectron microscopy has proved valuable for the visualization of certain viral agents. This procedure is accomplished by extracting material, such as feces, and mixing the extract with specific viral antibodies. The resulting viral aggregate can then be obtained by centrifugation and the clumped virus observed with the electron microscope.

## TECHNIQUES FOR VIRAL ISOLATION

The scope of this text does not permit a discussion of research techniques which might be used to isolate previously unde-

**Table 42-1. Rapid Identification of Viruses by Immunofluorescence**

| Specimen | Virus |
| --- | --- |
| Brain (biopsy or PM) | Rabies |
| | Herpes simplex |
| | Measles (SSPE) |
| | Papovavirus (PML) |
| Corneal scraping | Herpes simplex |
| Vesicle scraping | Smallpox |
| | Varicella |
| | Herpes simplex |
| Nasopharyngeal aspirate | Respiratory syncytial virus |
| | Parainfluenza |
| | Influenza |
| | Measles |
| Blood leukocytes | Cytomegalovirus |
| | Measles |
| | Arboviruses |
| | Many others |
| Heart (PM) | Coxsackieviruses |
| Liver biopsy | Hepatitis B |

scribed viruses. Rather, we shall limit our remarks to known agents and shall suppose that the diagnostic laboratory is aware of which possible viruses it is trying to isolate, since cells and techniques for determining viral growth vary from one virus to another. In general, the following procedures should be done:

1. Clinical material (blood, throat washings, spinal fluid, feces, skin lesions, etc.) should be either inoculated into susceptible cells immediately or kept frozen until used. In most cases, such material is treated with a mixture of penicillin and streptomycin to destroy contaminating bacteria. If one is searching for a nonenveloped virus, the material can usually be treated with 10–15% ether to destroy other viruses and bacteria, or the material can be filtered to remove bacteria. This latter technique, however, also removes a considerable amount of virus.

2. The type of tissue culture cells, animal, or fertile egg embryo chosen for inoculation will depend upon the virus for which you are searching. For example, if suspected rubella virus were inoculated into African green monkey kidney cells, little or no cytopathogenesis would occur. The virus must, therefore, be located by the ability of infected cells to adsorb red blood cells (hemadsorption) or by the observation that, following infection, cells become resistant to further infection and cytopathic effect by enteroviruses. On the other hand, inoculation of rubella virus onto a continuous cell line such as BHK-21 (baby hamster kidney) would result in an observable cytopathic effect occurring over a period of seven to ten days. Suspected influenza virus, however, would be inoculated into the amniotic cavity of fertile chick embryos and growth determined by hemagglutination.

So, you can see that for the routine diagnostic viral isolation, the laboratory must know which viruses could be expected in order to grow and find the viral agent. Table 42-2 lists the cell cultures used for the cultiva-

**Table 42-2. Cell Cultures Used for Cultivation of Animal Viruses Commonly Studied in the Laboratory**

| Virus | Culture Used |
|---|---|
| DNA VIRUSES | |
| *Parvovirus* | |
| Subgenus A | Rat embryo |
| Subgenus B (AAV) | Human embryo kidney, KB (both coinfected with adenovirus) |
| Papovaviridae | |
| Polyoma virus | Mouse embryo, 3T3 |
| SV40 | African green monkey kidney, rabbit kidney, BSC-1 |
| *Adenovirus* | |
| Human | African green monkey kidney, human embryo kidney, WI-38, HeLa, HEp-2, KB |
| Avian | Chick embryo kidney |
| *Herpesvirus* | |
| Herpes simplex virus | African green monkey kidney, human embryo kidney, chick embryo, WI-38, HeLa, HEp-2 |
| Pseudorabies virus | Rabbit kidney, baby hamster kidney, RK13 |
| Cytomegalovirus | African green monkey kidney, human embryo kidney, rabbit kidney, WI-38 |
| *Iridovirus* | |
| Frog virus 3 | Chick embryo, baby hamster kidney, FHM |
| *Poxvirus* | |
| Vaccinia | Chick embryo, HeLa, L929, KB |
| | |
| RNA VIRUSES | |
| Picornaviridae | |
| *Enterovirus* | African green monkey kidney, human amnion, WI-38, HeLa |
| *Rhinovirus* | African green monkey kidney, human embryo kidney, WI-38, HeLa, KB |
| *Aphthovirus* | Bovine embryo kidney, pig kidney, BHK |
| *Cardiovirus* | Mouse embryo, HeLa, L929 |
| Togaviridae | |
| *Alphavirus* | Chick embryo, mouse embryo, BHK, Vero, HeLa |
| *Flavivirus* | BHK, Vero, HeLa |
| Rubella virus | RK13, Vero, WI-38, BHK |
| *Orthomyxovirus* | |
| Influenza A virus | Chick embryo, calf kidney |
| *Paramyxovirus* | |
| Newcastle disease virus | Chick embryo, hamster kidney, HeLa, KB, Vero |
| *Rhabdovirus* | |
| Vesicular stomatitis virus | Chick embryo, BHK, HeLa, L929 |

Table 42-2. Cell Cultures Used for Cultivation of Animal Viruses Commonly Studied in the Laboratory (continued)

| Virus | Culture Used |
|---|---|
| *Leukovirus* | |
| Avian (including Rous sarcoma virus) | Chick embryo |
| Murine | Mouse embryo, 3T3 |
| *Reovirus* | |
| Reovirus type 3 | Human kidney, WI-38, L929 |
| *Orbivirus* | |
| Bluetongue virus | Bovine embryo kidney, lamb kidney |

Abbreviations: primary cultures, abbreviations not used; diploid strain: WI-38, human embryonic lung; heteroploid lines: BHK, baby hamster kidney cell line BHK-21; FHM, fat head minnow (fish); HeLa, HEp-2, and KB, human carcinoma, cervical, epidermoid, and nasopharyngeal, respectively; L929 and 3T3, lines of mouse fibroblasts; RK13, line of rabbit kidney cells; Vero and BSC1, lines of African green monkey kidney cells.

tion of animal viruses commonly studied in the laboratory.

## IDENTIFICATION OF ISOLATED VIRUSES

Since a serologic reaction with known antiserum is the major method used for the specific identification of a virus, the diagnostic virologist must know the limitations of possible choices. For example, one would not use influenza antiserum to identify a virus isolated from spinal fluid, nor western equine encephalitis antiserum to react with a virus obtained from throat washings. Thus, the virologist must be aware of the source of the clinical specimen and by the use of an educated guess limit the possibilities to a workable number. Once this decision is made, one or more of the following reactions should result in a specific diagnosis.

Complement fixation (CF) has an advantage in that many viruses within a specific group will share CF fixing antibodies. Thus, a single serum would react with the group-specific antigen of the orthomyxoviruses, another with polioviruses, or reoviruses, adenoviruses, poxviruses, and so forth, allowing one to determine the group to which the

unknown virus belongs. The big disadvantage of the CF test is that one must obtain sufficient virus free from interfering substances. This may be relatively simple for viruses grown in chick embryos or viruses that are released in high titer from infected tissue cells, but it may require cell disruption for those viruses that (for the most part) remain within the host cell.

The use of fluorescently-labeled antibody is also of value in determining in which group to place a virus. This can be accomplished by allowing an infected monolayer of cells to react with specific antibody and, after washing away excess antiserum, counterstaining the cells with fluorescently-labeled human anti-globulin. Infected cells which react with the specific antibody will be coated with human globulin and, after treatment with the labeled antihuman globulin, will fluoresce when viewed by microscope under ultraviolet light.

Hemagglutination-inhibition (HI) is a very effective and specific method which can be used to identify any of the many viruses that will agglutinate erythrocytes. Identification of an unknown virus is based on the fact that antibodies directed specifically against the viral hemagglutinin inhibit hemagglutina-

**Table 42-3. Specimens for Virus Isolation and Types of Serological Tests Employed for Diagnosis**

| Clinical Manifestations and Common Etiological Agents | SOURCE OF SPECIMEN FOR VIRUS ISOLATION | | SEROLOGICAL TESTS[4] | |
|---|---|---|---|---|
| | Clinical | Postmortem | Usual | (Special) |
| **UPPER RESPIRATORY TRACT INFECTIONS** | | | | |
| Rhinovirus | Throat swab or nasal secretions | — | NA | (Nt) |
| Mycoplasma | | | CF | |
| Parainfluenza | | | CF, HI | |
| Adenovirus | Throat swab and feces | — | CF, HI, Nt | (Nt, HI) |
| Enterovirus | | | NA | |
| Reovirus | | | HI, Nt | |
| **LOWER RESPIRATORY TRACT INFECTIONS** | | | | |
| Influenza | Throat swab and sputum | Lung, bronchus, trachea | CF, HI | |
| Adenovirus | | | CF, HI, Nt | |
| Parainfluenza | | | CF | |
| Mycoplasma | | | CF | |
| **PLEURODYNIA** | | | | |
| Coxsackievirus | Feces and throat swab | — | NA | (Nt) |
| **CUTANEOUS AND MUCOUS MEMBRANE DISEASES** | | | | |
| **VESICULAR** | | | | |
| Smallpox and vaccinia | Vesicle fluid and scrapings | Lung, liver, spleen, brain | CF, HI | (FA) |
| Herpes simplex | | | CF, Nt | (FA) |
| Varicella-zoster | | | CF | (FA) |
| Enterovirus | Vesicle fluid, feces, and throat swab | — | NA | (Nt, HI) |
| **EXANTHEMATOUS** | | | | |
| Measles | Throat swab | — | CF, HI | (Nt, FA) |
| Rubella | | | HI, CF | (Nt) |
| Enterovirus | Feces and throat swab | — | NA | (Nt, HI) |
| **CENTRAL NERVOUS SYSTEM INFECTIONS** | | | | |
| Enterovirus | Feces and cerebro-spinal fluid (CSF) | Brain tissue, intestinal contents | NA | (Nt, HI) |
| Herpes simplex | Throat swab and CSF | Brain tissue | CF | (Nt, FA) |
| Mumps | | | CF, HI | (Nt) |
| Lymphocytic choriomeningitis | Blood and CSF | Brain tissue | CF | (FA) |
| Arboviruses | | | | |
|   Western equine encephalitis | Blood and CSF | Brain tissue | CF, HI | (Nt) |
|   Eastern equine encephalitis | | | CF | (Nt) |

**Table 42-3. Specimens for Virus Isolation and Types of Serological Tests Employed for Diagnosis (continued)**

| Clinical Manifestations and Common Etiological Agents | SOURCE OF SPECIMEN FOR VIRUS ISOLATION | | SEROLOGICAL TESTS[A] | |
|---|---|---|---|---|
| | Clinical | Postmortem | Usual | (Special) |
| Venezuelan equine encephalitis | | | CF | (Nt) |
| California encephalitis | Usually not possible to isolate virus from clinical specimens | Brain tissue | CF | (Nt) |
| St. Louis encephalitis | | | CF | (Nt) |
| Japanese B encephalitis | | | CF | (Nt) |
| Rabies | Saliva | Brain tissue | Nt, FA | |
| **PAROTITIS** | | | | |
| Mumps | Throat swab | — | CF, HI | |
| **SEVERE UNDIFFERENTIATED FEBRILE ILLNESSES** | | | | |
| Colorado tick fever | Blood | Liver, spleen, lung, brain | CF | |
| Yellow fever | | | CF | |
| Dengue | | | CF | |
| **CONGENITAL ANOMALIES** | | | | |
| Cytomegalovirus | Urine and throat swab | Kidney, lung, other tissues | CF | (FA) |
| Rubella | Throat swab and CSF | Lymph nodes, lung, spleen, other tissues | HI, CF | (Nt, FA) |
| **HEPATITIS** | | | | |
| Virus B (HB$_s$Ag) | Agent not recoverable | Agent not recoverable | CF, CIEP, RIA | |

[A]Usual indicates types of serological tests commonly performed; (Special) indicates serological tests which may be used for special studies, not feasible for routine diagnosis. NA, Serological tests either not available or generally not feasible as routine diagnostic procedure; Nt, neutralization; CF, complement fixation; HI, hemagglutination inhibition; FA, flourescent antibody; CIEP, counterimmunoelectrophoresis; RIA, radioimmunoassay.

tion. The assay is both simple and rapid, and, can be carried out with very small amounts of virus. One merely mixes serial dilutions of known antiserum with the virus, and after 30 minutes incubation the appropriate erythrocytes are added. The absence of agglutination in the antiserum-treated virus as compared to untreated controls provides a definitive identification of the virus.

Neutralization tests are the most specific and sensitive of serologic tests used for viral identification, since kinetic evidence indicates that reaction of the virus with a single molecule of antibody will prevent infection. Thus, one needs only to mix dilutions of the unknown virus with known specific antiserum and (after an incubation of 30 to 60 minutes) infect cells, embryos, or animals with dilutions of the virus-antibody mixture. The absence of infection as compared to nontreated controls provides a positive identification of the unknown virus.

## SEROLOGIC DIAGNOSIS OF VIRAL DISEASES

By far, the majority of laboratory diagnoses of viral diseases are based on the measurement of an increase in antibody to a specific agent following recovery from the overt disease. All of these tests are essentially the reverse of those described for the serologic identification of an unknown virus, because in these cases one uses a known virus to react with antibodies that developed during convalescence. So, again, the virologist must use an educated guess to limit the number of possible reactions, but he or she is spared the decision of how, and on what, to grow an unknown agent.

Ideally, any serologic diagnosis should show a rise in antibody titer to a specific virus and therefore requires paired serum samples, i.e., an acute phase serum collected before antibody synthesis becomes measurable and a convalescent phase serum collected about two weeks later. As a general rule of thumb, at least a four-fold increase in antibody titer in the paired sera is necessary for a definitive diagnosis. On those occasions where only a convalescent phase serum is available, a diagnosis can be made by ascertaining whether the serum contains IgM antibodies to the specific agent. If present, the diagnosis is valid because IgM antibodies are short-lived, and their presence is evidence of a recent infection. They can be detected by using fluorescently-labeled anti-IgM to detect whether the patient's serum has reacted with virus-infected cells, or by determining a decrease in antibody titer after treatment of the serum with sulhydryl agents such as 2-mercaptoethanol to destroy IgM.

Neutralization, complement fixation, hemagglutination-inhibition, and the indirect immunofluorescence tests are all carried out as described for the identification of an unknown virus. Specific serologic tests such as counter-immunoelectrophoresis and radioimmune assay have been developed for the determination of the surface antigen for

hepatitis B (HB$_s$Ag), and they are described in Chapter 36. Table 42-3 summarizes the specimens which must be obtained from the patient for viral isolation and the types of serological tests that are employed for viral identification.

The presence of cellular immunity using skin tests to demonstrate a delayed-type hypersensitivity can be of value to ascertain if an individual has immunity to such viruses as mumps, herpes simplex, and a few other viruses. However, they are not totally reliable since the material used for skin testing is usually not pure and may induce hypersensitivity reactions in the absence of specific immunity. Furthermore, skin tests would be used primarily in situations where circulating antibody had already declined to unmeasurable levels.

## REFERENCES

Grillner, L., and O. Strannegard. 1976. Evaluation of the hemolysis-in-gel test for the screening of rubella immunity and the demonstration of recent infection. *J. Clin. Microbiol.* **3**:86–90.

Grist, N. R., C. A. C. Ross, and E. J. Bell. 1975. *Diagnostic Methods in Clinical Virology,* 2nd ed. Blackwell, Oxford.

Herrmann, E. C. 1974. New concepts and developments in applied diagnostic virology. *Progr. Med. Virol.* **17**:222–289.

Hsiung, G. D. 1973. *Diagnostic Virology.* Yale Univ. Press, New Haven, Connecticut.

Kurstak, E., and R. Morisset, eds. 1974. *Viral Immunodiagnosis.* Academic Press, New York.

Lennette, E. H., E. H. Spaulding, and J. P. Truant. 1974. *Manual of Clinical Microbiology,* 2nd ed. American Soc. for Microbiol., Washington, D. C.

McCracken, A. W., and J. T. Newman. 1975. The current status of laboratory diagnosis of viral diseases of man. *Critical Rev. Clin. Lab. Sci.* **5**:331–363.

Pursell, A. R., and J. R. Cole, Jr. 1976. Procedure for fluorescent-antibody staining of virus-infected cell cultures in plastic plates. *J. Clin. Microbiol.* **3**:537–540.

Schmidt, N. J., and E. H. Lennette. 1973. Advances in the serodiagnosis of viral infections. *Progr. Med. Virol.* **15**:244–308.

Symposium. 1972. Laboratory diagnosis of viral infections: Recent advances and their clinical application. *Amer. J. Clin. Pathol.* **57**:731–750.

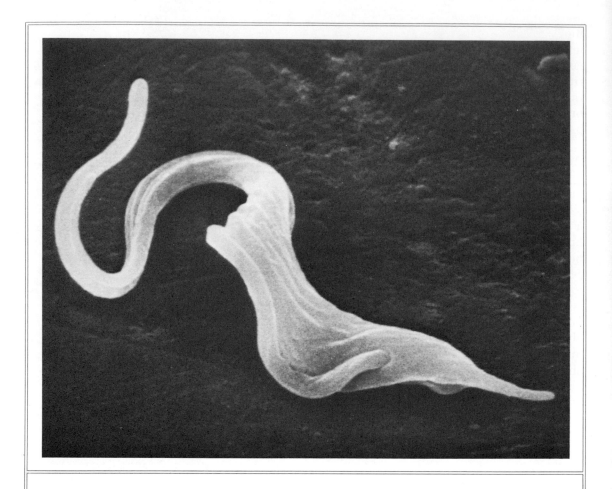

UNIT FIVE

# Medical Parasitology

One of the oldest disciplines in the field of microbiology is the study of the protozoan and animal parasites that infect humans. Such agents range from tapeworms with lengths of 10 meters to single-celled organisms only slightly bigger than a large bacterium. It is apparent, therefore, that wide-ranging diversity exists among the kinds of organisms included in the study of medical parasitology.

What do these organisms have in common? Actually not much, if one compares a round or flat worm with the protozoan that causes malaria. In fact, protozoa are no longer considered to be animals and are often placed in a separate kingdom, the Protista. Of course, both protozoa and animal parasites are composed of one or more eucaryotic cells. As a result, most parasites are not susceptible to treatment with the antibiotics effective against procaryotic cells, since they do not possess target structures such as a peptido-glycan cell wall, 70S ribosomes, or naked nucleic acid not surrounded by a nuclear envelope. In fact, elimination of a protozoan or animal parasite from an animal host is usually a compromise, with only a slim margin between the concentrations at which a drug is toxic to the parasite and to the host.

The organisms providing fodder for the vast field of medical parasitology can be separated into a number of phyla and classes; this text will consider them in two major groups: (1) the single-celled protozoa (Chapter 43), and (2) the helminths, in which the adult stage is a worm (Chapter 44).

Protozoa may be "merely" single-celled organisms, but the complexity of these cells far exceeds what we have seen among pro-caryotic organisms. Most are able to ingest solid particles of food, and some classes have special structures involved in the uptake of food particles and the elimination of waste products. Many are able to reproduce both asexually and sexually, and in some cases (such as the organisms causing malaria) the sexual cycle may be exceedingly complex.

Few have been grown in pure culture because it is seldom possible to provide their complicated requirements in a sterile environment. Thus, unlike bacteria, the metabolic characteristics of protozoa are usually not of importance to the diagnostic laboratory, and identification is based primarily on their appearance.

The parasitic worms infecting humans and other animals are given the general name "helminths." Infections by helminths are extremely prevalent, and it is estimated that over one-fourth of the world population is infected with one or more kinds of parasitic worms. Many of these organisms, such as the tapeworms, are confined to the small intestine. Unless heavily infected, an individual may show few signs or symptoms of their presence. Others may damage the liver, lungs, and brain, and some characteristically infect the lymphatics, eyes, skin, or muscles.

Most helminthic infections occur in regions of the tropics and in the Near and Far East where sanitary conditions are less than optimum. Nevertheless, the temperate climates and the Western Hemisphere are far from free of these creatures, as evidenced by the worldwide occurrence of amoebiasis, human trichinosis, ascariasis, hydatid disease, and pinworms. Moreover, the recent mobility of previously unexposed groups has resulted in the occurrence of parasitic infections such as malaria, trypanosomiasis, and schistosomiasis in populations where they had been previously unknown.

It will become apparent that in many regions of the world the infections and resulting misery caused by protozoa and parasitic worms are enormously more important than those diseases caused by the pathogenic bacteria and viruses that fill most of this book. This short unit makes no pretense of thoroughly covering the field of medical parasitology. It will, however, briefly describe the epidemiology and pathogenesis of the major protozoan and helminthic infections that occur in humans. The control of many of these infections is dependent upon an increased standard of living, manifested by better education and improved sanitation, nutrition, and medical care for the underprivileged peoples of the world.

## REFERENCES

Beck, J. W., and E. Barrett-Connor. 1971. *Medical Parasitology*. The C. V. Mosby Co., St. Louis.

Brown, H. W. 1975. *Basic Clinical Parasitology*. Appleton-Century-Crofts, New York.

Cheng, T. C. 1973. *General Parasitology*. Academic Press, New York.

Faust, E. C., P. C. Beaver, and R. C. Jung. 1975. *Animal Agents and Vectors of Human Disease*. 4th ed. Lea & Febiger, Philadelphia.

Faust, E. C., P. F. Russell, and R. C. Jung. 1970. *Clinical Parasitology*. 8th ed. Lea & Febiger, Philadelphia.

Garcia, L. S., and L. R. Ash. 1975. *Diagnostic Parasitology*. Clinical Laboratory Manual. The C. V. Mosby Co., St. Louis.

Markell, E. K., and M. Voge. 1976. *Medical Parasitology*. 4th ed. W. B. Saunders Co., Phildelphia.

Meyer, M. C., and O. W. Olsen. 1975. *Essentials of Parasitology*. 2nd ed. W. C. Brown Co., Dubuque, Iowa.

Olsen, O. W. 1974. *Animal Parasites: Their Life Cycles and Ecology*. 3rd ed. Univ. Park Press, Baltimore.

Schmidt, G. D., and L. S. Roberts. 1977. *Foundations of Parasitology*. The C. V. Mosby Co., St. Louis.

Taylor, A. E. R., and R. Muller. 1975. *Pathogenic Processes in Parasitic Infections*. Blackwell Scientific Publications, Oxford.

Taylor, A. E. R., and R. Muller, eds. 1973. *Chemotherapeutic Agents in the Study of Parasites*. Blackwell Scientific Publications, Oxford.

# 43

# Protozoa

It is generally agreed that protozoa are neither plants nor animals and instead belong in a separate kingdom. As a result, the designation of a phylum for all protozoa is being abandoned in favor of a kingdom, Protista, composed of a number of phyla. This belated recognition of the enormous diversity of the various groups has resulted from studies of the ultrastructure and biochemistry of the protozoa during the past decade. However, the brief presentation of the protozoa in this chapter does not permit a detailed discussion of the current status of their taxonomy; the reference list at the end of this chapter can provide additional information.

Morphologically, protozoa exhibit a wide variety of shapes and sizes. Some are oval or spherical, others elongate, and some may change shape as they move along a surface. Some species may be as small as 5 or 10 $\mu$m in diameter, whereas others will reach diameters of 1 to 2 mm and thus be visible to the unaided eye.

In general, the overall structure of a protozoan does not differ appreciably from that of other eucaryotic cells. A typical protozoan cell is enclosed by a cytoplasmic membrane, and many have an outer layer of cytoplasm, the ectoplasm, which can be visually differentiated from the inner part of the cytoplasm, the endoplasm. Within the cytoplasm are found one or two nuclei, mitochondria, food vacuoles, one or more contractile vacuoles that pump out excess water in freshwater forms, as well as numerous other eucaryotic organelles. Most protozoa also possess structures for motility. Accordingly, the term "simple" applies only to the cellular organization of protozoa, since a single protozoan cell carries on most of the activities usually ascribed to higher forms of life.

## LIFE PROCESSES OF PROTOZOA

For the most part, protozoa are aquatic, with habitats ranging from droplets of moisture around soil particles to large rivers and oceans. Some, however, live only as obligate parasites in animals and may produce chronic to acute diseases in humans.

### Nutrition

Unlike bacteria, which obtain nutrients by the transport of dissolved substances into the cell, most protozoa are holozoic; that is, they ingest food as solid particles through a mouth opening, or cytostome. The ingested food usually consists of bacteria, algae, or other protozoa. After ingestion, the food becomes enclosed in a food vacuole and enzymes are secreted into the vacuole to catalyze the degradation of complex materials into soluble substances. Once dissolved, nutrients can enter the cytoplasm to be used for the synthesis of cellular material or to be further metabolized to provide energy for the cell. Ingested material not dissolved in the vacuole is either expelled from the cell body through an anal pore or moved to the surface, where the vacuole breaks open to free the undigested material from the cell. Many members of one class of protozoa, the Apicomplexa, are unable to engulf solid particles of food, and these organisms obtain their nutrients by the transport of soluble nutrients into the cell in the same manner as bacteria.

### Reproduction

Many protozoa are able to reproduce both sexually and asexually. Asexually, most divide by splitting into two cells of equal size following nuclear division. Some protozoa divide by simple transverse fission (crosswise) while other classes divide longitudinally (lengthwise). Unequal fission, budding, or multiple fission is found in some species.

Sexual reproduction occurs when two morphologically different cells fuse (conjugate), resulting in the exchange of nuclear material before segregating into daughter cells. Some protozoa have complex reproductive cycles in which part of the life cycle must occur in humans or other vertebrates while another stage of the cycle must occur in a different host.

### Encystment

Under certain adverse environmental conditions certain protozoa may become encysted; that is, the cell assumes a fairly round or oval shape and secretes a protective coating around itself. At this stage the cell may sur-

vive a lack of food or moisture, adverse temperature changes, or contact with toxic chemical agents. The cyst is particularly valuable in permitting parasitic forms to survive outside the host until they can enter a new host. Under a return to favorable conditions water is absorbed into the cyst, and the organism emerges and resumes its growth.

In addition to the parasitic species, free-living forms are found in most classes of protozoa. In rare cases the protozoan exists in its host in a mutualistic relationship, one in which the host benefits from the presence of the guest and the guest benefits from the host. One notable example of mutualism is the termite, which could not live if its gut was not inhabited by a protozoan capable of digesting wood ingested by the termite. On the other hand, these protozoa are unable to live if they are removed from the intestine of the termite.

Many animals infected by protozoa are not this fortunate, and the results of infections may vary from chronic to acute diseases. Such dire infections are most common in tropical areas, where conditions seem to be more favorable for the growth and spread of parasites.

## CLASSIFICATION OF THE PROTOZOA

Of the approximately 40,000 species of protozoa that have been described, only a few cause disease in humans. These pathogenic species are distributed in all four classes (or, in some views, subphyla) of protozoa, and thus a study of the medically important species requires a general knowledge of each of the classes.

Amoebae form the class Sarcodina and are characterized by their ability to send out finger-like projections called pseudopodia (false feet), which serve both for motility and for the engulfment of food particles (see Figure 43-1). The cells do not contain complex organelles, nor do these organisms have a sexual mechanism of reproduction. Actively growing cells reproduce by binary fission, but under adverse conditions many species

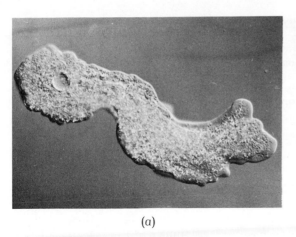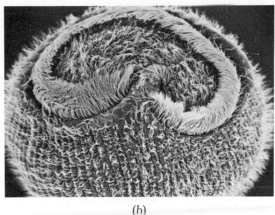

(a)                              (h)

**Figure 43-1.** *a. Amoeba proteus* (×154; Nomarski differential interference microscopy). *b.* Scanning electron micrograph of the ciliate *Stentor coeruleus* (×336).

may form a dormant cyst. When environmental conditions are favorable, the amoeba can emerge to become an active feeding cell, called a trophozoite. Most amoebic infections of humans are confined to the intestine, but they may at times be carried by the blood to other organs of the body, causing abscess formation in the liver, lungs, brain, pericardium, and spleen.

The class Ciliophora encompasses the ciliates. Most ciliates are free-living, and *Balantidium coli* is the single species causing disease in humans. The organisms in this class are characterized by the possession of cilia responsible for rapid movement through an aqueous environment (see Figure 43-1). Most divide by transverse fission, and many possess two nuclei, one a larger, less dense structure termed a macronucleus and the other a small, dense nucleus called a micronucleus. Sexual conjugation also occurs in many ciliates.

Organisms known as flagellates form the class Mastigophora and differ grossly from the ciliates by possessing long filamentous flagella. Although the fine structure is much the same, flagella are readily distinguished from cilia in that a flagellate usually possesses only one or several of these long, whip-like appendages. Ciliates, on the other hand, are covered with hundreds of cilia. A number of protozoan flagellates infect humans, causing intestinal, genital, and systemic diseases. All divide by longitudinal fission, and some also possess a sexual cycle of reproduction.

All members of the class Apicomplexa are parasitic for one or more animal species. The members of the Apicomplexa are unable to engulf solid food particles and must obtain their nutrients by the transport of soluble substances into the cytoplasm or, as in the species of *Plasmodium,* by endocytosis. Furthermore, these organisms normally lack obvious organs of locomotion, but all are probably motile at one stage of the life cycle. An amoeboid-type motility or gliding along the substrate using surface ridges or folds are found. The most unusual aspect of their reproductive cycles is the frequent requirement for two different animal hosts in order for the complete asexual and sexual cycles to occur. Malaria and toxoplasmosis are the major human diseases caused by the Apicomplexa.

Table 43-1 summarizes the major human diseases caused by some of the protozoa to be discussed in this chapter.

## SARCODINA

### Entamoeba histolytica

*Entamoeba* is the most prevalent genus of the Sarcodina found associated with humans.

## Table 43-1. Major Protozoa Causing Specific Human Diseases

| Parasites (Diseases) | Definitive Hosts | Intermediate Hosts | Important Reservoir Hosts | Transmission to Humans |
|---|---|---|---|---|
| *Entamoeba histolytica* (Amoebiasis) | Humans | None | Humans | By ingestion (mature cyst) |
| *Balantidium coli* (Balantidiasis) | Hogs, humans | None | Hogs, humans | By ingestion (mature cyst) |
| *Giardia lamblia* (Giardiasis) | Humans | None | Humans | By ingestion (mature cyst) |
| *Trichomonas vaginalis* (Trichomonad vaginitis) | Humans | None | Humans | By contact (flagellate) |
| *Trypanosoma gambiense* *Trypanosoma rhodesiense* (African sleeping sickness) | Humans, animals | Tsetse flies (*Glossina* species) | Humans, animals | By inoculation (bite of fly) |
| *Trypanosoma cruzi* (Chagas' disease) | Animals, humans | Reduviid bugs | Armadillos, opossums, humans | By contamination (infective feces of bug) |
| *Leishmania donovani* (Kala-azar) *Leishmania tropica* (Oriental sore) *Leishmania braziliensis*[a] (Espundia) | Humans, dogs | Sand flies (*Phlebotomus* species) | Dogs, humans | By inoculation (bite of fly; direct transmission possible) |
| *Plasmodium vivax* *Plasmodium falciparum* *Plasmodium malariae* *Plasmodium ovale* (Malaria) | Anopheline mosquitoes | Humans | Humans | By inoculation (bite of mosquito; also by transfer of infected blood) |

[a]Dogs and other animals have been implicated in the life cycles of *Leishmania donovani* and *L. tropica,* but the part played by hosts other than humans in the case of *L. braziliensis* is yet questionable. Naturally infected dogs have been found in South America.

Most species of *Entamoeba* appear to exist in the human intestine as commensals much like our other normal flora, but one species, *Entamoeba histolytica,* is potentially a human intestinal pathogen.

Human infections with *Entamoeba histolytica* occur with or without clinical symptoms, and all such infections are referred to as amoebiasis. Overt intestinal disease, however, is termed amoebic dysentery. The active amoebae, called trophozoites, move by extruding pseudopodia, with the remaining cytoplasm flowing into the pseudopodium. During a usual asymptomatic infection the amoebae colonize on the intestinal wall and feed on bacteria and other amoebae present in the intestine. In cases of amoebic dysentery, however, the trophozoites invade the intestinal mucosa, and examination of stool specimens may reveal ingested red blood cells in the amoebae. Since *E. histolytica* is essentially the only parasitic amoeba to engulf red blood cells, their presence within the amoeba provides strong evidence for its identification.

Trophozoites of *E. histolytica* reproduce by binary fission. In a specimen stained with hematoxylin the nucleus appears as a granular structure containing a small dense mass of chromatin (called a karyosome) in its center (see Figure 43-2).

The cyst stage of the life cycle of E. histolytica occurs as trophozoites are scraped from the intestinal wall and carried down the colon with the fecal mass. During cyst formation the amoebae usually excrete their ingested food particles, shrink to form rounded, nonmotile cells, and begin to secrete a thin, refractile covering. As this structure, known as a precyst, moves down the intestine, the nucleus undergoes two divisions, resulting in the formation of a mature cyst containing four small, identical nuclei. Reserve food particles in the form of bars that stain with Gomori's trichrome stain or iron hematoxylin are normally seen in the one or two-nucleated precysts, but the majority of the mature four-nucleated cysts will not possess them. Because of their staining properties, these bars are referred to as chromatoidal bars. Trophozoites of E. histolytica can thus be identified by observing the granular appearance of the nuclear chromatin and, in some cases, by the presence of ingested red blood cells. Mature cysts are characterized by the presence of four identical nuclei (all containing karyosomes) and by the occasional presence of chromatoidal bars within the cytoplasm.

SYMPTOMATOLOGY AND PATHOGENESIS OF AMOEBIC DYSENTERY. Approximately 90% of all infections by Entamoeba histolytica are asymptomatic and undiagnosed. For the remaining 10% of infected individuals, intestinal dysentery or colitis are the most common symptoms. In a typical case of amoebic dysentery the organisms first penetrate the intestinal mucosa. The resulting lesions may be minor and the symptoms confined to a few daily loose stools containing flecks of blood and mucus. In acute cases there may be numerous intestinal ulcers, and these may coalesce and become secondarily infected with bacteria. When this happens, an individual may have severe diarrhea characterized by the presence of considerable blood and mucus.

In occasional severe cases the intestinal ulcers may erode into adjoining blood vessels, causing intraluminal bleeding and permitting the spread of the amoebae to the liver. Painful hepatic abscesses can develop, and may erode through the diaphragm into the lung, causing bronchial abscesses. Other organs may also be infected, but such sequelae are extremely rare.

EPIDEMIOLOGY OF AMOEBIC DYSENTERY. The presence and frequency of amoebic dysentery can be correlated with the sanitary conditions prevailing within a given area. The disease is considerably more prevalent in tropical and subtropical areas than in temperate latitudes. It has been estimated that 1–5% of individuals in the United States are infected with E. histolytica, contrasted with an infection rate of 50–80% in some tropical regions.

Paradoxically, the spread of Entamoeba histolytica is usually not caused by individuals with acute cases of amoebic dysentery

**Figure 43-2.** *Entamoeba histolytica.* *a.* Trophozoite containing red blood cells. *b.* Binucleated cyst containing chromatoid bars. *c.* Mature tetranucleated cyst.

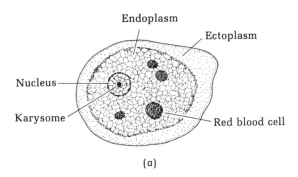

(a)

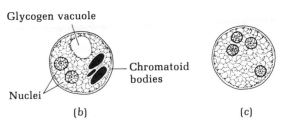

(b)                        (c)

but, rather, by asymptomatic chronic carriers of the organisms. In explanation, individuals with the acute disease pass actively growing trophozoites in their stools, and this form of the organism has a short survival time outside the host. The chronic carrier, on the other hand, excretes primarily the cyst form of the organism, and cysts are much more resistant to external conditions. In addition, it is extremely unlikely that the fragile trophozoites would withstand normal gastric acidity long enough to pass through the stomach into the intestinal area, and thus it is probably the ingestion of the cyst form of *E. histolytica* that causes disease. Figure 43-3 schematically summarizes the various courses that can occur in amoebiasis.

DIAGNOSIS OF INFECTIONS.    A definitive diagnosis requires that the parasite be identified in feces or infected tissues. Feces must be examined soon after voiding, because the

**Figure 43-3.** Possible courses of infection occurring during amoebiasis.

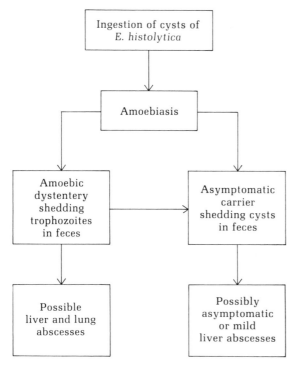

trophozoites have a rather short survival time outside the host. Trophozoites containing ingested red blood cells, showing invasion of the intestinal mucosa, are indicative of active disease. Trophozoites without ingested red blood cells are characteristically observed from individuals with asymptomatic amoebiasis. In many countries of the world such persons are not treated. Stained cysts over 10 μm in diameter that possess four nuclei also indicate an *Entamoeba histolytica* infection.

CONTROL AND TREATMENT OF INFECTIONS. Control of amoebic dysentery is essentially synonomous with adequate sanitation. Most sporadic cases in the Western Hemisphere occur in rural areas and in the lower socioeconomic groups. Breaks in the normal sanitation chain resulting in fecally contaminated drinking water or food bring about occasional epidemics. Normal chlorination procedures used for the treatment of municipal water sources are generally effective in eliminating the cysts of *E. histolytica*. Control in tropical and Third World countries will require increased health education to bring about improved methods of fecal disposal.

A number of effective drugs are available for the treatment of amoebic dysentery. Most of these drugs, such as dehydroemetine, diiodohydroxyquin, chloroquin (Aralen), or metronidazole, exhibit varying degrees of toxicity and should be taken only under the supervision of an experienced physician.

**Nonpathogenic *Entamoeba***

A number of species of the genus *Entamoeba* are of worldwide distribution but do not appear to cause disease. A knowledge of these species is of value in differentiating the harmless commensals from the potentially pathogenic *E. histolytica*. One amoeba usually considered to be nonpathogenic is *Entamoeba hartmanni*. This organism is differentiated from *E. histolytica* primarily on the basis that both its trophozoites and its cysts are smaller than those of E. histolytica. The absence of ingested red blood cells in E. hartmanni also may be of value in distinguishing between these two species.

Entamoeba coli is another widely dispersed nonpathogenic amoeba which is difficult to differentiate from E. histolytica. The trophozoites are described as sluggish organisms exhibiting a nondirectional motility and, like other nonpathogenic amoebae, do not contain ingested red blood cells. The nucleus of Entamoeba coli contains peripheral chromatin irregularly distributed on the nuclear envelope. Cysts of Entamoeba coli are somewhat easier to identify, since they routinely possess eight nuclei within a granular cytoplasm.

Other nonpathogenic amoebae such as Entamoeba polecki and Entamoeba gingivalis can also be confused with E. histolytica. E. polecki is an intestinal parasite, and E. gingivalis can be found in pyorrheal pockets between the teeth and gums and in the crypts of the tonsils. There are no data, however, suggesting that Entamoeba gingivalis is the etiologic agent of oral lesions, and it is generally assumed that both are present only as secondary invaders.

Dientamoeba fragilis is a small amoeba that is found as an intestinal parasite. This organism does not form cysts and can be recognized only by staining the trophozoites occurring in fresh stool specimens. The trophozoites are usually differentiated from other intestinal amoebae by the possession of two nuclei within the cell. Infections with Dientamoeba fragilis are usually asymptomatic, but some persons may experience a mild, persistent diarrhea along with gastrointestinal distress.

### Primary Amoebic Meningoencephalitis

In recent years, strains of the free-living amoeboflagellate Naegleria fowleri have been isolated from patients with meningoencephalitis. These organisms are characterized by a life cycle in which the amoeboid phase alternates with organisms possessing two or four flagella.

Naegleria fowleri is widespread in fresh water and is also found in moist soils, decaying vegetation, and fecal wastes. Cases of human meningoencephalitis occur during the summer months and usually become manifested within a week after swimming in contaminated water; however, since both lakes and swimming pools are apparent sources of infection, the use of the phrase "contaminated water" does not necessarily imply foul or brackish waters.

The dramatic clinical course is characteristic of a typical fulminating meningoencephalitis and almost invariably ends with the death of the patient within three to six days after the initial symptoms.

Little is known about the pathogenesis of this infection, but it is believed that the nasal mucosa may provide the portal of entry. Diagnosis is based on the observation of the motile amoebae in unstained preparations of spinal fluid and at autopsy by finding stained amoebae in sections of the brain.

Treatment has been exceedingly disappointing, and none of the usual amoebicidal drugs appear to be effective. Initial reports, however, suggest that amphotericin B possesses clinical potential for the treatment of amoebic meningoencephalitis.

### CILIOPHORA – BALANTIDIUM COLI

This extremely large class of ciliated protozoa is composed largely of free-living organisms, and Balantidium coli is the only species that causes disease in humans.

Balantidium coli may attain a length of 200 μm and is the largest of the parasitic protozoa that may be found in the human intestine. The organisms reside primarily in the lumen of the intestine and obtain food by the ingestion of bacteria. Occasionally, however, Balantidium coli may cause a bloody diarrhea not unlike the acute episodes of amoebic dysentery.

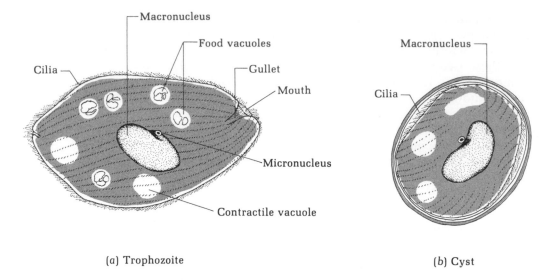

(a) Trophozoite　　　　　　　　　　(b) Cyst

**Figure 43-4.** *Balantidium coli.* a. Trophozoite. b. Cyst.

Trophozoites of the organism are oval in shape and are covered with cilia (see Figure 43-4). Like other ciliates, *B. coli* possesses two nuclei, a macronucleus and a micronucleus. The micronucleus functions in sexual reproduction of the cell and the macronucleus controls the metabolic activities within the organism. *Balantidium coli* forms a cyst approximately 60–70 μm long. The cyst is covered with a thin, refractile covering, and in newly formed cysts the ciliated organisms can be seen within the cyst wall.

*Balantidium coli* appears to be routinely present in swine, and it seems possible that humans become infected by the ingestion of water or food contaminated with cysts present in swine feces. Overt disease, however, is quite rare, and it seems that most infections produce no demonstrable symptoms. Spread of the organisms to the liver, lymph nodes, and lungs has been reported, but such complications are exceedingly rare. Treatment with oxytetracycline, carbarsone, or diodoquin appears to be effective for the elimination of this potential parasite.

## MASTIGOPHORA

The parasitic flagellated protozoa fall into two categories with respect to the type of disease produced in humans. One group, commonly called the intestinal flagellates, is found only in the digestive or genital tracts. These organisms may produce infections varying from asymptomatic to severe disease. Members of the second group, the hemoflagellates, are transmitted by blood-sucking insects to humans, where they produce severe and frequently fatal infections.

## INTESTINAL FLAGELLATES

### Giardia lamblia

*Giardia lamblia* is the only flagellated protozoan that produces frank intestinal disease. It is easy to recognize because the trophozoites are bilaterally symmetrical. Each organelle and structure is paired as shown in Figure 43-5a. *Giardia* possess two nuclei, each containing a central karyosome, and four pairs of flagella, which impart an erratic motility and result in a slow oscillation around its long axis. Cysts of *Giardia lamblia* are ovoid structures approximately 8 by 12 μm in size, containing four nuclei and numerous refractile threads in the cytoplasm.

Infections in adults may be asymptomatic, and for many years the organism was considered to be a nonpathogen. It is now amply demonstrated, however, that this organism can cause an intestinal disease (particularly in children) that varies in severity. It is likely that the majority of overt cases of intestinal infections by *Giardia* are manifested by diarrhea and abdominal cramps, but severe cases may also be accompanied by malabsorption deficiencies in the small intestine.

*Giardia lamblia* is of worldwide distribution, and its occurrence in the United States is similar to that of *Entamoeba histolytica* in that it is most frequent in rural and lower socioeconomic areas. (An outbreak in Aspen, Colorado, during the 1966 ski season hardly fits this geographical definition, but this epidemic occurred when sewage from defective pipes leaked into a well supplying drinking water.) Infections can be effectively treated with quinacrine hydrochloride.

### Chilomastix mesnili

This organism is not known to cause symptomatic disease in humans, but since it is found throughout the world as an intestinal parasite, it must be differentiated from organisms such as *Giardia*. The organism possesses several anterior flagella and a single large anterior nucleus. (Note that *Giardia* has two nuclei and four pairs of flagella.) Cysts of *Chilomastix mesnili* are lemon-shaped and contain a single large nucleus.

### Trichomonas hominis

This protozoan appears to exist only as a commensal in the intestinal tract of humans and, along with *Trichomonas vaginalis,* possesses the dubious honor of being the only flagellate parasitizing humans that does not form cysts. Morphologically, it is characterized by four anterior flagella plus a posterior flagellum that forms the outer edge of an undulating membrane (see Figure 43-5b). The organism appears to be an obligate parasite of the intestinal tract, and its presence elsewhere is, therefore, a result of recent fecal contamination.

### Trichomonas vaginalis

*Trichomonas vaginalis* is morphologically similar to *T. hominis,* but is larger with a shorter undulating membrane (see Figure

**Figure 43-5.** Flagellates infecting the human genital and intestinal tract. *a. Giardia lamblia* trophozoite. *b. Trichomonas hominis* trophozoite. *c. T. vaginalis* trophozoite.

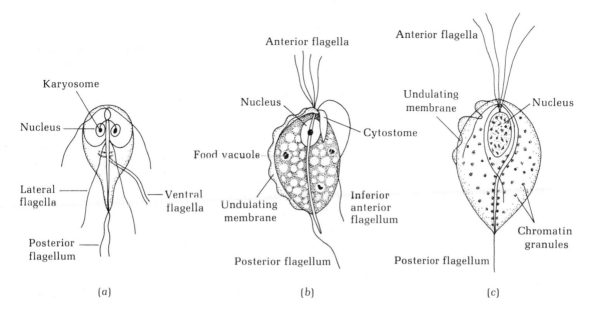

(a)  (b)  (c)

43-5c). Moreover, *T. vaginalis* is found only in vaginal secretions, whereas *T. hominis* is never observed in this area of the body.

The organism appears to be spread as a venereal disease, infecting both men and women. In the latter, a thin watery vaginal discharge is the most prominent symptom, although many cases are also accompanied by burning and itching. Infection in males is usually asymptomatic except in cases involving the prostate and seminal vesicles.

Metronidazole is normally effective for the elimination of the parasite. Since the infection is venereal in nature and frequently asymptomatic in the male, both male and female partners should receive treatment.

## HEMOFLAGELLATES

Flagellated protozoa transmitted to humans by the bites of infected, blood-sucking insects are referred to as the hemoflagellates. These organisms can be found in the blood, lymph, and cerebrospinal fluid and as intracellular parasites in various organs of the body.

Hemoflagellates are classified in either the genus *Trypanosoma* or *Leishmania*, and it is believed that they were originally parasites of insects that later acquired the ability to propagate in humans and other animals. This is supported by the observation that some genera are still exclusively insect parasites, and even those species that infect higher animals undergo part of their developmental cycle in the insect.

Cells of *Leishmania* and *Trypanosoma* pass through similar morphologic stages during their life cycle in vertebrate and invertebrate hosts (see Figure 43-6). As shown, the trypomastigote form characteristically possesses an undulating membrane composed of a thin protoplasmic extension along the entire length of the organism. A single flagellum forms the outer edge of this membrane and, in usual circumstances, will extend anterior to the cell where it functions as an organ of locomotion. The undulating membrane of the epimastigote stage originates in the central part of the cell anterior to the nucleus, while

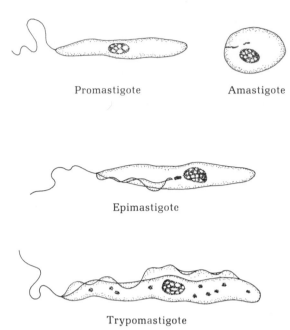

Promastigote            Amastigote

Epimastigote

Trypomastigote

**Figure 43-6.** Morphologic forms occurring in the hemoflagellates.

the promastigote form lacks an undulating membrane but is motile by a single flagellum inserted in the anterior end of the cell. Amastigote forms appear as rounded, nonmotile organisms. Of the major pathogens we shall discuss, *Trypanosoma gambiense* grows as a trypomastigote form in a vertebrate host but is seen in both the trypomastigote and epimastigote forms in an invertebrate host. On the other hand, all four stages are seen when *T. cruzi* grows in the vertebrate host, but only the trypomastigote and epimastigote forms are in the invertebrate host. All species of *Leishmania* grow only in the amastigote form in the vertebrate and the promastigote form in the invertebrate host. It is therefore obvious that there is no sharp anatomical dividing line between the genera *Trypanosoma* and *Leishmania*.

### Trypanosomiasis

*Trypanosoma gambiense* is the etiologic agent of a West African sleeping sickness sometimes referred to as Gambian trypanosomiasis. A more virulent form of this disease is seen in Central and Eastern Africa, where it is called East African sleeping sickness or Rhodesian trypanosomiasis. The etiologic agent of this latter form has been named *Trypanosoma rhodesiense.* Although there is no dispute concerning the difference between the severity of these two diseases, the two trypanosomes are indistinguishable morphologically and serologically. A third hemoflagellate, *Trypanosoma brucei,* produces a severe infection in domestic animals but is not known to infect humans. Oddly, this species is also indistinguishable from *T. gambiense* and *T. rhodesiense,* and many parasitologists considered these to be subspecies of *T. brucei.*

WEST AFRICAN SLEEPING SICKNESS (GAMBIAN TRYPANOSOMIASIS). Following the bite of an infected tsetse fly, there is usually a period of two to three weeks before the occurrence of overt symptoms. In some cases, an ulcer may develop at the site of the bite, but this will normally heal after one to three weeks. During the incubation period trypanosomes can be seen in small numbers in blood smears, but the attacks of fever do not begin until the organisms invade the lymph nodes. At this time the number of trypanosomes in the blood stream and lymph nodes increases dramatically. After several days to a week, the fever subsides, and the patient is asymptomatic for several weeks before the occurrence of a subsequent, similar episode. These intermittent attacks may continue over a period of several months, normally causing the face to swell and often leading to heart damage. As the disease progresses, the trypanosomes invade the central nervous system, causing a meningoencephalitis frequently manifested by slurred speech and difficulty in walking. Later stages are characterized by convulsions, paralysis, and mental deterioration. The central nervous system symptoms may last for many months before the individual finally becomes comatose and dies.

The pathogenesis and epidemiology of the disease are moderately well understood.

*Trypanosoma gambiense* is not known to infect other vertebrate hosts, and thus the cycle of infection is from human to tsetse fly and back to human (see Figure 43-7). For many years the most puzzling aspects of this disease were the unexplained, recurrent, febrile attacks and the apparent absence of an effective immune response to the trypanosomes, in spite of the presence of high titers of IgM antibodies to trypanosomal antigens. An explanation for this paradox became available from experimental infection of animals with *Trypanosoma brucei.* These experiments showed conclusively that during an infection trypanosomes undergo surface changes with the formation of new surface antigens. Moreover, the experimental data support the hypothesis that the variant glycoproteins secreted by the trypanosomes during an infection are not the result of mutant selection but rather the repression of the genes for one surface antigen and the sequential derepression of genes producing a new antigen. Curiously, when the tsetse fly becomes infected, the organisms undergo several changes in their surface antigens before infecting the salivary glands of the tsetse fly, and the initial infection of a human from the bite of an infected tsetse fly always yields organisms with identical surface antigens. Thus, it appears that in the tsetse fly, the trypanosomes secrete a surface glycoprotein that can be considered a "basic antigen."

Although trypanosomes are able to infiltrate most organs in the body, including the central nervous system, the cause of death from such infections has been difficult to explain. One provocative hypothesis proposes that each time the trypanosomes are cleared from the blood, the host undergoes an immunological shock resembling an Arthus reaction (see Chapter 16). This concept proposes that the pathological changes occurring during trypanosomiasis may, in large part, be due to an immunological hypersensitivity. Also, it has been proposed that the trypanosomes liberate a series of kinins that cause increased vascular permeability, a fall in blood pressure, and eventually heart failure.

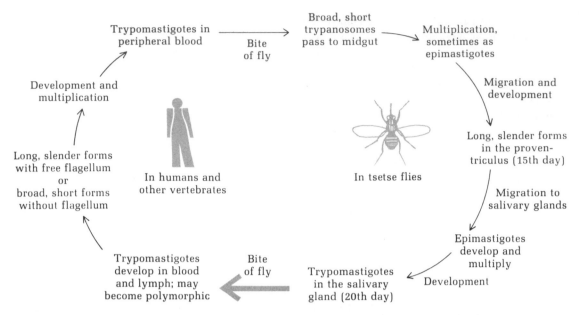

**Figure 43-7.** Life cycle of *Trypanosoma gambiense* and *Trypanosoma rhodesiense*.

The diagnosis of trypanosomiasis is dependent upon observation of the parasites in blood, lymph nodes, or spinal fluid, or by the demonstration of IgM antibody directed toward the basic antigen of the trypanosome. The presence of this antibody in spinal fluid provides a definitive diagnosis for trypanosomal meningoencephalitis. The organisms can be grown on a concentrated blood agar, but continuous cultivation is presently too difficult to be of practical value as a diagnostic technique. Good growth does occur, however, on the chorioallantoic membrane of the chick embryo.

Control is directed toward the elimination of the vectors, *Glossina palpalis* and *Glossina tachinoides*. These species of tsetse flies normally inhabit the banks of shaded streams near human habitation, and the use of insecticides plus the clearing of streamside brush provides effective control.

A variety of drugs can be used for the successful treatment of trypanosomiasis, although the more effective ones exhibit some toxicity to the host. Pentamidine isothionate or melarsoprol are the usual therapeutic agents for the treatment of Gambian trypanosomiasis.

EAST AFRICAN SLEEPING SICKNESS (RHODESIAN TRYPANOSOMIASIS). *Trypanosoma rhodesiense*, the etiologic agent of Rhodesian trypanosomiasis, is morphologically and serologically indistinguishable from *T. gambiense*, but the corresponding disease is more severe than its West African counterpart. The pathogenesis is similar to Gambian trypanosomiasis, but the disease progresses more rapidly and death frequently occurs prior to the development of meningoencephalitis. When encephalitis does occur, central nervous system involvement takes place earlier than in Gambian trypanosomiasis.

The vector of Rhodesian sleeping sickness is also a tsetse fly (*Glossina morsitans*) but this vector usually becomes infected from feeding on wild animals. Thus, unlike *T. gambiense*, the etiologic agent of Rhodesian trypanosomiasis infects a number of wild animals; although the disease tends to occur sporadically, control is more difficult than in the West African variety.

The treatment of choice is a drug called suramin; however, the high toxicity of this drug for the host may require the use of drugs normally used in the treatment of Gambian trypanosomiasis.

AMERICAN TRYPANOSOMIASIS (CHAGAS' DISEASE). Chagas' disease is also caused by a trypanosome, *Trypanosoma cruzi*, but its epidemiology and pathogenesis are different from African trypanosomiasis, as shown in Figure 43-8.

The disease occurs in the southern United States, Central America, and as far south as Argentina. The reservoir for the trypanosomes includes a wide variety of wild animals —particularly rodents, opossums, and armadillos. The vector may be any one of a number of species of infected reduviid bugs (also called triatomids). These vectors characteristically inhabit houses; trypanosomes grow in the gut of the bug and are passed in its feces. Humans become infected because the bug habitually defecates while feeding, and the trypanosomes are introduced into the site of the bite from the fecal contamination of the infected vector.

*Trypanosoma cruzi* differs from the other trypanosomes we have discussed in that it is unable to multiply extracellularly in a vertebrate host. Instead, the organisms undergo a morphological change in which they round-up and lose their undulating membrane and flagellum. This morphologic stage, depicted in Figure 43-6, is called an amastigote form, and it is this form of *T. cruzi* that multiplies intracellularly in essentially every organ of the body.

Ordinarily, an erythematous (red, due to an infiltration of red blood cells) lesion develops at the site of infection. The organisms infect the regional lymph nodes and from there are spread via the blood stream to other organs of the body. The liver and macrophages in the spleen are commonly infected, but the organ most characteristically affected is the heart. Growth of the amastigote forms within the heart induces an inflammatory response and an enlarged heart with typical electrocardiographic changes due to Chagas' disease. Central nervous system involvement resulting in a fatal meningoencephalitis is not

**Figure 43-8.** Life cycle of *Trypanosoma cruzi*. The electron micrograph shows a thin section through the epimastigote form (×3,740).

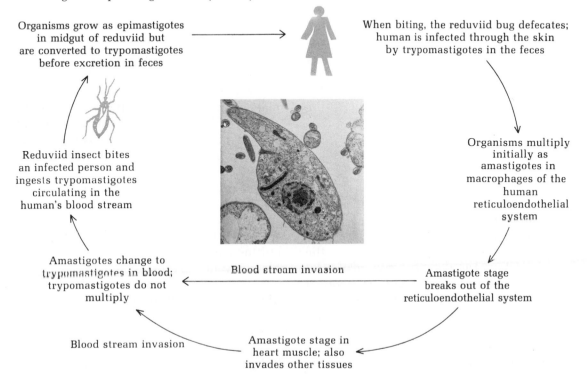

Organisms grow as epimastigotes in midgut of reduviid but are converted to trypomastigotes before excretion in feces

When biting, the reduviid bug defecates; human is infected through the skin by trypomastigotes in the feces

Reduviid insect bites an infected person and ingests trypomastigotes circulating in the human's blood stream

Organisms multiply initially as amastigotes in macrophages of the human reticuloendothelial system

Amastigotes change to trypomastigotes in blood; trypomastigotes do not multiply

Blood stream invasion

Amastigote stage breaks out of the reticuloendothelial system

Blood stream invasion

Amastigote stage in heart muscle; also invades other tissues unusual in infants. However, older children and adults may show few or no signs of encephalitis, and these infections are most often characterized by myocarditis (an inflammation of the muscular tissue of the heart). In fact, most fatal infections occur in children under the age of five, and the disease may be chronic in older children and adults.

Chagas' disease can be diagnosed early in the infection by observing the trypanosomes in blood smears. During later stages of the disease the organisms can be grown from blood cultures. A fluorescently-labeled antibody is also successfully used in diagnosis. A rather unusual technique, called xenodiagnosis, is occasionally employed for the diagnosis of this disease. This method involves the use of uninfected reduviid bugs that are allowed to feed on a suspected case. The bugs are examined at a later date for the presence of trypanosomes.

It is exceedingly difficult to control the spread of Chagas' disease. Success will, undoubtedly, require an improvement in housing and the elimination of reduviid bugs (which include at least 40 species of the family Reduviidae) within the house.

The drugs used for the treatment of African trypanosomiasis are of no value against the American variety. The only treatment of any value goes by the trade name of Bayer 2502, with the chemical name of 3-methyl-4 (5'-nitrofurfurylidenamino)-tetrahydro-(1,4)-thiazine-1,1-dioxide.

### Leishmaniasis

The taxonomic classification of the genus *Leishmania* seems to be an almost unsurmountable problem. The situation is confusing because there are no obvious morphological differences among any of the leishmanias, and apparently a myriad of serological types produce essentially identical infections. There are, however, a few general properties true for all leishmanial infections. All species of *Leishmania* are transmitted from one animal to another (including humans) by the bite of infected sandflies belonging to the genus *Phlebotomus*. Each species of parasite has an extreme host specificity for a particular species of sandfly, and if more than one serological species of *Leishmania* exists in a given area, each will be transmitted by a different species of *Phlebotomus*. Additionally, each *Leishmania* exists in two different morphological forms. The organisms introduced by the bite of the sandfly exist as flagellated promastigote forms (see Figure 43-6). The parasites then transform into a nonmotile, ovoid cell (amastigote form), and this stage proliferates within the host's macrophages and endothelial cells. When a sandfly acquires the parasites from an infected host, the organisms proliferate in the insect's gut as motile promastigotes, which eventually accumulate in the pharynx and buccal cavity in a position to infect a new host.

The diseases caused by members of the genus *Leishmania* occur as two major types, cutaneous leishmaniasis and visceral leishmaniasis. We shall see, however, that the cutaneous variety can be manifested by different species of *Leishmania* as a dermatotrophic form producing skin lesions and as a mucocutaneous variety producing ulcers on the oral or nasal mucosa. It is important to note that all forms of leishmaniasis are intracellular infections of the reticuloendothelial system (fixed phagocytic cells scattered throughout the body, especially in the liver, spleen, bone marrow, and lymph nodes) and that the different types of this disease are really manifestations of the invasive properties of the parasite. It would seem, therefore, that the cutaneous infections are caused by a species of low invasive power in which the parasites are confined to the reticuloendothelial cells in the skin and subcutaneous area of the body. On the other hand, the organisms causing visceral leishmaniasis are able to invade the reticuloendothelial system throughout the body, particularly the reticuloendothelial cells of the spleen and liver.

CUTANEOUS LEISHMANIASIS. Numerous serological variants of *Leishmania* serve as the etiologic agents of cutaneous leishmaniasis.

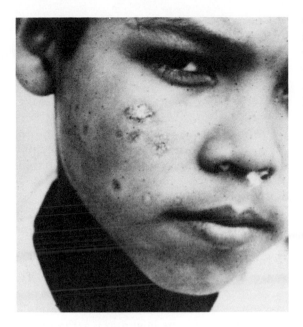

**Figure 43-9.** Oriental sores resulting from cutaneous leishmaniasis.

Because of the similarity of these parasites, they are usually classified as *Leishmania tropica* or are referred to by some parasitologists as the *L. tropica* species complex.

The prototype of the cutaneous ulcer is called an "oriental sore" (see Figure 43-9); the disease occurs primarily in the Near East, the Mediterranean region, Africa, southern Russia, and southern Asia. As in all cases of leishmaniasis, the parasites are transmitted to the host by the bite of an infected sandfly. After an incubation period varying from several weeks to several months, a papule eventually evolves into an ulcer at the site of the bite. Routinely, the ulcer is also the site of a secondary bacterial infection. The lesion usually heals in about a year, leaving a disfiguring and depigmented scar. Immunity is solid, and since an endemic area is usually infested with only one serological type of *L. tropica,* it is not unusual for parents to infect their children intentionally in a part of the body where the resulting scar will not normally be visible.

Dermal leishmaniasis occurs also in Central and South America, and some investigators have given new species names to these variants of American leishmaniasis. A mild cutaneous infection occurring in the mountainous areas of Peru is called "uta," and the causative agent is frequently referred to as *L. peruviana.* A similar infection prevalent in the Brazilian forest region is called "chiclero's ulcer," and many persons have used the name of *L. mexicana* for the etiologic agent of this disease.

The normal reservoir for *L. tropica* varies from one endemic area to another. For example, in India the dog seems to be the only reservoir of infection for humans. Elsewhere rodents serve this role, and in some regions gerbils and ground squirrels provide the source of parasites from which the sandflies become infected.

Diagnosis is usually based upon the observation of the parasites in stained scrapings from infected areas; however, the intradermal injection of a killed suspension of promastigotes (called the Montenegro test) will give a delayed-type skin reaction in a large percentage of infected individuals.

Treatment with arsenical compounds is usually effective. Currently, the most effective therapeutic agent is antimony sodium glutamate (Pentostam), although the antibiotic amphotericin B is also reported to yield good results.

MUCOCUTANEOUS LEISHMANIASIS. This disease is a variant of the cutaneous variety, but it is considered by most investigators to be sufficiently distinct to warrant the naming of a new species, *Leishmania braziliensis,* as its causative agent. Particularly prevalent in Brazil, the disease is frequently fatal.

The infection normally begins as a dermal lesion similar to that described for cutaneous leishmaniasis. The lesion heals and after an interval of months to years the organisms reappear, causing lesions in the mucous membranes of the nasopharyngeal area. If untreated, the nasal septum, the lips, and the soft palate may be destroyed. Death is usually the result of secondary bacterial infections.

The major reservoir of infection for American leishmaniasis seems to be a large number of rodents inhabiting the forest regions of South America, although occasional other animals such as dogs and opossums have been implicated. As with other leishmanial infections, the sandfly appears to be the vector in the spread of these organisms from animals to humans.

The diagnosis and the treatment of mucocutaneous leishmaniasis is essentially the same as that described for the cutaneous variety; however, the mucocutaneous type is somewhat unresponsive to therapy, and a drug known as cycloguanyl pamoate is frequently used for the treatment of this disease.

VISCERAL LEISHMANIASIS. This disease, caused by *Leishmania donovani,* is more commonly known by its Indian name of kala-azar. It is seen in the Near and Far East, southern Russia, the Mediterranean area, in parts of Africa, and in Central and South America.

Humans acquire the parasites from the bite of an infected sandfly (see Figure 43-10); the onset is gradual. The incubation period may vary from several weeks to more than a year but is commonly several months. The initial complaint is usually abdominal swelling, and

examination will reveal gross enlargement of the spleen and liver as a result of the increased size of the parasitized reticuloendothelial system. *L. donovani* is found also in this system in the skin and subcutaneous areas; except for the African form of the disease, the ulcerative lesions characteristic of *L. tropica* are not characteristic for kala-azar. Skin lesions (which heal as depigmented areas) may, however, occur after apparent recovery from the systemic aspects of kala-azar. It is estimated that as high as 90% of untreated cases of visceral leishmaniasis terminate in death about two years after the onset of the initial symptoms.

In urban areas humans and dogs apparently serve as the vertebrate reservoir for *L. donovani,* whereas the reservoir in rural sections is rodents and other wild animals. As in the cutaneous leishmanias, the organisms grow intracellularly in the vertebrate host as nonflagellated amastigote forms but multiply in the midgut of the sandfly as a flagellated promastigote form. The diagnosis of the human disease is dependent upon the demonstration of the parasites. Biopsies of liver and spleen are frequently done, and

**Figure 43-10.** Life cycle of *Leishmania donovani* (Kala-azar).

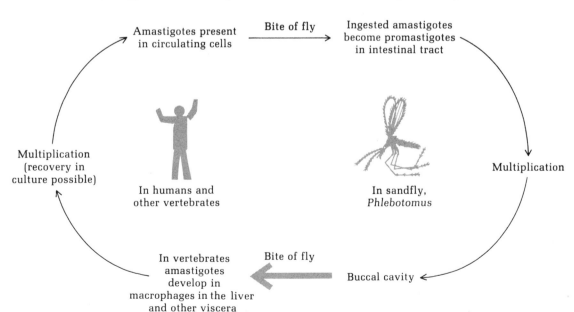

cultures of blood or sternal bone marrow aspirates may reveal the organisms. Also, since hamsters are particularly susceptible to infection by *L. donovani*, material can be injected intraperitoneally into these animals and after several weeks the hamster sacrificed and its spleen examined for the presence of *L. donovani*.

Treatment is similar to that described for cutaneous leishmaniasis, and antimony sodium gluconate is usually the drug of choice. A drug known as Lomidine (pentamidine isethionate) also may be used to treat kala-azar.

## DINOFLAGELLATES

Dinoflagellates are flagellated protozoa that characteristically grow as photosynthetic organisms. Human illness does not occur as an infection but rather from a toxic reaction following the ingestion of the organisms.

Two pigmented dinoflagellates, *Gonyaulax catanella* and *Gymnodinium brevis*, occasionally multiply to very high concentrations in coastal waters. This phenomenon, known as a "red tide," is a potential danger to humans because of toxic reactions following the ingestion of shellfish that have fed on the dinoflagellates. Muscle weakness is the most characteristic symptom, and, in the event of paralysis of the respiratory muscles, the toxemia may terminate in death.

In the United States the red tide appears on the Pacific Coast and in the Gulf of Mexico and occasionally invades the coastal waters of New England and eastern Canada. During such outbreaks shell fishing on the affected areas is banned. Thus, this photosynthetic protozoan also causes a severe economic loss to the shellfish industry in addition to the health hazard.

## APICOMPLEXA

Members of the class Apicomplexa are obligate parasites of animal hosts. Human diseases include the systemic infections malaria and toxoplasmosis and an intestinal disease caused by members of the genus *Sarcocystis* (previously designated as *Isospora*). In all cases the life cycles of the Apicomplexa are considerably more varied than that described for other pathogenic protozoa, and a new vocabulary is required to describe the stages in the incredibly complex life cycles of these parasites.

## Malaria

Four species of Apicomplexa are recognized as etiologic agents of human malaria: *Plasmodium vivax*, *P. ovale*, *P. malariae*, and *P. falciparum*. The clinical picture in humans varies somewhat with each species, but the usual symptoms are chills and fever at more or less regular intervals followed by profuse sweating. *Plasmodium vivax* produces an infection known as benign tertian or vivax malaria, in which these paroxysms occur approximately every 48 hours. The symptoms caused by *P. ovale* are similar to those of *P. vivax*. In infections by *P. malariae*, or quartan malaria, symptoms occur at 72-hour intervals, while in falciparum malaria, produced by *P. falciparum*, the chills and fever have a tendency to appear every 36 to 48 hours. The infection caused by *P. falciparum* is the most serious because of the continual growth of the parasites in red blood cells in the internal organs. As a result, the paroxysms differ in that the periodic chills are less pronounced, and the fever stage is usually not followed by sweating and tends to be continuous. Since these organisms become localized in the red cells in different organs, the clinical picture of an infection by *P. falciparum* may resemble that of a number of other diseases; the symptoms may vary from gastrointestinal manifestations to brain invasion resulting in coma and death.

The source of human infections is the bite of an infected female *Anopheles* mosquito. There are over 200 species of *Anopheles*, and about 60 of these are known to be vectors of malaria. Humans constitute the usual reser-

Preerythrocytic and exoerythrocytic cycle in liver cells

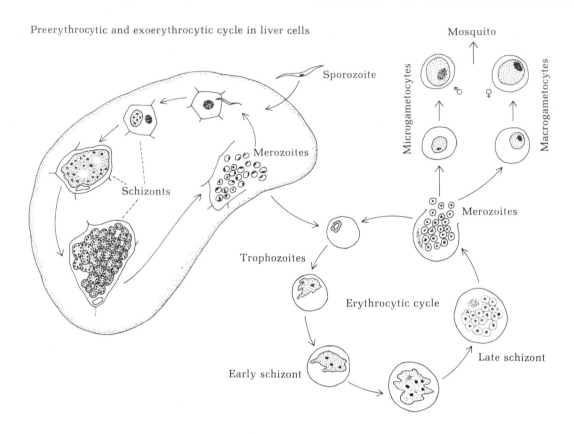

**Figure 43-11.** Asexual reproduction of malaria parasites in humans.

voir for infecting the mosquito, although *P. malariae* has been found in higher apes. The incubation period is about 14 days for *P. vivax* and *P. ovale,* about 30 days for *P. malariae,* and about 12 days for *P. falciparum* infections.

The life cycle of the malarial parasites is complex, and variations exist among the different species, particularly involving their asexual reproduction. Other differences include the size and the number of asexual parasites produced within a host cell and, in the case of *P. falciparum,* the range of host cells infected. The following description, however, will describe the general stages in the life cycles of these parasites.

PATHOGENESIS.   We shall return to the developmental cycle of the malaria parasite within the mosquito; suffice it at the moment to say that an individual becomes infected when

the sporozoite form of the parasite is injected into the bloodstream by the bite of an infected mosquito. The sporozoites immediately invade the parenchymal cells of the liver, where, depending upon the species, they undergo one or more cycles of asexual reproduction before being liberated back into the bloodstream (see Figure 43-11). This stage of infection is called the preerythrocytic cycle. While *P. falciparum* appears to undergo only one preerythrocytic cycle of reproduction before invasion of red cells, the other species may continue to reproduce in the liver cells (exoerythrocytic reproduction) concurrently with red blood cell invasion. After entering a liver cell, the filamentous sporozoite rounds up to form a trophozoite which continues to enlarge for approximately a week, varying for each species of *Plasmodium.* When mature, the nucleus of the trophozoite begins to divide to form thousands of nuclear masses. During this stage the parasite is called a schizont. A cytoplasm and membrane surrounds each nucleus to form a merozoite, after which the infected host cell ruptures to release the merozoites, which then either infect red blood cells or begin a new round of asexual reproduction in liver cells.

The erythrocytic cycle begins when a merozoite infects a red blood cell. The general sequence of events occurring during the erythrocytic cycle is similar to that described for the preerythrocytic cycle. The merozoite first differentiates into an immature trophozoite, which appears as a round or crescent-shaped structure called a ring stage. This structure continues to expand to form a large compact trophozoite. The nucleus of the mature trophozoite begins to divide (schizogony) to form 12 to 28 nuclear masses (depending upon the species of *Plasmodium*) and, as in the preerythrocytic cycle, the parasite is termed a schizont. After a membrane and a cytoplasm surround each nucleus, the red cell ruptures, releasing the merozoites which can then infect additional red blood cells.

It is at the time of red cell rupture that an individual undergoes the paroxyms of chills, fever, and sweating. Although the cycle is not entirely synchronous, the rupture of the red cells and the release of the merozoites usually occur within a short time interval.

After one or more cycles of asexual reproduction in the red cells, some of the merozoites will not divide but will instead form male or microgametocytes and female or macrogametocytes. In humans these forms are the end of the line, and unless ingested by a mosquito they will degenerate within 6–12 hours or be destroyed by the host's immune system. Recurrent cycles of schizogony in the red cells periodically replenish the gametocytes, which are essential for the transmission of the parasite to mosquitoes. When the gametocytes are ingested during a blood meal by a mosquito, they are converted to male and female gametes and sexual fusion occurs within the stomach of the mosquito (see Figure 43-12). The resulting zygote undergoes a developmental stage to become an ookinete; this rounds up outside the stomach to become an oocyst, within

**Figure 43-12.** Sexual reproduction of malaria parasites in mosquito.

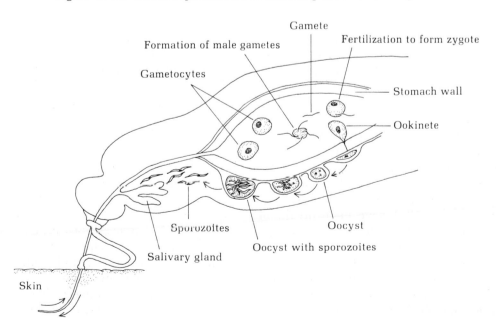

which are formed hundreds of spindle-shaped sporozoites. When the sporozoites are liberated from the oocyst, they become dispersed throughout the mosquito's body, and many reach the salivary glands. This chain of events requires 10–12 days. Once the sporozoites are liberated, the mosquito is capable of transmitting the infection during its next blood meal.

In the human, recurrent attacks result in a significant anemia. If untreated, attacks may continue for three to six weeks, after which the parasites can no longer be found in the blood. Relapses are not uncommon for a year or more after the initial infection. This suggests that the parasites can exist in an exo-erythrocytic stage during these periods of latency. After a year or two, the organisms may die, and if not reinfected, the patient may be permanently cured. The species *P. malariae* can, however, cause relapses for many years. *P. falciparum* does not persist in the liver phase, but malaria caused by *P. falciparum* is considered the most dangerous because the merozoites from this species may penetrate up to 30% of all erythrocytes and cause them to become sticky, resulting in plugged capillaries and internal hemorrhages in the brain, lungs, and kidneys.

DIAGNOSIS AND CONTROL. The diagnosis of malaria requires the visualization of the parasites in a stained blood smear as shown in Figure 43-13. Thick smears frequently are used, since the number of red cells infected at any one time may be meager. Fluorescently-labeled antibody is also used to detect the presence of the parasites in a blood film.

Control is directed toward finding and treating infected persons to render them noninfective and to the elimination of adult mosquitoes and their breeding places. Insecticides such as DDT have been invaluable, but as so frequently occurs, some strains of mosquitoes have acquired a resistance to the usual insecticides. The eradication of breeding places for the mosquito has been effective in some areas, but the disease is still prevalent in many of the tropical regions of

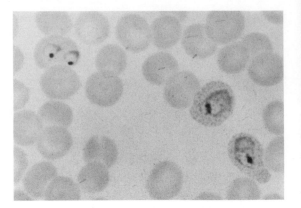

Figure 43-13. *Plasmodium vivax* in red blood cells. One cell has two rings, and two other cells contain growing trophozoites.

the world. Interestingly, the process of selection appears also to have been an important factor in the control of human malaria. A large majority of American and African blacks are resistant to infection by *Plasmodium vivax*, and it is now known that this resistance is attributable to the lack of a specific membrane factor on their erythrocytes to which the parasite must bind to invade and multiply intracellularly. Moreover, it has also been shown that people with hemoglobin AS (sickle-cell anemia trait—restricted to blacks) have a survival advantage in regions where *Plasmodium falciparum* is endemic. The mechanism of this resistance is unknown, but it seems quite probable that malaria has exerted a considerable influence on the proportions of various alleles for hemoglobin synthesis in the black populations.

TREATMENT. Quinine was used for many years to suppress the growth of the blood parasites, but during the last several decades synthetic drugs have been developed to suppress and, for some species, cure the disease. A few of these are quinacrine (Atabrine), chloroquin (Aralen), amodiaquine (Camoquin), pyrimethamine, and primaquine. As with antibiotic resistance in bacteria, many malarial parasites have developed forms resistant to one or more of these drugs. It is also worth noting that some drugs are effective only on the asexual erythrocytic phase and do not affect the exoerythrocytic reproduction of the parasites. In such cases, subsequent relapses are frequent. Thus, the occurrence of drug resistance and the fact that a single drug is usually not effective against all of the stages of the particular malarial parasite necessitates the use of a combination of drugs for successful treatment. The combination depends upon the species of *Plasmodium* involved and the properties of the current local strains.

### Toxoplasmosis

*Toxoplasma gondii,* the etiologic agent of toxoplasmosis, is one of the most widespread of the parasites that infect vertebrate hosts. Serologic tests indicate that over 50% of adults in the United States have been infected, and in some countries the infection rate exceeds 90%. Since the disease in humans is frequently mild or asymptomatic, many readers of this text may have never heard of toxoplasmosis. This mildness, however, holds only in adults and children past the neonatal period. When the infection is acquired congenitally by the human embryo or occurs in newborn infants who acquired the organism late in fetal development, the infection is frequently very severe. Central nervous system involvement (encephalomyelitis), resulting in mental retardation, and vascular changes in the retina (which may also occur in adults), leading to severe visual impairment and blindness, are two of the more common sequelae; however, fever, convulsions, and an enlarged liver are also commonly observed.

EPIDEMIOLOGY OF TOXOPLASMOSIS.   Since the disease is widespread throughout the animal kingdom, a common source of infection for adult humans is the ingestion of undercooked or raw meat containing the trophozoites or cysts of *Toxoplasma gondii*. During an inap-

parent infection, the trophozoites can be transmitted transplacentally to produce the severe effects described above. Interestingly, as illustrated in Figure 43-14, the parasite will undergo its sexual reproductive cycle only in the intestinal cells of members of the cat family, Felidae (which includes domestic cats). Here, the organisms produce schizonts and gametocytes which, after sexual fusion, form oocysts that are passed in the feces. Ingestion by another animal (including humans) of the oocysts releases the enclosed sporozoites, which then multiply in epithelial cells, leukocytes, the reticuloendothelial system, and the central nervous system. In vertebrates other than the cat, however, only the actively multiplying trophozoites or cysts enclosing a large number of rounded parasites are found.

DIAGNOSIS AND TREATMENT OF TOXOPLASMOSIS.   The inoculation of infected tissue into mice will usually result in the intraperitoneal occurrence of intracellular proliferative trophozoites. This is rarely done, however; the usual diagnosis is based upon serological tests. One such test, the Sabin-Feldman dye exclusion test, requires living

**Figure 43-14.** Life cycle of *Toxoplasma gondii.*

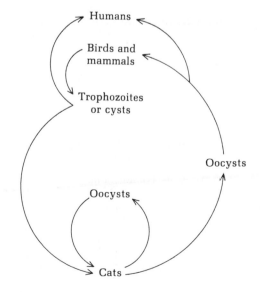

organisms of the genus *Toxoplasma* and is carried out by staining the parasites with alkaline methylene blue in the presence of the patient's serum. In the absence of specific antibodies, the organisms are stained by the dye. If antibodies are present, the dye is excluded from the organisms. Routinely, complement fixation and fluorescently-labeled antibodies are used as additional diagnostic aids.

Treatment of toxoplasmosis with pyrimethamine in combination with trisulfapyrimidines or sulfadiazine is the only effective chemotherapy.

### Intestinal Infections by Apicomplexa

Two species, until recently classified in the genus *Isospora* (*I. belli* and *I. hominis*), may cause human intestinal infections. It has, however, now been reported that these organisms are actually two species of *Sarcocystis* whose sexual cycle occurs in humans; one species (*I. hominis*) utilizes the cow as an intermediate host and the other uses the pig. Humans presumably become infected by eating undercooked flesh.

Human infections are characterized by diarrhea, fever, and nausea. Most cases are mild, lasting for only about a month; the disease may, however, become chronic with periodic relapses occurring for as long as one year. The diagnosis is made by observing the sporocysts in freshly passed feces.

### REFERENCES

Anderson, K., and A. Jamieson. 1972. Primary amoebic meningoencephalitis. *Lancet* **2**:379.

Barbour, A. G., C. R. Nichols, and T. Fukushima. 1976. An outbreak of giardiasis in a group of campers. *Amer. J. Trop. Med. Hyg.* **25**:384–389.

Carter, R. F. 1970. Description of a *Naegleria* sp. isolated from two cases of primary amoebic meningoencephalitis, and the experimental pathological changes induced by it. *J. Pathol.* **100**:217–244.

Coatney, G. R. 1976. Relapse in malaria—an enigma. *J. Parasitol.* **62**:3–9.

Durfee, P. T., J. H. Cross, Rustam, and Susanto. 1976. Toxoplasmosis in man and animals in South Kalimantan (Borneo), Indonesia. *Amer. J. Trop. Med. Hyg.* **25**:42–47.

French, F. F. 1976. Visceral leishmaniasis in the Mediterranean. *J. Trop. Med. Hyg.* **79**:85–88.

Frenkel, J. K. 1973. Toxoplasma in and around us. *Bioscience* **23**:343–352.

Goodwin, L. G. 1970. The pathology of African trypanosomiasis. *Trans. R. Soc. Trop. Med. Hyg.* **64**:797–812.

Herrer, A., and H. A. Christensen. 1976. Natural cutaneous leishmaniasis among dogs in Panama. *Amer. J. Trop. Med. Hyg.* **25**:59–63.

Hübsch, R. M., A. J. Sulzer, and I. G. Kagen. 1976. Evaluation of an autoimmunity type antibody in the sera of patients with Chagas' disease. *J. Parasitol.* **62**:523–527.

Jeffery, G. M. 1976. Malaria control in the twentieth century. *Amer. J. Trop. Med. Hyg.* **25**:361–371.

Kimball, A. C., B. H. Kean, and F. Fuchs. 1971. Congenital toxoplasmosis: a prospective study of 4,048 obstetric patients. *Amer. J. Obstet. Gynecol.* **111**:211–218.

Mahmoud, A. A. F., and K. S. Warren. 1976. Algorithms in the diagnosis and management of exotic diseases. XVII Amebiasis. *J. Infect. Dis.* **134**:639–643.

Manson-Bahr, P. E. 1964. Variations in the clinical manifestations of leishmaniasis caused by *L. tropica*. *J. Trop. Med. Hyg.* **67**:85–87.

Moore, G. T., W. M. Cross, D. McGuire, C. S. Mollohan, N. N. Gleason, G. R. Healy, and L. H. Newton. 1969. Epidemic giardiasis at a ski resort. *New Engl. J. Med.* **281**:402–407.

Padilla y Padilla, C. A., and G. M. Padilla, eds. 1974. *Amebiasis in Man.* Charles C. Thomas, Springfield, Ill.

Peters, W. 1974. Recent advances in antimalarial chemotherapy and drug resistance. *Adv. in Parasitol.* **12**:69–114.

Price, E. W., and M. Fitzherbert. 1965. Cutaneous leishmaniasis in Ethiopia. *Ethiopian Med. J.* **3**:57–83.

Shaw, J. J., and R. Lainson. 1976. Leishmaniasis in Brazil: XI. Observations on the morphology of *Leishmania* of the *Braziliensis* and *Mexicana* complexes. *J. Trop. Med. Hyg.* **79**:9–13.

Wallace, G. D. 1976. The prevalence of toxoplasmosis on Pacific islands, and the influence of ethnic group. *Amer. J. Trop. Med. Hyg.* **25**:48–53.

World Health Organization. 1972. Trypanosomiasis. *Bulletin of the World Health Organization* **47**:685–820.

# 44

---

# Helminths

The multitude of invertebrates that parasitize humans and other animals is enough to stagger the imagination, and descriptions of the life cycles and pathogenesis of these parasites fill textbooks. This chapter, however, will introduce no more than a few of the most important and representative examples to illustrate their general characteristics.

Helminths (Gr. *helmins,* worm) are often classified in the phyla Platyhelminthes, or flatworms, and Aschelminthes, or roundworms. Many live only in the intestinal tract of a parasitized host, while others invade internal organs such as the liver, lungs, blood, subcutaneous tissue, and brain, and yet others are free-living and nonparasitic. Most are macroscopic, but identification frequently requires a microscopic examination of their eggs.

Three parasitic classes will be described: the Cestoda and the Trematoda—both flatworms—and the Nematoda, a group of roundworms.

## Platyhelminthes

The flatworms are the most primitive of the helminths in that they characteristically have either no digestive tract or only a rudimentary one. They are flat, in rough terms shaped like a leaf or a measuring tape, and are in most examples hermaphroditic (both male and female organs occur in the same animal). Many of the parasitic species have complicated life cycles that require an alternation of hosts. Humans frequently are the definitive host for the adult worm, while other animals are the intermediate hosts for larval stages.

### INTESTINAL CESTODES OF HUMANS

The habitat of the adult cestode (tapeworm) is the intestinal tract, and the animal in which the larval stage develops into an adult worm is termed the definitive host. Animals in which the eggs develop into the larval stage are called intermediate hosts.

Adult tapeworms are usually long and ribbon-like and divide into segments called proglottids (see Figure 44-1). The scolex (head) at the anterior end is provided with

612

suckers and, in some cases, hooks that attach the worm to the intestinal wall. Posterior to the scolex is a neck region, followed by immature proglottids, mature proglottids containing male and female sex organs, and fertilized segments, called gravid proglottids, containing fertilized eggs.

We shall not attempt to divide the class Cestoda taxonomically. Rather, we shall characterize selected important tapeworms and the ways in which humans become infected.

### Taenia saginata

Humans are the only definitive host for *Taenia saginata*, or beef tapeworm. The infection is acquired by the ingestion of raw or rare beef infected with the larval stage. After reaching the small intestine, the worm head emerges from the larva and attaches itself to the intestinal mucosa. The mature worm may reach a length of 8–12 meters and contain as many as 2,000 proglottids. The posterior gravid proglottids are filled with fertilized eggs, and as these break off they are passed in the feces.

Cattle and allied animals become infected from grazing on contaminated soil. After the fertilized eggs hatch in the animal's intestine, the embryos disseminate throughout the body of the intermediate host via the lymphatics and blood stream, terminating in the muscles. There they develop into a larval stage, the cysticercus, which is a fluid-filled bladder containing an invaginated scolex. If not eaten by the definitive host (humans), the cysticercus will die in about nine months. Thus, as depicted in Figure 44-2, *T. saginata* would cease to exist if humans did not eat undercooked infected beef and cows did not eat food contaminated with human feces.

In humans beef tapeworms commonly occur singly, and their presence is ascertained by the occurrence of gravid proglottids and embryonated eggs in the feces. The proglottids average 6 by 20 mm in size and can easily be mistaken for small adult worms. Surprisingly, most infected individuals show no symptoms, although anemia and malnutrition, weight loss, abdominal pain, and loss of appetite can occur. Many concoctions have been used to treat this infection, but the current drug of choice is niclosamide.

**Figure 44-1.** Major morphologic parts of an adult tapeworm.

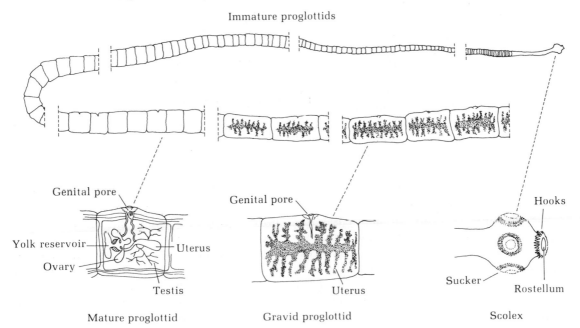

Immature proglottids

Genital pore

Yolk reservoir
Ovary
Uterus
Testis

Mature proglottid

Genital pore

Uterus

Gravid proglottid

Hooks
Sucker
Rostellum

Scolex

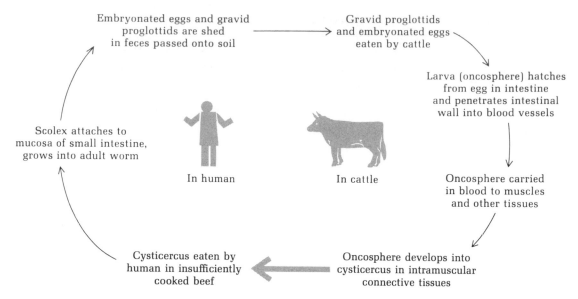

**Figure 44-2.** Life cycle of the beef tapeworm, *Taenia saginata.*

### Taenia solium

Many similarities exist in the life cycle and epidemiology of beef and pork tapeworms. Humans are the only known definitive hosts for the pork tapeworm, *Taenia solium*; however, the cysticerci of pork tapeworms can also develop in humans as they do in the normal intermediate host, the pig. A life cycle is presented in Figure 44-3.

The adult pork tapeworm may reach a length of 2–3 meters and normally consists of less than 1000 proglottids. When the pig ingests eggs on fecally contaminated food, larvae develop and disseminate throughout the musculature where they may survive for several years. Humans become the definitive host for the adult worm by eating infected raw or uncooked pork. In general, symptoms are few or absent.

The situation is much different if a person ingests eggs instead of larvae through contaminated food or drink. In such cases the eggs hatch in the small intestine, and the liberated larvae (also called onchospheres) are disseminated throughout the body, where they form cysticerci. This condition is called cysticercosis, and symptoms vary according to the number and location of the cysticerci.

Thus, in muscle or subcutaneous tissue, a light infection may be asymptomatic, whereas involvement of the central nervous system can cause epilepsy and death.

The diagnosis of an intestinal pork tapeworm infection requires the identification of the eggs or egg-filled gravid proglottids passed in the feces. In human cysticercosis, however, diagnosis is usually based upon biopsies or X-rays of characteristic calcified cysticerci. Niclosamide is used for the chemotherapy of the intestinal infection, but there is no satisfactory treatment for cysticercosis.

### Diphyllobothrium latum

This tapeworm enjoys a wide variety of definitive hosts, but in endemic areas the disposal of human sewage into fresh water maintains the cycle.

In the infected definitive host (for example, a human) fertilized eggs are discharged from gravid proglottids into the intestine. After reaching fresh water, the life cycle of the worm requires two different intermediate hosts before it can infect the definitive host. The sequence of events, as diagrammed in Figure 44-4, occurs as follows: (1) the egg must first hatch in fresh water to form a motile

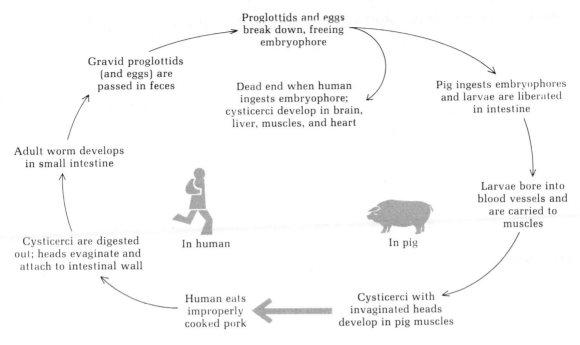

**Figure 44-3.** Life cycle of the pork tapeworm, *Taenia solium*.

**Figure 44-4.** Life cycle of *Diphyllobothrium latum*.

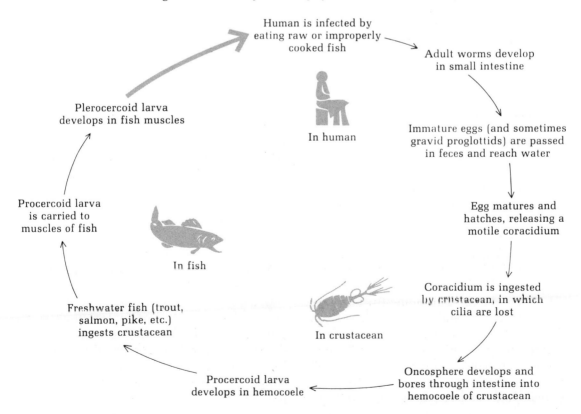

embryo (coracidium) before it becomes infective; (2) this form is ingested by a crustacean where it penetrates the intestine and forms an elongated stage (called a procercoid larva) within the crustacean body; (3) when the crustacean is ingested by a suitable fish (pike, salmon, trout, whitefish, turbot), the larvae are disseminated throughout the body of the fish where they are transformed into a spindle-shaped larval stage (plerocercoid); (4) the definitive host becomes infected from eating raw or inadequately cooked infected fish. In the definitive host, the adult worm attaches to the intestinal wall, where it may reach a length of 10 meters and contain 3000–4000 proglottids.

Symptoms may be mild or absent, but *Diphyllobothrium latum* appears to possess an unusually high affinity for vitamin $B_{12}$. If the worm is attached high in the small intestine, it will absorb essentially all of the vitamin $B_{12}$ ingested by the host, producing pernicious anemia; this does not occur when the worm is farther down in the intestinal tract.

Diagnosis is usually based on case histories plus the finding of typical eggs in the feces. Niclosamide is considered the therapy of choice.

### Hymenolepis nana

The definitive hosts for this cestode are humans, mice, or rats, and no intermediate host is required. Humans are the major reservoir for this cestode, known also as the dwarf tapeworm. Infection occurs under conditions of poor sanitation—usually by the direct transfer of fertilized eggs from hand to mouth. After reaching the intestine the embryos hatch from the eggs, enter the mucosa, and develop into a larval stage, the cysticercoid. These larvae subsequently enter the intestinal lumen and develop into adult worms.

Symptoms routinely are limited to mild abdominal discomfort unless the infection is heavy, in which case they may include abdominal pain, nausea, diarrhea, and headaches. Diagnosis is made by observing typical eggs in the feces. Niclosamide is used for therapy.

## EXTRA-INTESTINAL INFECTIONS OF HUMANS BY CESTODES

### Echinococcus granulosus

As described for *Taenia solium,* a tapeworm infection in which the larvae are distributed throughout the body of the intermediate host causes symptoms very different from those that occur in the definitive host where the adult worm is confined to the intestinal tract.

Humans may serve as hosts for several other larval cestodes in addition to *Taenia solium,* but our discussion will include only one common species, namely *Echinococcus granulosus.* The usual intermediate hosts of this worm are sheep, cattle, and other herbivores. Humans almost always acquire the infection from dogs, although wolves, coyotes, and foxes also serve as definitive hosts.

After the ingested eggs hatch, the liberated larvae (onchospheres) penetrate the intestinal wall and are disseminated throughout the body via the lymphatics and blood stream. The liver is the organ most frequently infected, but the larvae may also settle in the lungs, kidneys, bone, or brain. Each larva forms a fluid-filled bladder—a hydatid cyst—which continues to increase in size and to form secondary interior cysts known as brood capsules. The primary and secondary cysts contain countless scolices, and each scolex may develop into an adult worm when ingested by a dog. Rupture of the hydatid may release thousands of scolices into the surrounding tissues. The life cycle is summarized in Figure 44-5.

Usually in humans a single cyst develops, and it frequently impairs organ function by pressure on the surrounding tissues. An inflammation develops, mediated in part by a hypersensitivity response to the scolices, and adjacent tissues either atrophy or undergo pressure necrosis.

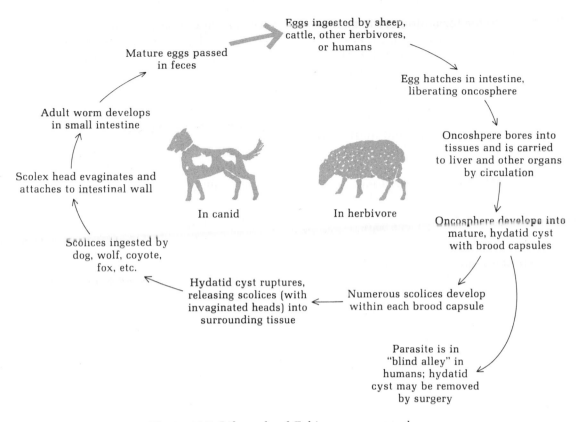

**Figure 44-5.** Life cycle of *Echinococcus granulosus*.

The diagnosis of hydatid disease is commonly based on finding a tumor mass, usually in the liver, and a history of association with dogs in an endemic area. X-rays may reveal a calcified cyst wall. The diagnosis can be confirmed by the demonstration of brood capsules and scolices in the fluid of the surgically removed cyst.

Most human cases of hydatid disease occur in grazing countries where an intimate association between humans and dogs is common, and the disease is occasionally seen in the United States, particularly in California. Infections follow a hand-to-mouth transfer of the eggs from contaminated soil or dog fur. Drugs are ineffective for the chemotherapy of hydatid disease, and treatment must rely upon the surgical removal of the hydatid cyst. Control is directed at the prevention of the infection in dogs; dogs should not be fed uncooked viscera from slaughtered animals.

Dogs in endemic areas should be treated periodically with atabrine or niclosamide.

## TREMATODES

Trematodes are also referred to as flukes. Adult worms may vary in size from one millimeter to several centimeters, and all exhibit suckers used for attachment to host tissue.

Trematodes are of world-wide distribution and may be found any place that one finds the snails required as intermediate hosts by the species of these parasites. Most human infections, however, occur in the Far and Near East (particularly in areas with rice paddies), Africa, Latin America, and other tropical areas.

Comprehension of the epidemiology of trematode infections requires a general knowledge of the complex events that occur between the excretion of the egg of the definitive host and the formation of the final larval stage. During this period four different larval forms occur (except in the blood flukes, which have only three). (1) The hatching of the egg usually occurs only in fresh water. Within the egg is formed a miracidium, a small, ciliated larva. The miracidium escapes from the egg and swims about until it finds a snail, its first intermediate host. (2) After finding the specific species of snail required for its species of trematode, the miracidium bores into the tissues of the snail. (3) The larva then loses its cilia and undergoes a metamorphosis to form a long, tubular larva called a sporocyst. (4) The sporocyst migrates to the hepatic tissue of the snail where it continues to form masses of germ cells within a sac-like structure. With the exception of certain flukes such as schistosomes, the sporocyst then undergoes another morphological change to become a more differentiated larva possessing a mouth and a rudimentary digestive tract. This stage is called a redia. (5) Within each redia, germ cells develop into more rediae, but, eventually, a final larval change occurs when cercariae begin to develop within the redia. A cercaria resembles the adult worm, possessing suckers and a rudimentary digestive and excretory system. It also possesses a tail for locomotion after leaving the snail. The cercaria can infect a new intermediate host. This host may be a freshwater fish, a crab, another snail, or aquatic vegetation. In any case, following infection the cercaria loses its tail and secretes a cyst wall around the larva. This cyst form is called a metacercaria, and, except for the schistosomes, humans are infected *only* by the ingestion of metacercariae. These stages are reviewed in Figure 44-6.

The life cycle of the schistosomes differs from that of most other trematodes in that they do not form rediae; the results of asexual reproduction within the sporocysts are motile cercariae. The cercariae of schistosomes do not encyst, but rather infect by burrowing directly through the unbroken skin of the definitive host.

We are now ready to consider the trematodes that infect humans. These parasites are usually divided into the intestinal flukes, the liver flukes, the lung flukes, and the blood flukes.

## THE INTESTINAL FLUKES

Intestinal flukes are basically parasites of other animals, and humans become accidental hosts during their development.

### Fasciolopsis buski

This fluke normally parasitizes pigs in Southeast Asia, although the incidence of infection in humans may reach 100% in some areas. After leaving the snail, the cercariae attach themselves to various types of vegetation, where they develop into metacercariae. Humans become infected by eating contaminated plants such as water chestnuts, bamboo, and water hyacinths (see Figure 44-7).

The metacercariae evolve into adult worms that attach to the mucosa of the small intestine. Symptoms will vary according to the degree of infection. In small children heavy infections may be particularly severe, occasionally resulting in death. Diagnosis is confirmed by the presence of characteristic eggs in the feces. Both hexylresorcinol and tetrachloroethylene are effective for treatment.

### Metagonimus yokogawai and Heterophyes heterophyes

The metacercariae of these flukes are formed under the scales of freshwater fish. Dogs and cats serve as the usual definitive hosts in Asia, and humans become infected by eating raw fish.

The adult worms attach to the mucosa of the small intestine, and symptoms are usually mild. Eggs are occasionally carried by the lymphatics to the heart or central nervous system, which can cause severe reactions. Hexylresorcinol is an effective treatment, as is tetrachloroethylene.

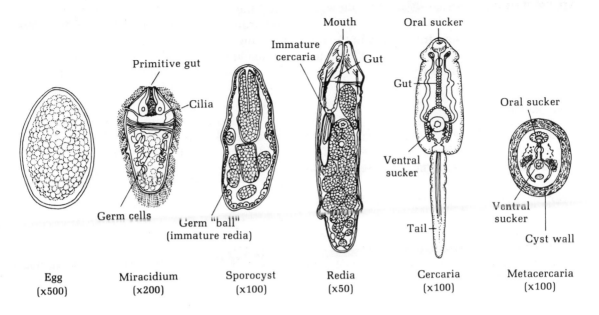

Egg
(x500)

Miracidium
(x200)

Sporocyst
(x100)

Redia
(x50)

Cercaria
(x100)

Metacercaria
(x100)

**Figure 44-6.** Immature stages of flukes that infect humans.

**Figure 44-7.** Life cycle of the intestinal fluke, *Fasciolopsis buski.*

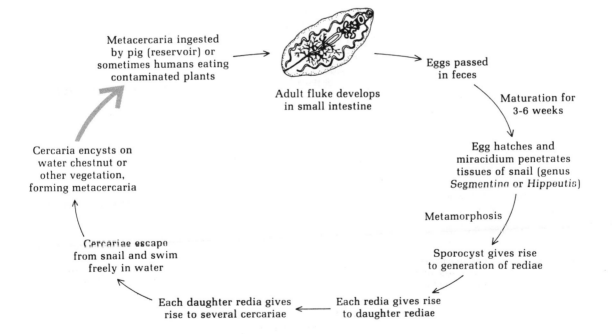

## LIVER FLUKES

Flatworms that mature into adults in the bile ducts of the definitive host are commonly referred to as liver flukes.

### Fasciola hepatica

Sheep and to a lesser extent cattle constitute the usual hosts for this parasite. Human infections occur in many parts of the world, and cases have been reported from southern France, Algeria, Cuba, and the Latin American countries.

. Fertilized eggs pass via the common bile duct into the intestinal tract. If they reach water that contains the appropriate snails, the miracidia will infect this intermediate host, and motile cercariae will be released at the end of larval development. The cercariae encyst on local vegetation (such as grass or watercress) to form metacercariae. Sheep, cattle, and occasionally humans become the definitive host following the ingestion of metacercariae on contaminated vegetation.

In the definitive host, the metacercariae penetrate the intestine and migrate from the peritoneal cavity to infect the liver parenchyma and, eventually, the bile ducts. There they produce mechanical and toxic injuries which, in severe infections, terminate with cirrhosis. Eggs entering the intestines from the common bile duct are passed and re-initiate the larval cycle.

Bithionol is currently the drug of choice for the treatment of infections caused by these liver flukes.

### Clonorchis sinensis

This parasite, also known as the Chinese liver fluke, exists primarily in the Far East. The intermediary larval stages in the snail are as described for trematodes in general; the definitive hosts (usually dogs and cats but also humans) become infected from eating raw fish infected with the metacercariae (see Figure 44-8).

Symptoms vary considerably, depending upon the degree of infection. Light infections

**Figure 44-8.** Life cycle of the liver fluke, *Clonorchis sinensis*.

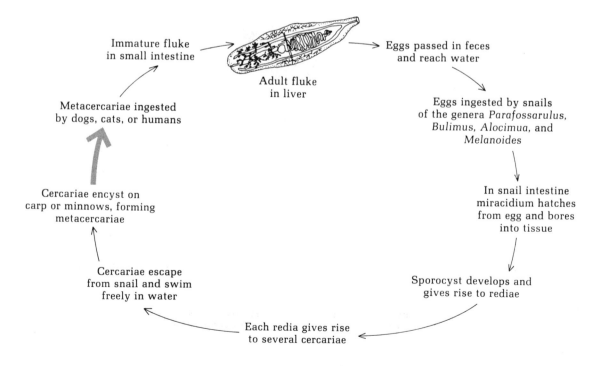

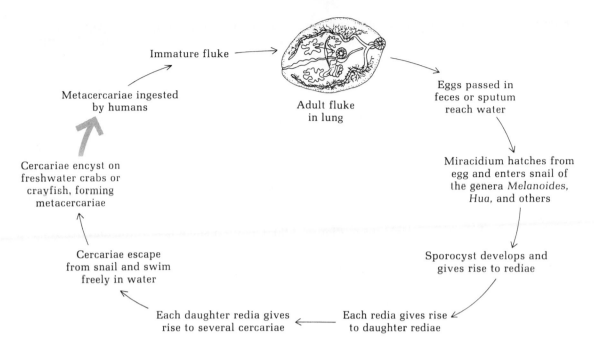

**Figure 44-9.** Life cycle of the lung fluke, *Paragonimus westermani.*

may be asymptomatic, while heavy and repeated ingestion of the larvae may cause abscesses and liver impairment.

Two other liver flukes that occasionally infect humans are *Opisthorchis felineus* and *Opisthorchis viverrini.* Cats and, to a lesser extent, dogs comprise the primary definitive hosts for the adult stage of these parasites.

Experimental drugs are under trial in the Far East, but there is no effective therapy available in the United States for infections by *Clonorchis* or *Opisthorchis* species.

## LUNG FLUKES

### *Paragonimus westermani*

This fluke causes a major disease, paragonimiasis, in which the adult worm parasitizes the lungs. It is restricted to the Far East. Other species of *Paragonimus* are responsible for human infections in Africa and South America.

After leaving the snail, the cercariae infect crabs or crayfish (in which they become en-

cysted) as second intermediary hosts. Humans become infected by eating raw or improperly cooked crabs or crayfish containing metacercariae (see Figure 44-9).

Following ingestion the cercariae leave the small intestine and migrate from the peritoneal cavity through the diaphragm into the bronchioles, where a fibrous capsule forms around the larva. After the development of the adult worm the capsule ruptures into the bronchioles, releasing eggs which are coughed up and expectorated or swallowed. In fresh water the eggs hatch into miracidia and infection of the appropriate snails starts the cycle over again.

Symptoms are absent or restricted to occasional coughing of rusty sputum, depending upon the number of parasites in the lungs.

Paragonimiasis responds to the oral administration of bithionol. This drug, however, may cause side effects such as skin rashes, nausea, diarrhea, headaches, and dizziness. It can also induce a contact dermatitis, and, because bithionol was at one time incorporated into a number of medicated soaps and shampoos, patients should be checked for hypersensitivity reactions before using this drug.

## BLOOD FLUKES

The human blood flukes belong to the genus *Schistosoma*. The life cycle of these parasites differs from that of the tremodes previously described in the following ways: (1) The adult worms are not hermaphroditic and exist as two separate sexes. The sexes can easily be differentiated because the male worm is much larger than the female (see Figure 44-10). (2) Schistosomes do not require a secondary intermediate host and, hence, do not form metacercariae; animals, including humans, become infected by the direct penetration of the cercariae through the skin.

In general, after penetrating the skin the cercariae migrate through the heart and the lungs, eventually reaching the intrahepatic part of the portal system. Here they mature and mate, after which (depending upon the species) they migrate together to the mesenteric venules where the fertilized eggs are deposited.

**Figure 44-10.** Adult schistosomes. The larger male is coupled with the slender female worm.

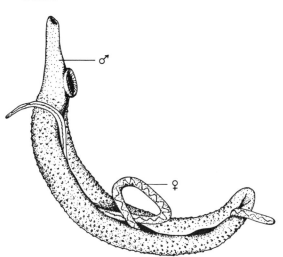

Human schistosomiasis occurs in three fairly distinct stages. (1) The invasion, unless overwhelming, is usually asymptomatic. This stage also includes the migration of the cercariae (referred to as schistosomula after losing their tails following penetration) to the hepatic veins. (2) The acute stage occurs with the start of egg laying after the mature worms have migrated to the mesenteric veins. This stage is characterized by diarrhea, fever, malaise, and general discomfort. Most of the symptoms of this second stage appear to be due to hypersensitivity reactions to the eggs. (3) The final stage is chronic and occurs as a tissue reaction to the eggs. Eggs are passed in the urine or feces and may be deposited in various organs of the body, particularly the liver. In these cases of deposition a tissue reaction is manifested by walling off of the foreign material to form granulomas not unlike the tubercles that occur in tuberculosis.

Three species of *Schistosoma* constitute the major causes of disease in humans, namely S. *mansoni*, S. *japonicum*, and S. *haematobium*. Each of these is tightly restricted to the genus of snail that it can use for its intermediate host. They also vary in the body location of the adult stage (a period that may last as long as 30 years).

### Schistosoma mansoni

These parasites are found in Africa, as well as in South America, the West Indies, and Puerto Rico. In human infections the parasites characteristically leave the liver and the adult worms take up permanent residence in the inferior mesenteric veins of the large intestine. In this environment they deposit eggs in the wall of the intestine; the eggs eventually break through the mucosa into the lumen and are passed with feces. After reaching fresh water the eggs hatch, and, if the appropriate species of snail is present, the miracidia enter the intermediate host to become cercariae that will initiate a new cycle of human infection (see Figure 44-11).

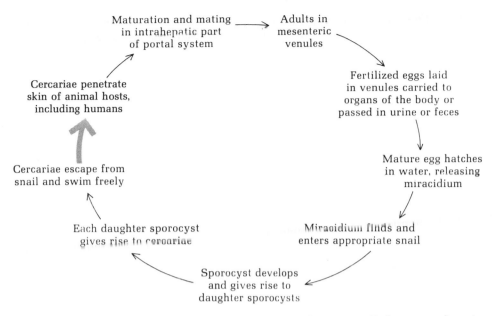

**Figure 44-11.** Life cycle of the blood flukes in the genus *Schistosoma*. Refer to text for minor differences among species.

### Schistosoma japonicum

This species occurs exclusively in the Far East, and its definitive hosts include, in addition to humans, horses, cattle, pigs, dogs, cats, rodents, and water buffalo.

The life cycle and pathogenesis of *S. japonicum* is as described for *S. mansoni*. The final residence for the adult worms is found in the superior mesenteric veins of the small intestine. The eggs break through the wall into the lumen and are passed with the feces. *S. japonicum* is the most prolific egg layer of the parasites causing human schistosomiasis, and it is common for the eggs to be carried to the liver and other organs of the body, including the central nervous system. As a result, both cirrhosis and brain lesions are more commonly associated with this species than with the other schistosomes.

### Schistosoma haematobium

Large areas of Africa, the Nile River Valley, and the Near East are endemic for this pre-dominately human parasite. The adult worms characteristically migrate into the rectal vessels and eventually reach veins surrounding the bladder. Unlike the other schistosomes, the eggs of *S. haematobium* penetrate the bladder mucosa and are passed in the urine. Ulceration of the bladder causes numerous small hemorrhages, and the passage of blood in urine is not rare.

### Diagnosis, Therapy, and Control of Schistosomal Infections

The diagnosis of all schistosomal infections is based upon a history of exposure to an endemic area and upon the finding of eggs in the urine or stools of the infected individual.

Success of therapy varies among the species, with *S. haematobium* the most readily cured and *S. japonicum* the most difficult to eradicate. The successful drugs contain trivalent antimony; all of these are quite toxic, and considerable effort has been expended to produce less toxic chemotherapeutic agents. Oral drugs used with some success include agents such as leucanthone hydrochloride, 1-diethylaminoethylamino-4-methylthiaxanthone hydrochloride (Miracil-D), and niridazole (Ambilhar). Currently, stibophen is the drug choice for treatment of infections by *S. mansoni,* and antimony potassium tartrate is used for *S. japonicum* infections.

Efforts to control schistosomal infections (estimated by the World Health Organization to be second only to malaria as a cause of morbidity and mortality in the tropics) are directed toward the elimination of the snails acting as intermediate hosts and the protection of water from human fecal contamina-tion. A number of chemicals, such as copper sulfate, can be used to kill snails, but the migration of snails from untreated areas frequently neutralizes this method of control. In the Far East the task is further complicated by the commonplace use of human feces as a primary source of fertilizer. It would seem that the only hope for controlling schisto-somiasis lies in a program of education designed to teach methods for the sanitary disposal of feces and urine; however, such programs alone have not been effective to date.

# Nematoda

Nematodes are round, elongate worms; the sexes are separate, and, unlike the flatworms, adult nematodes possess complete digestive systems that include both a mouth and an anus (see Figure 44-12). Human infections caused by these roundworms are usually divided into two large categories, the intestinal roundworms and the blood and tissue roundworms.

## INTESTINAL NEMATODE INFECTIONS IN HUMANS

Roundworms that exist in the intestine during their adult stage are generally considered as intestinal nematodes. We shall see, however, that the larval stages of some intestinal species may be widely distributed throughout the body of an infected individual.

### Trichinella spiralis

*Trichinella spiralis* is the etiologic agent of trichinosis, a disease disseminated in carnivorous animals. Human infections occur worldwide, and as recently as the 1930's incidence in the United States was estimated to include 20% of the population (control measures have now reduced this to approximately 4%). Human infections almost invariably result from the ingestion of im-properly cooked pork containing the encysted larvae; however, bear meat has also been implicated in the northwestern United States. Following ingestion, the cysts reach the intestine where larvae are liberated and develop into adult worms. After copulation the male worms are passed in the feces and the female penetrates the intestinal mucosa, where she will produce as many as 1500 larvae over a period of one to three months. The larvae enter the blood stream, primarily via the lymphatics, following which they penetrate the skeletal muscles and become encysted (see Figure 44-13).

As with many helminthic infections, the symptoms are in large part dependent upon the magnitude of the initial infection. Light infections are normally asymptomatic, but the ingestion of large numbers of encysted larvae may cause a severe disease culminating in the death of the patient. Initial symptoms, occurring within one to three days after infection and resulting from the intestinal activities of the adult worms, characteristically include diarrhea, malaise, and fever. This stage may be mild to severe but persists for only about a week. The second stage of the infection, involving the migration of the larvae into skeletal muscle, begins about one week after the initial infection, and in cases of moderate to heavy infection

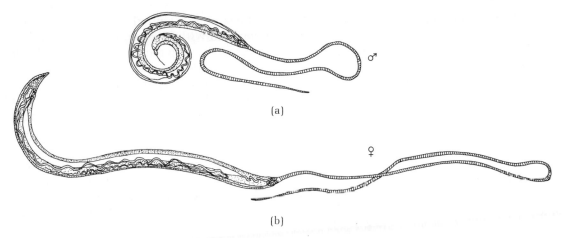

**Figure 44-12.** The nematode *Trichuris trichiura. a.* Male. *b.* Female.

muscular pain throughout the body may be prominent. Moreover, although encystment occurs only in muscle, the larvae may infect other organs of the body, including the lungs, heart, eyelids, meninges, and brain. Massive invasion of these latter organs may result in death during the early weeks of the infection. The usual pathogenic effects, however, result from the destruction of striated muscle fibers and occur during the encystment and subsequent calcification of the larval cysts.

Barring reinfection, major symptoms subside in several months, but weakness, rheumatic pain, and loss of dexterity may persist for long periods.

There are several laboratory tests for the diagnosis of trichinosis, but the only definite one is the observation of the larvae or larval cysts in biopsies of infected muscles. Complement fixation and a skin reaction using an antigen prepared from *Trichinella* are used to support a tentative diagnosis.

**Figure 44-13.** Life cycle of *Trichinella spiralis.*

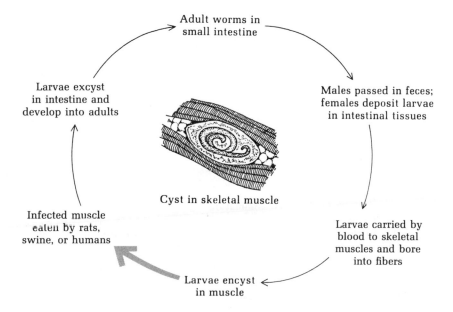

Adult worms in small intestine

Larvae excyst in intestine and develop into adults

Males passed in feces; females deposit larvae in intestinal tissues

Cyst in skeletal muscle

Infected muscle eaten by rats, swine, or humans

Larvae carried by blood to skeletal muscles and bore into fibers

Larvae encyst in muscle

Thiabendazole appears to be effective against the intestinal phase of this parasite, but its efficacy against larvae in muscles is not clearly established. In severe cases, steroids are given to lessen the extent of inflammation and to provide symptomatic relief. Since ingestion of undercooked infected meat provides the only mechanism of infection, it would seem possible to eliminate this disease from domestic animals. However, the major reservoir for *Trichinella spiralis* occurs in cannibalistic brown and black rats, and it is essentially impossible to completely control this source of infection for pigs. Laws requiring sterilization of garbage to be used for feeding hogs are in force throughout the United States, and such measures, plus the thorough cooking of pork or freezing, which also destroys the encysted larvae, have done much to decrease the incidence of trichinosis.

### Trichuris trichiura

Trichuriasis, or whipworm disease, is caused by the nematode *Trichuris trichiura*. This disease occurs extensively in the tropics and, occasionally, in lower socioeconomic areas in the southern United States. It is a disease associated with filth and is seen primarily in children. Its prevalence is indicated by the estimate that about 500 million persons are infected with this parasite.

The adult worm lives mainly in the human cecum attached to the intestinal mucosa, where it will continue to produce eggs for a period of six to eight years. The eggs are passed in the feces, and in a moist, warm environment infective larvae will develop within the eggs in three to six weeks. Ingestion of the mature eggs, either directly from the soil or through contaminated food and water, initiates a new cycle—shown in Figure 44-14—during which the larvae will develop into mature adults in the cecum.

Heavy infections are usually accompanied by chronic diarrhea. Abdominal pain, vomiting, constipation, headache, and anemia may also accompany whipworm infections.

The observation of the barrel-shaped eggs in the feces provides a definitive diagnosis for trichuriasis. Adult worms are rarely seen in the feces, for they normally remain attached to the intestinal mucosa. By proctoscopy heavy infections of worms can be observed attached to the rectal mucosa.

**Figure 44-14.** Life cycle of *Trichuris trichiura*.

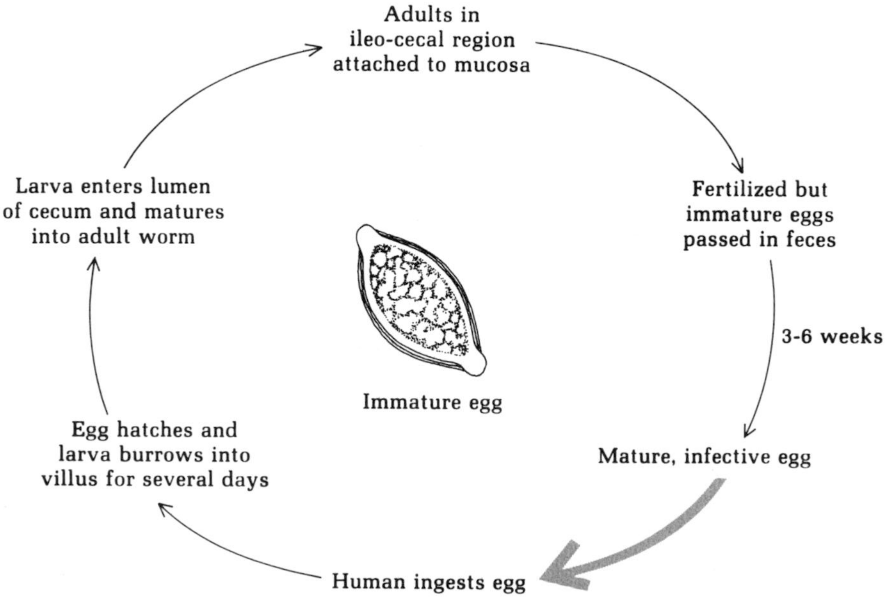

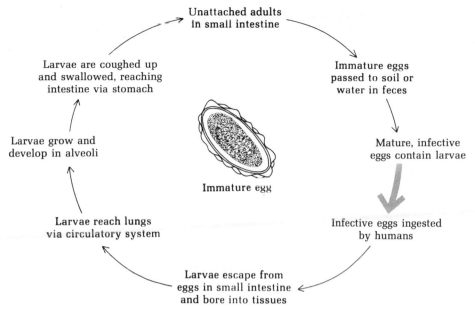

Unattached adults
in small intestine

Larvae are coughed up
and swallowed, reaching
intestine via stomach

Immature eggs
passed to soil or
water in feces

Larvae grow and
develop in alveoli

Immature egg

Mature, infective
eggs contain larvae

Larvae reach lungs
via circulatory system

Infective eggs ingested
by humans

Larvae escape from
eggs in small intestine
and bore into tissues

**Figure 44-15.** Life cycle of *Ascaris lumbricoides*.

The drug mebendazole is an effective treatment when given orally for several days. Enemas containing hexylresorcinol were previously used to treat heavy infections. The major effective control is directed toward the sanitary disposal of human feces. Secondary measures involve thorough sanitary procedures such as the washing of hands before meals and the complete cleansing of uncooked vegetables before consumption.

### Ascaris lumbricoides

This worm may attain a length of 20–30 centimeters and is the largest nematode that parasitizes humans. It occurs most frequently in young children in the tropics and, to a lesser extent, in certain areas of the southern United States. It is estimated that over 900 million persons are infected and that about one million of these live in the mountainous regions of the southern United States.

Second-stage larvae develop within the eggs while in the soil and humans are infected by the ingestion of the infective eggs (see Figure 44-15). After reaching the intestine, the larvae hatch, penetrate the intestinal mucosa, and (after being picked up in the portal circulation and passing through the heart and liver) eventually reach the lungs. There they undergo additional differentiation and are coughed up, swallowed, and returned to the intestine.

Adult worms remain unattached in the small intestine and, in the absence of a heavy infection, symptoms are mild or absent. Heavier infections cause abdominal pain, and complications may occasionally occur as a result of invasion of the liver, bile ducts, gallbladder, and appendix by adult worms. Hypersensitivity reactions occurring during the pulmonary migration of larvae in subsequent infections may result in an asthma-like condition known as Loeffler's syndrome.

Since the adult female is capable of producing over 20 million eggs at the rate of 200,000 per day, not many females are required to cause the excretion of large numbers of *Ascaris* eggs. The primary technique employed in the diagnosis of ascariasis is the visualization and identification of the eggs voided in the feces.

Pyrantel pamoate is the therapy of choice, and a single administration will cure most infections; however, piperazine citrate is also effective as well as inexpensive and

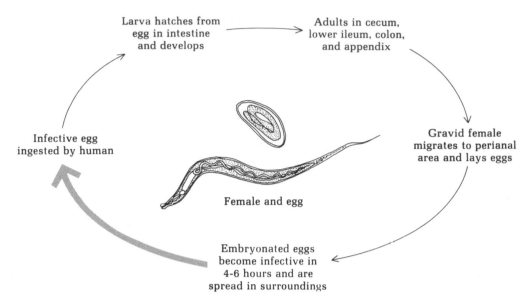

Larva hatches from
egg in intestine
and develops

Adults in cecum,
lower ileum, colon,
and appendix

Infective egg
ingested by human

Gravid female
migrates to perianal
area and lays eggs

Female and egg

Embryonated eggs
become infective in
4-6 hours and are
spread in surroundings

**Figure 44-16.** Life cycle of the pinworm, *Enterobius vermicularis.*

relatively nontoxic to the host. As with parasitic infections in which humans are the major reservoir, control is dependent upon the sanitary disposal of human feces.

### Enterobius vermicularis

Humans are the only known host of *Enterobius vermicularis,* or, as the organisms are frequently called, pinworms. Contrary to popular belief, dogs and cats do not carry this human parasite.

Humans—frequently children—become infected by the ingestion of the fertilized eggs. The adult worms live and copulate in the cecum. When gravid, the female will migrate to the anus where she deposits her eggs in the perianal area, usually at night. On rare occasions, such eggs may gain re-entry into the intestine but infections ordinarily result from the ingestion of fertilized eggs. Their presence in the anal area causes an intense itching; the subsequent scratching contaminates the hands, leading to reinfection via a hand-to-mouth contact or by the contamination of such materials as food, drink, bed linen, and towels, where the eggs may survive for weeks. Most infections are asymptomatic and, barring reinfection, a cure is spontaneous after

all the females have died. A schematic cycle is shown in Figure 44-16.

Since eggs are not deposited in the feces, a diagnosis is made by recovering eggs from the perianal skin. If a piece of scotch tape looped over a microscope slide is firmly pressed into the anal area, the eggs will attach and be visible when the scotch tape is examined microscopically. In addition, an examination of the anus during periods of intense itching—usually occurring shortly after retiring for the night—will frequently reveal the presence of adult female worms.

A number of therapeutic drugs can be used to treat pinworm infections. A single dose of pyrantel pamoate (Antiminth) or pyrvinium pamoate (Povan) is ordinarily effective. Piperazine is also effective, but it must be given over a period of a week. Treatment should be repeated after two weeks. If one can prevent scratching and the subsequent reinfection, spontaneous recovery normally occurs after several months.

### Strongyloides stercoralis

This parasite is unique among nematodes in that it is capable of having a free-living generation and a parasitic generation, as diagrammed in Figure 44-17. The parasites exist worldwide but are most commonly found in tropical climates that provide a warm, damp environment for the free-living stage of the parasite.

In most cases the infective larvae in the soil enter humans by penetration of the skin (direct cycle). They then pass through the heart via the venous circulation, eventually reaching the lungs. After penetration of the alveoli, the larvae are coughed up, swallowed, and gain entrance to the mucosa of the small intestine where they develop into adult parthenogenetic females. The progeny of these worms pass in the feces as first-stage larvae (rhabditiform) which then develop into infective filariform larvae.

In other cases it appears that larvae in the soil can develop into adult males and females that copulate and produce fertilized eggs (indirect cycle). Larvae infective for humans may develop in the soil from these eggs. This cycle requires a suitable warm, moist environment.

Still a third life cycle called internal autoinfection occurs in which the larvae undergo partial development in the intestine. They then penetrate the intestinal mucosa to enter the venous circulation, complete the entire developmental cycle in the lungs, and are coughed up and swallowed again, reaching the intestine without leaving the host.

Most infections are light and asymptomatic, but vomiting and diarrhea may occur. Heavy infections can cause anemia, weight loss, and chronic diarrhea. Fatal cases seem to follow extensive dissemination of the larvae throughout the body as a result of massive autoinfection.

The observation of the larvae in freshly passed stools provides the most definite diagnosis. Since the larvae may be in extremely small numbers, special techniques (such as examination of duodenal fluid) are often required for detection. Thiabendazole is the treatment of choice. Since contaminated human feces are the major source of infection, the only effective control is the sanitary disposal of human sewage.

**Figure 44-17.** Life cycle and various means by which humans may become infected with *Strongyloides stercoralis.*

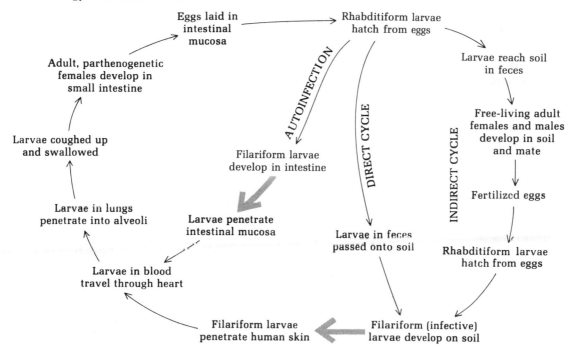

### Necator americanus and Ancylostoma duodenale

These two nematodes are the major etiologic agents of human "hookworm disease." Neither the larval stages nor the eggs can be differentiated from each other, and, since their life cycles, treatment, and control are essentially identical, it is usually not necessary to complete a diagnosis beyond determining that it is a hookworm infection.

Both species are widespread in tropical areas, but *A. duodenale* also occurs extensively in Europe. On the other hand, *N. americanus* was brought from Africa by slaves, and it is now the major hookworm species in the United States. As a result, infections by *A. duodenale* are sometimes referred to as Old World hookworm, while those caused by *N. americanus* are called New World hookworm.

As diagrammed in Figure 44-18, the eggs of both species are passed in the feces and hatch into first stage larvae (rhabditiform) that feed on bacteria and vegetation in the soil. After five days they become longer, more slender forms called filariform larvae. The filariform larvae gain access to the host by penetrating the skin, usually on the foot or between the toes. The larvae migrate via the blood to the lungs, where they break through the alveoli and are coughed up and swallowed. The adults reside in the small intestine attached to the mucosa.

Symptoms may be mild, although the simultaneous passage of many larvae through the lungs may cause headaches, fever, and nausea and result in production of sputum containing blood. The primary intestinal symptoms are diarrhea, vomiting, and fever. Heavy infection causes a significant anemia through the loss of blood from the intestine due to the feeding activities of the worms.

Recovery and identification of eggs from the voided feces provide for the only definitive diagnosis. Since anemia is a prominent feature of heavy infections, treatment with iron, vitamins, and a high-protein diet will frequently alleviate the symptoms. Pyrantel pamoate and mebendazole are the drugs of choice, although tetrachlorethylene is an effective drug for *Necator* and has been used for many years. Control requires the sanitary disposal of human feces plus protection from

**Figure 44-18.** Life cycle of the hookworms, *Necator americanus* and *Ancylostoma duodenale.*

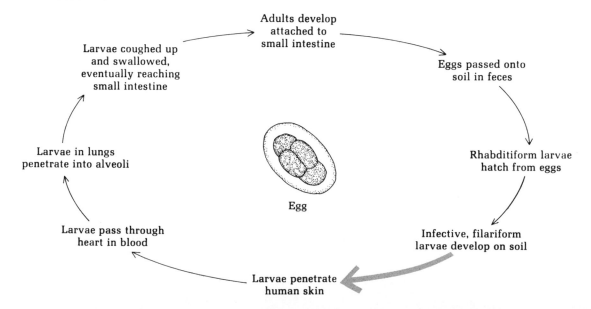

Adults develop attached to small intestine

Larvae coughed up and swallowed, eventually reaching small intestine

Eggs passed onto soil in feces

Larvae in lungs penetrate into alveoli

Rhabditiform larvae hatch from eggs

Egg

Larvae pass through heart in blood

Infective, filariform larvae develop on soil

Larvae penetrate human skin

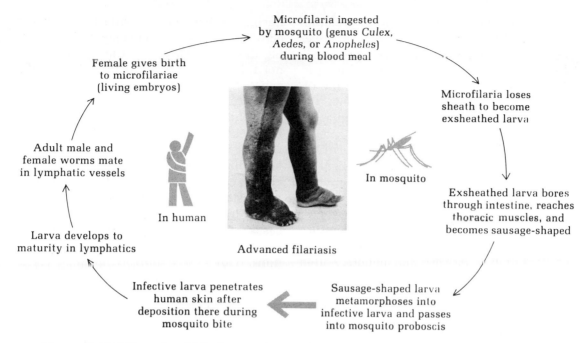

Microfilaria ingested
by mosquito (genus *Culex,
Aedes,* or *Anopheles*)
during blood meal

Female gives birth
to microfilariae
(living embryos)

Microfilaria loses
sheath to become
exsheathed larva

Adult male and
female worms mate
in lymphatic vessels

In mosquito

In human

Advanced filariasis

Exsheathed larva bores
through intestine, reaches
thoracic muscles, and
becomes sausage-shaped

Larva develops to
maturity in lymphatics

Infective larva penetrates
human skin after
deposition there during
mosquito bite

Sausage-shaped larva
metamorphoses into
infective larva and passes
into mosquito proboscis

**Figure 44-19.** Life cycle of *Wuchereria bancrofti.* The photo demonstrates an advanced case of filariasis caused by blockage of the lymphatics in both legs of a child by this parasite.

infection by such means as wearing shoes in endemic areas.

## BLOOD AND TISSUE NEMATODE INFECTIONS IN HUMANS

Unlike intestinal roundworm infections, nematodes infecting blood and tissue are not spread via fecal contamination. Most of these latter parasites are carried from human to human by the bite of an arthropod vector.

With one exception, the worms to be discussed in this section belong to the superfamily Filarioidea, and a resulting human infection is called filariasis. Adult worms generally range from 2 to 30 centimeters in length, with the female about twice the size of the male. One property distinguishing the filariae from other nematodes is that the female does not lay eggs but, instead, gives birth to prelarval forms called microfilariae. As we shall see, the ingestion of the microfilariae by blood-sucking insect vectors provides for the transmission of filariae from one person to another.

### *Wuchereria bancrofti*

Bancroftian filariasis (a cause of elephantiasis) is seen extensively in the Pacific islands as well as in much of Africa. Sporadic cases occur in European countries bordering the Mediterranean Sea, and the disease is also found scattered throughout the Near and Far East and in Central and South America.

*Wuchereria bancrofti* is transmitted to humans by the bite of an infected mosquito—a species of *Culex, Aedes,* or *Anopheles* (see Figure 44-19). The mosquito, however, provides more than a mere mechanical vector for transmission; the ingested microfilariae must undergo transformation within the mosquito to form larvae infective for the definitive host, i.e., humans. This development requires about ten days, after which time infective larvae enter the proboscis of the mosquito and are transmitted to a human during the next blood meal.

Within the human the larvae enter the lymphatic vessels and nodes where they develop into adult worms during the ensuing six months. The worms appear to preferentially infect the lymphatics of the lower extremities, and pathologic changes occur most frequently in the groin and genital areas. Once ensconced, mating occurs and the resulting microfilariae migrate through the walls of the lymphatics into the adjacent blood vessels.

Symptoms result from the presence of the adult worms in the lymphatics, but light infections are often unnoticed, with the only physical signs being slightly enlarged lymph nodes, particularly in the groin. However, in endemic areas where frequent exposure occurs, attacks are characterized by fever, chills, vomiting, malaise, and tender, swollen lymph nodes. Such attacks last several days and may result in the formation of draining ulcers in the lymph nodes or along the lymphatic vessels. Surprisingly, the major symptoms seem to be the result of a hypersensitivity reaction directed against antigens present in the adult worms. In rare cases, multiple exposure to the filariae results in the proliferation of fibrous tissue around the dead worms, leading to an obstruction of lymphatic flow and causing extensive edema (swelling due to the accumulation of fluid) in the legs, scrotum, female genitalia, or breasts. This obstructive filariasis, more commonly called elephantiasis (shown in Figure 44-19), is fortunately rare even in endemic areas and occurs only after repeated infections and many years of chronic filariasis.

The physical signs of inflamed lymph vessels (lymphangitis), swollen, tender lymph nodes (lymphadenitis), and edema of the extremeties, genitalia, or breasts (elephantiasis) occurring in an endemic area are sufficient to make a tentative diagnosis of chronic filariasis. An unequivocal diagnosis, however, requires the observation of the microfilariae in the blood. This may prove difficult for two reasons: (1) very few microfilariae are present during the chronic stage, and (2) with the exception of the South Pacific strain, the microfilariae show a definite periodicity in which very few are present in the blood during daylight hours while the patient is active but large numbers may be found during the night. This nocturnal periodicity is not fully understood, but it could be influenced by an increased partial pressure of oxygen in the lungs during normal activity. This phenomenon necessitates collection of blood samples between 10 PM and 2 AM. Diethycarbamazine (Hetrazan) kills the microfilariae of W. bancrofti, but it is not always effective in eliminating adult worms. Antihistamines and steroids are used to decrease hypersensitivity reactions. Advanced cases of elephantiasis, however, usually require surgery to correct lymphatic obstructions. This may require removal of an enlarged scrotum or the anastomosis (joining together) of the deep and superficial lymphatics in the legs.

Control can be directed toward two vulnerable stages in the life cycle of the filariae: (1) the elimination of the mosquito, as was achieved against yellow fever, and (2) the mass administration of diethylcarbamazine to all individuals within an endemic region. This latter procedure destroys the microfilariae and has proved successful in several isolated island areas such as the Virgin Islands and Tahiti.

### Brugia malayi

Brugia malayi, the etiologic agent of Malayan filariasis, differs slightly in morphology from Wuchereria bancrofti but shares many life cycle characteristics. In addition, the clinical and pathological features of Malayan filariasis are similar to those described for the bancroftian variety.

The Malayan Peninsula comprises one of the major endemic areas, although the parasites are seen also in India, Vietnam, Indonesia, Thailand, and Ceylon. The microfilariae can develop in the same mosquito species as can W. bancrofti, but the principal mosquito vector for B. malayi is a mosquito belonging to the genus Mansonia. Unlike W. bancrofti, for which humans comprise the only known reservoir, B. malayi has been found in monkeys, dogs, and cats; it is assumed that there may be any number of mammalian hosts able to serve as reservoirs for this nematode.

Laboratory diagnosis requires the visualization of the microfilariae in a blood smear. As described for W. bancrofti, microfilariae from most strains also exhibit a nocturnal periodicity, but some strains have been reported to lack this periodicity.

Treatment and control employ essentially the same procedures as for the bancroftian variety. The major vectors, mosquitoes of the genus Mansonia, breed in ponds heavily populated with the water plant Pistia stratiotes, an essential component of the life cycle of these mosquitoes. As a result, herbicides such as sodium methyl chlorphenoxyacetate provide effective control.

## Loa loa

The scientific designation for this species of nematode is derived from its African name. It is found only in Africa, and a common name is "the African eye worm."

The transmission of loiasis, the disease resulting from an infection of Loa loa, is much the same as with diseases from other filarial parasites, except that here the vector is one of several species of mango or deer flies (genus Chrysops). The microfilariae undergo development within the fly and are transmitted to humans by the bite of an infected fly. Monkeys and humans appear to be the only definitive hosts.

Following infection, the larvae develop into adult worms, which migrate throughout the subcutaneous tissues of the definitive host. The infection is generally asymptomatic, although occasional inflammatory reactions known as Calabar swellings occur at irregular intervals. These swellings are thought to result from hypersensitivity reactions and normally disappear within a week. The disquieting and somewhat painful manifestation of a Loa infection occurs when

adult worms migrate into the facial area. There they can frequently be seen (and removed) as they pass over the bridge of the nose or migrate through the subconjunctival tissue of the eye. Untreated, the infection may last for many years without major apparent damage to the host. Chronic loiasis sometimes results in an allergic dermatitis in which abscesses may form following secondary bacterial infections.

The occurrence of Calabar swellings, in an endemic zone, suggests a Loa loa infection; however, a definitive diagnosis of loiasis is based on finding the microfilariae in the blood or observing the adult worms beneath the conjunctiva. The oral administration of diethylcarbamazine is very effective for eliminating adult worms and microfilariae. Also, the worms can be removed surgically, but since chemotherapy is effectual, this procedure is probably unwarranted.

Prevention is directed at eliminating the carriers by mass treatment with diethylcarbamazine in endemic sections; nets, screens, and repellants are also used to ward off infected flies.

## Onchocerca volvulus

Most infections by Onchocerca volvulus are found in Central Africa, but they also are present in restricted areas of Central America and northern South America. Larvae are transmitted to humans by the bites of infected black flies (genus Simulium). The adult worms occur in the subcutaneous tissue of the definitive host. There the male and female worms routinely become enclosed in fibrous capsules that can be seen grossly as small nodules under the skin (see Figure 44-20). Microfilariae migrate from the capsules and move throughout the dermis and connective tissue; these microfilariae induce the major, pathologic lesions of onchocerciasis. The most serious lesions occur following the migration of the microfilariae into the eyes. Ocular lesions may be caused, in part, by toxic products, but it is generally thought that

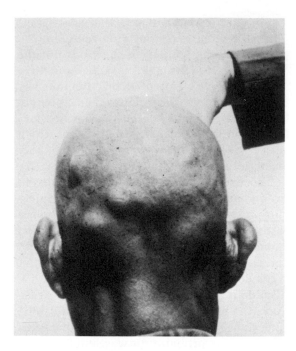

**Figure 44-20.** Skin nodules containing the filarial parasite, *Onchocerca volvulus.*

the chief destructive changes are the effect of allergic reactions to the invading microfilariae. The severity of the damage can be emphasized by statistics obtained from some endemic regions of Africa, revealing that 30% of the population have impaired vision and that approximately 10% are blind as a result of onchocerciasis.

Skin inflammation is also a frequent manifestation of this disease. Onchodermatitis, which is the result of an allergic reaction to the microfilariae in the skin, may after long-established, chronic disease be seen as thick, wrinkled, hyperpigmented skin. In extreme cases a sac of tissue may hang down to the knees due to loss of elasticity in the skin. This elephantiasis, however, is not the result of lymphatic obstruction as described for bancroftian elephantiasis.

The appearance of characteristic skin nodules, in endemic areas, is highly suggestive of onchocerciasis, but a definitive laboratory diagnosis requires detection of the

microfilariae. As they do not occur in the blood, skin biopsies or superficial snips of the skin are examined for the presence of the microfilariae. Microfilariae can be destroyed by the administration of diethylcarbamazine; this is not, however, effective against the adult encapsulated worms. The superficial nodules containing the adult parasites can be removed surgically, but if this procedure fails to eradicate the infection, a highly toxic drug called suramin can be used. In all cases, chemotherapeutic drugs must be administered with caution, since the massive killing of either the microfilariae or the adults can trigger a highly destructive hypersensitivity reaction in the host.

Prevention is directed toward the elimination of the disease in humans (the only definitive host from which the vector becomes infected with the microfilariae) and the eradication of the vector itself. The latter procedure involves the addition of insecticides to local waters to destroy the aquatic developmental stages of the black flies.

### *Dracunculus medinensis*

These parasites, known as guinea worms, are believed to be the "fiery serpents" that, according to the Old Testament, infected the Israelites during one of their earlier ventures into the Sinai Peninsula. *Dracunculus medinensis* is found in Africa and large areas of Asia, and it is estimated that approximately 48 million persons are currently infected. In the past these worms have been observed in the West Indian islands and in Brazil, but they are no longer believed to cause human disease in the Western Hemisphere.

Unlike other nematodes infecting blood and tissue, guinea worm infections are acquired by drinking water that contains the intermediate host for this parasite, infected copepods (minute freshwater and marine crustaceans). When a person digests the copepods, the ingested larvae penetrate the intestinal wall and move via the lymphatics to the deep, subcutaneous tissues. Here they develop into adult worms. After mating, the male worm is believed to die, and about a year after the initial infection the female (which may exceed a length of one meter) migrates to a position just beneath the skin. A local ulcer develops, exposing a loop of the worm's uterus which, on contact with water, will discharge huge numbers of motile larvae. When ingested by an appropriate copepod, these larvae undergo metamorphosis and are able to initiate a new cycle of human infection in about three weeks.

Systemic symptoms of vomiting, diarrhea, hives, and shortness of breath seem to be more from an allergic reaction than from direct toxicity of the parasite. Symptoms may last for several weeks while the female discharges her larvae, after which the worm may be expelled or may again penetrate to deeper tissues before dying. Local healing occurs at this time, and subsequent X-rays reveal calcified lesions surrounding the remains of the dead worms.

The intracutaneous injection of an extract of the worms will induce a delayed-type skin reaction, but the appearance of the worm just under the skin provides the most common means of diagnosis.

Diethylcarbamazine is an effective drug if used early before the larvae develop into mature worms; however, niridazole is currently the drug of choice for the adult parasite. This latter drug is quite toxic and may cause a number of severe side reactions.

The most common technique for removing the adult guinea worm is to insert a stick into the ulcer beneath the worm and slowly turn it to wind the worm around the stick. This must be done very carefully so as not to rupture the parasite and cause secondary infections. Each day only a few centimeters of the worm may be wound about the stick, and, as one can imagine, considerable time is necessary to extract a worm one meter in length.

The life cycle of D. medinensis could be easily interrupted by using protected springs or wells as sources of drinking water. Water supplies may be rendered noninfectious by boiling or filtering to remove infected copepods.

## REFERENCES

Ansari, N., ed. 1973. *Epidemiology and Control of Schistosomiasis.* S. Karger, Basel, and University Park Press, Baltimore.

Augustine, D. L. 1933. Effects of low temperatures upon encysted *Trichinella spiralis. Amer. J. Hyg.* **17:**697–710.

Beaver, P. C., and T. C. Orihel. 1965. Human infection with filariae of animals in the United States. *Amer. J. Trop. Med. Hyg.* **14:**1010–1029.

Blumenthal, D. S., and M. G. Schulz. 1976. Effects of *Ascaris* infection on nutritional status in children. *Amer. J. Trop. Med. Hyg.* **25:**682–690.

Dewhirst, L. W., J. D. Cramer, and W. J. Pistor. 1963. Bovine cysticercosis. I. Longevity of cysticerci of *Taenia saginata. J. Parasitol.* **49:**297–300.

Duke, B. O. L. 1972. Onchocerciasis. *Br. Med. Bull.* **28:**66–71.

Ecleson, J. F. B. 1972. Filariasis. *Br. Med. Bull.* **28:**60–65.

Emson, H. E., M. A. Baltzan, and H. E. Wiens. 1972. Trichinosis in Saskatchewan: An outbreak due to infected bear meat. *Can. Med. Assoc. J.* **106:**897–898.

Gould, S. E. 1971. The story of trichinosis. *Amer. J. Clin. Pathol.* **55:**2–11.

Hiatt, R. A. 1976. Morbidity from *Schistosoma mansoni* infections: An epidemiological study based on quantitative analysis of egg excretion in two Highland Ethiopian villages. *Amer. J. Trop. Med. Hyg.* **25:**808–817.

Katz, N., and J. Pellegrino. 1974. Experimental chemotherapy of schistosomiasis mansoni. *Adv. in Parasitol.* **12:**369–390.

Larsh, J. E., Jr., and N. F. Weatherly. 1975. Cell-mediated immunity against certain parasitic worms. *Adv. in Parasitol.* **13:**183–222.

Miyazaki, I. 1969. On the lung flukes causing paragonimiasis. *Jap. J. Trop. Med.* **10:**8–13.

Nourmand, A. 1976. Hydatid cysts in children and youths. *Amer. J. Trop. Med. Hyg.* **25:**845–847.

Sakamota, K., and Y. Ishii. 1976. Fine structure of schistosome eggs as seen through the scanning electron microscope. *Amer. J. Trop. Med. Hyg.* **25:**841–844.

Ruppanner, R., and C. W. Schwabe. 1973. Early records of hydatid disease in California. *Amer. J. Trop. Med. Hyg.* **22:**485–492.

Smithers, S. R., and R. J. Terry. 1976. The immunology of schistosomiasis. *Adv. in Parasitol.* **14:**399–422.

Strauss, G. W. 1962. Clinical manifestations of clonorchiasis: A controlled study of 105 cases. *Amer. J. Trop. Med. Hyg.* **11:**625–630.

Weller, T. H. 1976. Manson's schistosomiasis; frontiers *in vivo, in vitro,* and in the body politic. *Amer. J. Trop. Med. Hyg.* **25:**208–216.

World Health Organization. 1973. Schistosomiasis Control. Report of a WHO Expert Committee. *WHO Tech. Report* No. 515.

# Figure and Table Credits

## Unit-Opening Photos

Unit One. Section through a cell of *E. coli* B approximately 30 minutes after phage infection, showing a T2 virion adsorbed at the "12 o'clock" position and daughter particles at various stages of assembly within the cell. Note also the clear resolution of the gram-negative cell wall. Courtesy of L. D. Simon, Waksman Institute for Microbiology, Rutgers Univ., and T. F. Anderson, Institute for Cancer Research, Philadelphia.

Unit Two. Scanning electron micrograph of murine lymphocytes (round cells) and peritoneal macrophages (spreading cells) growing on a glass coverslip that was surgically implanted in the peritoneal cavity of a mouse. Courtesy of R. M. Albrecht and R. D. Hinsdill, The Univ. of Wisconsin, Madison.

Unit Three. Freeze-etch electron micrograph of a cell of the pathogenic fungus *Cryptococcus neoformans*. Courtesy of S. C. Holt, Dept. of Microbiology, Univ. of Massachusetts, Amherst.

Unit Four. Electron micrograph of negatively-stained particles of vesicular stomatitis virus. Courtesy of J. J. Cardamone, Jr., and J. S. Youngner, Dept. of Microbiology, Univ. of Pittsburgh School of Medicine.

Unit Five. Scanning electron micrograph of *Trypanosoma equiperdum*, a protozoan that causes a venereal disease of horses known as dourine. Courtesy of J. J. Paulin, Dept. of Zoology, Univ. of Georgia.

## Figures

1-1*a*. Bausch and Lomb, Rochester, N.Y.

1-3*a*. M. E. Doohan and E. H. Newcomb, Dept. of Botany, The Univ. of Wisconsin, Madison.

1-3*b*, 11-6. I. Carr, Dept. of Pathology, Univ. of Saskatchewan.

1-4, 2-1, 3-2, 3-5, 3-7, 3-12, 3-15, 6-1, 6-2, 26-1, 26-4*b*, 26-5*b*. S. C. Holt, Dept. of Microbiology, Univ. of Massachusetts, Amherst.

1-6. E. F. Lessel and J. G. Holt. 1970. In *Methods for Numerical Taxonomy,* W. R. Lockhart and J. Liston, eds. American Society for Microbiology, Washington, D.C.

2-2. N. S. Hayes, K. E. Muse, A. M. Collier, and J. B. Baseman, Dept. of Bacteriology and Immunology, School of Medicine, The Univ. of North Carolina at Chapel Hill.

3-1*a*, *b*, and *d*; 18-1. Z. Skobe, Forsyth Dental Center, Boston, Mass.

3-1*c* (top). L. M. Pope, Dept. of Microbiology, The Univ. of Texas at Austin.

3-1*c* (bottom), 3-13. T. J. Beveridge, Dept. of Bacteriology and Immunology, The Univ. of Western Ontario.

3-3*e*. W. L. Dentler, Dept. of Physiology and Cell Biology, Univ. of Kansas, Lawrence.

3-4. M. L. DePamphilis and J. Adler. 1971. *J. Bacteriol.* **105**:384–395.

3-6, 10-3, 10-4. J. L. Strominger. 1967. *Fed. Proc.* **26**:9.

3-9. O. Luderitz, et al. 1973. *J. Infect. Dis.* **128** (Supp.):S17–S29.

3-11. S. J. Singer and G. L. Nicolson. 1972. *Science*

175:720–731. Copyright 1972 by the American Association for the Advancement of Science.

3-14. P. Fitz-James and E. Young. 1969. *The Bacterial Spore,* G. W. Gould and A. Hurst, eds. Academic Press, N.Y.

6-3. A. K. Kleinschmidt, et al. 1962. *Biochim. Biophys. Acta.* **61**:857–864.

6-4. W. B. Wood. 1973. In *Genetic Mechanism of Development,* F. J. Ruddle, ed. Academic Press, N.Y.

6-5. A. H. Doermann. 1952. *J. Gen. Physiol.* **35**:645–656.

6-8, 31-5, 36-2. J. Griffith, Dept. of Biochemistry, Stanford Univ. School of Medicine.

7-4. R. Kavenoff and B. C. Bowen. 1976. *Chromosoma* **59**:89–101.

8-5. C. C. Brinton, Jr., and J. Chapman, Dept. of Life Sciences, Univ. of Pittsburgh.

9-1*b*. 3M Co.

9-3. Millipore Corp., Bedford, Mass.

11-1. R. Austrian. 1953. *J. Exp. Med.* **98**:21.

11-2, 11-3. D. F. Bainton. 1966. *J. Cell Biol.* **28**:277–301.

11-4. D. F. Bainton, Dept. of Pathology, Univ. of California, San Francisco.

11-7. E. L. Kaplan, T. Laxdal, and P. G. Quie. 1968. *Pediatrics* **41**:591–599.

11-8. R. K. Root, A. S. Rosenthal, and D. J. Balestra. 1972. *J. Clin. Invest.* **51**:649–665.

12-2. M. Z. Atassi. 1975. *Immunochem.* **12**:423–438.

12-3. A. Tiselius and E. A. Kabat. 1939. *J. Exp. Med.* **69**:119–131.

12-7. I. Roitt. 1974. *Essential Immunology,* 2nd ed. Blackwell, Oxford.

12-8. T. T. Wu and E. A. Kabat. 1970. *J. Exp. Med.* **132**:211–250.

12-9*b*. N. M. Green, National Institute for Medical Research, London, U.K.

12-10*b* and *c*. A. Feinstein, Institute of Animal Physiology, Agricultural Research Council, Cambridge, U.K.

13-4, 13-6, 13-7*a*. D. E. Normansell, Univ. of Virginia School of Medicine.

14-1, 14-2. H. J. Muller-Eberhard. 1975. *Annu. Rev. Biochem.* **44**:697–724.

14-3. R. Dourmashkin, Clinical Research Centre, Harrow Middx., U.K.

15-1. P. Ehrlich. 1900. *Proc. R. Soc. Lond., Biol.* **66**:424.

15-2. L. Pauling. 1949. *J. Am. Chem. Soc.* **62**:2643.

15-5. D. Metcalf and M. A. S. Moore. 1971. *Haemopoietic Cells.* American Elsevier, N.Y.

15-6. D. Mosier. 1967. *Science* **158**:1573–1575. Copyright 1967 by the American Association for the Advancement of Science.

15-7. A. A. Nordin, Gerontology Research Center, National Institute on Aging, Baltimore City Hospitals.

15-8. M. F. Greaves, Dept. of Zoology, University College London, U.K.

15-12, 15-13. A. J. Munro and M. J. Taussig. 1975. *Nature* **256**:103–106.

16-2. C. G. Cochrane and D. Koffler. 1973. *Adv. in Immunol.* **16**:185–264.

17-2. J. R. David. 1964. *J. Immunol.* **93**:264

17-3. M. Ohishi and K. Onoue. 1975. *Cellular Immunol.* **18**:220–232.

17-4. B. H. Waksman. 1974. In *Mechanisms of Cell-Mediated Immunity,* R. T. McCluskey and S. Cohen, eds. John Wiley and Sons, N.Y.

18-2, 18-3*a*. R. M. Krause. 1970. *Fed. Proc.* **29**:59–65.

18-3*b* and *c*. P. P. Cleary, Dept. of Microbiology, Univ. of Minnesota Medical School.

18-4. R. R. Facklam, Center for Disease Control, Atlanta.

18-5, 18-6*b*. C. A. Schnaitman, Univ. of Virginia School of Medicine.

18-6*a*, 19-2, 23-5, 24-5. L. J. LeBeau, Depts. of Pathology and Microbiology, Univ. of Illinois Hospital at the Medical Center, Chicago.

18-7, 26-2. American Society for Microbiology, Washington, D.C.

19-1*a*, 19-4, 20-5, 23-2, 24-2, 25-2*a*, 28-3, 28-4, 29-3*a*, 29-6*c* (bottom), 29-10, 29-11, 29-12, 29-13*b*, 29-14, 29-15, 29-17 (top), 29-18, 43-9, 43-13, 44-19 (center), 44-20. Photo-Art Resource Library, Instructional Media Division, Center for Disease Control, Atlanta.

19-1*b*, 19-5. J. S. Hook and D. Leith, Dept. of Microbiology and Immunology, Univ. of Oregon Health Sciences Center.

19-3. I. W. DeVoe and J. E. Gilchrist. 1974. *Infect. Immun.* **10**:872–876.

19-6. R. Rodewald and Keith Powell, Univ. of Virginia.

20-3. I. Snyder, Dept. of Microbiology, West Virginia Univ. Medical Center.

20-4. D. G. Evans, Program in Infectious Diseases and Clinical Microbiology, The Univ. of Texas Medical School.

20-6. E. T. Nelson, Dept. of Biological Sciences, Southeastern Louisiana Univ.

20-8, 20-9. R. L. Guerrant, Dept. of Internal Medicine, Univ. of Virginia School of Medicine.

21-2. M. J. Tufte, Dept. of Biology, Univ. of Wisconsin, Platteville.

21-3. *MMWR Annual Supplement—1972.* **21**:47.

21-4. D. J. Bibel and T. H. Chen. 1976. *Bacteriol. Rev.* **40**:633–651.

21-5. U.S. Army Medical Research Institute of Infectious Diseases, Fort Detrick, Frederick, Md.

22-1. F. L. A. Buckmire, Dept. of Microbiology, The Medical College of Wisconsin.

22-2. J. Mayhew, Milwaukee, Wis.

22-3. J. H. Morse and S. I. Morse. 1970. *J. Exp. Med.* **131**:1342–1357.

23-1. R. J. Heckly and E. Goldwasser. 1949. *J. Infect. Dis.* **84**:92–97.

23-3. V. R. Dowell, Center for Disease Control, Atlanta.

24-1. S. M. Gibson, General Bacteriology Lab., Texas Dept. of Health Resources, Austin.

24-4. R. J. Collier. 1975. *Bacteriol. Rev.* **39**:54–85.

25-1. R. W. Smithwick, Center for Disease Control, Atlanta.

25-4b. E. H. Runyon, Salt Lake City, Utah.

26-4a. W. Burgdorfer. 1970. *Infect. Immun.* **2**:256–259.

26-5a. D. Bromley, Dept. of Microbiology, West Virginia Univ. Medical Center.

27-1a. E. S. Boatman and G. E. Kenny. 1971. *J. Bacteriol.* **106**:1005.

27-1b, 27-2. M. G. Gabridge, Dept. of Microbiology, Univ. of Illinois, Urbana.

27-3. M. C. Shepard and D. R. Howard. 1970. *Ann. N.Y. Acad. Sci.* **174**:809–819.

27-4. S. Madoff (Dienes Collection), Dept. of Bacteriology, Massachusetts General Hospital, Boston.

28-1, 28-2. W. Burgdorfer, Rocky Mountain Lab., Hamilton, Mont.

28-5, 28-6. L. A. Page, National Animal Disease Center, Ames, Iowa.

29-1. J. J. Duda and J. M. Slack. 1972. *J. Gen. Microbiol.* **71**:63–68.

29-2, 29-3b. J. M. Slack and M. A. Gerencser. 1975. *Actinomyces, Filamentous Bacteria: Biology and Pathogenicity.* Burgess, Minneapolis.

29-4, 29-9. J. T. Sinski. 1974. *Dermatophytes in Human Skin, Hair and Nails.* Charles C. Thomas, Springfield, Ill.

29-5a, 29-6a and c (top), 29-7, 29-8. © Carroll H. Weiss, RBP, 1978.

29-13a. C. T. Colan, et al. 1975. *Atlases of Clinical Mycology II. Systemic Mycosis—Deep Seated.* American Society of Clinical Pathologists, Chicago.

29-16. C. T. Dolan, et al. 1975. *Atlases of Clinical Mycology I. Systemic Mycosis—Yeasts.* American Society of Clinical Pathologists, Chicago.

29-17 (bottom). F. Marsik, Dept. of Clinical Pathology, Univ. of Virginia School of Medicine.

30-2. Uricult, Medical Technology Corp., Hackensack, N.J.

30-3. G. P. Blundell. 1970. *Progress in Clinical Pathology,* Vol. III, M. Stefanini, ed. Grune and Stratton, N.Y.

31-1. R. W. Horne, et al. 1959. *J. Mol. Biol.* **1**:84–86.

31-4a. G. Wertz, Dept. of Bacteriology and Immunology, School of Medicine, The Univ. of North Carolina at Chapel Hill.

31-4b. J. W. Heine, Dept. of Medical Viral Oncology, Roswell Park Memorial Institute, Buffalo, N.Y.

31-6a, 33-1, 33-4. B. Roizman, Committee on Virology, The Univ. of Chicago.

31-6b. J. J. Cardamone, Jr., and J. S. Youngner, Dept. of Microbiology, Univ. of Pittsburgh School of Medicine.

32-4. J. S. Lazuick and W. S. Archibald, Vector-Borne Diseases Division, Center for Disease Control, Ft. Collins, Colo.

32-5. D. J. Muth and W. S. Archibald, Vector-Borne Diseases Division, Center for Disease Control, Ft. Collins, Colo.

32-6, 35-1, 37-4, 38-4, 38-7, 38-10, 39-1a, 39-6a, 39-7, 40-2. F. A. Murphy, Center for Disease Control, Atlanta.

32-7. Stephen Leech, Univ. of Virginia School of Medicine.

32-8. A. S. Huang. 1973. *Annu. Rev. Microbiol.* **27**:101–117.

33-3. P. Weary, Univ. of Virginia School of Medicine.

33-5. E.-S. Huang, Cancer Research Center, School of Medicine, The Univ. of North Carolina at Chapel Hill.

34-1a. R. C. Valentine and H. G. Pereira. 1965. *J. Mol. Biol.* **13**:13–20.

34-1b, 35-4, 38-1a. S. Dales and S. L. Wilton, Dept. of Bacteriology and Immunology, The Univ. of Western Ontario.

34-2. D. T. Brown and B. T. Burlingham. 1973. *J. Virol.* **12**:386–396.

34-3. J. K. McDougall, A. R. Dunn, and P. H. Gallimore. 1975. *Cold Spring Harbor Symposium on Quantitative Biology* **39**:591–600.

34-4. J. K. McDougall. 1975. *Progr. Med. Virol.* **21**:118–132. Copyright © 1970 by S. Karger AG, Basel.

34-5. R. C. Williams, Virus Laboratory, Univ. of California, Berkeley.

34-6. A. Z. Kapikian, et al. 1972. *J. Virol.* **10**:1075–1081.

34-7a. C. Garon and J. Rose, National Institute of Allergy and Infectious Diseases, Bethesda, Md.

34-7b, 38-5, 38-6. H. D. Mayor, Dept. of Microbiology, Baylor College of Medicine, Texas Medical Center, Houston.

35-2b. C. Morgan. 1976. *Science* **193**:591–592. Copyright 1976 by The American Association for the Advancement of Science.

35-3. World Health Organization, Geneva, Switzerland.

36-1. E. H. Cook, Jr., Phoenix Labs., Center for Disease Control, Phoenix.

36-3. D. Clayton and W. Robinson, Stanford Univ. School of Medicine.

37-1. D. T. Brown, M. R. F. Waite, and E. R. Pfefferkorn. 1972. *J. Virol.* **10**:524–536.

37-3. R. W. Schlesinger. 1977. *Dengue Viruses.* Virology Monographs, Vol. 16. Springer-Verlag, Vienna, New York.

38-1*b*. B. A. Phillips, Dept. of Microbiology, Univ. of Pittsburgh School of Medicine.

38-3. *MMWR.* Nov. 16, 1974.

38-8. N. M. Bartlett, et al. 1974. *J. Virol.* **14**:315–326. (Photos via A. R. Bellamy.)

38-9. A. Z. Kapikian, et al. 1974. *Science* **185**:1049. Copyright 1974 by the American Association for the Advancement of Science.

39-1*b*. W. G. Laver. 1973. *Advan. Virus Res.* **18**:62.

39-2. R. W. Compans and N. J. Dimmock. 1969. *Virology* **39**:499–515.

39-3. W. R. Dowdle, M. T. Coleman, and M. B. Gregg. 1974. *Progr. Med. Virol.* **17**:91–135. Copyright © 1974 by S. Karger AG, Basel.

39-4. W. G. Laver, Dept. of Microbiology, John Curtin School of Medical Research, The Australian National Univ., Canberra City.

39-5. R. G. Webster, C. H. Campbell, and A. Granoff. 1973. *Virology* **51**:149–162.

39-6*b*. R. W. Compans, et al. 1966. *Virology* **30**:411–426.

39-8. *MMWR.* Apr. 28, 1973.

39-9. F. L. Forrester, Center for Disease Control, Atlanta.

39-10. *MMWR.* Nov. 15, 1975.

40-1. N. Salomonsky, Dept. of Microbiology, Univ. of Virginia School of Medicine.

40-3. *MMWR.* July 27, 1974.

40-4. F. A. Murphy and S. G. Whitfield. 1975. *Bull. World Health Organ.* **52**:409–419.

40-5. K. M. Johnson, P. A. Webb, and G. Justines. 1973. In *Lymphocytic Choriomeningitis Virus and Other Arena Viruses,* F. Lehmann-Grube, ed. Springer-Verlag, New York.

41-1*a* and *b*, 41-6. G. H. Smith, Lab. Molecular Biology, National Cancer Institute, Bethesda, Md.

41-1*c*. N. Salomonsky and J. T. Parsons, Univ. of Virginia School of Medicine.

41-3. J. P. Bader, Chemistry Branch, National Cancer Institute, Bethesda, Md.

41-5. J. Tooze, ed. 1973. *The Molecular Biology of Tumour Viruses,* 2nd ed. Cold Spring Harbor Lab., Cold Spring Harbor, N.Y.

43-1*a*. D. L. Taylor, Dept. of Biology, Harvard Univ.

43-1*b*. J. J. Paulin and A. Steiner, Dept. of Zoology, Univ. of Georgia.

43-8 (center). J. J. Paulin, Dept. of Zoology, Univ. of Georgia.

43-11. J. W. Brown. 1975. *Basic Clinical Parasitology,* 4th ed. Appleton-Century-Crofts, N.Y.

## Tables

1-1, 21-1. After *Bergey's Manual of Determinative Bacteriology,* 8th ed. © 1974 The Williams and Wilkins Co., Baltimore.

1-2. After D. J. Brenner, G. R. Fanning, and A. G. Steigerwalt. 1972. *J. Bacteriol.* **110**:12–17.

9-1. J. G. Mulvany. 1969. In *Methods in Microbiology I,* J. R. Norris and D. W. Ribbons, eds. Academic Press, New York.

10-3. R. Benveniste and J. Davies. 1973. *Annu. Rev. Biochem.* **42**:471–506.

12-1. After K. Landsteiner and J. van der Scheer. 1936. *J. Exp. Med.* **63**:325–339.

12-2. After A. Nisonoff, J. E. Hopper, and S. B. Spring. 1975. *The Antibody Molecule.* Academic Press, New York.

12-3. T. B. Tomasi, Jr. 1970. *Annu. Rev. Med.* **21**:281–298.

13-1. After M. Heidelberger and F. E. Kendall. 1935. *J. Exp. Med.* **62**:697–720.

14-1, 14-2. After H. J. Muller-Eberhard. 1975. *Annu. Rev. Biochem.* **44**:697–724.

15-1. After D. Mosier. 1967. *Science* **158**:1573–1575.

15-2. After M. C. Raff and J. J. T. Owen. 1971. *Eur. J. Immunol.* **1**:27–30.

19-2. *MMWR.* Jan. 31, 1976.

19-3. *MMWR.* Oct. 11, 1975.

20-2. World Health Organization International Reference Centre for Salmonella, Pasteur Institute, Paris.

20-4, 20-5. O. R. Pavlovskis, L. T. Callahan III, and M. Pollack. 1975. In *Microbiology 1975,* D. Schlessinger, ed. American Society for Microbiology, Washington, D.C.

20-6. B. H. Iglewski and D. Kabat. 1975. *Proc. Nat. Acad. Sci. USA* **72**:2284–2288.

20-7. J. V. Bennett. 1974. *J. Infect. Dis.* **130** (Supp.):S4–S7.

21-2. *MMWR.* Sept. 24, 1976.

23-1. *MMWR.* June 22, 1974.

23-2, 37-1. B. D. Davis, et al. 1973. *Microbiology,* 2nd ed. Harper and Row, Hagerstown, Md.

24-1. *MMWR Annual Summary 1976.* Aug., 1977.

24-2. Data from Center for Disease Control, Atlanta, Ga.

25-1. After H. L. Arnold, Jr., and P. Fasal. 1973. *Leprosy: Diagnosis and Management,* 2nd ed. Charles C. Thomas, Springfield, Ill.

28-1. R. A. Ormsbee. 1974. In *Manual of Clinical Microbiology,* 2nd ed., E. H. Lennette, E. H. Spaulding, and J. P. Truant, eds. American Society for Microbiology, Washington, D.C.

29-3. After M. Saito, M. Enomoto, and T. Tatsuno. 1971. In *Microbial Toxins, Vol. VI,* A. Ciegler,

S. Kadis, and S. J. Ajl, eds. Academic Press, New York.

30-1. H. D. Isenberg and J. I. Berkman. 1966. *Progress in Clinical Pathology, Vol. I,* M. Stefanini, ed. Grune and Stratton, New York.

30-2, 30-6. H. D. Isenberg, J. A. Washington II, A. Balows, and A. C. Sonnenwirth. 1974. In *Manual of Clinical Microbiology,* 2nd ed., E. H. Lennette, E. H. Spaulding, and J. P. Truant, eds. American Society for Microbiology, Washington, D.C.

30-4, 30-5. V. L. Sutter and S. M. Finegold. 1973. In *Progress in Clinical Pathology, Vol. V,* M. Stefanini, ed. Grune and Stratton, New York.

33-1. Herpesvirus Study Group, International Committee for the Nomenclature of Viruses. 1973. *J. Gen. Virol.* **20:**417–419.

33-2. I. Davidsohn and J. B. Henry. 1969. *Clinical Diagnosis by Laboratory Methods,* 14th ed. W. B. Saunders, Philadelphia.

33-4. F. Rapp and R. W. Koment. 1974. In *Viruses, Evolution and Cancer: Basic Considerations,* E. Kurstak and K. Maramorosch, eds. Academic Press, New York.

34-1. After M. Green. 1970. *Annu. Rev. Biochem.* ,**39:**701–756.

36-1. *MMWR.* July 26, 1975.

36-2. *MMWR.* Dec. 23, 1972.

36-4. WHO. 1975. *Viral Hepatitis. Report of a WHO Meeting.* WHO Technical Report Series, No. 570. World Health Organization, Geneva.

37-2. *MMWR.* Apr. 16, 1976.

41-1, 41-2. J. Tooze. 1973. *The Molecular Biology of Tumour Viruses,* 2nd ed. Cold Spring Harbor Laboratory, Cold Spring Harbor, New York.

41-3. After P. C. Hageman, J. Calafat, and J. H. Daams. 1972. In *RNA Viruses and Host Genome in Oncogenesis,* P. Emmelot and P. Bentvelzen, eds. North-Holland, Amsterdam.

41-4. R. Hehlmann. 1976. *Current Topics Microbiol. Immunol.* **73:**141–215.

42-1. F. Fenner and D. O. White. 1976. *Medical Virology,* 2nd ed. Academic Press, New York.

42-2. F. Fenner, B. R. McAuslan, C. A. Mims, J. Sambrook, and D. O. White. 1974. *The Biology of Animal Viruses,* 2nd ed. Academic Press, New York.

42-3. E. H. Lennette, J. L. Melnick, and R. L. Magoffin. 1974. In *Manual of Clinical Microbiology,* 2nd ed., E. H. Lennette, E. H. Spaulding, and J. P. Truant, eds. American Society for Microbiology, Washington, D.C.

43-1. U.S. Navy. 1962. *Medical Protozoology and Helminthology.* U.S. Naval Medical School, National Naval Medical Center, Bethesda, Md.

# Index